Handbook of Research on Geriatric Health, Treatment, and Care

Barre Vijaya Prasad
Dharwad Institute of Mental Health and Neurosciences (DIMHANS), India

Shamsi Akbar
King George's Medical University, India

A volume in the Advances in Medical Diagnosis, Treatment, and Care (AMDTC) Book Series

IGI Global
DISSEMINATOR OF KNOWLEDGE

Published in the United States of America by
IGI Global
Medical Information Science Reference (an imprint of IGI Global)
701 E. Chocolate Avenue
Hershey PA, USA 17033
Tel: 717-533-8845
Fax: 717-533-8661
E-mail: cust@igi-global.com
Web site: http://www.igi-global.com

Library of Congress Cataloging-in-Publication Data

Names: Vijaya Prasad, Barre, 1981- editor. | Akbar, Shamsi, 1985- editor.
Title: Handbook of research on geriatric health, treatment, and care / Barre Vijaya Prasad and Shamsi Akbar, editors.
Description: Hershey PA : Medical Information Science Reference, [2018] | Includes bibliographical references.
Identifiers: LCCN 2017017345| ISBN 9781522534808 (hardcover) | ISBN 9781522534815 (ebook)
Subjects: | MESH: Geriatrics | Aging | Mental Disorders | Health Services for the Aged | Aged
Classification: LCC RC952.5 | NLM WT 100 | DDC 618.97--dc23 LC record available at https://lccn.loc.gov/2017017345

This book is published in the IGI Global book series Advances in Medical Diagnosis, Treatment, and Care (AMDTC) (ISSN: 2475-6628; eISSN: 2475-6636)

British Cataloguing in Publication Data
A Cataloguing in Publication record for this book is available from the British Library.

For electronic access to this publication, please contact: eresources@igi-global.com.

Advances in Medical Diagnosis, Treatment, and Care (AMDTC) Book Series

ISSN:2475-6628
EISSN:2475-6636

Mission

Advancements in medicine have prolonged the life expectancy of individuals all over the world. Once life-threatening conditions have become significantly easier to treat and even cure in many cases. Continued research in the medical field will further improve the quality of life, longevity, and wellbeing of individuals.

The **Advances in Medical Diagnosis, Treatment, and Care (AMDTC)** book series seeks to highlight publications on innovative treatment methodologies, diagnosis tools and techniques, and best practices for patient care. Comprised of comprehensive resources aimed to assist professionals in the medical field apply the latest innovations in the identification and management of medical conditions as well as patient care and interaction, the books within the AMDTC series are relevant to the research and practical needs of medical practitioners, researchers, students, and hospital administrators.

Coverage

- Disease Management
- Alternative Medicine
- Medical Procedures
- Experimental Medicine
- Critical Care
- Patient Interaction
- Diagnostic Medicine
- Internal Medicine
- Medical Testing
- Emergency Medicine

IGI Global is currently accepting manuscripts for publication within this series. To submit a proposal for a volume in this series, please contact our Acquisition Editors at Acquisitions@igi-global.com or visit: http://www.igi-global.com/publish/.

The Advances in Medical Diagnosis, Treatment, and Care (AMDTC) Book Series (ISSN 2475-6628) is published by IGI Global, 701 E. Chocolate Avenue, Hershey, PA 17033-1240, USA, www.igi-global.com. This series is composed of titles available for purchase individually; each title is edited to be contextually exclusive from any other title within the series. For pricing and ordering information please visit http://www.igi-global.com/book-series/advances-medical-diagnosis-treatment-care/129618. Postmaster: Send all address changes to above address.

Titles in this Series

For a list of additional titles in this series, please visit: www.igi-global.com/book-series

Complementary and Alternative Medicine and Kidney Health
Mayuree Tangkiatkumjai (Srinakharinwirot University, Thailand) Annalisa Casarin (The NIHR Research Design Service East of England, UK) Li-Chia Chen (University of Manchester, UK) and Dawn-Marie Walker (University of Southampton, UK)
Medical Information Science Reference • copyright 2018 • 308pp • H/C (ISBN: 9781522528821) • US $265.00 (our price)

Research-Based Perspectives on the Psychophysiology of Yoga
Shirley Telles (Patanjali Research Foundation, India) and Nilkamal Singh (Patanjali Research Foundation, India)
Medical Information Science Reference • copyright 2018 • 456pp • H/C (ISBN: 9781522527886) • US $225.00 (our price)

Sustainable Health and Long-Term Care Solutions for an Aging Population
Ben Fong (The Hong Kong Polytechnic University, Hong Kong) Artie Ng (The Hong Kong Polytechnic University, Hong Kong) and Peter Yuen (The Hong Kong Polytechnic University, Hong Kong)
Medical Information Science Reference • copyright 2018 • 441pp • H/C (ISBN: 9781522526339) • US $225.00 (our price)

Emerging Applications, Perspectives, and Discoveries in Cardiovascular Research
Ashim Malhotra (Pacific University, USA) and Shivani Soni (California State University, Fullerton, USA & Chapman University, USA & Alabama State University, USA)
Medical Information Science Reference • copyright 2017 • 439pp • H/C (ISBN: 9781522520924) • US $225.00 (our price)

Healthcare Community Synergism between Patients, Practitioners, and Researchers
Valerie C. Bryan (Florida Atlantic University, USA) and Jennifer Lynne Bird (Florida Atlantic University, USA)
Medical Information Science Reference • copyright 2017 • 348pp • H/C (ISBN: 9781522506409) • US $210.00 (our price)

Transformative Healthcare Practice through Patient Engagement
Guendalina Graffigna (Catholic University of the Sacred Heart, Italy)
Medical Information Science Reference • copyright 2017 • 382pp • H/C (ISBN: 9781522506638) • US $215.00 (our price)

IGI Global
DISSEMINATOR OF KNOWLEDGE

701 East Chocolate Avenue, Hershey, PA 17033, USA
Tel: 717-533-8845 x100 • Fax: 717-533-8661
E-Mail: cust@igi-global.com • www.igi-global.com

Handbook of Research on Geriatric Health, Treatment, and Care is an edited collection of 26 chapters on the epidemiology, factors, prevalence of disability, scope of research in diagnosis/management, and implementation strategies of ageing by scholars from the diverse disciplines. The chapters therein contain all the major elements and concepts related to the aspects of geriatric health based on the researchers' experiences, innovative research, practice and care giving in the field of Applied Gerontology. This comprehensive update of an excellent text is timely and relevant. The Editors, Dr. Barre Vijaya Prasad and Shamsi Akbar deserve appreciation for editing this volume. Readers and researchers will understand and apply key concepts and principles in ways that will not only create innovative higher-order thinking but will also enhance knowledge in the practicing aspect of Geriatric Medicine.

Akbar Husain
Aligarh Muslim University, India

With rapid strides in the health care technology and improving economy, there is an explosive rise in the population of elderly all over the world. Consequent to it, the health problems of the elderly are also proportionately rising. In some developed countries, just the population of elderly itself is a major public health concern. Hence it is essential to have a book on the health issues of geriatric population. There exist only few books on the topics dealing with health issues of the elderly. But the books dealing comprehensively with different topics of physical as well as mental health are still rarer here. I must congratulate the editors Dr Barre Vijaya Prasad and Shamsi Akbar for not just thinking of this idea but actually working on it and giving it a shape. I admire the patience and perseverance with which both kept working despite all odds. Hats off to the editors and their families. The proposed book contains 26 chapters, all written by well established authors. These are well organized in five sections arranged from basic aspects to the applied clinical topics. This step ladder arrangement helps the readers understand some complex topics very easily. I am sure that the postgraduate students, researchers, teachers as well clinicians would find this book not just useful but interesting too.

Happy reading!

Hitesh Khurana
Pandit Bhagwat Dayal Sharma Postgraduate Institute of Medical Sciences, India

The book entitled Handbook of Research on Geriatric Health, Treatment, and Care edited by Dr Barre Vijay Prasad and Shamsi Akbar is a necessary attempt to probe into the current research perspectives on not only the curative aspects of geriatric health but also the care. Gero-Psychology is the much sought after research area considering the increasing geriatric population worldwide thanks to advancements in science and medicine towards enhancement of longevity. The bio-psycho-social effects like disabilities, dependency and others are often seen to lead to a self-perception by the elders themselves and perception of others towards the elderly as the 'burdensome old'. It is thus the responsibility of learned professionals such as Psychologists, Social workers, Medical and para medical professionals, along with the family support to form Health teams to provide a holistic support to the elderly. This book provides a platform to illustrate the research relating to aspects of cure and care for the elderly. The four main sections with 26 chapters cover several subthemes and topics of contemporary relevance and importance. Thus it seeks to provide a panorama of research areas both from theoretical to applied perspectives. The editors are congratulated for this integrative vision and fusion of articles from across a wide array of fields. This combined presentation helps in creating a synthesis of areas focusing on the needs and necessities of the elderly showcasing a need for holistic support to the elderly.

G. Padmaja
University of Hyderabad, India

I thank the Editors Dr Barre Vijaya Prasad and Shamsi Akbar for asking to review and share my thoughts about this book. I appreciate the work of Dr Barre Vijaya Prasad, a devotee of excellence in the publishing work on various themes in Mental Health. To remind his previous book on chronic Mental illness was a commendable job, in continuum he has moved forward with new theme Research on geriatric Health treatment and care with focus on the Psychiatric and Psychological aspects of the Ageing. It is worth to note, World health Organization report on Ageing, Populations around the world is rapidly ageing. Hence ageing presents both challenges and opportunities. There is increase demand for primary health care and long-term care for ageing population. To meet the needs we require a larger and better trained workforce and intensify the need for environments to be made more age-friendly. Societies that adapt to this changing demographics and invest in Healthy Ageing, enable individuals to live both longer and healthier lives and for societies to reap the dividends". I think editors have fairly done justice to these aspects in the book by incorporating various issues highlighted by WHO in the research work. Twenty-six chapters organized into four sections on various themes, makes handy for the reader to choose his topic of interest. Very informative and interesting topics for reader would be topics on approach for promoting successful positive ageing, psychosocial and medical management of cognitive impairment which catches the special attention. Chapter on sleep related disorders in elderly needs special mention, less discussed topic is well presented, treatment aspects like sleep hygiene and cognitive behavioral therapies is noteworthy for a reader. Last thing but not the least, the book caught my attention was on suicide and sexual needs among the elderly. For any treating physician these are of low priority areas, editors have done justice by incorporating these chapters. The book is well researched, reads well, and represents theme, I hope difficult subject presented in simple language will catch the attention of all the stakeholders. I wish editors good luck for their commendable job, hoping to see this work at earliest in the bookshelves

Srinivas Kosgi
Dharwad Institute of Mental Health and Neurosciences (DIMHANS), India

Editorial Advisory Board

List of Contributors

Table of Contents

Section 4
Medical and Psychiatric Comorbidities in Ageing

Detailed Table of Contents

The present chapter will help in understanding the role of positive psychology and intervention in approaching towards a healthy aging. Aging is inevitable. The clock cannot be turned backwards. At first glance, it seems that generally the growing population enjoy what they face which is true to a certain extent but at the same time it is important not to overlook or discount the stresses they face when they start to age. How they age depends how they look at their life. Positive intervention has its effect in all ages. Taking the help of positive psychology as a primary prevention can help eliminating various effects of aging. In the same way, it can also help in reducing the exiting trouble occurring in elderly. By taking preventive steps, one can take care of the body and the mind, and that can help stave off some of the devastating illnesses associated with age and live a full, meaningful and energetic life. Elderly person must acknowledge that their roles in life will change as their former lifestyles are replaced by new schedules, approaches and relationships.

This chapter reviews the available literature on different aspects of spirituality and health in old age. Old age is marked with physical, mental and social dysfunctions whereas spirituality provides the way to overcome these difficulties. The Asian scriptures give a very clear evidence that spirituality is the way of life that has a meaning, a purpose and connectedness with others. In the Indian description, Vasudhaiv Kutubhkam, it points towards the spiritual interconnectedness. The spiritual practices give a meaning and purpose to life therefore instills a feeling of hope which can protect against mental disorders. The same also strengthen immune system protecting us from physical problems connectedness with others is the ultimate aim of spirituality. With increasing age and degenerative processing taking place in the body, spiritual practices by elderly, make them feel a part of community and improves physical health status.

The increase of human lifespans and the aging has brought increased attention to what factors contribute to aging healthy. People are not only interested in longevity but how to remain in the best health in their later years. Therefore, the aim of this chapter is to (a) understand the concept of positive aging (b) identifying the factors contributing to successful positive aging across health continuum (c) review strategies that promotes management healthy aging in elderly, and (d) identify future directions to promote successful population health management programs/interventions. The holistic approach, therefore provide an opportunity to improve the situation of older people in society.

The present chapter presents an intertwined view on aging, quality of life and social support. Aging is a sensitive process of transformation from a young age structure to old age. It is a pressing problem for many countries in this century. Therefore, attention to needs and problems of this age has an importance. The domains that need more attention in elderly is both quality of life and social support in their life. Though social support and quality of life have received much attention in studies of the psychological issues of older adults but still researches are needed in special attention at the intervention level.

This chapter is an attempt to highlight the numerous ways in which elders are abused in our society and the ways to support them. A concise account in ways elders are vulnerable and how they are exploited are discussed in the chapter as well as remedies to these problems. The chapter includes types of abuse faced by elders and the consequences they face due to it. It also discusses Social Support as the main remedy, social support as an acronym of 13 types of social support. The chapter concludes by recommendation of how elder abuse can be stopped or at least controlled.

Section 2
Cognition and Cognitive Impairment in Ageing and Clinical Outcome

This chapter describes how one of the challenging issues of clinical diagnosis is distinguishing between the cognitive deficits manifested in normal aging, depression, mild cognitive impairment (MCI) and dementia. The diagnostic challenge is that there is a great deal of overlap in the symptom constellations of these conditions. It is thus important to establish conceptual and clinical criteria with sufficient predictive validity to accurately identify differences and similarities in cognitive states to justify initiation of appropriate treatments.

This chapter focuses on cognitive functions and impairment in the elderly; its implications in daily functioning with inputs on differences in the existing literature. The chapter further focuses on the diagnostic and assessment issues and intervention strategies. Ageing is an inevitable phase of life and encompasses changes in physical, psychological and social realms of an individual. Concern with the dwindling health and presence of any medical issues make the geriatric population prone to develop mental health conditions. Poor memory and reduced functional ability is one of the common complaints from older adults coming to psychiatric or neurology clinics. Cognitive functions have been well documented regarding their role in daily functioning of an individual. With growing age of the brain; while some cognitive functions do slow down; some of the functions do evolve better with experience. In this context, it is important to differentiate between normal age related cognitive changes and symptoms of any degenerative disease.

This chapter describes how the world population is ageing with the advances in medical health technology. Longevity allows many humans to live beyond the sixth and seventh decade. With this comes the added medical co-morbidity that one sees with healthy ageing. Mild cognitive impairment (MCI) includes a heterogeneous group of persons who have declining deficits in cognitions with minimal impairment in doing complex activities with no deficits in daily activities and in the absence of dementia. The purpose of this chapter is to acquaint the readers with the concept of Mild Cognitive Impairment and the evolution of the diagnosis to its current nosological status. It will further elaborate on the assessment and management of patients with MCI.

This chapter describes how an individual progresses towards aging, several age-related cognitive declines are becoming an ever-increasing problem. Ageing causes changes to brain size, vasculature, and cognition. Protective factors that reduce cardiovascular risk, namely regular exercise, a healthy diet, and low to moderate alcohol intake, seem to aid the ageing brain as does increase cognitive effort in the form of education or occupational attainment. A healthy life both physically and mentally may be the best defense against the changes of an ageing brain. This chapter aims to characterize changes in brain structure with aging, and to investigate relationships between brain aging and cognitive decline. Along with these it will make and attempt to identify possible management, treatment and preventive measures for managing cognitive impairment in brain ageing and promoting cognitive reserve for healthy brain ageing.

This chapter describes how cardiovascular disease in industrialized nations the proportion is higher, reaching 90%. Ageing has a remarkable effect on the heart and arterial system, out of which leading to an increase in cardiovascular disease including atherosclerosis, hypertension, myocardial infarction, and stroke. Cardiovascular disease is one of the leading causes of Cardiovascular Disease morbidity and mortality today. Coronary heart disease accounts for 70 to 80 per cent of deaths in men and women in adults over 60 years of age. Congestive Heart Failure is the most common cause of hospitalization in the elderly. Since a significant proportion of the population is and will be elderly and the morbidity and mortality of cardiovascular disease in this population is so profound, it is important to understand the evaluation and treatment of cardiovascular disease in the elderly

This chapter describes how a stroke or 'brain attack' occurs when blood circulation to the brain fails. Although first recognized 2400 years ago by Hippocrates, the father of medicine, advances in treatment are made only in the last few decades. After a stroke, 8 out of 10 patients develop paralysis on the side of body opposite the side of brain damaged. There are other symptoms to look for such as drooping of face to one side, slurred or confused speech, sudden visual disturbance, sudden giddiness and imbalance

This chapter describes how sensory impairment is often regarded from a medical/disability point of view and its effects on mental health can be poorly recognized. Communication is a key issue for deaf and deaf-blind people and difficulties here underlie developmental, psychological and emotional problems and delay or prevent appropriate assessment and treatment. Sensory related issues are seen as medical problems and as disabilities. 95% of the information about the world around us comes from our sight and hearing. However, the main concerns of visual and hearing affected by the total or partial absence of sight and/or hearing are usually how to live, how to learn and how to communicate. Their difficulties are often as much to do with society's attitudes towards them as with the direct effect of sensory impairment.

Aging mirrors all the changes that occur over the period of life. It comes with various changes both positive and negative. Among all medical illnesses, Diabetes Mellitus is one of the most common and serious medical condition that has affected not only the aging population but also the young children and adults as well. Diabetes and its complications can contribute to aging process in a number of ways and the complications can speed up the aging process as well. For people with type 2 diabetes managing their emotional health can be as important as keeping their blood sugar under control. Patients with diabetes mellitus need psychological support throughout their life span from the time of diagnosis. However, provision of psychosocial support is generally inadequate due to its challenging nature of needs and demands on the healthcare systems. The present chapter will cover different aspects of diabetes mellitus and its impact on human life and also how with healthy coping mechanism one can prevent the distressing effect of diabetes on aging and vice versa.

This chapter describes the prevalence of obesity which is rising in all age groups. The World Health Organization declared obesity as a Global epidemic. There has been the abundance of research in all over the world that provides evidence for physical and mental health consequences of obesity. Obesity is considered as one of the leading cause of various non-communicable diseases. Higher body mass index and abdominal obesity are considered to be an independent risk factor that significantly contribute to the increased prevalence of Type 2 diabetes, cardiovascular diseases and hypertension, metabolic disorders along with various mental health problems among elderly. Geriatric obesity further affects the treatment process, outcome, quality and quantity of life older adults. It also increases the risk of disability among older adults.

Sleep complaints are prevalent among older adults. Sleep quality and quantity changes with advancing age. There are changes in sleep patterns that are normal with ageing but many changes are the sign of disordered sleep. Sleep can be divided into rapid eye movement (REM) sleep and non-rapid eye movement sleep (NREM). Each has unique characteristics that are differentiated by their waveforms on the electroencephalogram (EEG) and by other physiological signals; several physiological age-related changes are thought to produce alterations in circadian rhythms. While there are numerous psychological and social factors contributing to quality and quantity of sleep, specific sleep disorders more prevalent in old age are insomnia, sleep apnea, and rapid eye movement disorder. Non-pharmacological treatment is effective in management of sleep disorders. Cognitive behaviour therapy is most effective to tackle insomnia. Cognitive behavior therapy along with meditation is beneficial for other sleep disorders and a new technique is also emerging: mindfulness.

The World Health Organization has declared that the spread of tuberculosis is a global emergency. Despite the implementation of strong tuberculosis-control initiatives by WHO, this highly infectious disease continues to affect all vulnerable populations, including the elderly population. Adverse social factors and poor living conditions also affect the elderly much more than the young. The clinical characteristics of tuberculosis in older adults can be unusual and may be confused with age-related illnesses. Various factors related to old age can also cause complications in the diagnosis, treatment, and disease outcomes for tuberculosis patients. The contributory factors may be poor memory, deafness, mental confusion, or impairment of speech. In addition, therapy for tuberculosis in elderly individuals is challenging because of the increased incidence of adverse drug reactions. Hence, understanding the impact of these substantial aspects will help to overcome the problem of tuberculosis in the elderly population.

Thyroid disorders are highly prevalent, most frequently afflicting aging women. It is crucial to advance the means of diagnosing thyroid diseases, especially overt and subclinical hypothyroidism in elderly people, because thyroid-associated symptoms are very similar to symptoms of the normal aging process. Thyroid hormone production, metabolism, and action change with aging. The reference ranges for serum thyrotropin and thyroid hormones are derived mainly from younger populations. Thus, the prevalence of subclinical thyroid dysfunction is increased greatly in the elderly. There has been increasing interest in thyroid function in the elderly because of association of thyroid status with disability, cognitive function, cardiovascular disease risk, and longevity.

Alzheimer's disease (AD) is a worldwide epidemic. Multiple domains including memory, cognitive abilities, language, behaviour, and emotions are affected, resulting in significant disability and distress both for patients and caregivers. The management of patients with Alzheimer's disease is a significant public health problem. Different strategies have been applied to prevent/delay onset of Alzheimer's disease or at least to improve quality of life and health conditions of Alzheimer's disease patients and their caregivers. Given the limited effectiveness of pharmacological therapies combined with iatrogenic effects of drug treatments, the development of nondrug care has become a necessity. This chapter focuses on music therapy as an advanced intervention strategy for this population. Music therapy has evolved from a social science model to a neuroscience model of clinical practice and research. This paradigm shift has resulted in the formation of a new theory known as neurologic music therapy (NMT).

Estimated research findings suggest that almost two-thirds of adults with psychiatric conditions do not receive the required treatment services. This chapter enables readers to understand various aspects of ageing, how physical and mental health aspects are correlated, and which mental health conditions are most common in later life. The chapter also discusses major models of mental health in the context of ageing. Major psychiatric and psychological conditions that are most common in old age are outlined along with a major milestone of old age (i.e., retirement: a major lifestyle change that pushes older people towards psychological problems and adjustment issues with a new phase of life). A brief description is presented on the current status of psychiatric and psychological services for mental health issues of the elderly. The chapter concludes by summarizing the contents of discussed areas. Studies are presented throughout the chapter to accompany and enrich the discussion and validate the chapter content.

Ageing is related to problems in physical, emotional, and mental health. If we can delay the ageing process, we may be able to live more happily and successfully. Several factors are responsible for ageing: age, sleep, dietary habits, nutrition, physical activity, general health condition, emotional well-being, physical impairment, cultural factors, life events, social support, family well-being, financial resources, cognitive functioning, and diseases. The chapter is based on the above views and mainly focuses on the various factors that contribute to ageing.

Foreword

In these changing times, with an enormous rise in the stress levels, individuals need help in maintaining excellence and coping up with the demands. This stress impacts them the most when they turn old. The geriatric population has been increasing rapidly due to better lifestyle, availability of good healthcare facilities and other factors since 2009.

Globally, the population is ageing rapidly. Between 2015 and 2050, the proportion of the world's population over 60 years will nearly double, from 12% to 22%.

According to a recent projection by the World Health Organization, over three quarters of the deaths occurring in the developing world by the year 2020 will be due to non-communicable diseases, and mental health disorders form major chunk of it. There is a heavy burden of the Psychiatric illness in the elderly and the worst part is that they remain undetected and untreated. Mental illness in the geriatric population leads to a decline in social functioning leading to functional disability.

Multiple social, psychological, and biological factors determine the level of mental health of a person at any point of time. Older people are more likely to experience events such as bereavement, a drop in socioeconomic status with retirement, or a disability resulting in isolation, loss of independence, loneliness and psychological distress. Older adults are also vulnerable to elder abuse including physical, sexual, psychological, emotional, financial and material abuse.

The book titled *Handbook of Research on Geriatric Health, Treatment, and Care* targets professionals and researchers working in the field of Geriatric Medicine and Geriatric Mental Health including psychiatrists, neurologists, neurosurgeons, psychologists, social workers, psychiatric nursing, psychosocial rehabilitation therapists, mental health counsellors, general physicians and social scientists. It aims and focuses to provide with an individual's experience and innovative research, practice and care giving in the field of Geriatric Medicine and Geriatric Mental Health.

There are 26 chapters in this book and they are grouped into four main sections. Section1 contains five chapters that are focused on providing in-depth information on social and psychological factors in ageing. Section 2 contains four chapters which were focused on cognition and cognitive impairment in ageing and clinical outcome. In Section 3, medical morbidity in ageing consisting of 11 major chapters on physical and mental health aspects of diseases and ageing were emphasized in detail like cardiovascular disease in elderly and an early care: bio psychosocial perspective. In Section 4, medical and psychiatric co-morbidities in ageing are illustrated with six important chapters.

I have known Dr. Barre Vijaya Prasad since he was doing his second M.Phil in Clinical Psychology from one of the most reputed institutes in India, Institute of Human Behaviour and Allied Sciences (IHBAS) New Delhi. I have always appreciated his dynamism, flamboyance, modesty, and intellectual skills in almost all his works till date. Hence, this book shall emerge as a precious asset to people in desire to focus on geriatric mental health and I congratulate both the editors Dr. Vijaya Prasad Barre and Shamsi Akbar for this edited volume.

The book has been meticulously divided into four sections covering all the relevant geriatric mental health care required in practice. This book will be very helpful to all health professionals specifically mental health and who are dealing with geriatric population.

Prakash B. Behere
D. Y. Patil University, India

Preface

INTRODUCTION

Geriatric medicine is a specialty that focuses on health care of elderly people. It aims to promote health by preventing and treating diseases and disabilities in older adults. There is no set age at which patients may be under the care of a geriatrician or geriatric specialists, a specialist who specializes in the care of elderly people. Rather, this decision is determined by the individual patient's needs, and the availability of a specialist.

According to United Nations (n.d.), the older population has been growing at an unprecedented rate. In 1980, just prior to the convening of the First World Assembly on Ageing, there were 378 million people in the world aged 60 years or above. That figure has risen to 759 million over the past three decades and is projected to jump to 2 billion by 2050. The world's older population defined in the present context as those aged 60 years and above presently stands at around 760 million. Asia accounts for more than half of the total (414 million, including 166 million in China and 92 million in India). Europe is the region with the second largest number of older persons (nearly 161 million), followed by Northern America (65 million), Latin America and the Caribbean (59 million), Africa (55 million) and Oceania (6 million). Although the older population is growing in all parts of the world, most of the increase is taking place in the developing regions. On average, 29 million older persons will be added to the world's population each year between 2010 and 2025, with those in less developed countries accounting for more than 80 per cent of the total. As a result, the share of the older population residing in the developing world will increase from 65-80% by the year 2050.

According to a recent projection by the World Health Organization, over three-quarters of the deaths occurring in the developing world by the year 2020 will be due to non-communicable diseases. Communicable diseases and injuries together will account for the rest of the one-fourth. The ten most common diseases are: hypertension, cataract, osteoarthritis, chronic obstructive pulmonary disease, ischemic heart disease, diabetes, benign prostatic hypertrophy, dyspepsia, constipation and depression. The five most frequent causes of death in the elderly are bronchitis and pneumonia, ischemic heart disease, stroke, cancer and tuberculosis.

In addition, mental and physical disorders are common in old age but frequently remain undetected and untreated. Mental and physical disorders induce functional disability, disturb rehabilitation, burden the health system and impair life-quality of old patients and their relatives. Geriatric patients have a great need for both rehabilitation and for psychosocial services. Moreover, treatment of mental and physical disorders is decisive to prognosis of other somatic diseases. A large number of old patients are in need of treatment, even though a considerable proportion of clinically relevant psychiatric morbidity in the elderly does not meet common diagnostic criteria.

This book was examining research focused on new methodologies for identifying and diagnosing the epidemiological factors contributing for geriatric health issues and older adults in the community. It also discussed research related to psychopharmacological inventions and interventions for the care of older adults, disability due to multiple health complications. Further, it also focused on Treatment strategies at health care set ups, effectiveness of national policies/programmes and their outcomes across countries (South-East Asian, Europe, Australia, USA, Canada, Africa, etc.) in care of older adults and their acts across the world intended to protect the rights of older adults.

OBJECTIVE OF THE BOOK

Chapters on 26 methodological bases were included. We asked researchers to submit studies of the treatment and care in older adults. To look at the epidemiology, factors, prevalence of disability, scope of research in diagnosis/management, and implementation strategies of ageing. It also integrated the findings from the individual studies. We believe that research articles in the collection will make significant contributions to a currently under-researched aspect of geriatric health, and the collection as a whole will set an agenda at global level to guide ongoing re conceptualizations of the individual's experience and innovative research, practice and care giving in the field of Geriatric Medicine and Geriatric Mental Health.

TARGET AUDIENCE

The target audiences of this book were composed of professionals and researchers working in the field of Geriatric Medicine and Geriatric Mental Health including psychiatrists, neurologists, neurosurgeons, psychologists, social workers, psychiatric nursing, psychosocial rehabilitation therapists, mental health counselors, general physicians and social scientists. The book can also serve as a complementary textbook for advanced courses in the area of gerontology, medical sciences of various diseases, multidisciplinary courses designed to undergraduates, post graduates and doctorate research students in the field of Geriatric Medicine and Geriatric Mental Health. This book will be a referral book for academic purposes in various libraries. This publication also aims to guide administrative and policy matters for the care of older adults.

ORGANIZATION OF THE BOOK

There are 26 chapters in this book and the chapters are grouped into four main sections. The four sections assist the reader to be guided to a specific area of interest because each section is based on a particular theme.

The sections are divided as follows: Section 1 contains five chapters that are focused on providing in-depth information on social and psychological factors in ageing. Section 2 contains four chapters were focused on cognition and cognitive impairment in ageing and clinical outcome. Section 3 consists of 11 major chapters on physical and mental health aspects of diseases and ageing. Section 4 consists of six important chapters.

We hope these contributed chapters fulfilled the gap between research and subjects' aspects of physical and mental health issues in ageing and highlighted issues that could be taken up by further researchers. The description of each chapter is given below:

Section 1: Social and Psychological Factors in Ageing

Chapter 1: Positive Psychology and Ageing

"Positive Psychology and Ageing" is a chapter which deals with positive intervention has its effect in all ages. Taking the help of positive psychology as a primary prevention can help eliminating various effects of ageing and reducing the existing trouble occurring in elderly. By taking preventive steps, one can take care of the body and the mind, and that can help stave off some the divesting illness associated with age and live a full, meaningful and energetic life. Authors stress on elderly person to acknowledge that their roles in life will changes as their former lifestyles are replaced by new schedules approaches and relationships. Taking the help of positive psychology as a primary prevention can help eliminating various effects of ageing. In the same way it can also help in reducing the existing trouble occurring in elderly.

Chapter 2: Spirituality and Old Age – Spirituality and Ageing

"Spirituality and Old Age: Spirituality and Aging" deals with the fact that spiritual practices give a meaning and purpose to life therefore instills a feeling of hope which can protect against mental disorders. The same also strengthen immune system protecting us from physical problems connectedness with others is the ultimate aim of spirituality. With increasing age and degenerative processing taking place in the body, spiritual practices by elderly, make them feel a part of community and improves physical health status. The authors stressed upon the need for health care providers to effectively address the connection between spirituality and health is becoming broadly recognized as more people want spiritual content to their health care. An insight into the roots, nature, components and expressions of spirituality needs to be incorporated. Thus, there is clearly a long way to go before we sufficiently understand this ancient art of spiritual well-being to translate into health care practice.

Chapter 3: Promoting Successful Positive Ageing Across the Health Continuum – A Holistic Approach

This chapter focused on following objectives: (a) understand the concept of positive aging (b) identifying the factors contributing to successful positive aging across health continuum (c) review strategies that promotes management healthy aging in elderly, and (d) identify future directions to promote successful population health management programs/interventions. The holistic approach, therefore provide an opportunity to improve the situation of older people in society. Author emphasized that positive or active ageing requires ongoing participation in productive activity, with a particular emphasis on extending labor force involvement. It encourages individuals to accept responsibility for maintenance of health and economic activity so that older individuals may remain independent, thereby reducing the demand on health and social services. Further, it was suggested that those who are ageing in good health and are engaged in productive activities may benefit from increased opportunities if the strategies achieve their objectives. The strategies provide an opportunity to improve the situation of older people in society by drawing attention to the negative effects of age discrimination and exclusion from opportunities to participate. Successful aging is not only the absence of chronic illness, but the perceived life satisfaction of the elderly person. People with high levels of resilience, low rates of depression, few years of substance abuse, and a good social network are most likely to age successfully and, perhaps most importantly, report high levels of life satisfaction into their golden years.

Chapter 4: Ageing, Quality of Life, and Social Support

In this chapter authors focused on the concept of aging as a sensitive process of transformation from a young age structure to old age. It is a pressing problem for many countries in this century. Therefore, attention to needs and problems of this age has an importance. The present chapter presents an intertwined view on aging, quality of life and social support. Elderly people are not much satisfied with their life therefore they blame to their age which seems a big issue and number of elderly people are unsatisfied with their life. This can be reduced by providing them adequate social support. They suggested that physical and mental impairments have been known to significantly decrease quality of life in older adults, as many lose hope, become isolated or depressed, lose faith, and struggle to feel joy in everyday life. When care professionals identify factors such as depression, social isolation, or chronic medical illness in a client, immediate measures should be taken to address what can be done to improve quality of life; interventions to improve comfort level, happiness, social immersion, access to care, resources, support systems, etc., need to be explored. It is essential to identify and target the problem areas that may hamper the quality of life of elderly, and emphasis should be on creating and inventing positive interventions. They further suggested that people should try to sustain and encourage positive contributing factors to quality of life. Moreover, individual sense of purpose, environment for learning, self-expression, and promoting dignity and building connection with others should be encouraged. Further, elderly should be equipped with various stress management tactics and guided techniques to alter various conditions (mentally, emotionally, and physically). Individual quality of life of elderly could be meaningfully improved when they are cared effectively for unspoken, unaddressed areas of need.

Chapter 5: Management of Elder Abuse Through Social Support

In this chapter the authors are highlighted the importance of understanding the elder abuse at global scenario. This includes standard definitions and types of elder abuses. Major portion of the chapter explained identification and preventive measures of elder abuse. The key to prevention of elder abuse is the ability to recognize the warning signs of its occurrence. The authors stressed upon signs of elder abuse type of abuse the victim is suffering. Elder abuse can destroy an elderly person's quality of life. Therefore, part of intervention measures various supports systems were illustrated to management of elder abuse. Along with psychological, sociological, gender, legal, socio-economic and community perspectives in order to understand the meaning of this phenomenon

Section 2: Cognition and Cognitive Impairment in Ageing and Clinical Outcome

Chapter 6: Cognitive Functions in the Geriatric Population

In this chapter authors discussed about the challenging issues of clinical diagnosis in distinguishing between the cognitive deficits manifested in normal aging, depression, Mild Cognitive Impairment (MCI) and dementia. Further emphasis was put on importance to establish conceptual and clinical criteria with sufficient predictive validity to accurately identify differences and similarities in cognitive states to justify initiation of appropriate treatments. Authors suggested that it is important to divulge more into these surface level differences and explore and evaluate sub domain differences through detailed neuropsychological assessment. One useful approach in the context of cognitive impairment is to apply interventions that compensate for the compromised abilities. These interventions aim to reduce the symptoms, delay or prevent progression to dementia or increase the rate of conversion to normal cognition. Similar approaches to cognitive behavioural therapy and support groups have been helpful in facilitating problem solving and reducing negative affect among individuals with early dementia. Thus, developing guidelines for specific type of activities, defining degree of ability reflective of intact functioning would enhance sensitivity and specificity to diagnosis and holistic assessment.

Chapter 7: Cognition in Ageing Implications for Assessment and Intervention

This chapter focuses on aging as an inevitable phase of life which encompasses changes in physical, psychological and social realms of an individual. Concern with the dwindling health and presence of any medical issues make the geriatric population prone to develop mental health conditions. Poor memory and reduced functional ability is one of the common complaints from older adults coming to psychiatric or neurology clinics. With growing age of the brain; while some cognitive functions do slow down; some of the functions do evolve better with experience. In this context, the chapter focuses on cognitive functions and impairment in the elderly; its implications in daily functioning with inputs on differences in the existing literature and the diagnostic and assessment issues and intervention strategies. With ever increasing population of elder people across the world; managing this population which is on threshold of developing behavioural and emotional dysfunctional behaviour secondary to cognitive decline would be a challenging task. Authors further proposed that there could be certain markers that differentiate the normal ageing and MCI from each other. A thorough assessment of individuals brought into consultation to check these markers as well as early intervention could be the key for optimum functioning of the elderly individual.

Chapter 8: Mild Cognitive Impairment – Evolution of the Clinical Diagnosis

This chapter emphasis was to acquaint the readers with the concept of Mild Cognitive Impairment and the evolution of the diagnosis to its current nosological status. It also elaborated on the assessment and management of patients with MCI. It was suggested that in the future the diagnostic power of this clinical syndrome would have improved and patients that are bound to develop dementia are identified early and treated. Just like other non-communicable diseases like diabetes, hypertension, which can be screened for early and managed without any major deterioration in quality of life, one hopes that dementia also reaches this fate. It was anticipated that in the years to come, biomarkers are understood better so that asymptomatic patients can be identified and dementia may be prevented if possible.

Chapter 9: Brain Ageing and Cognitive Impairment – Implications, Treatment, and Care

"Brain Ageing and Cognitive Impairment: Implications, Treatment, and Care" suggested that a healthy life both physically and mentally may be the best defense against the changes of an ageing brain. The authors aim to characterize changes in brain structure with aging, and to investigate relationships between brain aging and cognitive decline. Along with these it will make and attempt to identify possible management, treatment and preventive measures for managing cognitive impairment in brain ageing and promoting cognitive reserve for healthy brain ageing. There is a lot we can do to take charge of our brain health and maintain our cognitive fitness, no matter how old we are. Many of the scourges of aging might be prevented if we followed the old-fashioned advice of eating right, staying active, and getting plenty of rest.

Section 3: Medical Morbidity in Ageing

Chapter 10: Cardiovascular Disease in Elderly an Early Care – Biopsychosocial Perspective

This chapter focuses on cardiovascular disease, risk factors and impact on ageing. Authors were highlighted many risk factors for heart diseases: age, gender, tobacco use, physical inactivity, excessive alcohol consumption, unhealthy diet, obesity, genetic predisposition and family history of cardiovascular disease, psychosocial factors, poverty and low educational status, and air pollution. However, many important cardiovascular risk factors are modifiable by lifestyle change, social change, drug treatment for example prevention of hypertension, hyperlipidemia, and diabetes. Further authors extended to the trend of gender differences in CVD, risk assessment followed by preventive measures were recommended like medical management, multidisciplinary team approach, social support and Comprehensive Cardiac rehabilitation etc. Although an unavoidable cardiovascular risk factors in ageing, may overcome all the other risk factors collectively. Therefore, understanding fundamental mechanisms that dictate the pace of aging could lead to significant advancements into both preventative and therapeutic treatments of CVD that of enhancing quality of life of elderly.

Chapter 11: Stroke in Geriatric Population

In "Stroke in Geriatric Population," the chapter author explained the concept, symptoms, aetiology and challenges related to stroke in old age. Further author/s mentioned that incidence of stoke increases with age and elderly people are more likely to have more severe stroke. In addition, elderly people will have multiple comorbidities which make management more difficult. After a disabling stroke, easing back to life requires a positive attitude to overcome difficulties. A physiotherapist can help restore the strength and reduce stiffness of muscles. Regular follow up with a physician or neurologist, taking medicines as prescribed is important to improve the outcome and prevent the recurrence of stroke. The authors concluded that management of elderly patients with stroke poses unique challenges due to associated comorbidities and factors specific for geriatric population. Clinical trials on stroke should include more and more elderly subjects to gain insight into the factors unique for geriatric population, which in turn will help in providing better treatment and care of such patients.

Chapter 12: Ageing and Cancer – The Epigenetic Basis, Alternative Treatment, and Care

Cancer is the disorder of immune system and is epigenetically controlled. As a person grows older the cells in their body becomes weaker. The defense system of the body and genetic repair mechanisms becomes more delicate. In this chapter authors discuss about explores the demographic changes, biological theories and clinical considerations that link cancer and ageing. It highlights the implications of these associations in the context of population and health system, with a focus on preventative strategies, research imperatives and delivery of cancer services. Furthermore, the chapter discusses how to best prepare the most junior of the medical profession to manage a growing number of senior cancer patients. Overall, it underscores how all elements in the relationship of cancer and ageing need to be considered and incorporated into a framework that facilitates a holistic approach to cancer control. Further author/s suggested scientific ways to prevent cancer to grow in individuals' body. They also emphasized that the research communities must acknowledge the fact that the war against cancer cannot be won using allopathic medicine system. Be it conventional or alternative or complementary, the war against cancer can only be won if and only if the best of all these three systems are combined to form an Integrated System of Medicine that will be personalized, more scientific and free from adverse effects. Because it's not the bits and pieces, it is the whole that matters.

Chapter 13: Ageing and Cancer – Intervention Strategies

This chapter is emphasized on the fact that the incidence of cancers increases with age. This increase incidence may be due to biological factors, prolonged exposure to carcinogens and incidence of mutations etc. Cancers in elderly may have poor biological vulnerability, presence of various co-morbidities and poor tolerance of therapy hence treatment got compromised. Elderly cancer patients also are neglected in various trials and strong data lacks for optimal management. They also stressed upon lack of emotional support, poor financial assistance and treatment monitoring etc. leading to various psychological problems related to cancer in elderly. They concluded by saying that older people need special attention regarding disease and treatment option, tailoring treatment according to comorbidities and performance status. Family members have great responsibilities of physical, mental and monitory support to this elderly population. Considering the severe nature of the illness a multimodality treatment is requiring with skilled professionals. Not only the patient but their family members also needs to be take into treating team to make the process realistically functional, although with advancement of treatment, treatment rule and regulation facilities physical, biological, economical, professional, legal needs had been taken care of.

Chapter 14: Sensory Impairments and Challenges in Ageing

In this chapter authors mentioned that sensory impairment is often regarded from a medical/disability point of view and its effects on mental health can be poorly recognized. Communication is a key issue for deaf and deaf-blind people and difficulties here underlie developmental, psychological and emotional problems and delay or prevent appropriate assessment and treatment. They suggested that the main concerns of visual and hearing affected by the total or partial absence of sight and/or hearing are usually how to live, how to learn and how to communicate. Their difficulties are often as much to do with society's attitudes towards them as with the direct effect of sensory impairment. They also focused on the fact that combined vision and hearing impairments have a greater effect on function than single sensory impairments and influence functional status independent of mental status and comorbid illness. With the increasing need for and use of health care services due to an ageing population, the major goal in public health and medicine is to keep elderly individuals living independently and to prevent institutionalization. Small improvements in vision and hearing impairment may enhance physical and psychological functioning in older adults.

Chapter 15: Diabetes Mellitus and Ageing

Among all medical illnesses, Diabetes Mellitus is one of the most common and serious medical condition that has affected not only the aging population but also the young children and adults as well. Diabetes and its complications can contribute to aging process in a number of ways and the complications can speed up the aging process as well. In chapter entitled "Diabetes Mellitus and Aging", author/s covers different aspects of diabetes mellitus and its impact on human life and also how with healthy coping mechanism one can prevent the distressing effect of diabetes on aging and vice versa. They emphasized on the fact that access to adequate health care plays an even stronger role in controlling diabetes, preventing the development of complications to aging. By doing few things a person can stop or decrease the devastating effects associated with age and diabetes and can live an energetic life. It requires a holistic approach. Social, psychological and economical determinants of health and diabetes need to be considered when focusing on improving diabetes outcomes.

Chapter 16: Obesity Physical and Mental Health Consequences in Ageing

In this chapter, the authors mentioned that the prevalence of obesity is on rise in all age groups and emphasized obesity as Global epidemic. Obesity is considered as one of the leading cause of various non-communicable diseases. Higher body mass index and abdominal obesity are considered to be an independent risk factors that significantly contributes to the increased prevalence of type 2 diabetes, cardiovascular diseases and hypertension, metabolic disorders along with various mental health problems among elderly. Geriatric obesity further affects the treatment process, outcome, quality and quantity of life older adults. It also increases the risk of disability among older adults. They suggested that research must focus more on determining behavioural treatment how these behavioural techniques can be best applied in a real-world setting. Behavioural treatment is an approach used to help individuals develop a set of skills to achieve a healthier weight. The behaviour change process is facilitated through the use of self-monitoring, goal setting, and problem solving.

Chapter 17: Sleep and Sleep Disorders in Old Age – Assessment and Non-Pharmacological Management

Sleep complaints are prevalent among older adults. Sleep quality and quantity changes with advancing age. There are changes in sleep patterns which are normal with ageing but many changes are the sign of disordered sleep. In this chapter author/s emphasized on numerous psychological and social factors contributing to quality and quantity of sleep. Specific sleep disorders more prevalent in old age are insomnia, sleep apnea, and rapid eye movement disorder. They focused on non-pharmacological treatment to be effective in management of Sleep disorders. Cognitive behaviour therapy is most effective to tackle Specifically Insomnia. Cognitive behaviour therapy along with meditation is beneficial for other sleep disorders and new technique is also emerging like, mindfulness. Focuses on preventive steps are needed to be adapted for wellbeing at least in terms of sleep. The establishment and maintenance of regular tight routine in both pre-bed time and sleep schedule may be an important preventive factor.

Chapter 18: Impact of Tuberculosis in Elderly Population

In this chapter authors focused on global scenario about tuberculosis and ageing. If we look at prevalence rate tuberculosis is a highly infectious disease and one of the top 10 causes of death worldwide in 2015, over 10 million people fell ill with TB and 1.8 million died from the disease. About one-third of the world's population has latent TB, which means people have been infected by TB bacteria but are not (yet) ill with the disease and cannot transmit the disease. Globally, six countries account for 60% of the total cases of TB, with India leading the count, followed by Indonesia, China, Nigeria, Pakistan and South Africa. Poor living conditions and poor socialization of patients has created a situation where the patients suffer from psychosocial affects along with the symptoms of the disease itself. Elderly are more prone to complications as ageing factors like memory loss, hearing or speech impairment and mental confusion can make it difficult to diagnose and treat symptoms affectively. Presence of Multi Drug Resistant TB (MDR-TB) is another risk for elderly patients as aggressive treatments have multi system impact in already frail patients. For these reasons, authors were suggested suitable recommendations for these special populations.

Chapter 19: Thyroid Disease in Ageing and Risk Factors

This chapter dealt with Thyroid disease in elderly and risk factors. Thyroid diseases regardless of age can be classified as functional disorders (hypothyroidism and hyperthyroidism), inflammatory conditions (thyroiditis) and neoplastic conditions (nodules and carcinomas). Further, the authors focused hypothyroidism, hyperthyroidism causes, consequences and management issues were addressed systematically. The highlights of the section are quoted previous research on thyroid disease. Several studies have investigated the role of thyroid function in the aging process. There is convincing evidence that higher levels of TSH are associated with longevity. The process of aging affects both the prevalence and clinical presentation of hypo- and hyperthyroidism. Importantly, subclinical disturbances of thyroid function are more frequent than overt diseases in general population, as well as in elderly people. In addition to this thyroidiosm and other risk factors like thyroid nodules, thyroid cancer and management issues were elaborated with suitable studies. Older patients with thyroid disorders require special attention to gradual and careful treatment, and, as always, require lifelong follow-up.

Chapter 20: Music Therapy – An Intervention in Alzheimer Disease

Alzheimer's disease (AD) is a progressive neurodegenerative disorder. With characteristic neuro pathological and neurochemical features characterized by symptom complex in which there is disturbance of multiple higher cortical functions, including memory, thinking, orientation, comprehension, calculation, learning capacity, language and judgment. The chapter discusses different strategies have been applied to prevent/delay onset of Alzheimer's disease or at least to improve quality of life and health conditions of Alzheimer's disease patients. And music therapy is an established health profession in which music is used within a therapeutic relationship to address physical, emotional, cognitive, and social needs of individuals. As mentioned by the authors music therapy is a goal directed process in which the therapist helps the patients to improve, maintain or restore a state of well-being. In this chapter the authors discussed the importance of music/music therapy is an effective intervention when dealing with patients with dementia. Hence, the need to discuss the scope of music therapy as an intervention in AD.

Section 4: Medical and Psychiatric Comorbidities in Ageing

Chapter 21: Ageing and Mental Health – A Psychological Aspect of Later Life

Geropsychology is a branch of psychology that deals with ageing as it relates to mental health. While awareness is growing, almost two-third adults with psychiatric conditions do not receive the required treatment. Manifestation of age related symptoms like physical illnesses often leads to psychological issues or vice versa. Various mental health models can project and predict psychological issues in later years like the Aging Psychodynamic model that analyzes based on events and conditions in the younger years or the Eriksonian Psychosocial Development model that uses developmental challenges as an analysis tool. The Cognitive Behavioral model emphasizes the importance of thoughts and belief system to maladaptive behaviors and negative emotions. A range of mental health issues can be observed as one ages. The author emphasized how these psychiatric and psychological conditions can be triggered by transition phases and events that one has to go through like retirement or the wedding of an offspring. The identification of mental health issues in the elderly has been a first step in improving the conditions and remedial services available for these populations.

Chapter 22: Factors Contributing of Ageing – Factors in Ageing

This chapter explores the cause and effects of relationships in some of the factors on ageing and over all wellbeing. Author aimed at how these factors that contributes to ageing. Those factors were such as biological, life style, social, psychological, spiritual, and cognitive and the diseases in the old age. Followed by ageing and health care measure were discussed for fine tuning of understanding about those factors influencing on ageing. Though Ageing is an unavoidable reality that everyone faces. The effects of aging appear in different people based on a wide variety of factors, not the least of them is race and ethnicity and the impact of social, psychological, and emotional factors on ones over all wellbeing. Some external factors like diet and nutrition and physical activity can be controlled while others like genetic predisposition to ailments become impossible to cope with.

Chapter 23: Ageing and Suicide

This chapter deals with cause and dynamics of suicidal behavior among elderly are quite different from the younger suicides. There have been different multidisciplinary theories proposed for it, among all mental disorders, depressive disorders are particularly associated with suicidal behavior. Alcohol use, social isolation, financial difficulties are few unique factors that identify a suicidal elderly. Physical illnesses particularly those marked with pain increase the chances of suicide. Psychiatric illness particularly depressive illness is commonly associated with the suicidal behavior. However, both physicians as well as community need to be sensitized for its identification. Isolation, financial and relationship problems also contribute to the suicidal behavior among elderly. These may set up a vicious circle with depressive symptoms leading to suicidal attempt by the victim. Authors suggested that prevention requires a multidisciplinary approach involving community, adequate and appropriate health services near to the place of victim, legal restrictions on the methods used for suicide such as availability of fire arm and insecticides, public policies to take care of the elderly are recommended. Religious and spiritual practices increase cohesiveness and prevent against suicide.

Chapter 24: Ageing and Sexuality

Sexual problems are more frequently found in elderly. This review describes briefly about the various causes of sexual dysfunction, assessment, and management of sexual problems in elderly. Author/s emphasized on healthy sexuality and its importance for elderly, and contrary to popular beliefs, elderly people continue to be sexually active, albeit with reducing frequency. Negative attitude towards old age sexuality are prevalent in laymen and in healthcare professionals alike, and negatively affect the help seeking behavior. They suggested that active screening for the sexual dysfunctions should be the integral part of medical evaluation. Patients with sexual dysfunctions like ED should be screened for cardiovascular risks, and modifying these risks may in turn improve sexual functioning. Appropriate use of non-pharmacological and pharmacological treatment processes may help in restoration of normal sexual functioning in elderly.

Chapter 25: Comorbidity of Medical and Psychiatric Disorders in Geriatric Population – Treatment and Care

This chapter author focused on the fact that with the advancement in health care facilities and better availability of health services, the geriatric population is gradually on raise. But, this group of population is at increased risk of developing both physical and psychological co-morbidities due to the age-related factors and changes in the social circumstances. The chapter proposes the concept and issues related to co-morbidity in geriatric population and their effective treatment regime and care/management in relation to geriatric population was addressed. Author emphasized on proper assessment and screening which enhances effective diagnosis is the need of the hour to manage several co-morbidities associated with old age. Also health plans used for administrative data for planning prevention and disease management programs, programs that often range in intensity from reminder letters for health screening to case management are required. For populations' identified, as in this chapter, medical needs might be assessed and variations in health practices could be explored such as adherence with medications and health screening rates. Economic factors, ethnic variations, and geographical differences, as examples, may differentially affect patients who vary in the combinations of chronic conditions they have to manage.

Chapter 26: Disability Issues in Ageing and Preventive Measures

The ageing population is now encompassing developing countries too. Population ageing has profound social, economic and political implications for a country. The increasing number of older persons put a strain on health care and social care systems in the country. In the chapter were discusses various disability in old age. Old age comes with lot of ailment and diseases like blindness, low vision, cerebral palsy, leprosy, leprosy cured, hearing impairment, locomotor disability, mental illness, and mental retardation as well as multiple disabilities. Researchers have theorized roughly ten percent of the world's population; suffer from some form of physical, sensory or mental handicap. Elderly in India suffer from cardio-vascular illnesses, circulatory diseases, cancer, arthritis, hyper tension, osteoporosis, communicable diseases, high blood pressure, kidney problems, vision problems, diabetes. This chapter focuses on the prevention of disability. It is understood that prevention is better than cure. Hence, different stake holders in government level and non- government level need to put efforts to create preventable diseases could yield better results and help elderly population.

Barre Vijaya Prasad
Dharwad Institute of Mental Health and Neurosciences (DIMHANS), India

Shamsi Akbar
King George's Medical University, India

REFERENCES

United Nations. (n.d.). *World population ageing 2009*. Retrieved from www.un.org/esa/population/publications/WPA2009/WPA2009_WorkingPaper.pdf

Acknowledgment

It's my privilege to acknowledge the important people who worked for this book. I would like to express my sincere thanks to all authors and reviewers who worked and part of this book. Thank you for all your valuable contribution and make this book a reality. I felt, my nobility to work this title at an early stage of my professional career towards elderly and I inspired by people who already serving in the field of Geropsychology. Further, it is an honor to acknowledge, mostly I learnt and influenced by my teachers Prof. T. B. Singh, Prof. G. Padmaja and Prof. Suvashisa Rana for their valuable suggestions and guidance.

My sincere thanks goes to Prof. Srinivas Kosgi, who always available for helping me during the seminal and completion of the work and I consider him as an architect of this book. I owe a huge thanks to Prof. Hitesh Khurana who has an ear to hear me like a young scholar when I seek out his help. No doubt his scientific knowledge in the field without mentioning is incomplete of his myriad support. My special thanks to other eminent person Prof. Akbar Hussian he is a back bone of every aspects of editorial and technical communication made us to reach beyond reachable. I am indebted to thanks to Pratima Kaushik, who is technically devoted many hours of her attention during the process of proof reading and final submission of this manuscript.

I would like express my thanks to Fazal Naqvi- Director Enterprise solutions and Ashwini R. Patil during midst of the time they helped us to review the chapters of the book. I am thankful to my friend Manjunath R. Bajantri and Gayatri Hegade, who provide feedback and support during the process of this book. I sincerely, thank and acknowledge faculty, staff and colleagues from DIMHANS, who have directly or indirectly considered this effort.

I would like to show my gratitude to L. Sam. S. Manickam, who is a moderator of Indian Clinical Psychologists yahoo groups. I thank him for call for chapters were heavily forward to the professional as fast as possible.

Thank you doesn't seem sufficient but it is said thank you parents for their support and unconditional love. Words would never say how grateful I am to both of you.

Last, but definitely not least, I'd like to thank Marianne Caesar, Assistant Development Editor IGI and IGI community for giving me opportunity to bring this work fruitfully.

Barre Vijaya Prasad
Dharwad Institute of Mental Health and Neurosciences (DIMHANS), India

Shamsi Akbar
King George's Medical College, India

Section 1
Social and Psychological Factors in Ageing

Chapter 1
Positive Psychology and Aging

Jyoti Mishra Pandey
Government Medical College and Hospital Chandigarh, India

Shobit Garg
SMI Medical College and Hospital, India

ABSTRACT

The present chapter will help in understanding the role of positive psychology and intervention in approaching towards a healthy aging. Aging is inevitable. The clock cannot be turned backwards. At first glance, it seems that generally the growing population enjoy what they face which is true to a certain extent but at the same time it is important not to overlook or discount the stresses they face when they start to age. How they age depends how they look at their life. Positive intervention has its effect in all ages. Taking the help of positive psychology as a primary prevention can help eliminating various effects of aging. In the same way, it can also help in reducing the exiting trouble occurring in elderly. By taking preventive steps, one can take care of the body and the mind, and that can help stave off some of the devastating illnesses associated with age and live a full, meaningful and energetic life. Elderly person must acknowledge that their roles in life will change as their former lifestyles are replaced by new schedules, approaches and relationships.

INTRODUCTION

Aging is a gradual and slow process and generates significant changes in one's life. A person completes all the responsibility that comes in their way, completes education, work, raises children, retire from work and so on. At first glance, it seems that generally they enjoy what they face which is true to a certain extent but at the same time it is important not to overlook or discount the stresses they face when they start to age. Many a times these changes can be discouraging and may lead to feelings of insecurity and loss of self-worth. How they age depends how they look at their life. Positive psychology has its significant role to play in the process of aging and helps in overcoming various challenges that they face. Elderly person must acknowledge that their roles in life will change as their former lifestyles are replaced by new schedules, approaches and relationships.

DOI: 10.4018/978-1-5225-3480-8.ch001

Worldwide, the population is ageing rapidly. World Health Organization (WHO), (2016) report says that between 2015 and 2050, the proportion of the world's population over 60 years will nearly double from 12% to 22%. The share of India's population aged 60 and above is projected to rise from 8% in 2010 to 19% in 2050, according to the United Nations Population Division (United Nations, 2011). This phase comes not only as an additional number to a persons' life but as a chapter with significant contributions from the surroundings. The higher the positive environmental inputs, the better the outcomes. There is a slow decline in the overall functioning of the body system as the person ages. They are more likely to experience several changes and disabilities at the same time (WHO, 2015). In 2011, approximately 22.7 million (62%) of community-dwelling older adults in the United States aged ≥65 years had at least one basic functional disability (National Center for Health Statistics, 2013).It is that life-cycle stage where individuals are forced to face life's most stressful experiences. They become more sensitive to criticism, become emotionally weak and dependent. However, there are some factors like lack of economic security, loneliness, loss of loved ones and limited social interactions that adversely affect aging process. However, positive psychology contributes significantly to the outcome of aging process. It focuses on the potentials and optimal functioning of human beings. The approach of positive psychology is not towards fixing problems, instead focuses on exploring things that make life worth living. This is not a distinct field, but rather a distinct way of viewing the human conditions. It focuses on people as having the potential to thrive given the right skills, strengths and social context (Kashdan & Ciarrochi, 2013.

It consists of interventions for promoting resilience, positive emotions, engagement, meaning, curiosity and social connectedness (Ciarrochi & Kashdan, 2013; Parks & Biswas-Diener, 2013).

The Gerodynamics/ Branching theory of aging explains about the branching behavior of an individual at the psychological, biological or social level of functioning. As an example, traumatic life events may result in lower order structures and a healthy life style may result in higher order structures, and consequently higher and lower probabilities of dying respectively. However, it may not hold true for everyone. There are exceptions. Some people are strengthened by illness, and divorce may have a positive rather than a negative effect on mental health in terms of life expectancy and quality of life for some people (Schroots, 1996). Similarly, in a theoretical continuum, with severe mental illness on the left and optimal human thriving on the right, Seligman pointed out that previous research had focused on the left half of the curve and that the right side of the curve mostly had been neglected. He focuses on more to mental health than the absence of mental illness. This field is dedicated to the rigorous scientific study of "strengths, well-being and optimal functioning" (Duckworth et al., 2005) and flourishing (Keyes & Haidt, 2003). Thus, aging with positive psychology helps a person to live a healthy life with a healthy approach.

AGING PROCESS

Tornstam (1989) suggested that the process of living into old age that is human aging visualizes a general potential towards gerotranscendence: that is a shift in metaperspective from a materialistic and rational vision towards a more cosmic and transcendent vision. This is normally followed by an increase in life satisfaction. Thus, there is a need to understand the basic requirements of elderly. This phase of aging has become much more a social phenomenon rather than merely a being a biological one. This process depends upon various components. It is a multidimensional construct where self-perception and attitude plays an essential role. The term "self-perceptions of aging" has been increasingly used to refer to adults' subjective aging experiences (Kleinspehn-Ammerlahn et al., 2008; Kotter-Grühn et al., 2009; Kotter-Grühn & Hess, 2012). It is related with both positive and negative age-related experiences (Wurm et al., 2007). A study conducted in-depth interviews with adults aged 50 to 80 years and identified five major dimensions of positive and negative aging experiences. These five dimensions described aging as: (1) a natural and gradual process; (2) a period of life evaluation, philosophical reflection, or increased wisdom and maturity; (3) a period of increased freedom, new interests, and fewer demands; (4) a period of physical health difficulties and health concerns; and (5) a period of losses, including interpersonal and job-related losses (Keller et al., 1989). Another important construct is "attitude towards aging" (Bennett & Eckman, 1973). It refers to both societal as well as individual attitudes and includes affective, cognitive, and evaluative components of behavior towards older adults as an age group and towards the process of aging as a personal experience (Hess, 2006). Bennett and Eckman (1973) pointed that attitude towards aging are considered critical for older people's adjustment and survival in the process of aging. It contributes to their adaptive and maladaptive behaviors and reinforces how individuals in younger age groups view and approach their own aging process. However, negative attitudes toward older adults are quite pervasive, and that older adults' views of their own behavior often reflect the societal beliefs and stereotypes about aging (Hess, 2006; Levy, 2009). They are often based on cultural images of aging and are developed from early childhood experiences. Attitudes toward one's own aging have also been referred to as self-related attitudes (Hess, 2006) to indicate the focus of the attitudes as studies have shown that older adults have more negative views about their memory than younger or middle-aged adults (Hertzog & Hultsch, 2000; Hess, 2006). Several studies have also shown that older adults who have more positive attitudes about their own aging tend to perform better on memory tasks (Levy, 1996; Levy & Langer, 1994), are more likely to engage in positive life styles (Levy & Myers, 2004), show less decline in disablement processes (Levy et al., 2012), and live longer (Levy et al., 2002). Studies show substantial positive associations with adults' health (Wurm et al., 2007) and preventive health behaviors (Levy & Myers, 2004; WurmTomasik & Tesch-Römer, 2010). However, a large body of work documented the association between negative age stereotypes and older adults' maladaptive behavior, such as lower cognitive functioning and poorer functional health behaviors that are very much associated with the vulnerabilities of old age (Hummert, 2011; Levy, 1996, 2003).

This is a stage where one requires assistance in their activities of daily living because of their physiological decline due to the aging process. When they fail in meeting physiological needs it results in psychological decline. A study reported that among the elderly population 47.8% reported an unmet need with one or more activities of daily livings (ADLs) or instrumental activities of daily livings (IADLs). Significant adjusted correlates of unmet assistance need included greater number of ADL and IADL difficulties and lower levels of social support (Schure et al., 2015). Research has identified several factors associated with an increased risk for unmet assistance need among adults including greater number of ADL limitations, greater morbidity, dementia, lower income, younger age, and living alone (Allen & Mor, 1997, Desai et al., 2001; Kennedy, 2001; LaPlante et al., 2004; Lima & Allen, 2001; Newcomer et al., 2005; Sands et al., 2006; Williams et al., 1997). This population with an unmet assistance need have been shown to have an increased likelihood of experiencing weight loss, dehydration, falls, burns (LaPlante et al., 2004), increased number of emergency room and hospital visits (Allen & Mor, 1997), increased number of hospitalizations and nursing home placements (Sands et al., 2006), and higher mortality rates (Blazer et al., 2005).

In this process, the psychological experience of old age group leads to increased introspection, search for meaning of life and of the very existence, questions of identity and sense of privacy. It is important to notice that, while the young have shorter pasts and longer futures, older people have longer pasts and shorter futures. It is a time of loss: the loss of spouse, friends, jobs, standard of living, and health. Increased psychological well-being is a significant protective factor from the occurrence of future episodes of major depression (Wood & Joseph, 2010; Sin & Lyubomirsky, 2009). Positive mental health is different from merely the absence of psychological distress (Keyes, 2002). Thus, aging process not only involves additional number to their age but various other significant factors that hinders the healthy process of aging. Therefore, increasing well-being and positive intervention might not only increase positive factors but also reduce negative states and psychopathology.

EFFECTS AND FACTORS CONTRIBUTING TO AGING

The aging population may be most aware of their new gray hairs and wrinkles, but this is just the external manifestation of aging. Changes are taking place throughout in the entire body. Poor diet, inactivity, weight gain, and a slower metabolic rate all set the stage for circulatory problems and cardiovascular disease. Blood pressure tends to rise with age, visual acuity diminishes, and difficulty seeing things, decrease hearing ability and sense of taste may become affected as well. Diabetes, obesity, and hypertension are all also reported to be higher among American Indians than the general population (Indian Health Service, 2014). There are various neuropsychological changes that take place in aging such as the slow decline in information-processing speed, dual task, task shifting, encoding, storage and retrieval of memory, deterioration in intellectual capacity. The old person finds it difficult to remember names and location. The psychomotor activity becomes very slow and they take more than usual time to complete a particular task. Dementia and Alzheimer's disease hinders their normal functioning significantly. However, some changes that have long been thought of as normal aging can be, in fact, the signs of a potential disease for example, sudden changes in personality. A common belief is that people become cranky, depressed, and withdrawn as they get older. But an analysis of long-term data from the Baltimore Longitudinal Study of Aging (BLSA) showed that an adult's personality generally does not change much after age 30. People who are cheerful and assertive when they are younger will likely be the same when they are age 80. Their findings suggest that significant changes in personality are not due to normal aging, but instead may be early signs of disease or dementia (National Institute of Aging, 2008).

Stressful life events have detrimental effects on physical and mental health in elderly (Cohen et al., 2007; Pearlin et al., 2005; Thoits, 2006). It results in various neuropsychiatric disorders that account for 6.6% of the total disability for this age group. Approximately 15% of adults aged 60 and over suffer from a mental disorder. The most common neuropsychiatric disorders in this age group are dementia and depression. Anxiety disorders affect 3.8% of the elderly population, substance use problems affect almost 1% and around a quarter of deaths from self-harm are among those aged 60 or above. Substance abuse problems among the elderly are often overlooked or misdiagnosed and mental health problems are under-identified by health-care professionals and older people themselves, and the stigma surrounding mental illness makes people reluctant to seek help (WHO, 2016). In India, in the year 2014, 7107 males and 2654 females (Total 9761) aged 60 years and above committed suicide. This comprises 7.4% of total number of suicides in the country (National Crime Record Bureau, 2014). Retirement is another phase which is inescapable. One person can see retirement as a phase of relaxation and freedom from responsibility and other can take it as stress and threat to financial condition and dependency on others. Limited social involvement is also a significant contributor. A systematic review of studies has shown that in industrialized countries, limited social connectedness is associated with suicidal ideation, non-fatal suicidal behavior and suicide in later life (Fassberg et al., 2012).

Elder mistreatment is another stressful life event that may lead to psychological distress in the victims. Several cross-sectional studies have shown that older adults who were mistreated had higher levels of psychological distress than those who had no such experience (Comijs et al., 1999; Mouton, 2003). Clinical studies suggest other effects of elder mistreatment, including feelings of learned helplessness, alienation, guilt, shame, fear, anxiety, denial, and posttraumatic stress syndrome (Wolf, 2000). At least 1 in 10 older adults suffers some form of elder abuse, and many in repeated forms (Government Accountability Office, 2011). Another very important factor in elderly is the sexual relationships. A study found that sexual pleasure and the need for intimacy continue to be important for older women, but that changing sexual abilities and sexual health needs, such as the reduction of sexual desire, as well as increased painful intercourse due to menopause-associated vaginal drying, were persistent barriers to sexual fulfillment and satisfaction (Taylor et al., 2016). Cultural and social factors contribute significantly to these changes. Sexual activity in old age is perceived as a social stigma in Indian society. In Indian culture sex in later life is a taboo and a shameful act. It is a kind of suppressing id and overpowering super ego. Old people suppress their desires and avoid talking about their sexual life because of this social stigma.

Functional limitations and health problems are the additional factors that also increase the risk for isolation and the need for social support in elderly (Langford et al., 1997). A study reported negative relationship between depression and social support for both American Indian adults and older adults (Roh et al., 2014; Whitbeck et al., 2002). However, despite fewer network ties, evidence suggests that different types of social support may increase with age, for example, instrumental support in conducting activities of daily living (Van Tilburg, 1998). Women generally report higher levels of social support and social network ties than men (Antonucci & Akiyama, 1987). It was significantly associated with excellent or good self-reported health status, especially for women (Richmond et al., 2007). A study of persons aged ≥65 years reported that functional decline and death due to acute heart failure at 12 months were predicted by low baseline scores of social support in men, but no effects were seen in women (Berard et al., 2012). Social support withdrawal with age stresses a potential concern that older adults are more at risk of low social support during a time when their need is high (Richmond et al., 2007). Experimental and longitudinal studies have found that increased positive emotions lead to social, occupational, and health benefits (Lyubomirsky et al., 2005). Correlational evidence also links higher reported focus on engaging and meaningful activities to greater occupational success and higher incomes (Schueller & Seligman, 2010).

EMPTY NEST CONCEPT

Successful agers are able to enjoy higher levels of well-being in spite of deteriorations in various domains of life because they have more spiritual, social and psychological resources mainly the positive attitude and approach towards healthy life changes. A high level of life satisfaction and positivity is achieved only when the aging population utilizes the above resources and applies existential coping policies of acceptance in the life. With aging these major sources of personal meaning, such as family, work, social status, and activities start shrinking, giving rise to question of 'Why to live?'. According to the "Empty Nest" concept of aging, in early phase of life whole family lives together. As the children grow they move away from their parental nest for further education and career and then get settled with their own families. Parents stay alone with their companion. They want their near and dear ones around. The situation gets worse when they lose their spouses. They already suffer from the biological changes and deterioration in their body which worsen by the addition of these environmental and emotional factors. This fatal combination gives rise to various psychiatric and psychological issues. The adverse conditions of physical and mental health can influence the elderly sense of life satisfaction (Pinto et al., 2016). Additionally, Ericksons' psychosocial theory (1959) explains old age as exemplified by integrity vs. despair. In this stage there is a question of existentialism of the self. Erikson believed that the last stage involves much of reflection of past life. As older people, some can look back with a feeling of integrity; a contentment and fulfillment, having led a meaningful life and did valuable contribution to the society. Others may have a sense of despair during this stage, reflecting upon their experiences and failures, feel guilty about the past, or feel that they did not accomplish their life goals, they become dissatisfied with life. Dissatisfaction and despair in life gives rise to many psychiatric and psychological problems. Depression, anxiety and loneliness become very common when the aging result in despair from life. This phase often leads to decrease in social activities and interaction. They prefer to stay within a very closely-knit environment, with family members, close relatives and very close friends. Many a times the youth find it very uninteresting to spend time with their elderly. This gives the elderly a feeling of being unwanted. A feeling of loneliness and sadness gradually sets in. Loneliness is highly prevalent among older persons with depressive symptoms (Van Beljouw et al., 2014). Community-based studies have identified a variety of risk factors for loneliness/isolation including widowhood, no (surviving) children, living alone, deteriorating health, and life events. Certain situational factors heighten the risk for increased loneliness. These include low socioeconomic status, marital discord, infrequent contact with friends and family, few social roles, lack of participation in voluntary organizations, physical health symptoms, and physical limitations (Hawkley et al., 2008; Santini Koyanagi et al., 2015). Apart from this, loss of loved ones, separation and retirement are also contributing factors causing isolation and depression in old age. Dealing with the issues of life changes and acceptability with positive approach and intervention helps in preventing its various devastating effects on aging.

EFFICACY OF POSITIVE INTERVENTION

Seligman (2004), proposes three pillars of positive psychology, that is: 1) study of positive emotions like checking satisfaction with the past, happiness in the present moment and the hope for the future; 2) study of the qualities/positive traits especially strengths and virtues such as: flexibility, self-control, courage and wisdom and; 3) study of positive institutions e.g. school, family, community. Similarly, searching meaning through inner and spiritual resources is a promising way of transcending personal losses and despair in old age (Wong, 1998). One way of seeing these changes can be positive approach mainly positive intervention. This is an intervention or therapy aimed at increasing positive feelings, positive behaviors, or positive cognitions, as opposed to ameliorating pathology or fixing negative thoughts or maladaptive behavior patterns (Sin & Lyubomirsky, 2009). Exercises like "Three Good Things," a gratitude exercise, outperformed the "You at Your Best" intervention, where participants are asked to describe a time in the past when they were at their best (Seligman et al., 2005). For example: The "Best Future Self" exercise instructs participants as follows:

Think about your life in the future. Imagine that everything has gone as well as it possibly could. You have worked hard and succeeded at accomplishing all of your life goals. Think of this as the realization of all of your life dreams. Now, write about what you imagined (King, 2001).

Positive interventions along with exercises are designed to promote kindness, generosity, and mindfulness (Layous et al., 2011). With aging these components can help in having a different perspective and approaches while aging. In a randomized control trials, a 7-week loving-kindness meditation workshop was shown to increase positive emotions, which in turn predicted increases in psychological, cognitive, social, and physical resources, which went on to increase life satisfaction and decrease depression (Fredrickson et al., 2008). Similarly, a meta-analysis of 51 randomized controlled studies of positive interventions of individuals who were healthy and of individuals who suffered from depression showed increase in well-being and decrease in depression (Sin & Lyubomirsky, 2009).

Ciarrochi et al. (2016) focus on two components of positive psychology interventions; Content and context -focused positive interventions. Content-focused positive interventions is defined as those that focus on altering the content of people's thinking, that reinforce the notion that a certain way of thinking is inherently good, and that tend to underemphasize or ignore the role of context. These interventions often seek to increase positive mental content or diminish negative mental content. For example, theorists have argued that positive emotions cause people to "broaden and build" (Fredrickson, 2001), optimism and grit cause people to succeed (Seligman, 2002; Duckworth& Gross, 2014), and a lack of positive thinking or the presence of negative thinking causes failure and unhappiness (Byrne, 2006; Peal, 2012). On the other hand, Context-focused positive interventions refer to situational and historical events that exert an organizing influence on behavior" (Hayes et al., 2011). It refers to influence that comes from the immediate antecedents and consequences of behavior, the historical context and the multiple groups and structures within which a person is nested, e.g., social class, culture, family group, friendship group (Bronfenbrenner & Ceci, 1994). Context-focused positive interventions help in treating the causes of behavior as largely residing within the environment. However, even contextual interventions can be done in a content-focused way. For example, mindfulness interventions can be treated as a universal way to reduce stress.

Long before positive psychology, the great philosophers (Socrates, Plato, Aristotle) and psychological thinkers (Freud, Jung, Adler, Frankl, Rogers, Maslow) articulated theories of the good life, pleasure, wholeness, purpose, health, and actualization (Duckworth et al., 2005; Ryff, 2003). In addition, empirical work existed on adaptation, resilience, thriving, spirituality, and growth (Aspinwall & Tedeschi, 2010). There are subsets of positive interventions, a self-administered without professional administration, such as "positive activity interventions" defined as "relatively brief, self-administered, and non-stigmatizing exercises that promote positive feelings, positive thoughts, and/or positive behaviors, rather than directly aiming to fix negative or pathological feelings, thoughts, and behaviors" (Layous et al., 2011). Lazarus criticized positive psychology for taking an overly simplistic approach to the complexities of human emotion and the harsh realities of human life (Lazarus, 2003). However, consistent findings suggest that stronger social relationships reduce mortality and help us cope with life stressors (Holt-Lunstad et al., 2010) Furthermore, psychological well-being in general and positive emotion in particular, appear to promote meaning-making in stressful situations, which in turn leads to more effective coping (Tugade & Fredrickson, 2004).

SOLUTIONS AND RECOMMENDATIONS

Acceptance and healthy welcome of aging can prevent various difficulties which one face during this process. Dependency on anyone makes a person handicap in dealing or adjusting with the life changes. The humans have a tendency to plan everything in advance to secure healthy and safe life. However, fails to plan a very essential aspect of life i.e. *"Old Age"*. Here are few recommendations along with positive interventions which can help a person in having a healthy approach towards aging;

- Plan aging before it comes and takes preventive measures to avoid the devastating effect of aging. For example, post retirement financial plan can prevent various psychiatric and medical conditions in an aging persons' life.
- There should be a policy of primary, secondary and tertiary management for aging population. Primary prevention should focus on a healthy lifestyle like exercise, yoga, meditation, healthy eating and sleeping habit, good interpersonal and social relations etc. In short, holistic bio-psycho-social management focusing on healthy aging. Secondary prevention should focus on early identification of factors that can further contribute to various medical and psychological complications to aging. These factors could be the unhealthy life style, personality traits, initial identification of illness and unhealthy environment etc. Tertiary prevention should focus on to decrease the impact of factors contributed to unhealthy aging, such as, psychotherapeutic psychosocial and pharmacological management etc.
- Have a good social support system as evidences report that older men and women having social support experience better health and decreased mortality (Hessler et al., 1995). Social support may play a more important role in moderating the relationship between their risk factors and poor health outcomes (Arthur, 2006).
- Existential approach to positive aging because there is no point having more time and live longer if not optimizing the appropriate conditions to live more fully.
- Positive psychotherapy is a novel and distinct therapy technique that focuses on positive emotions, engagement, and meaning rather than targeting negative states and depressive symptoms (Seligman et al., 2006).
- Internet and mobile Apps make it more convenient to take help of the online positive intervention programs (Seligman, 2002). These techniques might be less stigmatizing than other interventions that deal with difficulties and deficits. The "three good things exercise" was even integrated into Facebook through an application that provided users with tools to complete the gratitude journaling online and share with friends in their network (Munson et al., 2010).
- Targeting negative schemas with cognitive behavior therapy and tackling environmental issues mainly interpersonal with interpersonal therapy can also be useful in improving positive health in elderly.
- Having a positive and confident attitude has been identified as a protective factor for loneliness (Grenade & Boldy, 2008).

CONCLUSION

Aging is inevitable. We all will face it one day. The clock cannot be turned backwards. Our smooth skin will start wrinkling. Hands will start shaking, voice will tremble. The telomerase enzyme (which prevents cells from aging) will deplete. Prakriti (Nature) works in that way. We all want a happy ending in order to achieve that we need to plan early. We have to choose to face it and not to avoid it. How we deal with it is what makes the difference. Aging should be thought of as a spiritual journey. Positive intervention has its effect in all ages. Taking the help of positive psychology as a primary prevention can help eliminating various effects of aging. In the same way, it can also help in reducing the exiting trouble occurring in elderly. By taking preventive steps one can take care of the body and the mind, and that can help stave off some of the devastating illnesses associated with age and live a full, meaningful and energetic life.

वासांसजिीर्णानयिथावहिायनवानगिृह्णातनिरोपराणाि
तथाशरीराणविहिायजीर्णान्यन्यानसिंयातनिवानदिही।।

Death is but a change of attire in an uninterrupted continuity of immortality. (The Bhagwad Gita Chapter 2 V: 22.)

REFERENCES

Allen, S. M., & Mor, V. (1997). The prevalence and consequences of unmet need. Contrasts between older and younger adults with disability. *Medical Care*, *35*(11), 1132–1148. doi:10.1097/00005650-199711000-00005 PMID:9366892

Antonucci, T. C., & Akiyama, H. (1987). An examination of sex differences in social support among older men and women. *Sex Roles, 17*(11–12), 737–749. doi:10.1007/BF00287685

Arthur, H. M. (2006). Depression, isolation, social support, and cardiovascular disease in older adults. *The Journal of Cardiovascular Nursing*, *21*(Suppl. 5), 2–7. doi:10.1097/00005082-200609001-00002 PMID:16966925

Aspinwall, L. G., & Tedeschi, R. G. (2010). The Value of Positive Psychology for Health Psychology: Progress and Pitfalls in Examining the Relation of Positive Phenomena to Health. *Annals of Behavioral Medicine*, *39*(1), 4–15. doi:10.1007/s12160-009-9153-0 PMID:20091429

Bennett, R., & Eckman, J. (1973). Attitudes toward aging: A critical examination of recent literature and implications for future research. In C. Eisdorfer, & M.P. Lawton (Eds.), The psychology of adult development and aging. (pp. 575–597). Washington, DC: American Psychological Association doi:10.1037/10044-018

Berard, D. M., VanDenKerkhof, E. G., Harrison, M., & Tranmer, J. E. (2012). Gender differences in the influence of social support on one-year changes in functional status in older patients with heart failure. *Cardiology Research and Practice*, *2012*, 1–10. doi:10.1155/2012/616372 PMID:22957296

Blazer, D. G., Sachs-Ericsson, N., & Hybels, C. F. (2005). Perception of unmet basic needs as a predictor of mortality among community-dwelling older adults. *American Journal of Public Health, 95*(2), 299–304. doi:10.2105/AJPH.2003.035576 PMID:15671468

Bronfenbrenner, U., & Ceci, S. J. (1994). Nature-nutureeconceptualized in developmental perspective: A bioecological model. *Psychological Review, 101*(4), 568–586. doi:10.1037/0033-295X.101.4.568 PMID:7984707

Byrne, R. (2006). *The Secret*. New York, NY: Atria Books.

Ciarrochi, J., Atkins, P. W. B., Hayes, L. L., Sahdra, B. K., & Parker, P. (2016). Contextual Positive Psychology: Policy Recommendations for Implementing Positive Psychology into Schools. *Frontiers in Psychology, 7*, 1561. doi:10.3389/fpsyg.2016.01561 PMID:27777564

Ciarrochi, J., & Kashdan, T. (2013). The foundations of flourishing. In J. Ciarrochi (Ed.), *Mindfulness, Acceptance, and Positive Psychology*. Oakland, CA: Context Press.

Cohen, S., Janicki-Deverts, D., & Miller, G. E. (2007). Psychological stress and disease. *Journal of the American Medical Association, 298*(14), 1685–1687. doi:10.1001/jama.298.14.1685 PMID:17925521

Comijs, H. C., Penninx, B. W., Knipscheer, K. P., & Van Tilburg, W. (1999). Psychological distress in victims of elder mistreatment: The effects of social support and coping. *Journal of Gerontology Series B: Psycholical Science and Social Science, 54*(4), 240–245. doi:10.1093/geronb/54B.4.P240 PMID:12382593

Desai, M. M., Lentzner, H. R., & Weeks, J. D. (2001). Unmet need for personal assistance with activities of daily living among older adults. *The Gerontologist, 41*(1), 82–88. doi:10.1093/geront/41.1.82 PMID:11220818

Duckworth, A., & Gross, J. J. (2014). Self-Control and Grit: Related but Separable Determinants of Success. *Current Directions in Psychological Science, 23*(5), 319–325. doi:10.1177/0963721414541462 PMID:26855479

Duckworth, A. L., Steen, T. A., & Seligman, M. E. P. (2005). Positive psychology in clinical practice. *Annual Review of Clinical Psychology, 1*(1), 629–651. doi:10.1146/annurev.clinpsy.1.102803.144154 PMID:17716102

Erikson, E. H. (1959). *Childhood and society*. New York: Norton.

Fässberg, M. M., Van Orden, K. A., Duberstein, P., Erlangsen, A., Lapierre, S., & Bodner, E. (2012). A systematic review of social factors and suicidal behavior in older adulthood. *International Journal of Environmental Research and Public Health, 9*(3), 722–745. doi:10.3390/ijerph9030722 PMID:22690159

Fredrickson, B. L. (2001). The role of positive emotions in positive psychology -The broaden-and-build theory of positive emotions. *The American Psychologist, 56*(3), 218–226. doi:10.1037/0003-066X.56.3.218 PMID:11315248

Fredrickson, B. L., Cohn, M. A., Coffey, K. A., Pek, J., & Finkel, S. M. (2008). Open Hearts Build Lives: Positive Emotions, Induced Through Loving-Kindness Meditation, Build Consequential Personal Resources. *Journal of Personality and Social Psychology, 95*(5), 1045–1062. doi:10.1037/a0013262 PMID:18954193

Government Accountability Office. (2011). Elder justice: Stronger federal leadership could enhance national response to elder abuse. Retrieved from http://aging.senate.gov/events/hr230kb2.pdf

Grenade, L., & Boldy, D. (2008). Social isolation and loneliness among older people: Issues and future challenges in community and residential settings. *Australian Health Review*, *32*(3), 468–478. doi:10.1071/AH080468 PMID:18666874

Hawkley, L. C., Hughes, M. E., Waite, L. J., Masi, C. M., Thisted, R. A., & Cacioppo, J. T. (2008). From social structural factors to perceptions of relationship quality and loneliness: The Chicago health, aging, and social relations study. *The Journals of Gerontology. Series B, Psychological Sciences and Social Sciences*, *63*(6), 375–384. doi:10.1093/geronb/63.6.S375 PMID:19092047

Hayes, S. C., Strosahl, K., & Wilson, K. (2011). *Acceptance and Commitment Therapy: The Process and Practice of Mindful Change* (2nd ed.). New York, NY: The Guilford Press.

Hertzog, C., & Hultsch, D. F. (2000). Metacognition in adulthood and old age. In F. I. M. Craik & T. A. Salthouse (Eds.), *The handbook of aging and cognition* (2nd ed., pp. 417–466). Mahwah, NJ: Erlbaum.

Hess, T. M. (2006). Attitudes toward aging and their effects on behavior. In J. E. Birren & K. W. Schaie (Eds.), *Handbook of the psychology of aging* (6th ed., pp. 379–406). San Diego, CA: Academic Press. doi:10.1016/B978-012101264-9/50020-3

Hessler, R. M., Jia, S., Madsen, R., & Pazaki, H. (1995). Gender, social networks and survival time: A 20-year study of the rural elderly. *Archives of Gerontology and Geriatrics*, *21*(3), 291–306. doi:10.1016/0167-4943(95)00669-C PMID:15374205

Holt-Lunstad, J., Smith, T. B., & Layton, J. B. (2010). Social relationships and mortality risk: A meta-analytic review. *PLoS Medicine*, *7*(7). doi:10.1371/journal.pmed.1000316 PMID:20668659

Hummert, M. L. (2011). Age stereotypes and aging. In K. W. Schaie & S. L. Willis (Eds.), *Handbook of the psychology of aging* (7th ed., pp. 249–262). San Diego, CA: Academic Press. doi:10.1016/B978-0-12-380882-0.00016-4

Indian Health Service. (2014). Indian health disparities. Retrieved from www.ihs.gov/newsroom/includes/themes/newihstheme/display_objects/documents/factsheets/Disparities.pdf

Kashdan, T. B., & Ciarrochi, J. (2013). *Mindfulness, Acceptance, and Positive Psychology: The Seven Foundations of Well-being*. Oakland, CA: Context Press.

Keller, M. L., Leventhal, E. A., & Larson, B. (1989). Aging: The lived experience. *International Journal of Aging & Human Development*, *29*(1), 67–82. doi:10.2190/DEQQ-AAUV-NBU0-3RMY PMID:2628349

Kennedy, J. (2001). Unmet and undermet need for activities of daily living and instrumental activities of daily living assistance among adults with disabilities: Estimates from the 1994 and 1995 disability follow-back surveys. *Medical Care*, *39*(12), 1305–1312. doi:10.1097/00005650-200112000-00006 PMID:11717572

Keyes, C. L. (2002). The mental health continuum: From languishing to flourishing in life. *Journal of Health and Social Behavior*, *43*(2), 207–222. doi:10.2307/3090197 PMID:12096700

Keyes, C. L. M., & Haidt, J. (2003). *Flourishing: positive psychology and the life well-lived.* Washington, DC: American Psychological Association. doi:10.1037/10594-000

King, L. A. (2001). The health benefits of writing about life goals. *Personality and Social Psychology Bulletin, 27*(7), 798–807. doi:10.1177/0146167201277003

Kleinspehn-Ammerlahn, A., Kotter-Grühn, D., & Smith, J. (2008). Self-perceptions of aging: Do subjective age and satisfaction with aging change during old age? *The Journals of Gerontology. Series B, Psychological Sciences and Social Sciences, 63B*(6), 377–385. doi:10.1093/geronb/63.6.P377 PMID:19092041

Kotter-Grühn, D., & Hess, T. M. (2012). The impact of age stereotypes on self-perceptions of aging across the adult lifespan. *The Journals of Gerontology. Series B, Psychological Sciences and Social Sciences, 67*(5), 563–571. doi:10.1093/geronb/gbr153 PMID:22367710

Kotter-Grühn, D., Kleinspehn-Ammerlahn, A., Gerstorf, D., & Smith, J. (2009). Self-perceptions of aging predict mortality and change with approaching death: 16-year longitudinal results from the Berlin Aging Study. *Psychology and Aging, 24*(3), 654–667. doi:10.1037/a0016510 PMID:19739922

Langford, C. P., Bowsher, J., Maloney, J. P., & Lillis, P. P. (1997). Social support: A conceptual analysis. *Journal of Advanced Nursing, 25*(1), 95–100. doi:10.1046/j.1365-2648.1997.1997025095.x PMID:9004016

LaPlante, M. P., Kaye, H. S., Kang, T., & Harrington, C. (2004). Unmet need for personal assistance services: Estimating the shortfall in hours of help and adverse consequences. *Journal of Gerontology: Psychological Sciences and Social Sciences, 59*(2), S98–S108. doi:10.1093/geronb/59.2.S98 PMID:15014097

Layous, K., Chancellor, J., Lyubomirsky, S., Wang, L. H., & Doraiswamy, P. M. (2011). Delivering Happiness: Translating Positive Psychology Intervention Research for Treating Major and Minor Depressive Disorders. *Journal of Alternative and Complementary Medicine (New York, N.Y.), 17*(8), 675–683. doi:10.1089/acm.2011.0139 PMID:21721928

Lazarus, R. S. (2003). Does the positive psychology movement have legs? *Psychological Inquiry, 14*(2), 93–109. doi:10.1207/S15327965PLI1402_02

Levy, B. (1996). Improving memory in old age through implicit self-stereotyping. *Journal of Personality and Social Psychology, 71*(6), 1092–1107. doi:10.1037/0022-3514.71.6.1092 PMID:8979380

Levy, B. (2009). Stereotype embodiment: A psychological approach to aging. *Current Directions in Psychological Science, 18*(6), 332–336. doi:10.1111/j.1467-8721.2009.01662.x PMID:20802838

Levy, B., & Langer, E. (1994). Aging free from negative stereotypes: Successful memory in China and among the American deaf. *Journal of Personality and Social Psychology, 66*(6), 989–997. doi:10.1037/0022-3514.66.6.989 PMID:8046582

Levy, B. R. (2003). Mind matters: Cognitive and physical effects of aging self-stereotype. *The Journals of Gerontology. Series B, Psychological Sciences and Social Sciences, 58B*(4), 203–211. doi:10.1093/geronb/58.4.P203 PMID:12878645

Levy, B. R., & Myers, L. M. (2004). Preventive health behaviors influenced by self-perceptions of aging. *Preventive Medicine, 39*(3), 625–629. doi:10.1016/j.ypmed.2004.02.029 PMID:15313104

Levy, B. R., Slade, M. D., Kunkel, S. R., & Kasl, S. V. (2002). Longevity increased by positive self-perceptions of aging. *Journal of Personality and Social Psychology*, *83*(2), 261–270. doi:10.1037/0022-3514.83.2.261 PMID:12150226

Levy, B. R., Slade, M. D., Murphy, T. E., & Gill, T. M. (2012). Association between positive age stereotypes and recovery from disability in older persons. *Journal of the American Medical Association*, *308*(19), 1972–1973. doi:10.1001/jama.2012.14541 PMID:23168819

Lima, J. C., & Allen, S. M. (2001). Targeting risk for unmet need: Not enough help versus no help at all. *Journal of Gerontology: Psychological Sciences and Social Sciences*, *56*(5), 302–310. doi:10.1093/geronb/56.5.S302 PMID:11522812

Lyubomirsky, S., King, L., & Diener, E. (2005). The benefits of frequent positive affect: Does happiness lead to success? *Psychological Bulletin*, *131*(6), 803–855. doi:10.1037/0033-2909.131.6.803 PMID:16351326

Mouton, C. P. (2003). Intimate partner violence and health status among older women. Psychological Well-being Among Older Adults: Exploring the Role of Psychosocial Resources and Deficits. *The Journals of Gerontology. Series B, Psychological Sciences and Social Sciences*, *66B*(2), 217–229. doi:10.1093/geronb/gbq096

Munson, S., Lauterbach, D., Newman, M., & Resnick, P. (2010). Happier Together: Integrating a Wellness Application Into a Social Network Site. doi:10.1007/978-3-642-13226-1_5

National Center for Health Statistics. (2013). *Health, United States, 2012: With special feature on emergency care*. Hyattsville, MD: Author.

National Crime Record Bureau. (2014). Accidental deaths & suicide in India. Ministry of home affairs, Government of India. Retrieved from http://ncrb.nic.in/StatPublications/ADSI/ADSI2014/chapter-2%20 suicides.pdf

National Institute of Aging. (2008). Healthy aging: Lessons from the Baltimore Longitudinal Study of Aging. Retrieved from www.nia.nih.gov/health/publication/healthy-aging-lessons-baltimore-longitudinal-study-aging/why-study-aging

Newcomer, R., Kang, T., Laplante, M., & Kaye, S. (2005). Living quarters and unmet need for personal care assistance among adults with disabilities. *Journal of Gerontology: Psychological Sciences and Social Sciences*, *60*(4), S205–S213. doi:10.1093/geronb/60.4.S205 PMID:15980296

Parks, A., & Biswas-Diener, R. (2013). Positive interventions: past, present, and future. In J. Ciarrochi (Ed.), *Mindfulness, Acceptance, and Positive Psychology: The Seven Foundations of Well-being*. Oakland, CA: New Harbinger.

Peal, N. (2012). *The Power of Positive Thinking*. New York, NY: Random House.

Pearlin, L. I., Schieman, S., Fazio, E. M., & Meersman, S. C. (2005). Stress, health, and the life course: Some conceptual perspectives. *Journal of Health and Social Behavior*, *46*(2), 205–219. doi:10.1177/002214650504600206 PMID:16028458

Pinto, J. M., Fontaine, A. M., & Neri, A. L. (2016). The influence of physical and mental health on life satisfaction is mediated by self-rated health: A study with Brazilian elderly. *Archives of Gerontology and Geriatrics*, *65*, 104–110. doi:10.1016/j.archger.2016.03.009 PMID:27017415

Richmond, C. A., Ross, N. A., & Egeland, G. M. (2007). Social support and thriving health: A new approach to understanding the health of indigenous Canadians. *American Journal of Public Health*, *97*(10), 1827–1833. doi:10.2105/AJPH.2006.096917 PMID:17761564

Roh, S., Burnette, C. E., Lee, K. H., Lee, Y. S., Easton, S. D., & Lawler, M. J. (2014). Risk and protective factors for depressive symptoms among American Indian older adults: Adverse childhood experiences and social support. *Aging & Mental Health*. doi:10.1080/13607863.2014.938603 PMID:25070293

Ryff, C. D. (2003). Corners of Myopia in the Positive Psychology Parade. *Psychological Inquiry*, *14*(2), 153–159.

Sands, L. P., Wang, Y., McCabe, G. P., Jennings, K., Eng, C., & Covinsky, K. E. (2006). Rates of acute care admissions for frail older people living with met versus unmet activity of daily living needs. *Journal of the American Geriatrics Society*, *54*(2), 339–344. doi:10.1111/j.1532-5415.2005.00590.x PMID:16460389

Santini, Z. I., Koyanagi, A., Tyrovolas, S., & Haro, J. M. (2015). The association of relationship quality and social networks with depression, anxiety, and suicidal ideation among older married adults: Findings from a cross-sectional analysis of the Irish Longitudinal Study on Ageing (TILDA). *Journal of Affective Disorders*, *179*, 134–141. doi:10.1016/j.jad.2015.03.015 PMID:25863909

Schroots, J. J. F. (1996). Theoretical Developments in the Psychology of Aging. *The Gerontologist, 36*(6), 742-748. Retrieved from http://gerontologist.oxfordjournals.org/content/36/6/742.full.pdf

Schueller, S. M., & Seligman, M. E. (2010). Pursuit of pleasure, engagement, and meaning: Relationships to subjective and objective measures of well-being. *The Journal of Positive Psychology*, *5*(4), 253–263. doi:10.1080/17439761003794130

Schure, M. B., Conte, K. P., & Goins, R. T. (2015). Unmet Assistance Need Among Older American Indians: The Native Elder Care Study. *The Gerontologist*, *55*(6), 920–928. doi:10.1093/geront/gnt211 PMID:24451895

Seligman, M. E. (2004). *Authentic Happiness: Using the New Positive Psychology to Realize Your Potential for Lasting Fulfillment*. New York: The Free Press.

Seligman, M. E., Rashid, T., & Parks, A. C. (2006). Positive psychotherapy. *The American Psychologist*, *61*(8), 774–788. doi:10.1037/0003-066X.61.8.774 PMID:17115810

Seligman, M. E. P. (2002). *Authentic happiness: using the new positive psychology to realize your potential for lasting fulfillment*. New York: Free Press.

Seligman, M. E. P., Steen, T. A., Park, N., & Peterson, C. (2005). Positive psychology progress -Empirical validation of interventions. *The American Psychologist*, *60*(5), 410–421. doi:10.1037/0003-066X.60.5.410 PMID:16045394

Sin, N. L., & Lyubomirsky, S. (2009). Enhancing well-being and alleviating depressive symptoms with positive psychology interventions: A practice-friendly meta-analysis. *Journal of Clinical Psychology, 65*(5), 467–487. doi:10.1002/jclp.20593 PMID:19301241

Taylor, T. N., Munoz-Plaza, C. E., Goparaju, L., Martinez, O., Holman, S., Minkoff, H. L., ... Wilson, T. E. (2016). The Pleasure Is Better as I've Gotten Older": Sexual Health, Sexuality, and Sexual Risk Behaviors Among Older Women Living With HIV. *Archives of Sexual Behavior.* PMID:27220311

Thoits, P. A. (2006). Personal agency in the stress process. *Journal of Health and Social Behavior, 47*(4), 309–323. doi:10.1177/002214650604700401 PMID:17240922

Tornstam, L. (1989). Gero-transcendence: A meta-theoretical reformulation of the disengagement theory. *Aging, 1*, 55–63. PMID:2488301

Tugade, M. M., & Fredrickson, B. L. (2004). Resilient individuals use positive emotions to bounce back from negative emotional experiences. *Journal of Personality and Social Psychology, 86*(2), 320–333. doi:10.1037/0022-3514.86.2.320 PMID:14769087

United Nations Population Division (UN). (2011). World Population Prospects: The 2010 Revision. In Population Reference Bureau. Retrieved from http://www.prb.org/pdf12/TodaysResearchAging25.pdf

Van Beljouw, I. M., van Exel, E., de Jong Gierveld, J., Comijs, H. C., Heerings, M., Stek, M. L., & van Marwijk, H. W. J. (2014). Being all alone makes me sad": Loneliness in older adults with depressive symptoms. *International Psychogeriatrics, 9*, 1–11. doi:10.1017/S1041610214000581 PMID:24717770

Van Tilburg, T. (1998). Losing and gaining in old age: Changes in personal network size and social support in a four-year longitudinal study. *The Journals of Gerontology. Series B, Psychological Sciences and Social Sciences, 53*(6), S313–S323. doi:10.1093/geronb/53B.6.S313 PMID:9826973

Whitbeck, L. B., McMorris, B. J., Hoyt, D. R., Stubben, J. D., & LaFromboise, T. (2002). Perceived discrimination, traditional practices, and depressive symptoms among American Indians in the upper midwest. *Journal of Health and Social Behavior, 43*(4), 400–418. doi:10.2307/3090234 PMID:12664673

Williams, J., Lyons, B., & Rowland, D. (1997). Unmet long-term care needs of elderly people in the community: A review of the literature. *Home Health Care Services Quarterly, 16*(1-2), 93–119. doi:10.1300/J027v16n01_07 PMID:10168492

Wolf, R. (2000). Introduction: The nature and scope of elder abuse. *Generations (San Francisco, Calif.), 24*, 6–11.

Wong, P. T. P. (1998). Spirituality, meaning, and successful aging. In P. T. P. Wong & P. Fry (Eds.), *The human quest for meaning: A handbook of psychological research and clinical applications* (pp. 359–394). Mahwah, NJ: Erlbaum.

World Health Organization WHO. (2015). Aging and Health. Retrieved from http://www.who.int/mediacentre/factsheets/fs404/en/

World Health Organization WHO. (2016). Mental health and older adults. Extracted from http://www.who.int/mediacentre/factsheets/fs381/en/)

Wurm, S., Tesch-Römer, C., & Tomasik, M. J. (2007). Longitudinal findings on aging-related cognitions, control beliefs, and health in later life. *The Journals of Gerontology. Series B, Psychological Sciences and Social Sciences*, *62B*(3), 156–164. doi:10.1093/geronb/62.3.P156 PMID:17507583

Wurm, S., Tomasik, M. J., & Tesch-Römer, C. (2010). On the importance of a positive view on ageing for physical exercise among middle-aged and older adults: Cross-sectional and longitudinal findings. *Psychology & Health*, *25*(1), 25–42. doi:10.1080/08870440802311314 PMID:20391205

KEY TERMS AND DEFINITIONS

Aging: A process of becoming older.
Life Changes: Change in one's life or circumstances in a substantial way.
Positive Psychology: An applied approach to optimal functioning.
Satisfaction: Fulfilment of needs.
Successful Aging: It refers to physical, mental and social well-being in older age.

Chapter 2
Spirituality and Aging

Surendra Kumar Mattoo
Postgraduate Institute of Medical Education and Research, India

Vikas Punia
Institute of Mental Health, India

Lipika Malik
Institute of Mental Health, India

Hitesh Khurana
Pandit Bhagwat Dayal Sharma Post Graduate Institute of Medical Sciences, India

ABSTRACT

This chapter reviews the available literature on different aspects of spirituality and health in old age. Old age is marked with physical, mental and social dysfunctions whereas spirituality provides the way to overcome these difficulties. The Asian scriptures give a very clear evidence that spirituality is the way of life that has a meaning, a purpose and connectedness with others. In the Indian description, Vasudhaiv Kutubhkam, it points towards the spiritual interconnectedness. The spiritual practices give a meaning and purpose to life therefore instills a feeling of hope which can protect against mental disorders. The same also strengthen immune system protecting us from physical problems connectedness with others is the ultimate aim of spirituality. With increasing age and degenerative processing taking place in the body, spiritual practices by elderly, make them feel a part of community and improves physical health status.

Do not dwell in the past, do not dream of the future, Concentrate the mind on the present moment (Buddha)

WHY HEALTH PROFESSIONALS NEED STUDY SPIRITUALITY

Over the last several decades, the concept of spirituality has come to the forefront of public and professional interest. With the dawn of a new century, spirituality has received increased coverage in the media and more discussion in the workplace, in politics, and in education (Messikomer & De Craemer, 2002). Spirituality has also become more apparent in health care, with increasing evidence that spiritual

DOI: 10.4018/978-1-5225-3480-8.ch002

factors are important components of health and well-being (Dossey, 2001). The need for health care providers to effectively address the connection between spirituality and health is becoming broadly recognized as more people want spiritual content to their health care. And in this regard Burkhardt and Nagai-Jacobson (2002) quoted Spirituality, "Spirituality is at the heart of caring for the whole person". Yet the lack of a clear definition or a concise conceptual framework, coupled with limited opportunities for spiritual training and professional development of health care providers, has resulted in the neglect of this aspect of patient care.

INTRODUCTION

The word "spirituality" has been derived from the Latin word "spiritus" meaning breath or life, with the Latin "spiritulis" meaning "of the spirit". The term, frequently cited in the Hebraic Old Testament (*ruach*) and the Greek New Testament (*pneuma*), has historically been referenced in the context of religion and is still both experienced and expressed by many through conventional religious understanding (Zinnbauer et al., 1997). There are several definitions of spirituality. It has been defined by theorists as "the human response to God's gracious call to a relationship with himself" (Benner, 1989), "a subjective experience of the sacred" (Vaughan, 1991), and "…that vast realm of human potential dealing with ultimate purposes, with higher entities, with God, with love, with compassion, with purpose…" (Tart, 1983). A popular definition of spirituality was proposed by Koenig and Carson, (2012), stated spirituality as the personal quest for understanding answers to the ultimate question of life about its meaning and relationship with the sacred or transcendent, which may (or may not) lead to or arise from development of religious rituals and the formation of a community. Spilka's, (1993) reviewed literature and concluded that most contemporary understandings of spirituality fall into one of three categories: 1) a God-oriented spirituality where thought and practice are subsumed in theologies, either broadly or narrowly conceived; 2) a world-oriented spirituality which stresses one's relationship with ecology or nature; or 3) a humanistic (or people-oriented) spirituality which stresses human achievement or potential. Thus, according to Spilka, spirituality should be viewed as a multidimensional construct.

NATURE OF SPIRITUALITY

Some of the viewpoints about the nature of spirituality is described in the following manner.

- **Spirituality as Being Innate:** Many authors view spirituality as the heart of human experience (McCarroll, O'Connor, & Meakes, 2005). It is not only believed that "each individual has spiritual needs" (Oldnall, 1996). It is also claimed that "human spirituality in a very real sense that unifies the whole person". Spirituality can thus be seen as a basic, innate and vital component of being human which means simply understanding that others are human too. They have equal rights with you and you should treat them as you wish they treat you.
- **Spirituality as Being Emotive:** Spirituality is essentially emotive because it touches people's hearts as it deals with the very essence of being. Therefore, it is imperative for people in positions of power to remember that they cannot be neutral and hence they must try to be objective in examining the concepts of spirituality and spiritual health. (Warren, 1988).

- **Spirituality as Being Subjective:** Spirituality has often been viewed as subjective, lacking much of the objective nature which is considered necessary for scientifically based studies. (Chapman, 1987). However, "If concepts such as self-worth, self-esteem, and self-actualization can be accepted, then it should be reasonable to explore... spirituality, for these concepts are equally as intangible and subjective as spirituality" (Jose & Taylor, 1986).In order to balance the objective and subjective nature of spirituality, Thatcher argued that there is a "crippling price to pay for misidentification of spirituality as subjective and we need to go beyond the inner search to fully understand spirituality" (Thatcher, 1991).
- **Spirituality as Being Dynamic:** Priestley has quoted "The spirit is dynamic. It must be felt before it can be conceptualized" (Priestley, 1985). In lieu with this terms like "spiritual growth" and "development" are used to express the dynamic nature of spirituality (Chapman, 1987). Studies have also shown that spirituality tends to increase during later adulthood. The spiritual expedition is like being on a voyage: If you think you've arrived, you haven't yet begun, or you are dead.

Spirituality

Its components, Oldnall (1996) formulates that the elements like self, others and `God' are central to the understanding of spirituality and the focus of spirituality is on the relationships between them. Hungelmann, Kenkel-Rossi, Klassen, and Stollenwerk (1985) stated that the interconnectedness of these three core elements is the heart of spirituality which is shown in Figure 1.

- **Self:** The conception and perception of self is an essential ingredient in approaching spirituality. Hay (1989) states that an individual's spiritual well-being results in enhancement of one's inner resources. Howden (1992) further states `innerness' or inner resources, and the discovering of wholeness to be essential components of spirituality.

Figure 1. A model of interconnectedness of components of spirituality

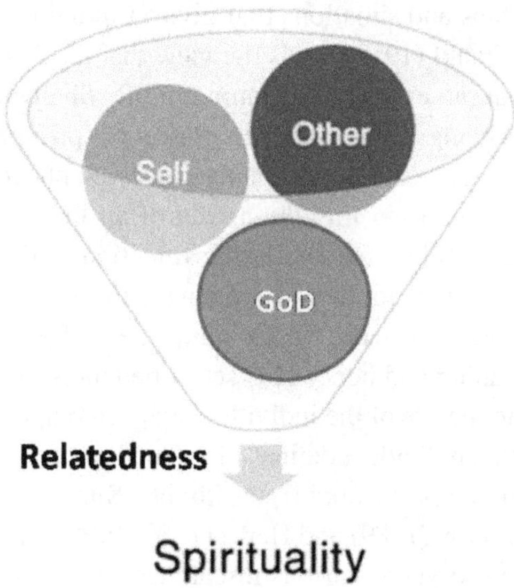

- **Others:** The community and society is another essential component while approaching the concept of spirituality. Hay (1989) noted that spirituality occurs in the context of the communities in which one is a part. Likewise, Liehr (1989) claims that spirituality may be relied upon on an individual's ability to give and receive human elements, such as touch, listening and committed presence in relationships with others. In this regard, Stoll (1979) has identified relationships of trust and mutuality as being one of the main sources of hope and strength. Sodestrom and Martinson (1987) further go on to state that having a common bond with others is a major part of the spiritual dimension and that this is achieved through one's relationships with others.
- **God:** Essential to spirituality is a relationship with "God". In this direction Stoll (1979) provides useful insights when she states that `whatever a person takes to be the highest value in life can be regarded as his "God". Clark (1987) further supports this broad view by hinting that spirituality is essentially based upon the `life principle' of a person. Hence it can be said the centrality of self, others and "God" and the relationships between these elements are well researched and remain important in the concept of spirituality.
- **Relatedness:** The above defined components of self, others and God cannot exist in isolation and hence a connectedness and relatedness between these components is essential. In this direction, Ley and Corless (1988), state that spirituality is `a state of connectedness to God to one's neighbor and to one's inner self. Several other theorists have also supported this view. Burkhardt (1989) has stated that sense of relatedness and connectedness is described in terms of harmony with the self, others and a sense of connection to `God'. Shelly and Fish (1988) have identified sources of love and relatedness with others; as being essential components of spirituality. Further, Lane (1987) has provided further directions by suggesting three forms of connectedness; first is the ability to engage in generative activities; second is the ability to belong to another; and third is the ability to achieve an inner sense of ultimate purpose. He further notes that when an individual utilizes these abilities they will experience a sense of fulfillment.
- **Meaning in Life:** While discussing elements like self, relationship with society and "God", the discussion leads to another essential component which is finding meaning in life. Howden (1992) proposes that purpose and meaning in life are critical attributes in spirituality and he includes in this a search for relationships and situations that give an individual sense of worth and a reason for living. In this regard, Frankl (1959) holds the view that man's primary concern is not to gain pleasure and avoid pain but rather to see a meaning in life. Shelly and Fish (1988), also perceive this search for meaning as being a important component of spirituality. However, meaning in life is subjective and can be recognized as a personally perceived phenomenon (Ellis, 1980).
- **Beliefs:** With respect to meaning in life, the aspect of an individual's particular belief system holds importance. Jourard (1971) provides further direction in this regard. He states that belief system which an individual hold helps him to explain the meaning of life. Clark, Cross, Deane and Lowry (1991) further places importance on the uniqueness of each individual's belief system in enabling them to have meaning and hope. This set of beliefs is said to emanate from the driving force that gives meaning to the life of the individual that can range from, their work, relationships with others, to whatever that individual defines his "God" to be.
- **Hope:** Finding meaning in life is essential in spirituality. Similarly, the concept of hope too is essential for spirituality. Nowotny (1989) and Herth (1989, 1990) maintained that hope is a spiritual need which is common to everyone. Various researches have tried to define hope. Owen (1989) has described it as a sense of energy which is exchanged between people and their environment.

> Miller and Powers (1988) have further stated that hope emanates from mutual affiliation and a sense of concern for others as well as oneself. Clark et al. (1991) also provide support for the view for this mutual affiliation by conveying that the source of hope has also been found to rest with relationships with others. Francis (1986) has also suggested that hope amasses a sense of relatedness to possibilities and powers beyond oneself and the present. To conclude it is defined that the majority of studies relating to spirituality have identified hope as a key component of spirituality.

Its expressions, in order to understand spirituality in its wholeness, it is essential to be sensitive towards its experience and thus its expression. If spirituality is said to be concerned with the self, others and `God', the spiritual expression can take a variety of forms. Many hold the view that art forms may provide an expression of spirituality. Cohen (1990) held the view that appreciation of music, food, wine, sex, literature and humor can all reflect spirituality. Burkhardt and Jacobson (1985) further recognize that spirituality is expressed in the context of connections with oneself, others, nature and `God'. Such connections may be expressed through happiness or crying (Lindholm & Eriksson, 1993), through relationships with others (Mayeroff, 1971) and through the expression of caring within those relationships exemplified through hugging and holding (Oliver, 1990).

Indian Model of Spirituality

The roots of spirituality in Asian subcontinent and particularly in India can be traced to the Bhagavad-Gita. The *Bhagavad-Gita* shows how our physical self is related to social self and work. It further goes on to explain how doing our prescribed work with the intention to achieve the fruits of our labor leads to a deep-rooted development of social self, but letting go of the expectation for the reward for our actions leads us toward the real self. This real self or the *atman* is the beaker which holds the promise of salvation. It is through the realization or connection with the *atman* that one can attain salvation. Hence the path of realization of our real self or *atman* is termed as spiritual. Therefore, the roots of spirituality in Indian context can be found in realization of our true self (Bhawuk, 1999).

The above model connecting self and work is derived from the *Bhagavad-Gita.* The model (see Figure 2) shows a strong tie between Self and one's duty (or *Svadharma*), which is cited in verses 2.31, 3.8, and 18.41-46. It is stated that an individual has a choice to do or not to do his or her duty, or work prescribed

Figure 2. A model of attainment of spirituality
Source: Adapted from Bhawuk (2000)

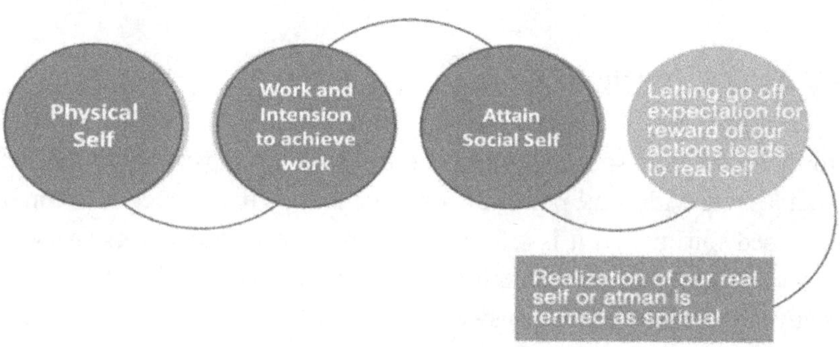

by one's caste and phase of life (*Varnashrama dharma*). According to the *varnashram dharma* human life is divided into four *ashrams* or phases, the student phase (or *brahmacarya ashram*), the householder phase (or *grihasthaashrama*), the forest dweller phase (or *vanaprasthaashrama*), and the monkhood phase (or *sanyasaashrama*). The four castes of *brahman, kshartriya, vaishya*, and *shudra* have their set duties of learning and teaching, protecting and fighting, trade and crafts, and service of the janitorial type, but everyone is supposed to follow the four phases of life. Thus, the caste bound work is only applicable to the first two phases of life when one is learning the trade and performing the duties. In the latter, two phases everyone should lead a spiritual life.

In verse 2.33 the negative consequences of not doing one's duties or work are cited, and thus one is encouraged to perform one's worldly duties. The positive aspects of performing one's duties or work are stated in verses 3.35, 18.47, and 18.48. If we decide to do our duties, then we face another crossroad, whether we should perform our duties with the expectation and intention to achieve the outcome of our work (or *sakama)*, or to work without concern for the outcome of our work (or *niskama)*. If we decide to pursue the work with the intention to enjoy the outcome of our effort, we follow a Path, which will lead to increased attachment to work and its consequences, or *Karmic* bondage. This is evident in verse 3.9. The nature of this Path is described in verses 2.41, 2.42-44, and 2.45. If we intend to work without being concerned with the outcome of our effort, or become detached from them, i.e., maintain balance in achieving or not achieving them, then we are following another path Path, which leads to liberation and salvation. This path is described in verses 2.38-40, 2.45, 2.48, 3.7, 3.9, 3.17, and 3.30.

Spiritual way of connectedness as the means to attain the goal of individual and social health was being practiced in ancient times in India. In the vedicera mental and spiritual well-being given priority over physical wellbeing of a person. They considered all ailments as the suffering of atman or soul. Thus, the body or any organ was not considered sick in isolation but the whole atman itself. Maha Upnishad proposed the doctrine of 'vasudhaivkutumbhkam' i.e. the whole world is a family. Just as one can't stay peacefully by disturbing peace of family similarly one cannot imagine himself healthy unless he is aware of suffering in the society(Bhasin and Kumari,2015) Thus the concept of 'vasudhaivkutumbhkam' is a spiritual way of attaining the goal of well-being through connectedness with others and also lays down the principles of ethical medicine (Seetharam,2013)The doctrine "live and let live" proposed by the King Ashoka the great (268-232 BC) is also an offshoot of this principle for attainment of social and individual wellbeing. There doesn't seem to be any parallel of this principle in the west, however, the doctrine 'voxpopulivoxdei' appears dictating the same. This doctrine broadly preaches the principles of democracy however it also seems to say that the social needs or the demands of the society are the ultimate and take priority over personal needs. This is again very similar to the principle of renunciation practiced in the vanprastha ashram of Hindu philosophy.

SPIRITUALITY AND RELIGIOSITY

Closely related to the concept of spirituality is the concept of religiosity. Both these concepts enjoy a complimentary status along with some points of convergence and divergence between both. Historically religiosity encompassed spirituality; it is only recently that the spirituality as an independent concept has sprung up. However, the question is; is spirituality and religiosity both independent concepts or are they the same? Many authors have tried to answer this question however no consensual answer has been reached. In this context, certain definitional criteria for religion and spirituality have been presented. Key concepts which are embedded within these criteria include: 1) the concept of the sacred, 2) a search process, 3) the concept of the non-sacred, and 4) the degree to which the search process is supported by a community (Hill et al., 2000).

Roads of Convergence

The terms spirituality and religiosity have been used complimentary and inconsistently by several authors. Miller and Martin (1988) frequently interchange the terms. Both the concepts can be defined in varied ways by different sets of individuals. Support for this statement has been found in the work of Pargament, Sullivan, Balzer, Van Haitsma, and Raymark (1995) where they assessed the meanings college students and clergy attribute to the word religiosity. Their findings indicated that different individuals attributed varied meanings to religiosity. For instance, religiosity meant church attendance, acts of altruism, or performing religious rituals. Likewise, popular publications such as the Newsweek and the Time reflect the views and attitudes of the individuals, and state that contemporary spirituality is also defined in several ways. Popular references to spirituality have included elements such as interest in angels, New Age interest in crystals and psychic readings, and evangelical or Pentecostal religious experiences (Hill et al, 2000).

Religious concepts are multidimensional in nature. For instance, LaPierre (2003) identifies the following components of spirituality: 1) a search for meaning in life; 2) an encounter with transcendence; 3) a sense of community; 4) search for ultimate truth 5) a respect and appreciation for the mystery of creation; 6) a personal transformation. Religion is likewise multidimensional. Marty and Appleby (1991), place emphasis on the multifaceted nature of religion. They state that religion is concerned with the ultimate concerns of people and provides personal meaning as well as social identity within the context of a cosmic or metaphysical background.

Religiosity and spirituality develop across lifespan. Many researchers have documented through both clinical (Rizzuto, 1991) and experimental research (Hood, Spilka, Hunsberger, & Gorsuch, 1996). There is prominence of spiritual and religious issues in psychological development across many cultures, even among individuals with little or no formal religious training. Religiosity and spirituality are found to be related to physical health status, especially in providing guidelines for religiously based norms that govern diet, sexual behavior, and health care behaviors (Levin & Vanderpool, 1992). Further, religiosity and spirituality has been recognized as having positive relationships with mental health. Religion and spirituality have been found to be essentially helpful among the aged (Koenig, 1994; McFadden, 1995), as it provides both a meaning to death and hope at the end of the life cycle (Glick, Weiss, & Parkes, 1974; Pruyser, 1986). Consequently, religiosity and spirituality have been shown to be efficient in coping with disability, illness, and negative life events (Pargament, 1997). Along these lines prayer too can be an especially effective coping mechanism (Poloma & Pendleton, 1989). In continuation of the above, religion and spirituality are increasingly recognized as having positive derivative social functions (Maton & Wells, 1995). It is reflected in the notion that many religious and spiritual practices teach that the individual and God should work cooperatively to prevent and cure illness, often relying upon prayer, meditation, or other forms of religiously and spiritually sanctioned healing practices (Pollner, 1989; Poloma & Gallup, 1990). Likewise, hedonistic outliers such as extramarital sexuality are negatively related with personal religious beliefs (Cochran & Beeghley, 1991).

Roads of Divergence

Definitions of religiosity historically included aspects like personal beliefs, such as a belief in God or a higher power, and institutional beliefs and practices such as church membership, church attendance and commitment to the belief system of a church or any organized religion. In contrast, spirituality was most often described in terms of personal or experiential beliefs, such as belief in (or having a relationship with) God or a higher power. Sheldrake (1992) noted that the recent diversion between religion and spirituality is the result of human knowledge and historical-cultural events that continually affect peoples' perceptions of the supreme. Consequently, each generation may be required to define what concepts such as "religion" and "spirituality" are meant to fathom. The effect of these changes during the 1960s and 1970s was that spirituality began to enjoy more highlighted meanings and more favorable connotations separate from religion (Turner, Lukoff, Barnhouse & Lu, 1995). This cultural differentiation has resulted in the present-day norm of perceiving spirituality as having positive connotations through its association with personal experiences of the transcendent (Spilka & Mclntosh, 1996), and to view religion with its demands of tradition in a much more negative light as a barrier to spiritual experience (Turner et al., 1995).

Religion historically was a "broad-band construct" (Pargament, 1999) that encompassed both individual and institutional elements, it is now however seen as a "narrowband construct" that has much more to do with the institutional alone (Zinnbauer, Pargament, & Scott, 1999). Conversely, spirituality appears to be the appropriate term to describe individual experience and is identified with such things as personal transcendence, supraconscious sensitivity, and meaningfulness (Spilka & Mclntosh, 1996). Providing evidence for the same, Pargament (1999) cites, "the term spiritual is increasingly reserved for the loftier/functional side of life". Religiosity, conversely is now more often identified with rigid, or "formally structured," religious institutions that often are often said to restrict or inhibit human potential (Pargament, 1997). Consequently, with respect to divergence between these constructs, many authors make a distinction between definition of religiosity and spirituality, preferring the term spirituality because it is more inclusive and universal (Moberg, 1979; Ley & Corless, 1988). In contrast, religiosity has been defined as 'participation in the particular beliefs, rituals and activities of traditional religion' (Elkins, Hedstrom, Hughes, Leaf & Saunders, 1988). It can thus, best serve as a 'nurturer and channel of expression' for spirituality (Elkins et al., 1988).

In this continuation, spirituality has been noted to be 'more basic' than religiosity (Elkins et al., 1988), being a 'subjective experience that exists both within and outside of traditional religious systems' (Vaughan et al., 1998). Religiosity, in contrast, is often described narrowly as formally structured and identified with religious institutions and authorized theology and rituals. As the term spirituality has become distinct from religiosity, it has been adopted by identifiable groups of believers. For instance, several of the 1,599 "baby boomers" studied by Roof (1993) had diverged from structured religion in the 1960s and 1970s. Roof also found an upheaval in "New-Age" religious participation, with its importance on direct spiritual experience over institutional religion, especially among "highly active seekers" who had discounted organized and structured religion and more traditional and conventional forms of worship in appreciation of a personal faith that they characterized as a "spiritual journey" or spiritual "quest."

In another study by Zinnbauer et al. (1997), a group of respondents who categorized themselves as "spiritual but not religious" were contrasted with a larger group of respondents who categorized themselves as "spiritual and religious." Findings of this study indicated that compared with the "spiritual and religious" group, the "spiritual but not religious" group was less probable to perceive religiosity in a positive light, less probable to engage in traditional and conventional forms of worship such as church attendance and prayer, less probable to hold orthodox or traditional Christian beliefs, more probable to be independent from others, more probable to participate in group experiences associated with spiritual growth, more probable to hold non-traditional "new age" beliefs, more probable to have had mystical and cosmic experiences, and more probable to distinguish religiosity and spirituality as distant and non-overlapping concepts. Remarkably, the "spiritual but not religious" group identified by Zinnbauer et al. (1997) correlates in several ways to the description of the "highly active seekers" within the baby boomer generation provided by Roof (1993).

Co-Occurrence

The discussion above suggests that spirituality is a central and pivotal function of religion. Therefore, spirituality and religiosity can (and often do) co-occur. Individual religions essentially those that are large, culturally heterogeneous, and have a long chronological record might have advocates who favour some spiritual core. For instance, Christians reverence Jesus Christ and view God as one entity incorporated in three persons. The religion itself is broad enough to accommodate people who also vouch distinctive spiritualties. For instance, desert spiritualties, evangelical spiritualties, feminist spiritualties, nature spiritualties. Hence, attempts to measure spirituality as a separate construct from religion are difficult. Beliefs and experiences that are considered to be an aspect of traditional religiousness i.e. prayer, church attendance, reading of sacred writings are also spiritual if they are fuelled by an individual's search for the sacred.

AGING

The last two decades have witnessed considerable changes in gerontology. Old age considered to be viewed negatively with increasing health problems. "This stage is characterized by physical debility, tardy movements, deterioration in sensory functions, depression, and irritability" (Alex & George, 2004). However, according to growth-oriented life span developmental models, the patterns of aging are more complex and differentiated (Erickson, 1963; Jung, 1971; Rybash, Roodin, & Santrock, 1991; Schaie & Willis, 1991). There are different dimensions to human development and some kind of growth is possible in every developmental stage. Spirituality in the elderly can be best understood from a life span perspective.

Different Dimensions of Aging

Aging involves following dimensions: chronological, biological, cultural, psychological and spiritual. Given the same level of chronological and biological aging, individuals may differ widely in terms of psychological aging. Rybash et al. (1991) define psychological age in terms of both adaptability and attitude: "Psychological age refers to the adaptive capacities of an individual - that is, an individual's ability to adapt to changing environmental demands as compared to the adaptability of other individuals of identical chronological age. Individuals adapt to their environments by drawing on various psychological characteristics: learning, memory, intelligence, emotional control, motivational strengths, coping styles, and so on. Therefore, individuals who display more of such psychological characteristics than their chronological age mates are considered "psychologically young"; while those who possess such traits to a lesser degree are "psychologically old". Spiritual aging refers to developmental changes on the spiritual dimension. For example, Fowler (1981) has proposed that faith progressing through different developmental stages. Similar to Flower and Tornstam (1999) offers a theory of "gerotranscendence" that argues for an age-related spirituality. Tornstam, (1999) postulates that seniors are more likely to be interested in the spiritual dimension, which includes a preoccupation with intergenerational relationship, the meaning of life and death.

Spirituality and Successful Aging

Normal aging refers to the natural process of growing old and successfully coping with debilitating effects of illness if any., while successful aging refers to the capacity to live a vital and productive life even in old age. Examples of successful agers in human history are Michelangelo, Picasso, Churchill, Rubenstein; Heifetz remained productive in their 80s. Bertrand Russell and George Bernard Shaw were still writing in their 90s. Grandma Moses was painting at 100. An increasing number of individuals maintain relatively good health and continue to engage in a productive life well into their 80s. Although successful aging means different things to different people, there is some consensus that we need to shift the emphasis from the medical model and physical components of aging to psychological and spiritual components. There is increasing recognition of the importance of meaning and spirituality in the psychological and physical well-being of the elders. Simply put, successful aging is 80% attitude and 20% everything else.

The notion that a spiritual perspective becomes increasingly important with aging adds a positive spin to the search for a 'spiritual journey' (MacKinlay & Trevitt, 2007). The concept of successful aging, which emerged from the 1990s McArthur Research Network on Successful Aging, brought about an interest in positive aging. Spirituality and religious participation are highly correlated with positive successful aging, as much as diet, exercise, mental stimulation, self-efficacy and social connectedness, stimulating an interest in the understanding of why spirituality has such positive effects on the quality of life and end of life.

Crowther et al. (2002) proposed that positive spirituality is defined by developing an internalized relationship with the sacred and transcendent world that is not bound by race, ethnicity, economics or class, and promotes the wellness and welfare of the self and others (Crowther et al., 2002). This attitude is more positive, and promotes self-enhancing behaviors and beliefs. Rogers claims that the universality of religion is based upon its social function during the later years of life, such as helping face inevitable losses and impending death, while also finding and maintaining meaningfulness of life (Rogers, 1976). Older adults who are more religious tend to demonstrate greater wellbeing than those who are not (McFadden, 1995). However, Seifert warns against the sentiment of assuming that spirituality automatically increases with age (Seifert, 2002).

In summary, spirituality appears to play an important and adaptive role in aging that seems to lead to a better quality of life and life satisfaction, as well as longevity in the older practitioners.

SPIRITUAL GROWTH DURING THE LAST STAGE OF DEVELOPMENT

In old age, there is an increase in interiority (Jung, 1971) and focus on achieving integrity (Erickson, 1963). Gutmann (1978) and Neugarten (1973) point out that increasing interiority reflects an age-related normative shift in personality. Successful aging depends on a person's capacity to maintain a meaningful life in spite of physical decline, personal losses, and ageism (Wong, 1989). This endeavor involves the integration of past experiences with current circumstances into a meaningful life story; it also involves a transition from achievements and external orientation toward an inner orientation (Neugarten, 1973; Wong, 1989). This shift from doing to being and from outer attachments to inner life facilitates spiritual growth. In 2000 Lou (Harris 1975) conducted a study of more than 3,000 adults for the National Council on the Aging. Sixty-seven percent of seniors in the study reported having a rich spiritual life. A large proportion of the subjects felt spiritual life being beneficial in late age (NCOA, 2002).

In the last two decades, gerontologists and psychologists have become increasingly aware of the importance of spirituality and religion to the well-being of seniors. Spirituality is primarily a personal and inward experience. In fact, aging is often referred to as a spiritual journey (Bianchi, 1997; Moberg, 2001). Personal growth on the spiritual journey often results in deepening relationships with God, faith communities, and loved ones. It always involves some kind of internal transformation, ranging from awakening, enlightenment, to changing priorities in life. Given the multidimensional nature of aging, one can still experience spiritual growth and psychological growth even when going through a period of physical decline. Furthermore, psychological and spiritual aging may have a positive impact on biological aging. However, there is a need to keep in mind the holistic view that "it is the whole person who is aging and aging. This wholeness is a blend of spiritual, physical, mental, emotional, and social dimensions of human growth and development" (Kimble, 1995).

In summary, the life-span perspective recognizes opportunities and challenges for personal growth in every stage of development till the very end of life. This is an important conceptual framework for the positive revolution in gerontology and for all the practitioners working with seniors.

The Developmental Context

It is notable, when one tries to consider the process of psychological development in old age that description of the psychological and spiritual dimensions of experience may start to become blurred. A number of psychological theories that consider developmental changes in later life touch upon the issues of an individual's changing sources of meaning and relationship to the world, in such a way that consideration of spiritual matters seems to become important. Two key theories informed the current literature review.

Erikson's (1982) model of psychosocial development attempts to bridge psychological and spiritual development. It suggests eight broad stages of psychosocial development, at each stage of which a person must resolve a key conflict in order to develop a particular quality or strength associated with that life stage. In 1989, Erikson, along with his wife and colleagues, revisited the later stages of his theory, considering older people's engagement with their lives and developmental tasks. They suggest that each life stage is re-addressed from the position of the current one. Hence it is proposed that, in the final stage, a process of life review occurs in which old conflicts and issues are revisited from a new perspective, achieving integrity as resolution is accomplished. They emphasize that the task for the final stage of life is paradoxical: to continue and develop a 'vital involvement' with life whilst facing and coming to terms with the 'necessary disinvolvements of old age'.

They suggest that the sense of a coherent and continuous identity is fundamentally threatened in old age and failure to manage this could lead to despair, disdain or dogmatism. The alternative, they suggest, is wisdom; that the sense of self transcends a time-bound identity such that one maintains a detached concern with life, in the face of death. More recently, Joan Erikson has offered a critique of the final stages of this model (Erikson, 1995, 1997). She advocated a ninth stage in which the task is to develop an attitude of retreat and retirement in relation to the world. She sees this as developing an increasingly spiritual perspective that is also described by the theory of gerotranscendence. Other writers have used Erikson's theory as a basis of thinking about spiritual development in old age. For example, McFadden (1999) draws attention to the seventh and eighth stages of Erikson's theory as representing two aspects of the spiritual life of older people. The penultimate stage, Generativity versus Stagnation, she sees as representing the 'outward turn of the self towards the world'. Whereas, the final stage of Integrity versus Despair is seen as representing an 'inward turn' and may be supported by meditative practices and the symbolic connections between humanity and the sacred offered by religion.

Tornstam (1989, 1996) is a Swedish gerontologist and his theory of gerotranscendence can be said to move on from where Erikson's theory ends. Tornstam suggests that a 'paradigm shift' occurs as people age, in which they move from a materialistic and rational perspective on life to one that is increasingly 'cosmic and transcendent'. This might be seen as a shift towards 'the sacred', in terms of the definition of spirituality. Tornstam's theory may seem to bear resemblance to the earlier theory of disengagement (Cumming & Henry, 1961) in which it was posited that older people naturally withdraw from society and the roles of earlier life. A notable difference is that the theory of gerotranscendence proposes a reorientation towards a new perspective and experience of life that could be understood as spiritual, rather than simply a withdrawal from the mainstream of life. Tornstam suggests that gerotranscendence may be speed up (for example by a terminal illness in a younger person) or inhibited (for example by dominant views in a society that are contrary to the transcendent trend). Gerotranscendence manifests on three levels: the cosmic level, the self, and social and individual relations (Tornstam, 1996). At the cosmic level, changes in perception of time and space occur, there is a sense of connection to earlier generations, fear of death disappears, the mysterious dimension of life is accepted and there is an experience of rejoicing in large and subtle aspects of life. At the level of the self there is the discovery of hidden aspects of self, decrease in self-centeredness, less concern with the body, increased altruism and the experience of ego-integrity. In terms of social and individual relations, relations take on changed meaning and importance, there is an increased need for solitude and an urge to abandon roles, and there is an understanding of the difficulty in separating right from wrong. Tornstam proposed these signs of gerotranscendence on the basis of qualitative interviews with a group of people aged 52–97. He suggests that the process of gerotranscendence is 'intrinsic and culture free' (Tornstam, 1989) but will be modified by specific cultural patterns.

Spirituality: Physical Health

There have been reviews of the evidence that links religion or spirituality to physical health (Ellison & Levin, 1998; Koenig & Cohen, 2002; Larson, Swyers, & McCullough, 1998; Thoresen, 1999). The reviews make strong claims for the broad health benefits of religion, and the reviews of the reviews raise concerns about selective attention to positive studies with methodological advantages.

Church/Service Attendance Protects Against Death

Eleven independent, longitudinal investigations of the relationship between church/service attendance and incidence of mortality were found. Of the nine studies of healthy participants, seven (78%) found a relationship after adjustment for demographic, socioeconomic, and health-related confounders, and six (66.6%) found a relationship after further adjustment for the established risk/protective factors of healthy lifestyle, social support, and depression. The strength of the relationship was, on average, approximately a 30% reduction in mortality after adjustment for demographic, socioeconomic, and health-related confounders and approximately a 25% reduction in mortality after adjustment for established risk factors. This evidence is strengthened by the fact that most of these studies were conducted on representative, population-based samples. Moreover, in two of these investigations (Hummer, Rogers, Nam, & Ellison, 1999), a dose–response relationship was found where increasing levels of churchgoing were associated with decreasing risk of mortality. Chatuvedi, (2007) also reported positive influence of spiritual practices near end of life. They found spirituality as the major determinant of health related quality of life.

Spirituality Protects Against Cardiovascular Disease

Cardiovascular disease includes diseases of the heart (myocardial infarction, angina pectoris), stroke, congenital cardiovascular defects, and congestive heart failure etc. Several prospective studies on spirituality and its impact on mortality due to various cardiovascular diseases have been conducted. For instance Hummer, Rogers, Nam, and Ellison, (1999) and Oman and Thoresen(2002), conducted studies on mortality purely due to coronary heart disease (Goldbourt, Yaari, & Medalie, 1993), and other studies have studied stroke incidence and its association with spirituality (Colantonio, Kasl, & Ostfeld, 1992). All these studies observed that church attendance/ service even at a weekly interval decreases the incidence of cardiovascular mortality Colantonio et al. (1992) studied the impact of several measures of religiousness on incidence of stroke in a community-based study of New Haven, Connecticut, elderly. The only variable that predicted seven-year events in unadjusted analyses was weekly church/service attendance (RR.0.86, *p.* 0.05). However, the associations were non-significant after adjustments for the confounders and protective factors.

Spirituality Protects Against Cancer Mortality

Oman and Thoresen (2002) studied a representative sample of 6,545 adults from Alameda County, California, who were followed for 31 years. Weekly church/service attendance was associated with a reduction in cancer mortality in analyses adjusted only for age and sex (RR _ 0.78, p _ 0.05), but this association was relegated to non-significance when adjustments were made for preexisting health conditions (RR _ 0.83, ns) and further adjustments were made for independent risk factors (RR _0.93, ns). Hummer et al. (1999) studied a national probability sample of 21,204 healthy adults and found a marginal association between weekly church/service attendance and cancer mortality after adjustment for age, sex, and race (RR _ 0.88, *p* _ 0.10) but no association after further adjustment for preexisting health status (RR _ 0.93, *ns*) or after further adjustment for both preexisting health status and independent risk factors (RR _ 0.90, *ns*).

Spirituality Protects Against Disability

Three well-controlled, prospective studies of the elderly that tested the relationship between religion (measured as church/service attendance or depth of religiousness) and disability (measured as activities of daily living or institutionalization). Two of these studies were with healthy participants (Goldman, Korenman, & Weinstein, 1995; Idler & Kasl, 1997), and one was with elderly post-stroke patients (Colantonio, Kasl, Ostfeld, & Berkman, 1993). None of these studies found any relationship between the religious variables and the development of disability.

One of these studies, however, deserves special mention. In the Idler and Kasl (1997) study of elderly New Haven, Connecticut, residents, the predictive relationship between church attendance assessed in 1982 and lowered risk for disability assessed repeatedly at various annual follow-up exams was, after adjustment for confounders and risk factors, significant at the 3-, 5-, and 6-year follow-up exams but not at the 1-, 2-, 4-, or 12-year follow-up exams. All associations were stronger among the subgroup that was disabled at baseline where significant reductions in risk for further disability were observed repeatedly at the fourth through the seventh annual follow-up exams. A more recent cross-sectional study of 3,851 elderly participants found that spiritual coping was more utilized by those having more severe diseases. They reported that people with severe disease prayed, meditated, or read the Bible daily in comparison with these with less severe disease who preferred were involved in spiritual activity on weekly basis (Haley, Koenig, & Bruchett, 2001). Although the temporal relationships in this study could not be disentangled, when it is taken together with the Idler and Kasl (1997b) study, the possibility is raised that private religious activity is a response to increasing physical disability.

In summary, the only supportive evidence for the hypothesis that religion or spirituality protects against disability is from one study in which attendance predicted disability inconsistently from one follow-up exam to another. However more consistency in prediction was expected had elderly with disability were followed up.

People Who Use Religion to Cope With Difficulties Live Longer

Krause (1998) tested religious coping both as a main effect and as an interaction effect with life events stress on mortality four years later and found, after adjustment for confounders, that religious coping was significantly associated with an increase in total mortality when it was examined as a main effect ($RR = 1.15$, $p < 0.05$) but with a reduction in risk when it was examined in interaction with the occurrence of stressful life events ($RR = 0.90$, $p < 0.05$). In the 266 participants with lower education, these effects were stronger (main effect: $RR = 1.32$, $p < 0.05$; interaction effect: $RR = 0.75$, $p < 0.001$). Krause (1998) also conducted a retrospective study that tested the same interactive model on the same nationally representative sample. In this case, however, the stressor was neighborhood deterioration, and the physical health outcomes were past changes in global self-reported health and past changes in functional disability and found the interaction between religious coping and stress to be significant for the more subjective outcome of self-reported health but non-significant for the more objective outcome of functional disability. This study is weakened by an inability to determine whether the religious coping affected health or health affected the religious coping and has not been considered further. Thus, there are inadequate data currently to evaluate the hypothesis that the use of religion to cope with difficulties results in a longer life. A viable hypothesis for future studies is that any coping effect of religion or spirituality on physical health may be stronger in people, such as those of lower educational attainment, who have more limited access to coping resources.

SPIRITUALITY AND MENTAL HEALTH

In the past couple of decades, a holistic approach to understanding individuals has paved the way for research to explore spirituality as one dimension of the cognitive, emotional, behavioral, interpersonal and psychological facets that make up a human being. In the eastern countries different religions and spiritual leaders found a significant link between mental health and religion. But in the West, this remained a controversial issue for long (King & Dein, 1998). The exploration of spirituality-mental health relationship had been multidimensional depending upon the theoretical frame work of the researchers. Researchers in a range of disciplines, including psychology, psychiatry, theology, nursing and gerontology, are exploring the connections between various elements of these two areas of human existence. Various sections of the community have expressed need for identifying the ways in which spirituality can contribute to mental health and wellbeing, mental illness and recovery (Foskett, Marriott, Wilson-Rudd, 2004; Barker, Buchanan-Barker, 2005).

Swinton, (2001) argues that spirituality is an intra-, inter- and trans-personal experience that is shaped and directed by the experiences of individuals and of the communities in which they live out their lives. In other words, there are internal, group, community and transcendent elements to spirituality. Thus, its interaction with a person's mental health is likely to be complex, interactive and dynamic. Although some research tends to look for a simple linear relationship between certain expressions of spirituality and narrowly-defined mental health outcomes, and several reports recognizes the value of an integrated approach to understanding a person's mental health and assumes that relationships between the two are likely to be bi-directional, interactive and open to influence from other factors. There is an inverse association between spiritual practices and severity of depressive symptoms (Cosar, Kocal, Arikan & Isik, 1997). This relationship is more prominent among those with intrinsic religious orientation based on internalized beliefs (Mickley, Carson & Soeken, 1995). Spirituality correlates with lower levels of general anxiety (Bergin, Masters & Richards, 1987) and with positive outcomes in coping with anxiety (Jahangir, 1995). Higher levels of spirituality among individuals recovering from substance abuse are related to optimism and resiliency against stress (Pardini, Plante & Sherman, 2001), and spiritual coping methods are found to have positive effects for persons diagnosed with schizophrenia (Walsh, 1995). Participation in spiritual and religious activities helps to integrate individuals into their families (MacGreen, 1997).

Several surveys showed a high prevalence of religious coping among patients with severe and persistent mental illness. Tepper, Rogers, Coleman and Malony, (2001) investigated 406 patients at one of thirteen Los Angeles County mental health facilities. More than 80% of subjects found religious activities or beliefs useful in managing daily life difficulties and frustrations. A majority of participants devoted as much as half of it was observed that those with severe symptoms (High SCL-90 scores) were using more religious prayers and readings to cope up and a lower GAF score (indicating greater impairment). The amount of time that participants devoted to religious coping was negatively related to reported levels of frustration and scores on the SCL-90 symptom subscales. The results of the study suggest that religious activities and beliefs may be particularly important for persons who are experiencing more severe symptoms, and increased religious activity may be associated with reduced symptoms over time. This is not only true in the United States but also in Europe. The findings of Tepper et al. (2001) have been replicated by Mohr, (2006) in Geneva, Switzerland. Semi-structured interviews focused on religious coping were conducted with a sample of 115 Religion was generally observed to give purpose and meaning to life by 71% of subject. Only few (14%) expressed spiritual despair. Patients also reported that religion lessened (54%) or increased (10%) psychotic and general symptoms. Religion was found to increase social integration (28%), although on occasion led to social isolation (3%). It reduced (33%) or increased (10%) the risk of suicide attempts, reduced (14%) or increased (3%) substance use, and fostered adherence to (16%) or was in opposition to (15%) psychiatric treatment. The findings suggest religious methods of coping having a potential for psychosocial interventions of for the patients with schizophrenia.

Huguelet, Mohr, Borras, Gillieron & Brandt (2006) from the same public psychiatric outpatient department in Geneva investigated spirituality and religious practices of outpatients (N = 100) with schizophrenia and compared them with their clinician's knowledge of patients' religious involvement. Audio-taped discussions about spirituality and religious coping were used for this study. The patient's clinicians (N = 34) were asked about their own beliefs and religious activities as well as their patients religious and clinical characteristics. Though, religion was considered important part of life by majority on the patients. But only few (36%) discussed it with their health care providers fewer clinicians were religiously involved, and, in half the cases, their perceptions of patient's religious involvement were inaccurate. Some patients found incompatibility of the treatment with their religious practices but the clinicians lacked this religious sensitivity.

Spirituality and Mental Health in Old Age

In everyday life, successful ageing can be described as coping well with the challenges and crises of growing old. Good mental health in old age depends on the absence of specific disease processes but, perhaps even more, on how we cope with any challenges that occur. Even with such devastating diseases such as severe depression or dementia, recovery or successfully coping with progressive disease depends on personal and interpersonal resources as well as specific treatment. Some of the most detailed work on the relationship between religious beliefs and mental health in old age has been carried out by Harold Koenig and associates at Duke University in the United States (Koenig 1994). They looked at self-reports relating to how important religion was to the individual and found those for whom religion had become increasingly important with ageing were less likely to be depressed (as scored on the observer-rated Hamilton Depression Scale and the self-rated Geriatric Depression Scale) and found around a third of men and two-thirds of women spontaneously mentioned religion as important for coping with the challenges of old age.

In other studies, strong religious affiliation was inversely related to levels of anxiety. Whether or not the association is directly causal it seems that, within North American culture, religious practice and coping styles are generally associated with less anxiety and depression. Methodologically sound research shows that over a six-year period among non-disabled elderly, lack of private religious activity (prayer) is associated with an increased risk of death (hazard ratio 1.6, 95 percent confidence internal 1.2-2.2) (Pargament et al., 2001). Not all religious belief is positive. For example, a two-year follow-up of medical inpatients showed those who believed God was punishing them, had abandoned them, did not love them, did not have the power to help or felt their church had deserted them, experienced 19-28 percent greater mortality (Pargament et al., 2001).

Negative religious coping involves beliefs and activities such as expressing anger at God, questioning God's power, attributing negative events to God's punishment, as well as discontent with religious communities and their leadership. Negative religious coping has been linked to greater affective distress, including greater anxiety, depression and lower self-esteem (Exline, Yali & Lobel, 1999). Religion becoming the reason for interpersonal conflicts and stains was more like to be associated with depression (Exline, Yali., & Sanderson, 2000). Feeling marginalized or rejected is commonly seen among those with negative religious experiences (Bussema & Bussema, 2000). Unfavorable religious convictions can intensify excesses of self-blame and perceptions of unredeemable sinfulness. These ideas are even more distressing if these have interwoven depressive or obsessive patterns. Many religious communities induce feelings of rejection mental disorders are perceived as moral or spiritual weakness. On the other hand compulsive religious prayers and rituals can become distressing and interfering in one;s daily functioning (Tepper et al., 2001). Finally, beliefs involving themes of divine abandonment or condemnation, unrelenting rejection, or powerful retribution may make recovery seem unattainable or unimportant (Exline, 2002).

A case series of two patients with dementia suggested beneficial role of Salvation Army meetings especially with involvement in singing. One of the authors knew a woman with moderate dementia who attended a (largely silent) Quaker meeting for workshop and others have written about the engagement of old people, including those with dementia, in religious activity (Jewel, 1986). Older people who are 'more religious' tend to reveals greater well-being than those who are not (McFadden, 1995), although less research has been directed towards a developmental understanding of spirituality in older people. . If increased spirituality is related to increased health or well-being, then it would be of benefit to understand how this dimension of life manifests and changes in later life. Seifert (2002) warns against the 'sentiment' of assuming that spirituality automatically increases with age and calls for such ideas to be supported by empirical study.

Spirituality as a Coping Mechanism

One could explain the urge to use religion / spirituality in coping by observing human being's existential condition in the world. Human beings are in fact from birth till death in a process of transition, negotiating change always and everywhere, negotiating relationships with oneself and others, yet facing the ongoing task of establishing and reestablishing a sense of continuity with self and others (Schlauch, 2006). Within these transitions in life, human beings become aware of their transitional position in life, in other words, of their temporality on earth, thus creating a deep existential fear of death (Arndt, Goldberg, Greenberg, Pyszczynski & Solomon, 2000). Human beings are therefore faced with this terror "to have emerged from nothing, to have a name, consciousness of self, deep inner feelings, an harsh inner yearning for life and self- expression and with all this yet to die" (Becker, 1973). Thus, a need for a "transitional object", a safe object, exterior to the individual but yet integral to him, is created in order to give the individual a sense of comfort and continuity. Those transitional objects have a special status by existing "outside" our transition, and therefore being immutable, eternal, revealing themselves in the space in which we live ("transitional space"), an "intermediate space" exiting between reality and fiction (Winnicott, 1971). Religion and spirituality as coping mechanisms therefore cannot be seen as purely psychological, social or physical coping processes that have little to do with religion itself. Since religion / spirituality are distinctive phenomena incorporating distinctive terminology using concepts such as infinitude, omnipotence, god, transcendence and more (Pargament, 2002).

Spiritual Care: Intervention to Alleviating Sufferings

Lunn, (2004) defines spiritual care in terms of "meeting people where they are and assisting them in connecting or reconnecting to things, practices, ideas, and principles that are at their core of their being- the breath of their life, making a connection between yourself and that person".

A Swedish national survey of hospital chaplains identified categories of questions posed to them by patients with terminal illness. Five main categories were identified, in order of frequency including: meaning; death and dying; pain and illness; relationships; and religious issues. Religious issues accounted for only 8% of the questions posed to chaplains. The authors concluded that physicians and other professionals should be able to address many of the questions posed to chaplains (Strang & Strang, 2002). A study of nurses' spiritual interventions found that the majority used the following five "therapies": holding a patient's hand, listening, laughter, prayer, and being present with a patient. More than 90% of 299 respondents indicated that they would offer, suggest, or provide spiritual help in the following situations: when a patient explicitly request spiritual support, is about to die, is grieving, or receives bad news (Grant, 2004). Some investigators (Chandler, 1999; Robinson, 2004) suggest that music and art may contribute to spiritual healing, particularly for those who are dying. The alternative modalities used in the service of spiritual care of the dying include acupuncture, therapeutic touch, biofeedback, relaxation, guided imagery, and aromatherapy (Chandler, 1999). Evaluation of the therapeutic efficacy of these modalities is largely descriptive and exploratory.

Cole and Pargament, (1999) describe a pilot psychotherapy program that integrates spiritual issues and resources for people diagnosed with cancer. The program aims to address four concerns including control, identity, relationships, and meaning. In psychotherapeutic groups, participants are encouraged to reflect on the four thematic spiritual issues and to draw on internal spiritual resources that support adaptive coping. The language used in the therapy sessions is overtly religious. For example, therapists encourage participants to visualize God's presence and to view God as partner in their group therapy work. Miller, Duckro, Videen and Chibnall (2001) have developed a supportive–affective program that focuses on three main areas: spirit, emotions, and relationships. The program targets adults experiencing heart or lung disorders, HIV/AIDS, cancer, or geriatric frailty, with a life expectancy of at least 6 months but likely not more than 24 months. Special attention is devoted to the needs of African American patients and their caregivers. Participants meet for monthly group discussions and are encouraged to raise issues related to spirituality, emotions, and relationships. The program is also designed to accommodate participants from diverse religious backgrounds and also for patients who do not participate in an organized religion. A randomized controlled trial demonstrated significant improvement on depression and measures of religious well-being but not existential well-being. Patients in the intervention groups were more likely to raise spiritual issues with their primary physicians.

Spiritual Issues as Psychoeducational Activities

The program was a seven-week semi-structured, psycho-educational intervention at the Department of Psychology, Bowling Green State University, Ohio (Phillips, Lakin & Pargament, 2002). Two doctoral students in clinical psychology served as ongoing facilitators for each group session (1.5 hours). Participants discussed religious resources, spiritual struggles, forgiveness, and hope. The intervention was designed to provide new information about spirituality to participants and to allow them to share experiences and knowledge. Spiritual topics were more discussed with those perceived severely mentally ill.

The subjects were selected through referral by community health workers. Potential members participated in individual interviews to determine whether their needs, expectations and level of functioning were appropriate for the group. One third of the group members reported a diagnosis of schizophrenia, one third indicated a diagnosis of depression, and one-third reported personality disorders as their primary diagnosis. In terms of religious affiliation, thirty percent identified themselves as Roman Catholic while all others were affiliated with Protestant denominations. Seventy percent indicated that they attend church on a weekly basis.

In conclusion, this intervention provided a safe environment for those with severe mental illness to discuss spiritual concerns. This unique intervention appeared to be highly valued by participants. Community mental health professionals may feel that it is not their place to employ a spiritual issues group in a publicly funded agency. Yet, Richards and Bergin, (1997) noted that some training in using spiritual practices in managing mental illness is required. However, there are no guidelines about it. Additionally, the existing guidelines do not prohibit in using/discussing spiritual methods with the patients. Rather it could be unethical to hurt patient's religious beliefs.

Bereavement and Loss

Grief is the emotional response which we feel when confronted with loss. There are many types of loss, as when we move away from our family home, or when a relationship comes to an end. People can experience grief at the loss of their health, or of their faith, or of their job. However, the loss of someone close through death is a particularly painful loss. The attachment we feel to those who are significant to us is a source of stability for us; these people, their presence and their love, are part of what Colin Murray Parks (2007) calls our "assumptive world" – they are part of how we make sense of life. Following the death of a patient, in several cultures one may seek to be supportive by allowing bereaved relatives to speak about the person who has died, or to express their own pain; may offer information, in writing or verbally, about the journey that lies ahead. Attention to detail such as in the performance of last offices, the giving of time for viewing and farewells, and the way property is returned, will all help the relatives start their bereavement journey. Relatives and caretakers will appreciate the fact that staffs are concerned for them, and they may be grateful for the opportunity, at the time or later, to ask questions and clarify their understanding of what has happened, which will help them begin to accept the reality of the death. And the process is called mourning (Parkes, 2007).

Mindfulness and Meditation

Mindfulness training with a skilled practitioner has been considered in the literature to have the potential to enhance the experience of old age (Nilsson, 2014). Engaging in mindfulness techniques, e.g., physical mindfulness (yoga, Tai Chi), mental mindfulness (meditation), existential mindfulness (resilience) and social mindfulness (cultivating empathy and compassion) has the potential to transform the experience of the older person from an illness experience to a wellness experience. Aligned with Buddhist philosophy, the practice of mindfulness techniques over the lifespan has been shown to have beneficial health-giving effects (Nilsson, 2014). For example, mindfulness meditation as part of a multicomponent spiritual care intervention has been shown to contribute to improved outcomes for community dwelling adults with cardiac disease (Delaney, Barrere, & Helming, 2011). Mindfulness techniques mentored by a skilled practitioner are well within the reach and scope of learning for older people living in residential aged care facilities and in the community. Meditation was considered to be an element of spiritual care in some papers. Two randomized controlled trials on adults with terminal disease studied the effects of meditation delivered by a qualified instructor and defined as involving an induced state of consciousness and delving into self-realization or meaning (Candy et al., 2012). The results found that meditation alone had no effect on well-being or quality of life. However, when combined with massage, reduced quality of life was prevented (Morgan, Simpson & Smith, 2015). A spirituality-based intervention piloted a combination of meditation techniques (Mindfulness/Self-Discovery Meditation, Relationship Meditation and Eco-Awareness Meditation) led to a significant improvement on quality of life (Delaney et al., 2011).

Prayer and Religious Rituals

Prayer is a powerful form of coping that helps people physically and mentally. Nearly 60% of Americans report praying daily (Mohr, 2006). Prayer is a communication or conversation with divine powers or a 'higher self.' Prayer is practiced by all Western theistic religions and several of the Eastern traditions (e.g., Hinduism, Sikkhism, Buddhism and Taoism). Group prayer is associated with a greater wellbeing and happiness, while solitary prayer is associated with depression and loneliness (Poloma & Pendleton, 1991). However, scientific validation of the efficacy of prayer, in terms of health outcomes, remains in its infancy when dealing with positive and negative biases. A number of studies report negative findings on the therapeutic effects of intercessory prayer, and illustrate the need for nonbiased experimental designs. Critics of prayer research have proposed that the benefits of prayer may be the results of a placebo effect (Jantos & Kiat, 2007). Open dialog and refining research methodology in studies of the health benefit of prayer can help discern potential health effects.

Worship and religious rituals are encouraged by most religions. Benson suggests that potentially therapeutic elements of worship include music, aesthetic surroundings, rituals, prayer and contemplation and opportunities to socialize with others (Benson, 1997). Bibliotherapy involves the use of literature to help gain insight into feelings and behaviors, and to assist with positive coping. All major world religions have a text that their followers view as holy, and use as a source of comfort, wisdom and guidance (Nigosian, 1994). All major theistic world religions teach that people should accept and forgive those who have harmed them and seek forgiveness from those whom they have harmed. Spiritual reading and practicing forgiveness and repentance are significant parts of any 12-step program (Galanter, 2008). Steps 4 and 5 of Alcoholic Anonymous involve public 'confessions', and recounting of one's wrongdoing. In medical settings, forgiveness and repentance are within the purview of a pastoral counselor and clergyperson (Latovich, 1995). Both prayer and bibliotherapy with sacred writings must be consistent with patients' needs and requests.

This chapter reviews the available literature on the health application aspects of spiritual practice. As depicted in Figure 3, spirituality has potential to improve all health dimensions.

CONCLUSION

Spirituality is a way of life that sees a positive meaning and purpose of life. It gives the person hope and feels connected with each other. Thus, spirituality at first sight seems to have a potential to ward off mental health problems. But spirituality does much more than that. Old age is specifically marked with physical mental and social disabilities. The available literature shows that spirituality helps in taking

Figure 3. Spirituality and its impact on health

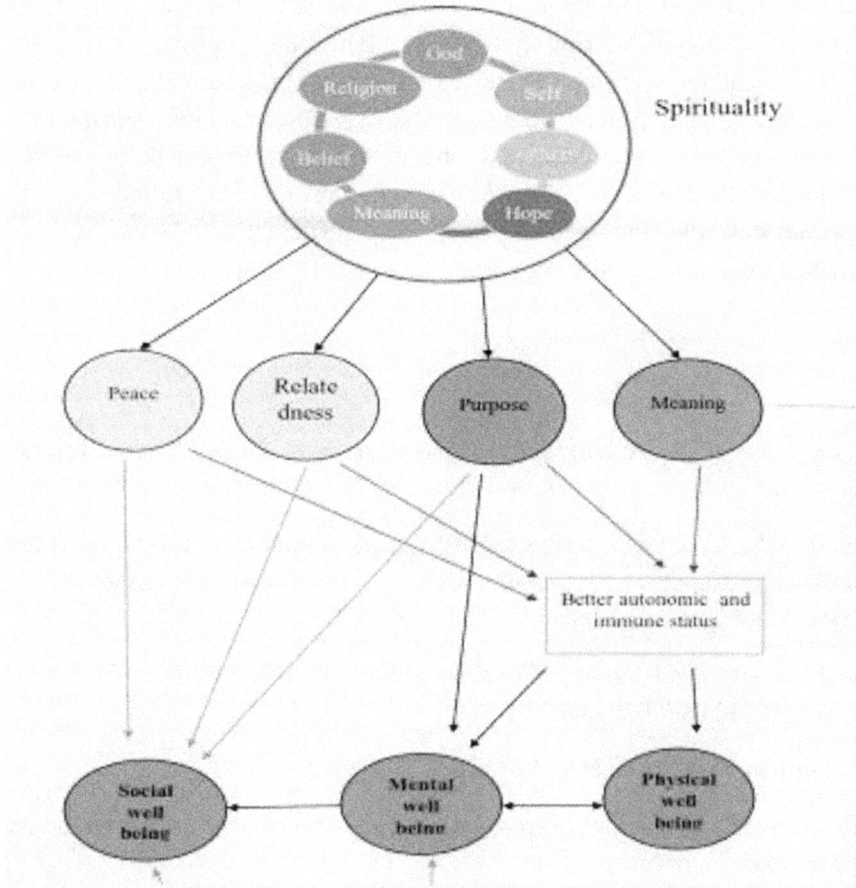

care of multiple old age-related problems such as cardiovascular disorders, malignancies, depression, loneliness etc. Despite marked positive effects in curing various diseases and promoting wellbeing, spirituality is sparingly being used as a branch of medicine. No empirical article or work of science is ever complete without mention of its strengths and weaknesses. Likewise, this chapter would not reach its pinnacle without mentioning its assets and flaws. The authors have tried the best to provide what is existing in literature. However, the strengths and the limitations of the literature are bound to creep in. Long term follow up studies on spirituality is a serious lacuna, which needs to be worked upon by the prospective researchers, especially from India. We didn't come across any culture free measure of spirituality, use of which could make studies comparable across the globe. Such tool is also an urgent need of the health care providers especially when spiritual well-being is increasing being recognized as an important dimension of health.

Keep in view these inadequacies we preferred to start with providing insights into the roots, nature, components and expressions of spirituality. Here too there we found no consensus about the definition of the term spirituality. In this context it becomes difficult to generate universally acceptable measures to spirituality. Different religions have viewed spirituality with subtle differences. However, the religious concept of spirituality needs a separate devoted chapter whereas we tried to focus upon spirituality with reference to the old age. The existing literature is also inadequate for suggesting any model to incorporate spirituality in the existing health care system. Do the health care providers need some training in spirituality before they can recommend it to the patient? What if the patient and the spiritual health care provider have different belief systems about spirituality? How to include spiritual leaders in the health care delivery system? And certainly, at this juncture we are short of making any kind guideline for integrating spirituality and general health care despite the former being an indispensable aspect of health care. Thus, there is clearly a long way to go before we sufficiently understand this ancient art of spiritual well-being to translate into health care practice.

REFERENCES

Alex, J. A., & George, P. O. (2004). Ageing: A Christian perspective. *Global Ageing: Issues and Action*, *2*, 36–43.

Arndt, J., Goldenberg, J. L., Greenberg, J., Pyszczynsky, T., & Solomon, S. (2000). In P. R. Duberstein & J. M. Masling (Eds.), (pp. 201–257). Washington, D.C., US: Psychodynamic Perspectives on Sickness and Health. Empirical Studies of Psychoanalytic Theories.

Barker, P. J., & Buchanan-Barker, P. (2005). *The Tidal Model: A guide for mental health professionals*. Psychology Press. doi:10.4324/9780203340172

Becker, E. (1973). *The denial of death*. New York: The Free Press.

Benner, D. G. (1989). Toward a psychology of spirituality: Implications for personality and psychotherapy. *Journal of Psychology and Christianity*.

Benson, P. (1997). Spirituality and the Adolescent Journey. *Reclaiming Children and Youth*, *5*(4), 206.

Bergin, A. E., Masters, K. S., & Richards, P. S. (1987). Religiousness and mental health reconsidered: A study of an intrinsically religious sample. *Journal of Counseling Psychology*, *34*(2), 197–204. doi:10.1037/0022-0167.34.2.197

Bhasin, B. B., &Kumari, R. (2015).Essence of 'preventive medicine and holistic health'.

Bhawuk, D. P. (1999). Who attains peace? An Indian model of personal harmony. *Indian Psychological Review*, *52*(3/4), 40–48.

Bianchi, E. (1997). *Aging as a spiritual journey*. New York: Crossroads.

Burkhardt, M. A. (1989). Spirituality: An analysis of the concept. *Holistic Nursing Practice*, *3*(3), 69–77. doi:10.1097/00004650-198905000-00011 PMID:2670980

Burkhardt, M. A., & Nagai-Jacobson, M. G. (1985). Dealing with spiritual concerns of clients in the community. *Journal of Community Health Nursing*, *2*(4), 191–198. doi:10.1207/s15327655jchn0204_3 PMID:3852858

Burkhardt, M. A., & Nagai-Jacobson, M. G. (2002). *Spirituality: Living our connectedness.* Cengage Learning.

Bussema, K. E., & Bussema, E. F. (2000). Is there a balm in Gilead? The implications of faith in coping with a psychiatric disability. *Psychiatric Rehabilitation Journal, 24*(2), 117–124. doi:10.1037/h0095109

Candy, B., Jackson, K. C., Jones, L., Leurent, B., Tookman, A., & King, M. (2012). Drug therapy for delirium in terminally ill adult patients. *Cochrane Database of Systematic Reviews, 9*(4), 285–288. PMID:23152226

Chandler, E. (1999). Spirituality. *The Hospice Journal, 14*(3/4), 63–74. doi:10.1300/J011v14n03_05 PMID:10839002

Chapman, L. S. (1987). Developing a useful perspective on spiritual health: Love, joy, peace and fulfillment. *American Journal of Health Promotion, 2*(2), 12–17. doi:10.4278/0890-1171-2.2.12 PMID:22208509

Clark, C., Cross, J., Deane, D., & Lowry, L. (1991). Spirituality: Integral to quality care. *Holistic Nursing Practice, 5*(3), 67–76. doi:10.1097/00004650-199104000-00012 PMID:2045441

Clark, F. (1987). Traditional Indian medicine/western medical measure hope. *Paper presented at Traditional Indian Medical conference*, Tucson, Arizona.

Cochran, J. K., & Beeghley, L. (1991). The influence of religion on attitudes toward nonmarital sexuality: A preliminary assessment of reference group theory. *Journal for the Scientific Study of Religion, 30*(1), 45–62. doi:10.2307/1387148

Cohen, M. (1990). Caring for ourselves can be funny business. *Holistic Nursing Practice, 4*(4), 1–11. doi:10.1097/00004650-199007000-00004 PMID:2365748

Colantonio, A., Kasl, S. V., & Ostfeld, A. M. (1992). Depressive symptoms and other psychosocial factors as predictors of stroke in the elderly. *American Journal of Epidemiology, 136*(7), 884–894. doi:10.1093/aje/136.7.884 PMID:1442754

Colantonio, A., Kasl, S. V., Ostfeld, A. M., & Berkman, L. F. (1993). Psychosocial predictors of stroke outcomes in an elderly population. *Journal of Gerontology, 48*(5), S261–S268. doi:10.1093/geronj/48.5.S261 PMID:8366275

Cole, B., & Pargament, K. (1999). Re-creating your life: A spiritual/psychotherapeutic intervention for people diagnosed with cancer. *Psycho-Oncology, 8*(5), 395–407. doi:10.1002/(SICI)1099-1611(199909/10)8:5<395::AID-PON408>3.0.CO;2-B PMID:10559799

Coşar, B., Kocal, N., Arikan, Z., & Işik, E. (1997). Suicide attempts among Turkish psychiatric patients. *Canadian Journal of Psychiatry, 42*(10), 1072–1075. doi:10.1177/070674379704201009 PMID:9469240

Crowther, M. R., Parker, M. W., Achenbaum, W. A., Larimore, W. L., & Koenig, H. G. (2002). Rowe and Kahn's model of successful aging revisited: Positive spirituality. The forgotten factor. *The Gerontologist, 42*(5), 613–620. doi:10.1093/geront/42.5.613 PMID:12351796

Cumming, E., & Henry, W. E. (1961). *Growing old, the process of disengagement.* Basic Books.

Delaney, C., Barrere, C., & Helming, M. (2011). The influence of a spirituality-based intervention on quality of life, depression, and anxiety in community-dwelling adults with cardiovascular disease: A pilot study. *Journal of Holistic Nursing*, *29*(1), 21–32. doi:10.1177/0898010110378356 PMID:20713655

Dossey, L. (2001). *Healing beyond the body* (pp. 10–22). Boston: Shambala.

Elkins, D. N., Hedstrom, L. J., Hughes, L. L., Leaf, J. A., & Saunders, C. (1988). Toward a humanistic-phenomenological spirituality: Definition, description, and measurement. *Journal of Humanistic Psychology*, *28*(4), 5–18. doi:10.1177/0022167888284002

Ellis, D. (1980). Whatever happened to the spiritual dimension? *The Canadian Nurse*, *76*(8), 42–43. PMID:6901632

Ellison, C. G., & Levin, J. S. (1998). The religion-health connection: Evidence, theory, and future directions. *Health Education & Behavior*, *25*(6), 700–720. doi:10.1177/109019819802500603 PMID:9813743

Erickson, E. H. (1963). *Childhood and society*. New York: Norton.

Erikson, E. H. (1982). *The life cycle completed*. New York, London: W. W. Norton & Company.

Erikson, E. H., Erikson, J. M., & Kivnic, J. (1989). *Vital involvement in old age*. New York, London: W.W. Norton & Company.

Erikson, J. M. (1995). *On old age 1: A conversation with Joan Erikson at 90*. California: Davidson Films.

Erikson, J. M. (1997). *The life cycle completed: Extended version with new chapters on the ninth stage of development*. New York, London: W.W. Norton & Company.

Exline, J. J. (2002). Stumbling blocks on the religious road: Fractured relationships, nagging vices, and the inner struggle to believe. *Psychological Inquiry*, *13*(3), 182–189. doi:10.1207/S15327965PLI1303_03

Exline, J. J., Yali, A. M., & Lobel, M. (1999). When God disappoints: Difficulty forgiving God and its role in negative emotion. *Journal of Health Psychology*, *4*(3), 365–379. doi:10.1177/135910539900400306 PMID:22021604

Exline, J. J., Yali, A. M., & Sanderson, W. C. (2000). Guilt, discord, and alienation: The role of religious strain in depression and suicidality. *Journal of Clinical Psychology*, *56*(12), 1481–1496. doi:10.1002/1097-4679(200012)56:12<1481::AID-1>3.0.CO;2-A PMID:11132565

Foskett, J., Marriott, J., & Wilson-Rudd, F. (2004). Mental health, religion and spirituality: Attitudes, experience and expertise among mental health professionals and religious leaders in Somerset. *Mental Health, Religion & Culture*, *7*(1), 5–22. doi:10.1080/13674670310001602490

Fowler, J. W. (1981). *Stages of faith: The psychology of human developmet and the quest for meaning*. San Francisco: Harper & Row.

Frankl, V. E. (1959). The spiritual dimension in existential analysis and logotherapy. *Journal of Individual Psychology*, *15*(2), 157.

Galanter, M. (2008). The concept of spirituality in relation to addiction recovery and general psychiatry. In Recent developments in alcoholism (pp. 125-140). Springer New York. doi:10.1007/978-0-387-77725-2_8

Glick, I. D., Weiss, R. S., & Parkes, C. M. (1974). The first year of bereavement following suicide: A review of the literature. *Current Psychological Research & Reviews*, *3*(2), 53–61.

Goldbourt, U., Yaari, S., & Medalie, J. H. (1993). Factors predictive of long-term coronary heart disease mortality among 10,059 male Israeli civil servants and municipal employees. *Cardiology*, *82*(2-3), 100–121. doi:10.1159/000175862 PMID:8324774

Goldman, N., Korenman, S., & Weinstein, R. (1995). Marital status and health among the elderly. *Social Science & Medicine*, *40*(12), 1717–1730. doi:10.1016/0277-9536(94)00281-W PMID:7660185

Grant, D. (2004). Spiritual interventions: How, when, and why nurses use them. *Holistic Nursing Practice*, *18*(1), 36–41. doi:10.1097/00004650-200401000-00007 PMID:14765691

Gutmann, D. (1978). Personal Transformations in the Post-Parental Period: A Cross-Cultural View.

Haley, K. C., Koenig, H. G., & Bruchett, B. M. (2001). Relationship between private religious activity and physical functioning in older adults. *Journal of Religion and Health*, *40*(2), 305–312. doi:10.1023/A:1012561909054

Harris, L. (1975). The Myth and Reality of Aging in America: Conducted for the National Council on the Aging.

Hay, M. W. (1989). Principles in building spiritual assessment tools. *The American Journal of Hospice Care*, *6*(5), 25–31. doi:10.1177/104990918900600514 PMID:2604991

Herth, K. (1990). Fostering hope in terminally-ill people. *Journal of Advanced Nursing*, *15*(11), 1250–1259. doi:10.1111/j.1365-2648.1990.tb01740.x PMID:2269747

Herth, K. A. (1989). The relationship between level of hope and level of coping response and other variables in patients with cancer. *Oncology Nursing Forum*, *16*(1), 67–72. PMID:2911529

Hill, P. C., Pargament, K. I., Hood, R. W., McCullough, M. E. Jr, Swyers, J. P., Larson, D. B., & Zinnbauer, B. J. (2000). Conceptualizing religion and spirituality: Points of commonality, points of departure. *Journal for the Theory of Social Behaviour*, *30*(1), 51–77. doi:10.1111/1468-5914.00119

Hood Jr, R. W., Spilka, B., Hunsberger, B., & Gorsuch, R. (1996). Religion, coping, and adjustment. *The psychology of religion: An empirical approach*, 377-405.

Howden, J. (1992). Development and psychometric characteristics of the Spirituality Assessment Scale [Doctoral dissertation].

Huguelet, P., Mohr, S., Borras, L., Gillieron, C., & Brandt, P. Y. (2006). Spirituality and religious practices among outpatients with schizophrenia and their clinicians. *Psychiatric Services (Washington, D.C.)*, *57*(3), 366–372. doi:10.1176/appi.ps.57.3.366 PMID:16524995

Hummer, R. A., Rogers, R. G., Nam, C. B., & Ellison, C. G. (1999). Religious involvement and US adult mortality. *Demography*, *36*(2), 273–285. doi:10.2307/2648114 PMID:10332617

Hungelmann, J., Kenkel-Rossi, E., Klassen, L., & Stollenwerk, R. M. (1985). Spiritual well-being in older adults: Harmonious interconnectedness. *Journal of Religion and Health*, *24*(2), 147–153. doi:10.1007/BF01532258 PMID:24306074

Idler, E. L., & Kasl, S. V. (1997). Religion among disabled and nondisabled persons II: Attendance at religious services as a predictor of the course of disability. *The Journals of Gerontology. Series B, Psychological Sciences and Social Sciences*, *52*(6), S306–S316. doi:10.1093/geronb/52B.6.S306 PMID:9403524

Jahangir, S. F. (1995). Third force therapy and its impact on treatment outcome. *The International Journal for the Psychology of Religion*, *5*(2), 125–129. doi:10.1207/s15327582ijpr0502_7

Jantos, M., & Kiat, H. (2007). Prayer as medicine: How much have we learned? *The Medical Journal of Australia*, *186*(10), S51. PMID:17516884

Jewell, A. (1999). *Spirituality and ageing*. Jessica Kingsley Publishers.

Jose, N., & Taylor, E. (1986). Spiritual health: A look at barriers to its inclusion in the health education curriculum. *The Eta Sigma Gamman*, *18*(2), 16–29.

Jourard, S. M. (1971). *Self-disclosure: An experimental analysis of the transparent self.* New York: Wiley-Interscience.

Jung, C. G. (1971). The stages of life. In *The portable Jung* (pp. 3-22).

Kimble, M. A. (1995). Pastoral care. In M. A. Kimble, S. H. McFadden, J. W. Ellor, & J. J. Seeber (Eds.), *Aging, spirituality, and religion: A handbook* (pp. 131–147). Minneapolis, MN: Fortress Press.

King, M. B., & Dein, S. (1998). The spiritual variable in psychiatric research. *Psychological Medicine*, *28*(6), 1259–1262. doi:10.1017/S003329179800703X PMID:9854267

Koenig, H., King, D., & Carson, V. B. (2012). *Handbook of religion and health.* US: Oxford University Press.

Koenig, H. G. (1994). Religion and hope. In *Religion in aging and health: Theoretical foundations and methodological frontiers* (pp. 18-51).

H. G. Koenig, & H. J. Cohen (Eds.). (2002). *The link between religion and health: Psychoneuroimmunology and the faith factor*. Oxford University Press. doi:10.1093/acprof:oso/9780195143607.001.0001

Krause, N. (1998). Neighborhood deterioration, religious coping, and changes in health during late life. *The Gerontologist*, *38*(6), 653–664. doi:10.1093/geront/38.6.653 PMID:9868846

La Pierre, L. L. (2003). JCAHO safeguards spiritual care. *Holistic Nursing Practice*, *17*(4), 219. doi:10.1097/00004650-200307000-00009 PMID:12889550

Lane, J. A. (1987). The care of the human spirit. *Journal of Professional Nursing*, *3*(6), 332–337. doi:10.1016/S8755-7223(87)80121-7 PMID:3429744

D. B. Larson, J. P. Swyers, & M. E. McCullough (Eds.). (1998). *Scientific research on spirituality and health: A report based on the Scientific Progress in Spirituality Conferences*. National Institute for Healthcare Research.

Latovich, M. A. (1995). The Clergyperson and the Fifth Step, in Spirituality and Chemical Dependency.

Levin, J. S., & Vanderpool, H. Y. (1991). Religious factors in physical health and the prevention of illness. *Prevention in Human Services*, *9*(2), 41–64. doi:10.1300/J293v09n02_03

Ley, D. C., & Corless, I. B. (1988). Spirituality and hospice care. *Death Studies*, *12*(2), 101–110. doi:10.1080/07481188808252227 PMID:10302346

Liehr, P. R. (1989). The core of true presence: A loving center. *Nursing Science Quarterly*, *2*(1), 7–8. doi:10.1177/089431848900200105 PMID:2648211

Lindholm, L., & Eriksson, K. (1993). To understand and alleviate suffering in a caring culture. *Journal of Advanced Nursing*, *18*(9), 1354–1361. doi:10.1046/j.1365-2648.1993.18091354.x PMID:8258592

Lunn, J. S. (2004). Spiritual care in a multi-religious context. *Journal of Pain & Palliative Care Pharmacotherapy*, *17*(3-4), 153–166. doi:10.1080/J354v17n03_23 PMID:15022959

MacGreen, D. (1997). Spirituality as a coping resource. *Behavior Therapy*, *20*, 28.

MacKinlay, E. B., & Trevitt, C. (2007). Spiritual care and ageing in a secular society. *The Medical Journal of Australia*, *186*(10), S74. PMID:17516891

Marty, M. E., & Appleby, R. S. (1991). *Fundamentalisms Observed*. Chicago: Univ.

Maton, K. I., & Wells, E. A. (1995). Religion as a community resource for well-being: Prevention, healing, and empowerment pathways. *The Journal of Social Issues*, *51*(2), 177–193. doi:10.1111/j.1540-4560.1995.tb01330.x

Mayeroff, M. (1971). *On caring*. New York: Perennial Library.

McCarroll, P., O'Connor, T., & Meakes, E. (2005). Assessing plurality in spirituality definitions. In *Spirituality and health: Multidisciplinary explorations* (pp. 43-61).

McFadden, S. H. (1995). Religion and well-being in aging persons in an aging society. *The Journal of Social Issues*, *51*(2), 161–175. doi:10.1111/j.1540-4560.1995.tb01329.x

McFadden, S. H. (1999). Religion, personality, and aging: A life span perspective. *Journal of Personality*, *67*(6), 1081–1104. doi:10.1111/1467-6494.00083 PMID:10637989

Messikomer, C. M., & De Craemer, W. (2002). The Spirituality of Academic Physicians: An Ethnography of a Scripture-based Group in an Academic Medical Center. *Academic Medicine*, *77*(6), 562–573. doi:10.1097/00001888-200206000-00017 PMID:12063205

Mickley, J. R., Carson, V., & Soeken, K. L. (1995). Religion and adult mental health: State of the science in nursing. *Issues in Mental Health Nursing*, *16*(4), 345–360. doi:10.3109/01612849509072529 PMID:7615381

Miller, D. K., Duckro, P. N., Videen, S. D., & Chibnall, J. T. (2001). Life threatening illness supportive±affective group experience: the LTI-SAGE program. *Supportive Care of the Dying*. Retrieved from www.CareOfDying.org/default.asp

Miller, J. F., & Powers, M. J. (1988). Development of an instrument to measure hope. *Nursing Research*, *37*(1), 6–10. doi:10.1097/00006199-198801000-00002 PMID:3340583

Miller, W. R., & Martin, J. E. (1988). *Behavior therapy and religion: Integrating spiritual and behavioral approaches to change*. Sage Publications, Inc.

D. O. Moberg (Ed.). (1979). *Spiritual well-being: Sociological perspectives*. University Press of America.

D. O. Moberg (Ed.). (2001). *Aging and spirituality*. New York: Haworth.

Mohr, W. K. (2006). Spiritual issues in psychiatric care. *Perspectives in Psychiatric Care*, *42*(3), 174–183. doi:10.1111/j.1744-6163.2006.00076.x PMID:16916420

Morgan, P., Simpson, J., & Smith, A. (2015). Health care workers' experiences of mindfulness training: A qualitative review. *Mindfulness*, *6*(4), 744–758. doi:10.1007/s12671-014-0313-3

Neugarten, B. L. (1973). Personality change in late life: A developmental perspective. In C. Eisdorfer & M. P. Lawton (Eds.), *The psychology of adult development and aging* (pp. 311–335). Washington, DC: American Psychological Association. doi:10.1037/10044-012

Nigosian, S. A. (1994). Islam. In World Faiths (pp. 417-457). Palgrave Macmillan UK.

Nilsson, H. (2014). A four-dimensional model of mindfulness and its implications for health. *Psychology of Religion and Spirituality*, *6*(2), 162–174. doi:10.1037/a0036067

Nowotny, M. L. (1989). Assessment of hope in patients with cancer: Development of an instrument. *Oncology Nursing Forum*, *1*(1), 57–61. PMID:2911528

Oldnall, A. (1996). A critical analysis of nursing: Meeting the spiritual needs of patients. *Journal of Advanced Nursing*, *23*(1), 138–144. doi:10.1111/j.1365-2648.1996.tb03145.x PMID:8708209

Oliver, N. R. (1990). Nurse, are you a healer? *Nursing Forum*, *25*(2), 11–14. doi:10.1111/j.1744-6198.1990.tb00843.x PMID:2235650

Oman, D., & Thoresen, C. E. (2002). 'Does religion cause health?': Differing interpretations and diverse meanings. *Journal of Health Psychology*, *7*(4), 365–380. doi:10.1177/1359105302007004326 PMID:22112748

Owen, D. C. (1989). Nurses' perspectives on the meaning of hope in patients with cancer: A qualitative study. *Oncology Nursing Forum*, *16*(1), 75–79. PMID:2911530

Pardini, D., Plante, T. G., & Sherman, A. (2001). Strength of religious faith and its association with mental health outcomes among recovering alcoholics and addicts. *Journal of Substance Abuse Treatment*, *19*, 347–354. doi:10.1016/S0740-5472(00)00125-2 PMID:11166499

Pargament, K. (1997). *The Psychology of Religion and Coping*. New York: Guilford Press.

Pargament, K. I. (1999). The psychology of religion and spirituality? Yes and no. *The International Journal for the Psychology of Religion*, *9*(1), 3–16. doi:10.1207/s15327582ijpr0901_2

Pargament, K. I. (2001). *The psychology of religion and coping: Theory, research, practice*. Guilford Press.

Pargament, K. I. (2002). Is Religion Nothing But...? Explaining Religion Versus Explaining Religion Away. *Psychological Inquiry*, *13*(3), 239–244. doi:10.1207/S15327965PLI1303_06

Pargament, K. I., Sullivan, M. S., Balzer, W. K., Haitsma, K. S., & Raymark, P. H. (1995). The Many Meanings of Religiousness: A Policy-Capturing Approach. *Journal of Personality*, *63*(4), 953–983. doi:10.1111/j.1467-6494.1995.tb00322.x

Parks, F. M. (2007). Working with narratives: Coping strategies in African American folk beliefs and traditional healing practices. *Journal of Human Behavior in the Social Environment, 15*(1), 135–147. doi:10.1300/J137v15n01_07

Phillips, R. E. III, Lakin, R., & Pargament, K. I. (2002). Brief report: Development and implementation of a spiritual issues psychoeducational group for those with serious mental illness. *Community Mental Health Journal, 38*(6), 487–495. doi:10.1023/A:1020832218607 PMID:12474936

Pollner, M. (1989). Divine relations, social relations, and well-being. *Journal of Health and Social Behavior, 30*(1), 92–104. doi:10.2307/2136915 PMID:2470806

Poloma, M. M., & Gallup, G. H., Jr. (1990). Religiosity, forgiveness and life satisfaction: An exploratory study. In *Proceedings of the annual meeting of the Society for the Scientific Study of Religion,* Virginia Beach, VA.

Poloma, M. M., & Pendleton, B. F. (1989). Exploring types of prayer and quality of life: A research note. *Review of Religious Research, 31*(1), 46–53. doi:10.2307/3511023

Poloma, M. M., & Pendleton, B. F. (1991). The effects of prayer and prayer experiences on measures of general well-being. *Journal of Psychology and Theology, 1*, 71–83.

Prati, G., & Pietrantoni, L. (2009). Optimism, social support, and coping strategies as factors contributing to posttraumatic growth: A meta-analysis. *Journal of Loss and Trauma, 14*, 364–388.

Priestley, J. G. (1985). Towards finding the hidden curriculum: A consideration of the spiritual dimension of experience in curriculum planning. *British Journal of Religious Education, 7*(3), 112–119. doi:10.1080/0141620840070303

Pruyser, P. W. (1986). Maintaining hope in adversity. *Pastoral Psychology, 35*(2), 120–131. doi:10.1007/BF01768711

Richards, P. S., & Bergin, A. E. (1997). A spiritual strategy for counseling and psychotherapy.

Rizzuto, A. M. (1991). Religious development: A psychoanalytic point of view. *New Directions for Child and Adolescent Development, 1991*(52), 47–60. doi:10.1002/cd.23219915205 PMID:1956547

Robinson, A. (2004). A personal exploration of the power of poetry in palliative care, loss and bereavement. *International Journal of Palliative Nursing, 10*(1), 32–39. doi:10.12968/ijpn.2004.10.1.12017 PMID:14966443

Rogers, T. (1976). Manifestations of religiosity and the aging process. *Religious Education (Chicago, Ill.), 71*(4), 405–415. doi:10.1080/0034408760710406

Roof, W. C. (1993). *A generation of seekers: The spiritual journeys of the baby boom generation.* Harper Collins.

Rybash, J. W., Roodin, P. A., & Santrock, J. W. (1991). Adult development and aging (2nd ed.). Dubuque, IA: Wm C. Brown Publishers.

Schaie, K. W., & Willis, S. L. (1991). Adult personality and psychomotor performance: Cross-sectional and longitudinal analyses. *Journal of Gerontology*, *46*(6), 275–P284. doi:10.1093/geronj/46.6.P275 PMID:1940082

Schlauch, C. R. (2006). Deeper affinities: Fundamental resonances between psychoanalysis and religion. *Pastoral Psychology*, *55*(1), 61–80. doi:10.1007/s11089-006-0032-3

Seifert, L. S. (2002). Toward a psychology of religion, spirituality, meaning-search, and aging: Past research and a practical application. *Journal of Adult Development*, *9*(1), 61–70. doi:10.1023/A:1013829318213

Sheldrake, P. (1992). *Spirituality and History: Christian living and the Doctrine of God*. New York: Marykmoll.

Shelly, J. A., & Fish, S. (1988). *Spiritual care: The nurse's role*. Inter Varsity Press.

Sodestrom, K. E., & Martinson, I. M. (1987). Patients' spiritual coping strategies: A study of nurse and patient perspectives. *Oncology Nursing Forum*, *14*(2), 41–46. PMID:3644298

Spilka, B. (1993). Spirituality: Problems and directions in operationalizing a fuzzy concept. In *Proceedings of the annual meeting of the American Psychological Association*, Toronto.

Spilka, B., & McIntosh, D. N. (1996). Religion and spirituality: The known and the unknown. *What is the difference between religion and spirituality*.

Stoll, R. I. (1979). Guidelines for spiritual assessment. *AJN The American Journal of Nursing*, *79*(9), 1574–1577. PMID:258568

Strang, S., & Strang, P. (2002). Questions posed to hospital chaplains by palliative care patients. *Journal of Palliative Medicine*, *5*(6), 857–864. doi:10.1089/10966210260499041 PMID:12685532

Swinton, J. (2001). *Spirituality and mental health care: Rediscovering a 'forgotten' dimension*. Jessica Kingsley Publishers.

Tart, C. T. (1983). Information acquisition rates in forced-choice ESP experiments: Precognition does not work as well as present-time ESP. *Journal of the American Society for Psychical Research*, *77*, 293–310.

Tepper, L., Rogers, S. A., Coleman, E. M., & Malony, H. N. (2001). The prevalence of religious coping among persons with persistent mental illness. *Psychiatric Services (Washington, D.C.)*, *52*(5), 660–665. doi:10.1176/appi.ps.52.5.660 PMID:11331802

Thatcher, A. (1991). A critique of inwardness in religious education. *British Journal of Religious Education*, *14*(1), 22–27. doi:10.1080/0141620910140105

Thoresen, C. E. (1999). Spirituality and health: Is there a relationship? *Journal of Health Psychology*, *4*(3), 291–300. doi:10.1177/135910539900400314 PMID:22021598

Tornstam, L. (1996). Gerotranscendence- a theory about maturing into old age. *Journal of Aging and Identity*, (1): 37–50.

Tornstam, L. (1999). Transcendence in later life. *Generations (San Francisco, Calif.)*, *23*(4), 10.

Turner, R. P., Lukoff, D., Barnhouse, R. T., & Lu, F. G. (1995). A culturally sensitive diagnostic category in the DSM-IV. *The Journal of Nervous and Mental Disease*, *183*(7), 435–444. doi:10.1097/00005053-199507000-00003 PMID:7623015

Vaughan, F. (1991). Spiritual issues in psychotherapy. *Journal of Transpersonal Psychology*, *23*(2), 105.

Vaughan, F., Wittine, B., & Walsh, R. (1998). Transpersonal psychology and the religious person. In P. Shafranske (Ed.), *Religion and the Clinical Practice of Psychology* (pp. 483–509). Washington, DC: American Psychological Association.

Warren, M. (1988). Catechesis and spirituality. *Religious Education (Chicago, Ill.)*, *83*(1), 116–132. doi:10.1080/0034408880830109

Winnicott, D. W. (1971). *Playing and reality*. Psychology Press.

Wong, P. T. (1989). Personal meaning and successful aging. *Canadian Psychology*, *30*(3), 516–525. doi:10.1037/h0079829

Zinnbauer, B. J., Pargament, K. I., Cole, B., Rye, M. S., Butter, E. M., Belavich, T. G., ... Kadar, J. L. (1997). Religion and spirituality: Unfuzzying the fuzzy. *Journal for the Scientific Study of Religion*, *36*(4), 549–564. doi:10.2307/1387689

Zinnbauer, B. J., Pargament, K. I., & Scott, A. B. (1999). The emerging meanings of religiousness and spirituality: Problems and prospects. *Journal of Personality*, *67*(6), 889–919. doi:10.1111/1467-6494.00077

KEY TERMS AND DEFINITIONS

Elderly: The ageing process is of course a biological reality which has its own dynamic, largely beyond human control.

Health: Health as a state of complete physical, mental and social well-being.

Mental Health: Mental health includes our emotional, psychological, and social well-being.

Old Age: Old age is the period of years towards the end of your life.

Religion: A religion is a particular system of belief in a god or gods and the activities that are connected with this system.

Spirituality: The quality or state of being concerned with religion or religious matters: the quality or state of being spiritual.

Well-Being: Someone's well-being is their health and happiness.

Chapter 3
Promoting Successful Positive Aging Across the Health Continuum:
A Holistic Approach

Pratima Kaushik
Amity University, India

ABSTRACT

The increase of human lifespans and the aging has brought increased attention to what factors contribute to aging healthy. People are not only interested in longevity but how to remain in the best health in their later years. Therefore, the aim of this chapter is to (a) understand the concept of positive aging (b) identifying the factors contributing to successful positive aging across health continuum (c) review strategies that promotes management healthy aging in elderly, and (d) identify future directions to promote successful population health management programs/interventions. The holistic approach, therefore provide an opportunity to improve the situation of older people in society.

INTRODUCTION

The older adult population is expanding, living longer, with multiple chronic conditions. Understanding and managing their needs over time is an integral part of defining successful positive aging. Population Health Management is used to describe the understanding, assessment, implementing holistic strategies and health outcomes of a population. Interventions promoting health across a continuum tend to be disease, risk, or health behavior specific rather than encompassing a global concept of health.

Positive Aging

Positive Aging is a way of living rather than a state of being in later life. It is an approach which recognizes how negative mental states (beliefs, thoughts, ideas, attitudes) can have a detrimental impact on

DOI: 10.4018/978-1-5225-3480-8.ch003

physical and emotional wellbeing as person ages. It focuses on the emotional and psychological aspects of aging. It understands that the 'mind' can have a big impact on our physical and emotional wellbeing. This term is used to describe the process of maintaining a positive attitude, feeling good about oneself, keeping fit and healthy, and engaging fully in life as you age. Aging is often associated with many rewarding experiences. It is however also a time when significant changes might occur. For example, some people experience changes in physical functioning, social networks, employment, and bereavement can become more common. Keeping a positive attitude toward aging is particularly important as it allows continuing to feel good and have a sense of control. As people age it is natural for them to move in and out of periods of positive aging. Those who age positively live longer and healthier lives, and enjoy a good quality of life (Martínez-Maldonado et al., 2016).

According to the World Health Organization and the United Nations (UN), population aging is both one of humanity's greatest triumphs and one of its greatest challenges. Notwithstanding further increases in life expectancy and healthy life expectancy in the coming decades, it has been proposed that the expected increase in the sheer numbers of people over the age of 65 years will lead to increased demands on our health and welfare services in particular. However, the WHO and UN also propose that it is how we plan for the aging of our population, how we choose to address the challenges and to maximize the opportunities, that will determine whether society can reap the benefits of the 'longevity dividend'. In essence, they propose that societies that are willing to plan can afford to grow old. Planning should focus on keeping people as healthy as possible for as long as possible. Planning should also focus on the positive opportunities provided by large numbers of healthy and active older people and of the significant contributions that they continue to make in society as consumers, workers, mentors, caregivers, child-minders and as volunteers.

Davey and Glasgow (2006) suggested several underlying themes can be identified in analyzing the Positive Aging Strategy (PAS) statement, encapsulating its core values:

...fostering a positive view of aging; promoting attitudes which respect and value older people; recognizing and supporting older people's participation and contribution; valuing self-reliance, independence, individual responsibility; acknowledging diversity among the older population.

Table 1, using direct quotations, shows how the first four themes identified in PAS are reflected in the National Strategy for an Aging Australia (Andrews, 2002) and the United Kingdom's Opportunity Age – meeting the challenges of aging in the 21st century (HM Government, 2005).

CHANGING MIND-SETS TO PROMOTE INCLUSION

Older people are often viewed as sick and disabled non-contributors to society and dependent on the welfare system. In recent years, another stereotype of older people has been emerging – one that portrays them as healthy, financially secure and taking advantage of state benefits that they can afford to pay for themselves. Neither of these portrayals properly captures the heterogeneity of the older population and of their contributions to all aspects of society. U.S. Census Current Population Report suggests that the older adult population (65 years and older) will almost double from 43.1 million in 2012 to 83.7 million in 2050 due to the aging Baby Boomers and increases in life expectancy (Ortman, Velkoff, & Hogan, 2014). This number also reflects a larger representation of minorities among older adults increasing

Table 1. Policy strategies for an ageing society: Underlying themes

Themes	New Zealand Positive Aging Strategy	National Strategy for an Aging Australia	Opportunity Age (UK)
Fostering a positive view of aging	Positive attitudes to aging and expectations of continuing productivity challenge the notion of older age as a time of retirement and withdrawal from society. (p.9)	Together we can ensure that the aging of our population is a positive experience. (p.v).	An older Britain is something to celebrate not fear. (p.3)
Promoting attitudes which respect and value older people	Older people are important members of society and have the right to be afforded dignity in their senior years. (p.9) Goal 8 – People of all ages have positive attitudes to aging and older people. (p.22)	Positive and informed attitudes to and by older Australians are fundamental to an aging nation. (p.x) A touchstone of a civilized society is that it values and provides support for older people … and respects their right to dignity. (p.8)	Older people … have the right not to be discriminated against. We will take steps to ensure that older people are able to maximize their potential, unhindered by prejudice. (p.31)
Recognizing and supporting older people's participation and contribution	The choice to work in later life is important in meeting the challenge of positive aging. (p.10) Flexible employment practices [will] support older people in the workforce. (p.13)	Ongoing engagement of mature age workers will be important to achieve sustained economic growth as the population ages. (p.x)	We must explode the myth that aging is a barrier to positive contribution to the economy and society, through work and through active engagement in the community. (p.v)

Source:(Davey & Glasgow, 2006)

from 20.7% in 2012 to 39.1% in 2050. The National Council on Aging (2014) reported that 92% of older adults have at least one chronic disease and 77% have at least two chronic diseases. The most common chronic conditions or diseases include hypertension, coronary heart disease, stroke, diabetes, and cancer (Ward & Schiller, 2013).

Health care utilization and support service needs are increasing among older adults. Due to the increasing population size and number of comorbidities among older adults, it is unrealistic to address their health needs solely on either an individual disease or condition-related basis; thus, a population strategy is required. The determinants and outcomes of population health are a function of three overarching domains of well-being: physical, psychological, and social well-being. Wellbeing is a subjective term that describes self-reported general life satisfaction and the positive and negative emotions associated with health status (Diener, 2000). Examples of determinants include physical activity, perceived social support, stress, depressive symptoms, cognition, and loneliness, and a sense of purpose. Examples of outcomes include self-rated health, medical services utilization and expenditures, and mortality. Rowe and Kahn (1987, 1997) first defined successful aging as the low probability of disease and disease-related disability, high cognitive and physical function capacity, and active engagement with life. Other researchers within the field expanded on successful aging theory to include additional factors such as adaptation, motivation, emotion, internal and external resources, and stress (Baltes & Baltes, 1990; Depp & Jeste, 2006; Kahana & Kahana, 1996). Health is more than just a condition or disease; it includes the psychosocial components as well. Successful aging reflects a combination of both objective and subjective measures of health, emphasizing its role in population health for older adults. Therefore, placing the "concept of health" across a continuum provides a framework in which both the subjective and objective health status indicators can be better understood. Furthermore, a continuum indicates that successful aging and health management can be implemented at multiple health stages (Depp & Jeste, 2006; Martin et al., 2015).

CONTINUUM OF POPULATION HEALTH

The field of population health has primarily focused on a medical model when placing individuals on a health continuum. Figure 1 illustrates the health of older adults is conceptualized on a population health continuum based on the numbers and severity of diagnosed chronic diseases (such as diabetes or heart disease), obtained from administrative claims databases. On one end of the continuum are the healthiest older adults whom we call healthy and active (disease-free, low health care expenditures). These older adults have no chronic health conditions or disease; staying healthy and active is critical to them. In the middle of the continuum are the majority of older adults who are classified into one of two groups: at risk but healthy or coping with disease (few and well-managed diseases, relatively low health care expenditures). Older adults in the at risk but healthy group are managing a chronic condition (such as hypertension) and their focus is to stay healthy, prevent the progression of their condition, and prevent future chronic conditions. Those in the coping with disease (multiple chronic conditions; higher health care expenditures) group may have multiple conditions or diseases and their focus is on slowing the progression of these conditions and/or reversing the damage. Finally, the very ill (high–very high health care expenditures) group consists of older adults who have had severe medical episodes and need constant or regular medical intervention.

CORRELATES OF WELL-BEING AND HEALTHY AGING

Healthy aging should ideally start in childhood and take a lifelong perspective. Yet it is never too late to start. Investing in prevention can have important benefits for the individuals involved. Well-being is a positive physical, social and mental state. It requires that basic needs are met, that individuals have a

Figure 1. The continuum of population health for older adults
Source: Tkatch et al., 2016

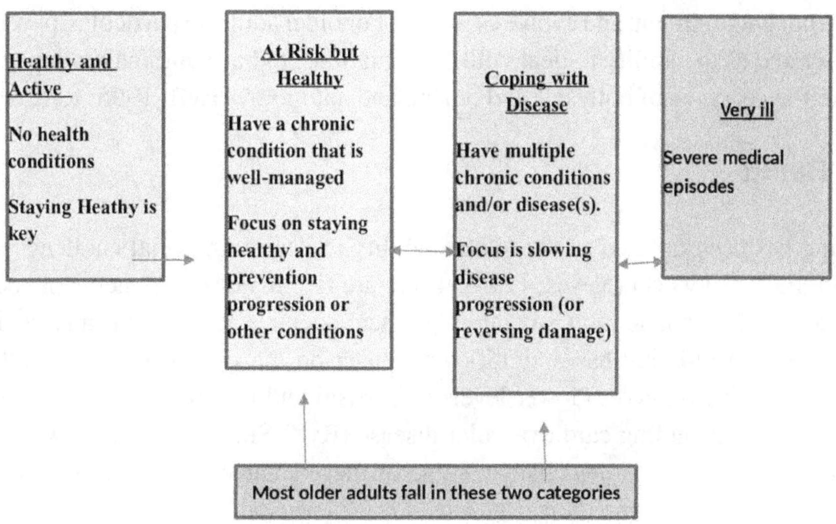

sense of purpose and feel able to achieve goals that are important to them and that they can participate in society and lives that they value. While there is no agreed definition of older people's wellbeing, current thinking associates it with the affirmative concepts of aging that have been developed internationally i.e. healthy, active, positive, productive and successful aging. Healthy aging is much more than increasing the number of healthy life-years without any activity limitation and disability or disease. It has been succinctly defined as the process of optimizing equal opportunities for health to enable older people to take an active part in society and to enjoy an independent and good quality of life (Swedish National Institute of Public Health, 2007).

The World Health Organization (WHO; 2007) defines health as "a state of complete physical, mental, and social well-being and not merely the absence of disease or infirmity." (p.1) The specificity of this definition has been criticized as it defines the majority of the population as "unhealthy" and lacks the subjectivity of health (Huber et al., 2011; Jadad & O'Grady, 2008). Health includes aspects defined by the individual and its meaning reflects individuals' ability to adapt to their environment and manage their well-being (Huber et al., 2011). Therefore, a holistic perspective on health that includes a more objective construct such as physical functioning and the more subjective constructs of psychological well-being, social well-being, and self-rated successful aging can provide a more accurate health description and a comprehensive perspective on the quality of life of older adults.

Physical Functioning

Physical functioning relies primarily on objective determinants and outcomes as it relates to issues that result as a function of a combination of age, illness, and mobility. The objective measures of age and chronic illness are particularly relevant as physical decline occurs (Holmes, Powell-Griner, Lethbridge Cejku, &Heyman, 2009; Hughes et al., 2001).

Psychological Well-Being

Psychological well-being is a multidimensional construct that personifies the human capacity to continue to grow, adapt to our environment, and evolve as we age. For older adults in particular, psychological well-being is characterized as the ability to deal with life situations, to have and maintain positive and close relationships, self-acceptance of both self and others, and autonomy (Ryff, 1995; Ryff & Keyes, 1995).

Social Well-Being

Social well-being has been defined as the relative ability to deal with social challenges and how well one functions in the social world (Keyes, 1998). There are five major components of social wellbeing: social integration, social contribution, social coherence, social actualization, and social acceptance (Keyes, 1998). Social well-being has a significant impact on the health of older adults, with higher levels of social well-being related to lower levels of cortisol and inflammatory factors that contribute to a number of diseases including cardiovascular disease (Ryff, Singer, & Love, 2004). As adults age, their social networks and social roles change; some of these changes enhance their social well-being and some detract from it.

Population Health Management

Programs and Research PHM programs promote health and well-being across the continuum of population health and have three basic goals: to improve health, improve the health care experience, or reduce health care costs (Berwick, Nolan, & Whittington, 2008). Primarily, PHM programs seek to keep healthy people healthy, reduce the progression of disease, and reduce the risk of future disease for those who have chronic conditions.

Core Principles of Healthy Aging

Many older people live a most meaningful life and are a resource for society. They contribute to society, work in a paid or unpaid capacity as volunteers, care for family members and friends, and carry out informal work in organizations and associations. Age discrimination is prohibited in certain EU legislation, but implementation and education are needed. Altgeld, Cohen, and Brussels (2012) proposed following four core principles of healthy aging:

It is Never Too Late to Promote Health

Evidence indicates that health promotion interventions can extend longevity and improve quality of life. Health promotion and prevention are possible even in groups of very high ages. Many preventive programs and health promotion interventions exclude older people.

Equity in Health

Tackling health inequalities in later life and improving the underlying socioeconomic determinants for older people should be at the core of any healthy-aging strategy and health promotion activity. Equity in health for older people explicitly includes non-discrimination of older people.

Autonomy and Personal Control

Autonomy and personal control are essential for human dignity and integrity throughout life. All individuals must have the opportunity for self-development and should take part in making decisions that concern them.

Heterogeneity

Heterogeneity among older people must be taken into account. It includes differences in gender, culture and ethnicity, sexual orientation, and variations in health, disability and socioeconomic status. The generation gaps among older people must also be taken into account. There are several generations between people aged 50 and those aged 100.

INTERVENTIONS TO PROMOTE SUCCESSFUL POSITIVE AGING

In order to manage positive aging across health continuum with aging is a challenging task. There are certain strategies which can help to achieve positive aging. There are a number of ways to prevent, delay or manage some of the physical, psychological, social and personal challenges people face as they age. Some of these studies have demonstrated success with small sample sizes and unknown long-term effects (LaMantia et al., 2015; Stefanacci, Reich, & Casiano, 2015). These are described below:

Maintaining a Positive Attitude

The way one feel about self and the aging process can affect one's view life and the extent to which they are involved in activities and the opportunities life offers.

Staying Connected

Social interaction and relationships with others are associated with positive aging and feeling optimistic about life. Maintaining social networks through membership of clubs, engaging in voluntary work and keeping in touch with family encourages interaction with others, prevents isolation and promotes good mental health and physical activity.

Keeping the Brain Active

Keeping the brain active, alert and flexible can promote good mental health and positive aging throughout the lifespan. Having an active mind can be as simple as reading a book, learning a new hobby or problem solving (e.g. doing crosswords). Learning new skills is exercise for the brain and makes it work a little harder.

Managing Stress

Stress is a natural part of life. While a little stress can be beneficial, when things become too much and usual methods of coping fail, stress may become unhealthy. The symptoms of stress vary greatly among different individuals. High levels of stress can produce emotional, behavioral, and even physical symptoms. In addition to affecting general wellbeing, stress can also impair the immune system and increase the risk of physical and mental health problems.

Volunteering or Seeking Part-Time Employment

Many older people find part-time employment or voluntary work rewarding and a chance to give something back to the community. Any type of work can help to keep your mind sharp and can provide a social network outside of the home and family.

Engaging in Physical Activity

Regular physical activity is vital for improved health and wellbeing. It is never too late to get moving - the human body responds to exercise, regardless of age. Exercise is a great way to maintain good health, helps you thinking positively, recover from illness and reduce the risk of disease. It has been demonstrated that physical fitness is more important than weight loss.

Having Regular Medical Checkups

Older people who have fewer medical conditions have a better quality of life, better mental health and are less restricted in their daily activities. By having regular medical check-ups, engaging in illness prevention (e.g. not smoking, drinking alcohol in moderation) and having regular tests or check-ups (e.g. blood pressure, dental) you can help to reduce the possible onset of chronic conditions.

Eating a Healthy Diet

Eating a healthy diet is important to maintaining a healthy weight, which will help to reduce the likelihood of developing conditions such as diabetes. A healthy weight will also improve energy levels and make it easier to participate in daily activities.

Seeking Psychological Help

Psychologists are trained to help people manage emotional stress and adjust to difficult life circumstances, as well as treat psychological disorders such as depression and anxiety. Psychologists can also support a person to maintain healthy behaviors, such as exercise, and change risky behaviors, such as smoking. Psychologists also work with individuals and their families affected by dementia by providing strategies to manage memory difficulties, initial support at the time of diagnosis and continued support as the condition progresses.

Lifestyle Behavior Interventions

The purpose of a lifestyle behavior intervention is to modify poor lifestyle behaviors to improve health, reduce risk of disease, or slow progression of disease (Glanz, Rimer, & Viswanath, 2008; Montaño & Kasprzyk, 2008). On the continuum of health, the majority of older adults already have chronic conditions and therefore lifestyle modification is of great significance. The three most relevant modifiable lifestyle behaviors are physical inactivity (or sedentary lifestyle), healthy diet, and tobacco usage. These lifestyle behaviors have strong associations with a number of diseases (Mokdad et al., 2003; Warburton, Nicol, & Bredin, 2006). Therefore, lifestyle behavior modifications can prevent older adults from moving further along the continuum of health.

Fall Risk Interventions

As the number of severity of chronic conditions or diseases increases across the continuum of health, so does the risk of falls. Falls are the leading cause of fatal and non-fatal injuries and have a significant impact on quality of life (Houry, et al., 2016). Although falls are considered a preventable health issue, it is estimated that about 40% of older adults fall every year, increasing health care utilization and costs (Houry et al., 2016). Predictors of falls and recurrent falls include gender (female), visual impairment, cognitive impairment, medications, poor physical functioning, poor balance, reduced gait, the need of a walking assistant (cane, walker), fear of falling, low body weight, and history of falls (Ambrose et al., 2013). The U.S. Preventive Service Task Force (Moyer, 2012) recommends exercise, physical therapy, and vitamin D to reduce the risk of falls.

Psychosocial Interventions

Several interventions aim to improve psychological or social well-being; however, these studies demonstrate mixed results (Hogan, Linden, &Najarian, 2002; Netz, Wu, Becker, & Tenenbaum, 2005). Physical activity and mindfulness training interventions have significant effects on psychological well-being (Penedo & Dahn, 2005). However, many mindfulness interventions are related to chronic pain or high levels of stress (Chiesa & Serretti, 2009). Interventions to improve social well-being for older adults have also shown some benefits (Dickens, Richards, Greaves, & Campbell, 2011).

Disease Management Interventions

Disease management (DM) programs were originally developed for high-cost patients dealing with a specific chronic disease such as diabetes, asthma, or congestive heart failure (CHF). Their purpose was to implement evidence-based practice to reduce cost by reducing emergency room visits and hospitalizations, improving quality of life, and improving clinical outcomes (Shelton, 2002).

Case Management (CM)/Care Coordination Interventions

Chronic DM becomes more complex as individuals move along the continuum of health to the very ill category. Multiple chronic conditions require a multidimensional approach to addressing the health needs of older adults, especially with concurrent medical episodes (Boyd et al., 2005). In CM programs, case managers help organize the health care needs of high-cost individuals by coordinating a multidisciplinary team to provide high-quality care, and thus help improve quality of life and reduce costs prior to and post hospitalization (Hickam et al., 2013).

Resilience Building Techniques

Resilience may be a latent characteristic in some individuals but will only manifest itself when they experience adversity. For older people that adversity may have been lifelong, in the case for example of a disability, may be a single life event for example the bereavement of a close friend, spouse or other family member or may be a long-term adversity experiences in later life for example the development of a chronic illness. The concept of resilience is closely related to the ideas of the origin of health- salutogenesis, outlines by Aaron Antonovsky in his 1979 book, Health, Stress and Coping. According to slutogenic theory, stressor will cause harm if they violate an individual's 'sense of coherence'. That sense of coherence is made up of three components: (1) Comprehensibility: a belief that things happen in an orderly and predictable fashion and a sense that one can understand events in once life and reasonably predict what will happen in the future, (2) Manageability: a belief that you have the skills or ability, the support, the help, or the resources necessary to take care of things, and that things are manageable and within once control; and (3) Meaningfulness: a belief that things in life are interesting and a source of satisfaction, that things are really worthwhile and that there is good reason or purpose to care about what happens. Resilience is the result of successful adaptation to adversity. It is relieved by an individual's ability to cope and recover from crises, sustain a sense of purpose and vitality, and emerge stronger from stressful experience. Resilience is a dynamic characteristic that may shift according to the circumstance. Although resilience is seldom associated with older adults they experience loss and decline, older adults actually have a higher level of subjective well-being than individuals in any other age group. "Resilience thinking" in older adults gives them the ability to recover from adversity, thrive with a sustains purpose, and grow in a world of turmoil, change, and chronic illness. It is a regenerative capacity that maintains health and function in the face of loss, disability, or disease. The level of resilience in older age may be associated with the level of overall health and well-being with those with a greater feeling of health and well-being being better able to cope with adversity (Gallacher et al., 2012; DePaula Couto et al., 2011; Gooding et al., 2012).

A number of studies link resilience in older age to the availability of social networks, social support and integration and connectedness within the community. Greater social connectedness is associated with improved resilience (Hardy et al., 2014; Netuveli et al., 2008; Hildon et al., 2010; Pentz et al., 2005; Moyle et al., 2010; Wells et al., 2010). Having a resilient personality has been shown to moderate the impact of ill-health on subjective well-being (Windel et al., 2010). Inherent resilience or 'hardiness' has been shown to be associated with life satisfaction, self-esteem and positive emotions (Beutel et al., 2010; Windel et al., 2010). Faigin and Pargament (2011) argue that the importance of religion increases with age and religion may serve as a source of grounding in the face of adversity. They cite a study of 338 elderly patients admitted to the hospital, who when asked an open-ended question regarding their coping resources, over 40% spontaneously cited religion. They examine qualitative research but provide no firm evidence of spirituality enhancing resilience and conclude there is a dearth of research on spiritual resiliency intervention with older adults. However, a San Diego based study of 1,973 older women concluded that spirituality had a role in promoting resilience to stressors, particularly for those with lower income and education levels, and this is confirmed by a number of smaller scale studies (Moyle et al., 2010; Ramsey & Bliezner, 2013; Cheung &Kam, 2012; Seidel et al., 2009). Improved resilience is associated with better health and well-being, so measures to bring about a general improvement in health and well-being for all people will also improve resilience. Resilience is crucially associated with the level of interpersonal relationships and social interaction so measures to enhance interpersonal relationships and social interaction, such as bus passes, or the ability to work part time beyond state retirement age, will help to promote resilience.

Mindfulness

Mindfulness practice includes a number of meditational techniques, such as activities focused on breath and physical awareness or using metaphors enlightening the essence of mindfulness. All these techniques have a common goal, which is expanding a subject's mindfulness – i.e., the ability to focus on the present moment and to perceive without any judgment or choice current internal or external impulses, which are emerging at a given moment of consciousness. Mindfulness thus allows one to stay "above" the particular content of thoughts, emotions, or imaginations and enables one to become aware of the process of consciousness itself (Kabat-Zinn, 2005).

Yoga and Meditation

Yoga and meditation are well-documented to have psychological, emotional and physical benefits for people at all stages of health, including_cancer patients. Now breakthrough research reveals yoga and meditation can positively affect DNA.The right combination of yogic practices can, to a large extent, correct most of the problems associated with aging. Certain asanas are particularly helpful in the prevention of aging, such as leg lock, cycling and leg rotations from a supine position, vajrasana, majariasana, hasta utthanasana, siddha/siddha yoni asana, shashankasana and, if health permits, suryanamaskara, sarvangasana, vipareetakarani asana and ekapadapranamasana (Saraswati, 2009).

Meditation techniques are considered to be specific cognitively stimulating activities. Western definitions emphasize that meditation is a self-regulatory technique focused on maintaining one's attention. However, in the spiritual tradition, meditation is perceived as a tool for spiritual development, the growth of inner peace, concentration, positive emotions, such as love and happiness, and on reduction of negative emotions, such as fear and anger. Walsh and Shapiro (2006) integrate those two views and propose a new definition. It characterizes meditation as a group of self-regulatory techniques focused on maintaining attention and awareness. The main goal is to achieve a greater rate of well-being, serenity, and concentration through the enhancement of control over spiritual processes.

Mindfulness practice includes a number of meditational techniques, such as activities focused on breath and physical awareness or using metaphors enlightening the essence of mindfulness. All these techniques have a common goal, which is expanding a subject's mindfulness – i.e., the ability to focus on the present moment and to perceive without any judgment or choice current internal or external impulses, which are emerging at a given moment of consciousness. Mindfulness thus allows one to stay "above" the particular content of thoughts, emotions, or imaginations and enables one to become aware of the process of consciousness itself (Kabat-Zinn, 2005). Mindfulness allows one's active approach, which can alter current categories and distinctions through focusing on new impulses, which would otherwise remain unconsciously unnoticed. This conscious processing of impulses impacts a person's behavior and supports a change of habitual behavioral patterns (Langer,1989).

Alexander et al. (1989) suggested a potentially positive impact of mindfulness meditation on cognitive decline in the elderly. A recent cross-sectional study (Prakash et al., 2012) compared cognitive skills between long-term meditating and non-meditating seniors. Meditating seniors showed significantly better results in all attentional tests. The study revealed that long-term meditation of Vihanagam yoga impacted positively on the extent of attention, the speed of processing, the ability of attentional shift, and performance in tests using distracting factors.

Aroma Related Therapies

Fragrance stimulation was shown to change physiological indices such as body temperature, blood pressures, and blood glucose through the control of autonomic nervous activity. It is considered that the sympathetic nervous activity due to stress can be decreased by the inhalation of a fragrance (Shibamoto et al., 2010). Smell stimulation is transmitted through the olfactory nerve to the cerebral limbic system, such as to the hippocampus and corpus amygdaloideum. The hippocampus and the corpus amygdaloideum are closely associated with cognitive disorders, and the hippocampus in particular shrinks remarkably in Alzheimer's disease (Jimbo & Urakami, 2008). A previous study has suggested that aromatherapy improves cognitive dysfunction, the major symptom of Alzheimer's disease, and patient quality of life. Jimbo et al. (2008) reported that disorientation in an aged patient at an elderly nursing home was improved by aromatic bathing. In addition, using a touch panel-type dementia evaluation standard, cognitive function was shown to be improved in patients with advanced Alzheimer's disease. Cognitive impairment in the sense of smell appears at an early stage of Alzheimer's disease. This may represent an effective index in the earlier detection of the progression of disease from slight to severe cognitive impairment (Kawai et al., 2007). Smell stimulation may be a useful method for the early detection and treatment of cognitive disorders.

By progressive use of various essential oils in accordance with time zone, sympathetic and parasympathetic balance can be controlled, and circadian rhythm can be adjusted. Many elderly subjects in geriatric health service facilities experience sleep disturbance and difficulties stemming from problems with circadian rhythm. Watanabe et al. provided treatment to the elderly in health services facilities using a mixed aroma of genuine lavender, geranium, and Anthemisnobilis, commonly known as Roman Camomile, for 30 minutes before they went to bed. Results showed an increase in sleeping time and an improvement in arousal patterns. Further, the 24-hour circadian rhythm cycle was strengthened (Watanabe & Imanishi, 2009).

In aging women, a decreased level of estrogen, induces various menopausal symptoms. With regard to perimenopausal symptoms, hormonal therapy plays a central role, but combined use of aromatherapy is also effective in the relief of symptoms during hormone treatment (Kawabata et al., 2000). Moreover, estrogen has effects on lowering serum LDL-cholesterol level, and increasing calcium absorption and bone formation. The development of osteoporosis in advance age is the single biggest problems in women. To live a fulfilling life until the end of life, it is important to prevent osteoporosis by using essential oils with hormonal effects, accompanied by nutrition therapy and therapeutic exercise (Sotozaki, 2008).

Panchkarma and Ayurvedic Technique

Much more than a purely medicinal technique, it represents an entire philosophy of life. It embraces the preventive and curative aspects of disease, together with the maintenance and promotion of health through one's lifestyle and dietary habits. Treatment has two broad components: Shodhana, purificatory or eliminatory and shaman, pacificatory (Vaidhya &Vaidhya, 1997; Datta et al., 2011). While describing aging, Ayurveda takes in consideration Prana (life energy that performs respiration, oxygenation and circulation). It governs two other subtle essence ojas and tejas. Ojas (the essence of the seven dhatus or bodily tissues) is responsible for the auto-immune system and mental intelligence, it is necessary for longevity. Displaced ojas creates the kapha-related disorders and decreased ojas creates vatarelated reactions. Thetridosha play a very important role in the maintenance of cellular health and longevity. Kapha maintains longevity on the cellular level. Pitta governs digestion and nutrition. Vata, which is closely related to pranic life energy, governs all life functions. Proper diet, exercise and lifestyle can create a balance among these three subtle essences, ensuring long life (Patwardhan & Bodeker, 2008). Ayurveda, the great Indian tradition also conceptual framework on various theories and concepts of aging process. Ayurveda also offers time tested therapies for healthy aging.

Positive Spirituality

Positive spirituality involves a developing and internalized personal relation with the sacred or transcendent that is not bound by race, ethnicity, economics, or class and promotes the wellness and welfare of self and others. Positive spirituality uses aspects of both religion and spirituality (Fetzer Institute, 1999; Shukla, 2015). Positive spirituality may reduce the sense of loss of control and helplessness that accompanies illness. Positive spiritual beliefs provide a cognitive framework that reduces stress and increases purpose and meaning in the face of illness. Spiritual activities like prayer and being prayed for may reduce the sense of isolation and increase the patient's sense of control over illness or disease. In Rowe and Kahn's (1998) model, as illustrated in Figure 2 maintains that model will enhance the percentage of older adults who age successfully by affirming an important and positive aspect in the lives, while in no way disenfranchising those to whom spirituality is not important. Furthermore, the theoretical incorporation of spirituality into models of successful aging represents an important scientific acknowledgement of the research findings of the past four decades. Rowe and Kahn's model has three components: (a) minimizing risk and disability, (b) engaging in active life, and (c) maximizing physical and mental activities. The three components of the model have the following characteristics: (a) each is a part of an overall system and each is therefore temporally related to the others, (b) the variables are activating characteristics that describe both weaknesses and strengths, and (c) each must consider both individual characteristics as well as contextual factors. We argue that positive spirituality is the missing component in the model; it addresses the interrelatedness between the older adults' beliefs and values, the community, and the efficacy of interventions focused on successful aging.

CONCLUSION

Positive or active aging requires ongoing participation in productive activity, with a particular emphasis on extending labor force involvement. It encourages individuals to accept responsibility for maintenance of health and economic activity so that older individuals may remain independent, thereby reducing the

Figure 2. Revised Rowe and Kahn Model of Successful Aging (Crowther et al., 2002)

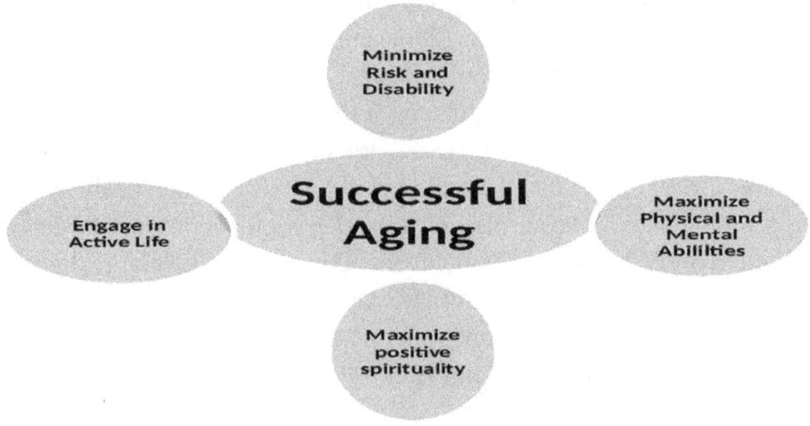

demand on health and social services. Those who are aging in good health and are engaged in productive activities may benefit from increased opportunities if the strategies achieve their objectives. The strategies provide an opportunity to improve the situation of older people in society by drawing attention to the negative effects of age discrimination and exclusion from opportunities to participate. Health plan organizations might also consider evidence-based, low-cost PHM to promote health and wellbeing and as a strategy to help manage health care costs for elderly. It is therefore, important to take a holistic view of what contributes to aging successfully. Those that are most likely to age well have good physical and psychological health as well as a social support network. Successful aging is not only the absence of chronic illness, but the perceived life satisfaction of the elderly person. People with high levels of resilience, low rates of depression, few years of substance abuse, and a good social network are most likely to age successfully and, perhaps most importantly, report high levels of life satisfaction into their golden years.

REFERENCES

Altgeld, T., Cohen, S., & Brussels, J. (2012). Healthy and active ageing. (A report commissioned by BundeszentralefürgesundheitlicheAufklärung (BZgA).). Euro Health Net.

Alexander, C. N., Langer, E. J., Newman, R. I., Chandler, H. M., & Davies, J. L. (1989). Transcendental meditation, mindfulness, and longevity: An experimental study with the elderly. *Journal of Personality and Social Psychology*, *57*(6), 950–964. doi:10.1037/0022-3514.57.6.950 PMID:2693686

Ambrose, A. F., Paul, G., & Hausdorff, J. M. (2013). Risk factors for falls among older adults: A review of the literature. *Maturitas*, *75*(1), 51–61. doi:10.1016/j.maturitas.2013.02.009 PMID:23523272

Andrews, H. K. (2002) National Strategy for an Ageing Australia: an older Australia, challenges and opportunities for all.

Antonovsky, A. (1979). *Health, Stress and Coping*. San Francisco: Jossey-Bass Publishers.

Baltes, P. B., & Baltes, M. M. (1990). Psychological perspectives on successful aging: The model of selective optimization with compensation. In P. B. Baltes & M. M. Baltes (Eds.), *Successful aging: Perspectives from the behavioral sciences* (pp. 1–34). New York, NY: Cambridge University Press. doi:10.1017/CBO9780511665684.003

Berwick, D. M., Nolan, T. W., & Whittington, J. (2008). The triple aim: Care, health, and cost. *Health Affairs*, *27*(3), 759–769. doi:10.1377/hlthaff.27.3.759 PMID:18474969

Beutel, M. E., Glaesmer, H., Wiltink, J., Marian, H., & Brahler, E. (2010). Life satisfaction, anxiety, depression and resilience across the life span of men. *The aging male: The official journal of the International Society for the Study of the Aging Male, 13*(1), 32-39.

Boyd, C. M., Darer, J., Boult, C., Fried, L. P., Boult, L., & Wu, A. W. (2005). Clinical practice guidelines and quality of care for older patients with multiple comorbid diseases: Implications for pay for performance. *Journal of the American Medical Association*, *294*(6), 716–724. doi:10.1001/jama.294.6.716 PMID:16091574

Cheung, C. K., & Kam, P. K. (2012). Resiliency in older Hong Kong Chinese: Using the grounded theory approach to reveal social and spiritual conditions. *Journal of Aging Studies*, *26*(3), 355–367. doi:10.1016/j.jaging.2012.03.004

Chiesa, A., & Serretti, A. (2009). Mindfulness-based stress reduction for stress management in healthy people: A review and meta-analysis. *Journal of Alternative and Complementary Medicine (New York, N.Y.)*, *15*(5), 593–600. doi:10.1089/acm.2008.0495 PMID:19432513

Crowther, M. R., Parker, M. W., Achenbaum, W. A., Larimore, W. L., & Koenig, H. G. (2002). Rowe and Kahn's Model of Successful Aging Revisited: Positive Spirituality—The Forgotten Factor. *The Gerontologist*, *42*(5), 613–620. doi:10.1093/geront/42.5.613 PMID:12351796

Datta, H.S., Mitra, S.K., Paramesh, R., & Patwardhan, B. (2011). Theories and Management of Aging: Modern and Ayurveda Perspectives. In *Evidence-Based Complementary and Alternative Medicine*. doi:10.1093/ecam/nep005

Davey, J., & Glasgow, K. (2006). Positive Ageing – A Critical Analysis. *Police Quarterly*, *4*(4), 21–28.

De Paula Couto, M. C., Koller, S. H., & Novo, R. (2011). Stressful Life Events and Psychological Well-being in a Brazilian Sample of Older Persons: The Role of Resilience. *Ageing International*, *36*(4), 492–505. doi:10.1007/s12126-011-9123-2

Depp, C. A., & Jeste, D. V. (2006). Definitions and predictors of successful aging: A comprehensive review of larger quantitative studies. *The American Journal of Geriatric Psychiatry*, *14*(1), 6–20. doi:10.1097/01.JGP.0000192501.03069.bc PMID:16407577

Dickens, A. P., Richards, S. H., Greaves, C. J., & Campbell, J. L. (2011). Interventions targeting social isolation in older people: A systematic review. *BMC Public Health*, *11*(1), 647. doi:10.1186/1471-2458-11-647 PMID:21843337

Diener, E. (2000). Subjective well-being: The science of happiness and a proposal for a national index. *The American Psychologist*, *55*(1), 34–43. doi:10.1037/0003-066X.55.1.34 PMID:11392863

Faigin, C. A., & Pargament, K. I. (2011). Strengthened by the Spirit: Religion, Spirituality, and Resilience Through Adulthood and Aging. In B. Resnick, L. P. P. Gwyther, & K. A. A. Roberto (Eds.), *Resilience in Aging: Concepts*. Research, and Outcomes. doi:10.1007/978-1-4419-0232-0_11

Fetzer Institute. (1999). Multidimensional measurement of religiousness/ spirituality for use in health research.

Gallacher, J., Mitchell, C., Heslop, L., & Christopher, G. (2012). Resilience to health related adversity in older people. *Emerald Quality in Ageing and Older Adults*, *13*(3), 197–204. doi:10.1108/14717791211264188

Glanz, K., Rimer, B. K., & Viswanath, K. (2008). Health behavior and health education: Theory, research, and practice. In K. Glanz, B. K. Rimer, & K. Viswanath (Eds.), *Health behavior and health education: Theory, research, and practice* (4th ed.). San Francisco, CA: Jossey-Bass.

Gooding, P. A., Hurst, A., Johnson, J., & Tarrier, N. (2012). Psychological resilience in young and older adults. *International Journal of Geriatric Psychiatry*, *27*(3), 262–270. doi:10.1002/gps.2712 PMID:21472780

Hardy, S. E., Concato, J.& Gill, T. H. (2014). Resilience of community-dwelling older persons. *Journal of the American Geriatrics Society, 52*(2), 257-262.

Hickam, D. H., Weiss, J. W., Guise, J.-M., Buckley, D., Motu'apuaka, M., Graham, E., & Saha, S. (2013). Outpatient case management for older adults with medical illness and complex care needs. Rockville, MD: Agency for Healthcare Research and Quality.

Hildon, Z., Montgomery, S. M., Blane, D., Wiggins, R. D., & Netuveli, G. (2010). Examining Resilience of Quality of Life in the Face of Health Related and Psychosocial Adversity at Older Ages: What is "Right" About the Way We Age? *The Gerontologist, 50*(1), 36–47. doi:10.1093/geront/gnp067 PMID:19549715

Government, H. M. (2005). *Opportunity Age: meeting the challenges of ageing in the 21st century.* London: HM Government.

Hogan, B. E., Linden, W., & Najarian, B. (2002). Social support interventions: Do they work? *Clinical Psychology Review, 22*(3), 381–440. doi:10.1016/S0272-7358(01)00102-7 PMID:17201192

Holmes, J., Powell-Griner, E., Lethbridge-Cejku, M., & Heyman, K. (2009). *Aging differently: Physical limitations among adults aged 50 years and over: United States, 2001-2007 (NCHS Data Brief No. 20).* Atlanta, GA: Centers for Disease Control.

Houry, D., Florence, C., Baldwin, G., Stevens, J., & McClure, R. (2016). The CDC injury center's response to the growing public health problem of falls among older adults. *American Journal of Lifestyle Medicine, 10*(1), 74–77. doi:10.1177/1559827615600137 PMID:26688674

Huber, M., Knottnerus, J. A., Green, L., van der Horst, H., Jadad, A. R., Kromhout, D., & Smid, H. (2011). How should we define health? *British Medical Journal, 343*(2), d4163. doi:10.1136/bmj.d4163 PMID:21791490

Hughes, V. A., Frontera, W. R., Wood, M., Evans, W. J., Dallal, G. E., Roubenoff, R., & Singh, M. A. F. (2001). Longitudinal muscle strength changes in older adults: Influence of muscle mass, physical activity, and health. *The Journals of Gerontology, Series A: Biological Sciences & Medical Sciences, 56*, B209-B217. doi:.B20910.1093/gerona/56.5

Jadad, A. R., & O'Grady, L. (2008). How should health be defined? *British Medical Journal, 337.* doi:.a290010.1136/bmj

Jimbo, D., & Urakami, K. (2008). Aromatherapy [in Japanese]. *Japanese Journal of Geriatric Psychiatry, 19*, 1365–1372.

Jimbo, D., & Urakami, K. (2008). Effect of aromatherapy on patients with severe Alzheimer's disease [in Japanese]. *Journal of Japanese Society of Aromatherapy, 7*, 43–48.

Kabat-Zinn, J. (2005). Bringing mindfulness to medicine: An interview with Jon Kabat-Zinn, PhD. Interview by Karolyn Gazella. *Advances in Mind-Body Medicine, 21*, 22–27. PMID:16170903

Kahana, E., & Kahana, B. (1996). Conceptual and empirical advances in understanding aging well through proactive adaptation. In V. L. Bengtson (Ed.), *Adulthood and aging: Research on continuities and discontinuities* (pp. 18–40). New York, NY: Springer.

Kawabata, K., Yoshii, Y., & Tamizu, S. (2000). *Medical aromatherapy using in the clinical*. Medicus Shuppan, Osaka Publisher Co. Ltd, in Japanese.

Kawai, M., Negoro, K., & Kanda, T. (2007). Olfactory disorder in the Alzheimer disease. [in Japanese.]. *Neurological Medicine*, *66*, 366–369.

Keyes, C. L. M. (1998). Social well-being. *Social Psychology Quarterly*, *61*(2), 121–140. doi:10.2307/2787065

LaMantia, M. A., Alder, C. A., Callahan, C. M., Gao, S., French, D. D., Austrom, M. G., & Boustani, M. A. (2015). The aging brain care medical home: Preliminary data. *Journal of the American Geriatrics Society*, *63*(6), 1209–1213. doi:10.1111/jgs.13447 PMID:26096394

Langer, E. J. (1989). Minding matters: The consequences of mindlessness mindfulness. *Advances in Experimental Social Psychology*, *22*, 137–173. doi:10.1016/S0065-2601(08)60307-X

Martin, P., Kelly, N., Kahana, B., Kahana, E., Willcox, B. J., Willcox, D. C., & Poon, L. W. (2015). Defining successful aging: A tangible or elusive concept? *The Gerontologist*, *55*(1), 14–25. doi:10.1093/geront/gnu044 PMID:24840916

Martínez-Maldonado, M. L., Vivaldo-Martínez, M., & Mendoza-Núñez, V. M. (2016). Comprehensive Gerontological Development: A Positive View on Aging. *Gerontology & Geriatric Medicin*, *2*, 1–6. PMID:28913371

Mokdad, A. H., Ford, E. S., Bowman, B. A., Dietz, W. H., Vincor, F., Bales, V. S., & Marks, J. S. (2003). Prevalence of obesity, diabetes, and obesity-related health risk factors, 2001. *Journal of the American Medical Association*, *289*(1), 76–79. doi:10.1001/jama.289.1.76 PMID:12503980

Montaño, D. E., & Kasprzyk, D. (2008). Theory of reasoned action, theory of planned behavior, and the integrated behavioral model. In K. Glanz, B. K. Rimer, & K. Viswanath (Eds.), *Health behavior and health education: Theory, research, and practice* (4th ed., pp. 67–96). San Francisco, CA: Jossey-Bass.

Moyer, V. A. (2012). Prevention of falls in communitydwelling older adults: US Preventive Services Task Force recommendation statement. *Annals of Internal Medicine*, *157*(3), 197–204. doi:10.7326/0003-4819-157-3-201208070-00462 PMID:22868837

Moyle, W., Clarke, C., Gracia, N., Reed, J., Cook, G., Klein, B., ... Richardson, E. (2010). Older people maintaining mental health well-being through resilience: An appreciative inquiry study in four countries. *Journal of Nursing and Healthcare of Chronic Illness*, *2*(2), 113–121. doi:10.1111/j.1752-9824.2010.01050.x

National Council on Aging. (2014). *Healthy aging: Fact sheet* (p. 2). Washington, DC: Author.

Netuveli, G., Wiggins, R. D., Montgomery, S. M., Hildon, Z., & Blane, D. (2008). Mental health and resilience at older ages: Bouncing back after adversity in the British Household Panel Survey. *Journal of Epidemiology and Community Health*, *62*(11), 987–991. doi:10.1136/jech.2007.069138 PMID:18854503

Netz, Y., Wu, M.-J., Becker, B. J., & Tenenbaum, G. (2005). Physical activity and psychological well-being in advanced age: A meta-analysis of intervention studies. *Psychology and Aging*, *20*(2), 272–284. doi:10.1037/0882-7974.20.2.272 PMID:16029091

Ortman, J. M., Velkoff, V. A., & Hogan, H. (2014). An aging nation: The older population in the United States. Retrieved from https://www.census.gov/prod/2014pubs/p25-1140.pdf

Patwardhan, B., & Bodeker, G. (2008). Ayurvedic genomics: Establishing genetic basis for mind-body typologies. *Journal of Alternative and Complementary Medicine*, *14*(5), 571–576. doi:10.1089/acm.2007.0515 PMID:18564959

Penedo, F. J., & Dahn, J. R. (2005). Exercise and well-being: A review of mental and physical health benefits associated with physical activity. *Current Opinion in Psychiatry*, *18*(2), 189–193. doi:10.1097/00001504-200503000-00013 PMID:16639173

Pentz, M. (2005). Resilience among older adults with cancer and the importance of social support and spirituality-faith. *Journal of Gerontological Social Work*, *44*(3-4), 3–22. doi:10.1300/J083v44n03_02

Prakash, R., Rastogi, P., Dubey, I., Abhishek, P., Chaudhury, S., & Small, B. J. (2012). Long-term concentrative meditation and cognitive performance among older adults. *Neuropsychology Developmental Cognitive Behaviour Aging Neuropsychological Cognition*, *19*(4), 479–494. doi:10.1080/13825585.2011.630932 PMID:22149237

Ramsey, J. L., & Blieszner, R. (2013). *Spiritual resiliency and aging: hope, relationality, and the creative self.* Amityville, NY: Baywood.

Rowe, J. W., & Kahn, R. L. (1987). Human aging: Usual and successful. *Science*, *237*, 143–149. doi:10.1093/geront/37.4.433 PMID:9279031

Rowe, J. W., & Kahn, R. L. (1997). Successful aging. *The Gerontologist*, *37*(4), 433–440. and doi:10.1093/geront/37.4.433

Rowe, J. W., & Kahn, R. L. (1998). *Successful aging*. New York: Pantheon/ Random House.

Ryff, C. D. (1995). Psychological well-being in adult life. *Current Directions in Psychological Science*, *4*(4), 99–104. doi:10.1111/1467-8721.ep10772395

Ryff, C. D., & Keyes, C. L. (1995). The structure of psychological well-being revisited. *Journal of Personality and Social Psychology*, *69*(4), 719–727. doi:10.1037/0022-3514.69.4.719 PMID:7473027

Ryff, C. D., Singer, B. H., & Love, G. D. (2004). Positive health: Connecting well-being with biology. *Philosophical Transactions of the Royal Society of London. Series B, Biological Sciences*, *359*(1449), 1383–1394. doi:10.1098/rstb.2004.1521 PMID:15347530

Saraswati, S. N. (1999, January). Yogic Management of Ageing.Magazine of Bihar School of Yoga. Retrieved from http://www.yogamag.net/archives/1999/ajan99/ageing.shtml

Seidel, D., Jagger, C., Brayne, C., Matthews, F. E., & Cfas, M. (2009). Recovery in instrumental activities of daily living (IADLs): Findings from the Medical Research Council Cognitive Function and Ageing Study (MRC CFAS*). Age and Ageing*, *38*(6), 663–668. doi:10.1093/ageing/afp128 PMID:19633320

Shelton, P. S. (2002). Disease management programs. *Disease Management & Health Outcomes*, *10*(8), 461–467. doi:10.2165/00115677-200210080-00001

Shibamoto, K., Mochizuki, M., & Kusuhara, M. (2010). Aroma Therapy in Anti-Aging Medicine. *Anti-Aging Medicine*, *7*(6), 55–59. doi:10.3793/jaam.7.55

Shukla, P. (2015). Spirituality and positive view of ageing in modern society. *Indian Journal of Positive Psychology*, *6*(1), 122–126.

Sotozaki, K. (2008). 'Fragrance' and 'healing' into the life. [in Japanese]. *Journal of Japanese Society of Aromatherapy*, *7*, 33–00.

Stefanacci, R. G., Reich, S., & Casiano, A. (2015). Application of PACE principles for population health management of frail older adults. *Population Health Management*, *18*(5), 367–372. doi:10.1089/pop.2014.0096 PMID:25647691

Swedish National Institute of Public Health (SNIPH). (2007). Healthy Ageing, A Challenge for Europe. Retrieved from www.healthyageing.eu)

Tkatch, R., Musich, S., MacLeod, S., Alsgaard, K., Hawkins, K., & Yeh, C. S. (2016). Population Health Management for Older Adults: Review of Interventions for Promoting Successful Aging Across the Health Continuum. *Gerontology & Geriatric Medicine*, *2*, 1–13. PMID:28680938

Vaidya, A. B., & Vaidya, R. A. (1997). Ancient insights and modern discoveries in the process of aging—an overview. *Indian Journal of Medical Sciences*, *51*, 10,349–363. PMID:9567510

Walsh, R., & Shapiro, S. L. (2006). The meeting of meditative disciplines and Western psychology: A mutually enriching dialogue. *The American Psychologist*, *61*(3), 227–239. doi:10.1037/0003-066X.61.3.227 PMID:16594839

Warburton, D. E., Nicol, C. W., & Bredin, S. S. (2006). Health benefits of physical activity: The evidence. *Canadian Medical Association Journal*, *174*(6), 801–809. doi:10.1503/cmaj.051351 PMID:16534088

Ward, B. W., & Schiller, J. S. (2013). Prevalence of multiple chronic conditions among US adults: Estimates from the National Health Survey 2010. *Preventing Chronic Disease*, *10*, 120203. doi:10.5888/pcd10.120203 PMID:23618545

Watanabe, S., & Imanishi, J. (2009). Aromatherapy. [in Japanese]. *Anti-Aging Igaku*, *5*, 375–379.

Wells, M. (2010). Resilience in older adults living in rural, suburban, and urban areas. *Online Journal of Rural Nursing and Health Care: the Official Journal of the Rural Nurse Organization*, *10*(2), 4554.

WHO. (2007). Age-Friendly Cities: A Guide.

Windle, G., Woods, R. T., & Markland, D. A. (2010). Living with Ill-Health in Older Age: The Role of a Resilient Personality. *Journal of Happiness Studies*, *11*(6), 763–777. doi:10.1007/s10902-009-9172-3

KEY TERMS AND DEFINITIONS

Health Continuum: The health continuum refers to an integrated system of health care that follows a patient through time or through a range of services. The goal of a health continuum is to offer a more comprehensive patient care.

Healthy Aging: Healthy aging is the development and maintenance of optimal mental, social and physical well-being and function in older adults. This is most likely to be achieved when communities are safe, promote health and well-being, and use health services and community programs to prevent or minimize disease.

Holistic Approach: Holistic medicine is a term used to describe therapies that attempt to treat the patient as a whole person. That is, instead of treating an illness, as in orthodox allopathy, holistic medicine looks at an individual's overall physical, mental, spiritual, and emotional wellbeing before recommending treatment.

Population Health Management: Population Health Management is the aggregation of patient data across multiple health information technology resources, the analysis of that data into a single, actionable patient record, and the actions through which care providers can improve both clinical and financial outcomes.

Successful Positive Aging: The attributes of successful aging concentrating on the positive scenarios. Highlighting techniques and policies that can help us to develop more resilience while strengthening our sense of fulfillment and control, despite the challenges that associated with growing older.

Chapter 4
Aging, Quality of Life, and Social Support

Garima Gupta
Arya Mahila Post Graduate College, India

Deepa Luxmi Sharma
Counselling Crux, India

ABSTRACT

The present chapter presents an intertwined view on aging, quality of life and social support. Aging is a sensitive process of transformation from a young age structure to old age. It is a pressing problem for many countries in this century. Therefore, attention to needs and problems of this age has an importance. The domains that need more attention in elderly is both quality of life and social support in their life. Though social support and quality of life have received much attention in studies of the psychological issues of older adults but still researches are needed in special attention at the intervention level.

INTRODUCTION

Aging is a global issue and continuously been increasing from the second half of the last century. It is a process where the proportion of old person increases than that of the proportion of children (Shettar, 2013). The World Health organization (WHO) defines people aged 60-74 years are elderly. In 1980, UN recommended 60 years as the age of transition for the elderly. Presently, India ranks with large elderly population amongst the countries of the world and researchers have come up with the statistics by United Nations (UN), 2011 that India's elderly population at age 60 and above shows an increase from about 105 million (or about 8% of total population) in 2011 to 376 million (or 22% of total population) in 2051 and to 622 million in 2100(or 37% of total population). The proportion of elderly persons in the population of India rose from 5.63% in 1961 to 6.58% in 1991 (Irudaya, Rajan, Mishra, & Sharma, 1999) and to 7.5% in 2001. It rose to 8 million by 21 million in 1991 from 1961 and 29 million in 2001. The growth rate among differences cohorts of elderly such as 60, 70, and 80 above during the decade 1991-2001 was much higher than the general population growth rate of 2% per annum during the same period.

DOI: 10.4018/978-1-5225-3480-8.ch004

DEFINITIONS OF AGING

There are several aspects that define aging from its own perspective. Aging actually is not a unidimensional concept and people can age in different ways giving rise to different sets of definitions of aging. The two most commonly used definitions are chronological age and functional age. Chronological age is based on time and refers to numbers of years, month or days passed by an individual since birth when used to demarcate limits for functions like voting, issuing driving hence, or for retirement. The underlying assumptions are that the chronological age is a barometer of the ability to perform certain functions. Functional age is a measure of how well a person can function in the physical and social environment as compared to other people of same age. It has three components: biological, psychological, and social. It is apparent that even though chronological age not is an indicator of an individual's level of functioning, yet it is linked with aspect of functional age in some way. Demographers and sociologists sometimes categorized the population in three groups (Carey, 2003) as follows: Aged 55-65 as young old (b) Aged 66-85 as old (c) Aged 85 years and above as oldest old. These categorizations have to be re-evaluated in different cultural contexts depending on the life expectancy for that specific cultural group.

AGING AND THEORIES OF AGING

Aging is a multi-dimensional change that includes changes within physical, psychological, as well as social aspects. It can be described as progressive deterioration of the physical and mental functions resulting in a simultaneous decline in both the capacity if the body to maintain homeostatic balance as well the adaptability of the individual to various stressors and thereby increasing the chances of illness and morality. However, not all individuals age in a similar way. In biological terms, aging is a dynamic process that represents the molecular, biochemical, physiological, and structural changes that take place in individual following the end of growth (Dey, 2003). Life is a continuous growth. It begins from infancy to old age and a process through childhood to adulthood and ultimately terminates with the death of an individual (Bhatia, 1983). In general, old age is related with deterioration of physical and mental capacities at a specific chronological age which is usually considered at the age of sixty. The truth about aging is that it is natural and universal process. It is not at all a crisis which hits us suddenly and abruptly in the middle age. It is a continuous unfolding cycle of change that begins to operate even before our birth (Oberoi & Dey, 1991). The process of aging is as old as life. According to the biological point of view, the wear and tear, the building (anabolic) and break down (catabolic) of cells (metabolic process) in the body starts early in the life, even in the prenatal period and continues all through life. However, in the later years of life, the replacement or repair gradually slows and become inefficient. The catabolism (debit) predominates over (credit). Wear and tear becomes more visible in its gross form. Though, Ramamurti (2008) has pointed out the factors, that contribute to ageing may be not only at the genetic level, but also in the body system, the metabolic process, the environment and life style or may be disease included.

Theories of Aging

Psycho-social theories, however, help in identifying the degree and the nature of psychosocial factors associated with changes across the adult life course as well as providing a measure of the extent of frustration and contentment with these change agents at various stages of life cycle of the individual. Some of the prevalent theories are being presented here.

Role Theory

Role theory was the earliest attempt in social gerontology to understand the adjustment of the aged individual. Cottrell (1942) was one of the first to propose a social theory of aging by applying the role theory to the adjustment of aged individual. Researchers were concerned with the problems of adjustment due to role changes in later life. Roles were viewed as a set of highly structured experience with aging, which were classified as being of two types. Role theory focuses on role changes that individuals experience with aging, which were classified as being of two types. One type of role change is role loss. For example, the relinquishment of social relationship and roles typical of adulthood, i.e. work roles.

Erickson's Stage Theory

Erickson's (1963, 1968) theory proposes eight-stages of psychological development and focuses more on how a positive state may be achieved in later years of life by resolving the crises and accomplishing the development tasks at earlier stages in an appropriate manner. Each stage has specific demands and poses specific crisis that is faced and needs to be adequately resolved. The more successfully people resolve these crises, the healthier their developments becomes. It describes old age as a period where there is a conflict of integrity vs. despair. Integrity means feeling at peace with oneself and the world and having no regrets or discriminations. The linking between the stages is perhaps clearer here. People are more likely to look back on their lives positivity and happily if they have left the world a better than they found it-in whatever way, to whatever extent and there lies integrity and acceptance. Despair and/ or disgust (i.e. rejection, denial or 'sour grapes' feelings towards what life might have been) represent the opposite disposition, i.e., feelings of wasted opportunities, regrets wishing to be able to turn back the clock and have a second chance. In the later years of life, beyond adulthood, it is the time for individuals to look back and retrospect. During the process of retrospection, if aged person feel that they have spent their life well, then a sense of satisfaction and integrity will be achieved. If the older adults had resolved many of the stages negatively, the retrospective glance is likely to yield gloom or despair.

Disengagement Theory

The disengagement theory based on expansive and intensive research was propounded by Cumming, Dean, Newell, and McCaffery (1960) and later elaborated by Cumming and Henry (1961). Cumming and Henry (1961) defined aging process as a state of "an inevitable mutual withdrawal or disengagement resulting in decreased interaction between the aging individual and other members of his social system". They further stated that this disengagement implies a loss of roles, restriction on social contacts and relationships, reduced commitment to social values as well as reduction in the activity levels and involvement, causing loss of morale. This theory of aging argues that as people get older, their abilities declines and hence, they seek to decrease their activities, assume more passive and societal roles. The proponents of these theories argue that gradual engagement is functional for society, which could otherwise be faced with disruption by sudden withdrawal of its members.

ISSUES AND PROBLEMS OF AGING

Aging has become the prominent problem during the last thirty years, for many countries especially for developing countries in the mid of 20th century. The disability, issues or problems that a person experiences during the ageing are several. For few, aging can contribute to life satisfaction while for others it can be difficult and problematic. Getting old not only provides an opportunity to relax, enjoy, and do things they always wanted (but never had the time for when they were young) but also causes physical, mental, and psychological disabilities. As age increases there seems to be various problems playing role in elderly life. For example, many of older faces economic crisis that can affect their well-being. Not only economic problems but older people may get prone to suffer from ill health and poor mental health. Failing health due to advancing age is complicated by non-availability to good quality, age-sensitivity, and health care for a large proportion of older persons in the country. It is known that aging is accompanied with various physical ailments and illness. The major conditions that affect people over 65 years are coronary heart disease, followed by stroke, cancer, pneumonia, and the flu. Accidents, particularly falls that result in hip fractures, are also unfortunately common in the elderly. Heart conditions (hypertension, vascular disease, congestive heart failure, high blood pressure and coronary artery disease), breathing problems, dementia, including Alzheimer's disease, Incontinence (urine and stool), Parkinson's disease, cancer, eye problems (cataracts, glaucoma, Macular Degeneration) and other psychiatric problem like depression. People over age 65 can experience depression that is triggered by life changes. At one hand, older adults often face health changes and challenges that can cause depression and on other hand a loss of independence can make people feel frustrated and depressed. Hereafter, aging comes with many physical changes.

Further, the needs of the aging population must be a critically considered in the provision of health care services. The older face difficulties in accessing health care services, e.g. problems in finding a family physician and/or a lack of treatment for particular medical conditions; they have limited benefits coverage of the health care system which may result in seniors having to pay for some medically-related and dental services; further, inadequate facilities and services for long-term care, complex continuing care, and rehabilitation; and inadequate community-based health care have been identified.

Another type of issues that most elderly faces is elder abuse which occurs in large part because of negative attitudes towards the elderly or their economic and social vulnerability. Since they are weak, they are vulnerable to abuse more both emotionally and mentally. Many older persons live in fear. Whether rational or irrational, this is a relevant problem face by the elderly that needs to be carefully and effectively addressed. Lowered self-esteem among older includes isolation, neglect, reduced responsibilities and decrease in values or worth by one-self, family and /or the society. A large number of people enter 'old age' with little, or no, awareness of what this entails. Based on the aforementioned studies, it can be said that elderly people have excessive probability of suffering from multiple health disorders because of reduced physical and mental functions. Loneliness, impaired sexual activity, and chronic metabolic disorders are some of causes can result in emotional disturbances (Figueira, Figueira, Mello, & Dantas, 2008) that can decrease the life quality of elderly. Poor economic, cultural, educational, health care conditions and inadequate social interactions results in poor quality of life in elderly people (Donmez, Gokkoca, & Dedeoglu, 2005; Gureje, Ogunniyi, Kola, & Afolabi, 2006; Mellor, Russo, McCabe, Davison, & George, 2008).In general, the issues that causes medical, social, and psychological problems can decrease the quality of elderly.

AGING AND QUALITY OF LIFE

Aging is a natural process of life that includes gradual changes in metabolic activity of organs and disability in regeneration capacity of cells (Massar & Khadi, 2016). Aging is commonly understood as the process of maturing or becoming older and includes numerous processes such as changes happening throughout the life, individual differences attributed to age and, the group of aged or older people (in comparison among those younger) (Birren, 1996). Across one's life there is an incessant balance among stability, gains, and declines especially when individual reaches to the third stage of life (Baltes, 1978). Balance includes bio-physical and psychological changes across life span. Bio-physical system includes lose efficiency, psychological characteristics maintain stability, show gains and declines depending not only on the biological organism but also on the socio-cultural context, and on the control individual exert through his/her behaviours (Bandura, 1978; 1997). Various factors such as heredity, life style, unhealthy diet, smoking and physical activity can effect the longevity of life. Not only these factors but there are several other factors or indicators of quality of life that also affect elderly. Quality of life (QOL) is a broad, dynamic, generic, and multidimensional parameter concept (see for a discussion of the construct "quality of life" Diener, 2005; The WHOQOL Group, 1998; Veenhoven, 2005). World health organization (WHO) defined it in terms of subjective perception of the individual's position in life, expectations, standards and concerns, of his/her physical and psychological health, as well as his/her social functioning and environmental and general life status (Malek et al., 2010; Farzian, Hosseini, Pirozi, & Shadi, 2012; Datta, Gangopadhyay, & Sengupta, 2013). Two different approaches have been emerged that defines objective and subjective evaluation of quality of life (Noll, 2000; 2010; Veenhoven, 2000). Objective quality of life is assessed by external observers by the extent to which a person has access to and command over relevant resources such as income, health, social networks, and competencies serve individuals to pursue their goals and direct their living conditions (Erikson, 1974). Therefore, it is a condition where person is having high income, good health, large and reliable social networks, and competencies as accomplished by high educational status. While, subjective quality of life is measured in terms of individual's perceptions and evaluations. It depends on the individual person and lies in the "eye of the beholder" (Campbell, Converse, & Rodgers, 1976). Broadly, Quality of life is defined by personal feelings, details, outlook, and day-to-day experiences how happy and positive one feels, how comfortable and secure, how productive and desired, how healthy and free an individual considers themselves, etc. Hereafter, subjective well-being means high life satisfaction on, strong positive emotions like happiness, and low negative emotions like sadness. Emotional maturity includes quality of life that favour social relationships, beyond the mere satisfaction of warmth, encouraging volunteer actions and demonstrating that besides serving one's own well-being, one must serve the community as well. In a survey on quality of life, elderly appraised their quality of life positively on the basis of comparison with others, social contacts especially with family and children, health, material circumstances and activities. While in making negative evaluations, they emphasised on dependency and functional limitations, unhappiness and reduced social contacts (death of friends and family members). On one hand, family, activities, and social contacts were found important factor for QOL while on other hand, various types of losses such as ill health and functional limitations were found making quality of life worse.

Similar to the above findings, Bowling and colleagues (2003) attempted to find out the concept of quality of life in a national survey of 999 individuals aged 65 years or more, living in England and Scotland. They used content analytical approach to responses to open-ended questions and identified constituent factors of quality of life as social relationships, social roles and activities, solo activities, health, psychological, home, and neighbourhood, financial circumstances, independence, miscellaneous and society/politics in the order frequency of mentioning. Moreover, health, home and neighbourhood emerged on the top as factors that can take away quality of life. In another study, Gabriel and Bowling (2004) reported that factors enhancing the quality of life were having good social relationships with children, family, friends and neighbours; neighbourhood social capital represented by good relationships with neighbours, nice and enjoyable neighbourhood, comfortable houses and good public services such as free transport facilities; psychological factors such as optimism and positive attitude, contentment, looking forward to things, acceptance and other coping strategies; being actively engaged in social activities for example, attending educational classes and volunteering, good health, financial security which brought enjoyment as well as empowerment and having not depend on others. In a recent study from Sweden, men and women aged more than 67 years were asked what quality of life was for them and findings revealed that for elderly living in own home and, in the context of severe illness, social relations were important for quality of life (Wilhemson, Andersson, Waern, & Allebeck, 2006).

Numerous factors are reported in researches that dramatically decrease quality of life such as abundance of hope, love, loneliness, lack of desire, negative reflection upon life, pessimistic approach to life, lack of satisfaction and control, chronic mental and physical diseases, physical, mental or spiritual deterioration, emotional and physical setbacks, inability, loss, negative affectivity, absence of successful intervention, fatigue, pain, fear, depression, absence of attention, feeling unwanted, inadequate, and unsuccessful, general insecurity, poor self-esteem, obesity, weight loss, etc. Further, minute details can cause major differences in one's quality of life and comfort level for example, food selections to meet personal preference and to encourage comfort and well-being, décor to meet personal preference and to encourage happiness and relaxation, spa accessibility (such as hair, skin, nails, and massage) to improve outward appearance, sense of well-being, and happiness, and improvements to overall living environment to promote comfort, healing, and well-being. These findings clearly reflect as quality of life is more than having good social relations, being active and able to participate in socially and personally meaningful activities and having no functional limitations are sometimes more important for older people (Fleck, Chachamovisch, & Trentini, 2003). Moreover, this understanding of quality of life crosses cultural boundaries. It is logical to wonder whether these perceptions are a result of older people living now having less health problems.

AGING AND SOCIAL SUPPORT

Aging takes place within a social context. At each phase of human cycle, the individual belongs to a variety of kinship and social groups. The extent to which an older person is enmeshed within a social network of kin, friends, and neighbours will greatly affect their experience of aging. Social support from various sources but especially from family has emerged as one of the strongest predictor of mental health and psychological well-being in studies on younger individuals but possibly its importance is manifold for the older people. However, in the current wave of social change, both family structure and family functions are under dramatic transformations. Social support is the physical and emotional comfort given by family, friends, co-workers and other and in general it has positive consequences for well-being. Social support is a mutual process. In the network of elderly, if they receive support from others, they feel needed and if they are able to provide support to others in reciprocation then they feel worthy because they can help others which in turn increases their self-confidence and self-esteem and contributes to positive mental health.

Social support is a concept that is generally understood in an intuitive sense help from other people in a difficult life situation. One of first definitions of social support was forward by Cobb (1976) according to whom it is the "individual belief that one is cared for and loved, esteemed and valued and belongs to network of communication and mutual obligations". He suggested four of the most frequently used defining attributes of social support, emotional, instrumental, informational and appraisal. Social network, social embeddedness, and social climate were identified as antecedent of social support. Social support consequences were subsumed under the general rubric of positive health states; the examples of which were personal competence, health maintenance behaviours, perceived control, sense of stability, recognition of self-worth, positive effect, psychological well-being, and decreased anxiety and depression. More recently, social support has been defined as 'the perceived availability of people whom the individual trust and who make one cared for and valued as a person' (Mindful, 2008).

STRUCTURE AND FUNCTIONAL SOCIAL SUPPORT

Cohen and his colleagues (Cohen & Syne, 1985; Cohen & Wills, 1985) proposed a distinction between structural and functional support measures. Structural support refers to measures describing the existence of and interconnections between social ties (e.g., marital status, number of relationships, or number of relations who know one another). Structural social support is related with the availability of prominent others (e.g., spouses, family members, friends, co-workers, social, and religious groups) irrespective of actual exchange of support. Structural support is also referred to as social integration (Cohen et al., 2000). One way of assessing social support has been to explore the social network of an individual without focusing on the nature of the support or its perception by the recipient. In structural terms, social support is the frequency with which individuals interact with members of their social networks. The number of interacting social contacts, or persons, that an individual can count upon or approach in times of need, constitutes his social support networks. When we think social support network structure, the term is considered as web of relationships that can be described along such dimensions as frequency of interaction among its members, its density and extensiveness, the reciprocity, disability and intensity of its interpersonal relationship (House & Kahn, 1985).

Birditt, Antonucci, and Tighe (2012) were studied how social ties support especially enacted social support (i.e., support actually provided during stressful events) in stressful life events in 152 adults (principal respondents; aged 50 to 69 years, 63% women) who had experienced three or more stressful life events in the last year and 180 of their identified supportive ties (core network members). Findings revealed that irrespective of high or low stress evaluation, higher quality relationships enact high levels of support while lower quality relationships enact greater support under higher stressful conditions. Similarly, Merz and Huxhold (2010) explored the relationship between different forms of support, support providers, and the well-being of the 1,146 elderly in Germany in an Ageing Survey conducted in 2002. The results demonstrated both emotional support from families and instrumental support from non-kin were associated positively with well-being. Instrumental support received from the families correlated negatively with well-being.

Further, progress is also being made in understanding the behavioural and biological correlates of positive psychological well-being in older adults. Physical activity is probably the most important link between psychological well-being and health. Regular physical activity at older ages is already recommended for the maintenance of cardiovascular health, muscle strength and flexibility, glucose metabolism, and healthy body weight, and is also consistently correlated with well-being (Windle, Hughes, Linck, Russell, & Woods, 2010). Positive well-being is found to be linked with lower cortisol output (Steptoe, Wardle, Marmot, 2005; Steptoe, O'Donnell, Badrick, Kumari, & Marmot, 2008). Not only positive affect is found to be related with reduced inflammatory and cardiovascular in stress but also with lower level of inflammatory markers such as C-reactive protein and interleukin 6 in older women, and huge amount of steroid hormone dehydroepiandosteronesulfat (Steptoe, Demakakos, De Oliveira, & Wardle, 2012). Not only India but the whole world is on the threshold of demographic transition with resulting massive changes in the age structure. Aging is a multidimensional change in physical, psychological as well social aspects of an individual. It can be describing as a progressive deterioration of the physical and mental functions resulting in a simultaneous decline in both the capacity of the body to maintain homeostasis balance as well as adaptability of the individual to various stressors consequently increasing the chances of illness and mortality.

Social support is the essential concept in gerontology. Empirical evidences based on relationship between, health, well-being, and quality of life in old age suggest that the amount and quality of individual's social relationships, and their interactions may affect their emotional as well as instrumental support that are associated with health, subjective well-being, and quality of life. Overall, it can be suggested that perceived social support can reduce loneliness amongst older people. Hence, it is essential to develop recreation programs that easily available to them, where they can have opportunity to get interact with other people. Facilitating meaningful connections among older can be an effective medium. As suggested by Forbes (1996) various activities such as adult education classes, involvement in community action schemes, and locally organized outings can be a potential way to alleviate loneliness amongst older people. Several prevention and intervention programs should be developed to alleviate loneliness which can be very effective in enhancing Quality of life among older adults. As reported by Kwag et al. (2011) who found that perceived social support had a negative influence on loneliness among older adults in Koreans. The older adults should also me made financially strong as being unsound from financial resources may prohibit older adults from participating in social activities (Cohen-Mansfield & Parpura-Gill, 2007).

CONCLUSION

In general, it was reported in literature that aging has found to have negative impact on the quality of life. Elderly people are not much satisfied with their life therefore they blame to their age which seems a big issue and number of elderly people are unsatisfied with their life. This can be reduced by providing them adequate social support. Elderly people seek time, attention, care, and support. They want someone to talk and to share their feelings. Therefore, in light of the aforesaid studies, social support is essential for enhancing the wellbeing and quality of life of elderly people. The thickness of an individual's social relationships, the degree to which he/she interacts with others and amount of affect one receives and gives, instrumental support, and/or services are all linked with health indicators, subjective well–being, and quality of life measures in elderly. Physical and mental impairments have been known to significantly decrease quality of life in older adults, as many lose hope, become isolated or depressed, lose faith, and struggle to feel joy in everyday life. When care professionals identify factors such as depression, social isolation, or chronic medical illness in a client, immediate measures should be taken to address what can be done to improve quality of life; interventions to improve comfort level, happiness, social immersion, access to care, resources, support systems, etc., need to be explored. It is essential to identify and target the problem areas that may hamper the quality of life of elderly, and emphasis should be on creating and inventing positive interventions. People should try to sustain and encourage positive contributing factors to quality of life. Moreover, individual sense of purpose, environment for learning, self-expression, and promoting dignity and building connection with others should be encouraged. Further, elderly should be equipped with various stress management tactics and guided techniques to alter various conditions (mentally, emotionally, and physically). Individual quality of life of elderly could be meaningfully improved when they are cared effectively for unspoken, unaddressed areas of need. More research should be encouraged, how aging can help older people to identify what is possible and how purpose, meaning, dignity, and fulfilment can be found.

REFERENCES

Baltes, P. B. (1987). Theoretical propositions of life-span developmental psychology: On the dynamic between growth and decline. *Developmental Psychology*, *23*(5), 611–626. doi:10.1037/0012-1649.23.5.611

Bandura, A. (1986). *Social foundation of thoughts and actions*. Englewood Cliffs, CA: Prentice Hall.

Bandura, A. (1997). *Self-efficacy: The exercise of control*. New York: Freeman and Co.

Bhatia, H. S. (1983). *Aging and society: A society: A sociological study of retired public servant*. Udaipur: Arya's Book Centre Publication.

Birditt, K. S., Antonucci, T. C., & Tighe, L. (2012). Enacted support during stressful life events in middle and older adulthood: An examination of the interpersonal context. *Psychology and Aging*, *27*(3), 728–741. doi:10.1037/a0026967 PMID:22308999

Bowling, A., Gabriel, Z., Dykes, J., Dowding, L. M., Evans, O., Fleissig, A., ... Sutton, S. (2003). Let's ask them: Definitions of quality of life and its enhancement among people aged 65 and over. *International Journal of Aging & Human Development*, *56*(4), 269–306. doi:10.2190/BF8G-5J8L-YTRF-6404 PMID:14738211

Campbell, A., Converse, P. E., & Rodgers, W. L. (1976). *The quality of American Life: Perceptions, evaluations and satisfactions*. New York: Russell Sage Foundation.

Carey, J. R. (2003). Life span: A conceptual overview. In J. R. Carey & S. Tuljapurkar (Eds.), *Life span evolutionary: Ecological and demographical perspectives, supplement to population and development review* (Vol. 29). New York: Population Council.

Chou, K. L., & Chi, I. (2001). Stressful life events and depressive symptoms: Social support and sense as mediator or moderators. *International Journal of Aging & Human Development*, *52*(2), 155–171. doi:10.2190/9C97-LCA5-EWB7-XK2W PMID:11352200

Cobb, S. (1976). Social support as moderator in life stress. *Journal of Psychosomatic Medicine*, *38*(5), 300–314. doi:10.1097/00006842-197609000-00003 PMID:981490

Cohen, S., Gottlieb, B. H., & Underwood, L. G. (2000). Social relationships and health. In S. Cohen, L. G. Underwood, & B. H. Gottlieb (Eds.), *Social Support measurement and intervention: A guide for health and social scientists* (pp. 3–25). Oxford: Oxford University Press. doi:10.1093/med:psych/9780195126709.003.0001

Cohen, S., & Syne, S. L. (1985). Issues in the study and application of social support. In S. Cohen & S. L. Syne (Eds.), *Social support and health* (pp. 3–22). New York: Academic Press.

Cohen, S., & Wills, T. A. (1985). Stress social support and buffering hypothesis. *Psychological Bulletin, 98*(2), 310–357. doi:10.1037/0033-2909.98.2.310 PMID:3901065

Corman, J.C., Lynch, S. M., Goldman, N., Weinstein, M., & Lin, H. (2004). Stability and change in perceived social support of older Taiwanese adults. *Journal of Gerontology: Series B: Psychological sciences and social sciences, 59*(6), 350-3357.

Cottrell, L. (1942). The adjustment of an individual to his age and roles. *American Sociological Review, 7*(5), 617–620. doi:10.2307/2085687

Cumming, E., & Henry, W. E. (1961). *Growing old: The process of Disengagement*. New York: Basic Book.

Cumming, E., Newell, D. S., & McCaffery, I. (1960). Disengagement: A tentative theory of aging. *Sociometry, 23*(1), 23–35. doi:10.2307/2786135

Datta, P. P., Gangopadhyay, N., & Sengupta, B. (2013). Association of psychological morbidity with socio-demographic characteristics among elderly: A cross-sectional study from Eastern Indian. *International Journal of Medicine and Public Health, 3*(2), 94–99. doi:10.4103/2230-8598.115172

Dey, A. B. (2003). *Aging in India: Situational analysis and planning for the future. Ministry of health and family welfare*. New Delhi: Ramko Press.

Donmez, L., Gokkoca, Z., & Dedeoglu, N. (2005). Disability and its effects on quality of life among older people living in Antalya city centre. *Turkey Archives of Gerontology and Geriatrics, 40*(2), 213–223. doi:10.1016/j.archger.2004.08.006 PMID:15680503

Erickson's, S. H. (1963). Childhood and society (2nd ed.). New York: W.W. Norton.

Erickson's, S. H. (1968). *Identity: Youth and crisis*. New York: W.W. Norton.

Farzian, P. F., Arab, M., Hosseini, S. M., Pirozi, B., & Shadi, H. (2012). Quality of life of the elderly residents in Marivan Evaluation of quality of life of the elderly population covered by healthcare centers of Marivan and the influencing demographic and background factors in 2010. *Iranian Red Crescent Medical Journal, 14*(11), 695–696. PMID:23397047

Figueira, H., Figueira, J., Mello, D., & Dantas, E. (2008). Quality of life throughout aging. *ActaMedicaLituanica, 15*, 169–172.

Figueira, H. A., Figueira, O. A., & Figueira, A. A. (2010). Elderly quality of life impacted by traditional Chinese medicine techniques. *Clinical Interventions in Aging, 5*, 301–305. doi:10.2147/CIA.S10615 PMID:21103400

Fleck, M. P. A., Chachamovisch, E., & Trentini, C. M. (2003). Projeto WHOQOL-OLD: Método e resultados de gruposfocais no Brasil. *Revista de Saude Publica*, *37*(6), 793–799. doi:10.1590/S0034-89102003000600016 PMID:14666311

Forbes, A. (1996). Education and debate, caring for older people: Loneliness. *BMJ (Clinical Research Ed.)*, *313*(7053), 352–354. doi:10.1136/bmj.313.7053.352 PMID:8760749

Gabriel, Z., & Bowling, A. (2004). Quality of life from the perspectives of older people. *Ageing and Society*, *24*(05), 675–691. doi:10.1017/S0144686X03001582

George, L. (1989). Stress, social support and depression over the life course.IN K. Markides & C. Cooper (Eds.), Aging, stress, social support and health (pp. 241-267). New York: John Wiley & Sons.

Graney, M. (1975). Happiness and social participation in aging. *Journal of Gerontology*, *30*(6), 701–706. doi:10.1093/geronj/30.6.701 PMID:1184930

Gureje, O., Ogunniyi, A., Kola, L., & Afolabi, E. (2006). Functional disability in elderly Nigerians: Results from the Ibadan study of aging. *Journal of the American Geriatrics Society*, *54*(11), 1784–1789. doi:10.1111/j.1532-5415.2006.00944.x PMID:17087709

Hawley, P. J., & Klaukev, M. R. (1988). Health practices and perception of social support in person over 60. *Journal of Gerontology*, *36*(1), 112–121.

House, J. S., & Kahn, R. L. (1985). Measures and concepts of social support. *See Cohen & Syme*, *1985*, 83–108.

Irudaya Rajan, S., Mishra, U. S., & Sarma, P. S. (1999). Review: India's Elderly: Burden or Challenge? *The Journal of Asian Studies*, *60*(2).

Lutz, W., Sanderson, W., & Scherbov, S. (2008). The coming acceleration of global population ageing. *Nature*, *451*(7179), 716–719. doi:10.1038/nature06516 PMID:18204438

Malek, A. H., Baradaran, E. M., Hejazi, F., Khojasteh, T., Noot, R. H., & Falahat, K. (2010). The effectiveness of educational intervention in the health promotion in elderly people. *Iranian Journal of Public Health*, *39*(2), 18–23. PMID:23113002

Massar, D., & Khadi, P. B. (2016). Quality of life of elderly of Northern Karnataka and Jaintia hills region. *Journal of Pharmaceutical Sciences*, *29*(4), 533–535.

Mellor, D., Russo, S., McCabe, M. P., Davison, T. E., & George, K. (2008). Depression training program for caregivers of elderly care recipients: Implementation and qualitative evaluation. *Journal of Gerontological Nursing*, *34*(9), 8–17. doi:10.3928/00989134-20080901-09 PMID:18795560

Merz, E. M., & Huxhold, O. (2010). Wellbeing depends on social relationship characteristics: Comparing different types and providers of support to older adults. *Ageing and Society*, *30*(05), 843–857. doi:10.1017/S0144686X10000061

Mindful. (2008). Indicators- Determinants of health-social and cultural environment-16, Social support-Metadata, Retrieved March, 16, 2009 from http://lib.stakes.fi/mindful/metadata150.htm

Noll, D. R., Degenhardt, B. F., Morley, T. F., Blais, F. X., Hortos, K. A., Hensel, K., ... Stoll, S. T. (2010). Efficacy of osteopathic manipulation as an adjunctive treatment for hospitalized patients with pneumonia: A randomized controlled trial. *Osteopathic Medicine and Primary Care, 4*(2).

Noll, D. R., Shores, J. H., Russell, G. G., Herron, K. M., & Swift, J. (2000). Benefits of osteopathic manipulative treatment for hospitalized elderly patients with pneumonia. *JAOA*, *100*(12), 776–782. PMID:11213665

Oberoi, K., & Dey, S. (1991). Satisfaction level of rural and urban aged persons for various need in Samastipur district (Bihar). *Indian Psychological Review*, *37*(7&8), 6–10.

Ontario Human Rights Commission [OHRC]. (2017). Specific issues facing older persons. Retrieved May 19, 2017 from http://www.ohrc.on.ca/en/consultation-paper-changing-face-ontario-discrimination-and-our-aging-population/specific-issues-facing-older-persons

Ramamurthi, P. V. (1970). Life Satisfaction in the older Years. *Indian Journal of Gerontology*, *2*, 68–70.

Ramamurthi, P. V. (1978). *The sixth decade and after. Tirupati.* S.V. University.

Ramamurti, P. V. (2008). Perspectives of Research on Aging in India. *Journal of Aging & Social Policy*, *15*(2-3). PMID:14696688

Shettar, S. C. (2013). Problems of Aged in Changing Indian Scenario. Retrieved May 21, 2017 from http://yojana.gov.in/problems-of-aged.asp

Singh, J. G., Singh, S., & Dawara, V. (1983). Adjustment problem of old people. *Indian Journal of Clinical Psychology*, *10*, 127–131.

Steptoe, A., Demakakos, P., De Oliveira, C., & Wardle, J. (2012). Distinctive biological correlates of positive psychological well-being in older men and women. *Psychosomatic Medicine*, *74*(5), 501–508. doi:10.1097/PSY.0b013e31824f82c8 PMID:22511728

Steptoe, A., O'Donnell, K., Badrick, E., Kumari, M., & Marmot, M. G. (2008). Neuroendocrine and inflammatory factors associated with positive affect in healthy men and women: Whitehall II study. *American Journal of Epidemiology*, *167*(1), 96–102. doi:10.1093/aje/kwm252 PMID:17916595

Steptoe, A., Wardle, J., & Marmot, M. (2005). Positive affect and health-related neuroendocrine, cardiovascular, and inflammatory processes. *Proceeding of the National Academy of Science United States of America*, *102*, 6508–6512. doi:10.1073/pnas.0409174102

Veenhoven, R. (2000). Wellbeing in the welfare state, level not higher, distribution not more equitable. *Journal of Comparative Policy Analysis*, *2*(1), 91–125. doi:10.1080/13876980008412637

Veenhoven, R. (2005). Average happiness in 90 nations in the early 2000s.World Database of Happiness, Distributional Findings in Nations (Rank report 2005/1). Retrieved from http://worlddatabaseofhappiness.eur.nl/hap_nat/findingreports/

WHOQOL Group. (1998). The World Health Organization Quality of Life Assessment (WHOQOL): Development and general psychometric properties. *Social Science & Medicine*, *46*(12), 1569–1585. doi:10.1016/S0277-9536(98)00009-4 PMID:9672396

Wilhemson, K., Andersson, C., Waern, M., & Allebeck, P. (2005). Elderly people's perspectives on quality of life. *Ageing and Society*, *25*(04), 585–600. doi:10.1017/S0144686X05003454

Windle, G., Hughes, D., Linck, P., Russell, I., & Woods, B. (2010). Is exercise effective in promoting mental well-being in older age? A systematic review. *Aging & Mental Health*, *14*(6), 652–669. doi:10.1080/13607861003713232 PMID:20686977

Zhang, Z., & Hayward, M. (2001). Childlessness and the psychological well-being of older persons. *The Journals of Gerontology. Series B, Psychological Sciences and Social Sciences*, *56B*(5), S311–S320. doi:10.1093/geronb/56.5.S311 PMID:11522813

KEY TERMS AND DEFINITIONS

Aging-Aging: Is defined as a biological process where gradual deterioration of physiological function with age took place. It is a progressive process of becoming older which is genetically determined and environmentally modulated.

Quality of Life: Quality of life (QOL) is the general well-being of individuals that includes negative and positive features of life. It is measured in terms of life satisfaction in various domains such as physical health, family, education, employment, wealth, religious beliefs, finance and the environment.

Social Support: Social support can be defined in terms of assistance available to the individual from other people or extent to which a person is nested in a social network. This support can be tangible, intangible, emotional, and informational etc.

Chapter 5
Management of Elder Abuse Through Social Support

Akbar Husain
Aligarh Muslim University, India

Nongzaimayum Tawfeeq Alee
Aligarh Muslim University, India

ABSTRACT

This chapter is an attempt to highlight the numerous ways in which elders are abused in our society and the ways to support them. A concise account in ways elders are vulnerable and how they are exploited are discussed in the chapter as well as remedies to these problems. The chapter includes types of abuse faced by elders and the consequences they face due to it. It also discusses Social Support as the main remedy, social support as an acronym of 13 types of social support. The chapter concludes by recommendation of how elder abuse can be stopped or at least controlled.

INTRODUCTION

The problem of elder abuse has driven through the world. Millions of older people were impacted by the elder abuse. In India elder abuse has caused suffering to many. The impact of elder abuse on older people is shocking. This disorder shakes up our faith on younger generation, family, and society. We wonder about the existence of God or another higher force and its justice why would it want millions of older people to suffer from this social disorder? Here is an attempt to manage the problem of elder abuse. Further, it is important to recognise what happens to the people of elder abuse at the physical and mental level, and how they respond to it. Elder abuse has a deep impact on the inner as well as outer state of older people. Elder abuse people can connect with their inner source of strength and wisdom to make life more meaningful.

DOI: 10.4018/978-1-5225-3480-8.ch005

ELDER ABUSE

Elder abuse (also called "elder mistreatment," "senior abuse," "abuse in later life," "abuse of older adults," "abuse of older women," and "abuse of older men") is "a single, or repeated act, or lack of appropriate action, occurring within any relationship where there is an expectation of trust, which causes harm or distress to an older person." (Action on Elder Abuse, n.d.). This definition has been adopted by the World Health Organization from a definition put forward by Action on Elder Abuse in the UK. The UK's Action on Elder Abuse, a voluntary organization, developed a definition, following consultation with its membership, which the International Network for the Prevention of Elder Abuse (INPEA) has subsequently adapted. The agreed version is 'Elder abuse is a single or repeated act or lack of appropriate action occurring within any relationship where there is an expectation of trust, which causes harm or distress to an older person' (Action on Elder Abuse, 1995; INPEA, 1997). The above definition explains the frequency of abuse (single or repeated act); that abuse (or neglect) might consist of a lack of necessary action (omission as well as commission); that there is some relationship between the parties consisting of at least an expectation of trust; and that the action causes some harm or distress to the elder.

The abuse of elders by caregivers is a worldwide issue. In 2002, the work of the World Health Organization brought international attention to the issue of elder abuse (Cook-Daniels, 2003b).In 2006 the International Network for Prevention of Elder Abuse (INPEA) designated June 15 as World Elder Abuse Awareness Day (WEAAD) and an increasing number of events are held across the globe on this day to raise awareness of elder abuse, and highlight ways to challenge such abuse (International Network for the Prevention of Elder Abuse, accessed June 26, 2007). Elder abuse is a violation of Human Rights and a significant cause of injury, illness, loss of productivity, isolation and despair. (WHO/INPEA, 2002a). In the *Encyclopedia of Positive Psychology*, Gottlieb (2009) defines social support as the social-psychological and interpersonal processes that maintain and promote health and well-being.

The purpose of this chapter is to describe what is elder abuse; types of abuse; health consequences and risk factors associated with elder abuse; and the role of social support in the management of elder abuse.

TYPES OF ABUSE

There are several types of abuse of older people that are generally recognized as being elder abuse, including: (Robinson, 2012; what is Elder Abuse, 2012).

- **Physical:** e.g. hitting, punching, slapping, burning, pushing, kicking, restraining, false imprisonment / confinement, or giving excessive or improper medication as well as withholding treatment and medication.
- **Psychological/Emotional:** e.g. humiliating a person. A common theme is a perpetrator who identifies something that matters to an older person and then uses it to coerce an older person into a particular action. It may take verbal forms such as yelling, name-calling, ridiculing, constantly criticizing, accusations, blaming, or non-verbal forms such as ignoring, silence, shunning or withdrawing affection.
- **Financial Abuse:** Also known as financial exploitation. e.g. illegal or unauthorized use of a person's property, money, pension book or other valuables (including changing the person's will to name the abuser as heir). It may be obtained by deception, coercion, misrepresentation, undue in-

fluence, or theft. This includes fraudulently obtaining guardianship or use of a power of attorney. Other forms include deprivation of money or other property, or by eviction / removal from their own home.

- **Scam by Strangers:** e.g. worthless "sweepstakes" that elderly persons must pay in order to collect winnings, fraudulent investment schemes, predatory lending, and lottery scams (Shilling, 2008).
- **Sexual:** e.g. forcing a person to take part in any sexual activity without his or her consent, including forcing them to participate in conversations of a sexual nature against their will; may also include situations where person is no longer able to give consent (dementia).
- **Neglect:** e.g. depriving a person of proper medical treatment, food, heat, clothing or comfort or essential medication and depriving a person of needed services to force certain kinds of actions, financial and otherwise. Neglect can include leaving an at-risk (i.e. fall risk) elder person unattended. The deprivation may be intentional (active neglect) or happen out of lack of knowledge or resources (passive neglect).
- **Hybrid Financial Exploitation (HFE):** e.g. financial exploitation that co-occurs with physical abuse and/or neglect. HFE victims are more likely to be co-habiting with abusive individual, to have fair/poor health, to fear the abusive individual, to perceive abusive individual as caretaker, and to have a longer duration of abuse (Jackson & Hafemeister, 2012).
- **Institutional Abuse:** Refers to physical or psychological harms, as well as rights violations in settings where care and assistance is provided to dependant older adults or others. More commonly, institutional abuses or neglect may reflect lack of knowledge, lack of training, lack of support, or insufficient resourcing. Institutional abuse may be the consequence of common practices or processes that are part of the running of a care institution or service. Sometimes this type of abuse is referred to as "poor practice," although this term reflects the motive of the perpetrator (the causation) rather than the impact upon the older person.

In addition, some U.S. state laws (Nursing Home Abuse Laws, 2017) also recognizes the abandonment, right abuse and self-neglect as elder abuse:

IDENTIFY AND PREVENTING ELDER ABUSE

The key to prevention of elder abuse is the ability to recognize the warning signs of its occurrence. Signs of elder abuse differ dependent on the type of abuse the victim is suffering. Each type of abuse has different signs associated with it (Signs and symptoms of elder abuse and neglect in care, 2012).

- **Physical Abuse:** Can be detected by visible signs on the body, including bruises, scars, sprains, or broken bones. More subtle indications of physical abuse include signs of restraint, such as rope marks on the wrist, or broken eyeglasses. Physical elder abuse is also in the form of inflicting physical pain, injury, or impairment. Such abuse includes not only physical assaults such as hitting or shoving but the inappropriate use of drugs, restraints, or confinement.
- **Emotional Abuse:** Often accompanies the other types of abuse and can usually be detected by changes in the personality or behavior. The elder may also exhibit behavior mimicking dementia, such as rocking or mumbling. Verbal forms of emotional elder abuse include intimidation through yelling or threats, humiliation and ridicule, and habitual blaming or scapegoating. Nonverbal psy-

chological elder abuse can take the form of ignoring the elderly person, isolating an elder from friends or activities, and terrorizing or menacing the elderly person (Bhatia, Srivastava, & Bansal, 2008).

- **Financial Exploitation:** Is a more subtle form of abuse, in comparison to other types, and may be more challenging to notice. Signs of financial exploitation include significant withdrawals from accounts, belongings or money missing from the home, unpaid bills, and unnecessary goods or services.
- **Sexual Abuse:** Like physical abuse, can be detected by visible signs on the body, especially around the breasts or genital area. Other signs include inexplicable infections, bleeding, and torn underclothing. Sexual elder abuse is contact with an elderly person without the elder's consent. Such contact can involve physical sex acts, but activities such as showing an elderly person pornographic material, forcing the person to watch sex acts, or forcing the elder to undress are also considered sexual elder abuse (Bhatia, Srivastava, & Bansal, 2008).
- **Neglect:** Is a type of abuse in that it can be inflicted either by the caregiver or oneself. Signs of neglect include malnutrition and dehydration, poor hygiene, non-compliance with a prescription medication, and unsafe living conditions. In addition to observing signs in the elderly individual, abuse can also be detected by monitoring changes in the caregiver's behavior. For example, the caregiver may not allow them to speak to or receive visitors, exhibit indifference or a lack of affection towards the elder, or refer to the elder as "a burden." Caregivers who have a history of substance abuse or mental illness are more likely to commit elder abuse than other individuals (Dong, 2005).
- **Healthcare Fraud and Abuse:** This type of elder abuse is carried out by unethical doctors, nurses, hospital personnel, and other professional care providers. Bhatia, Srivastava, and Bansal (2008, p. 151) listed a number of healthcare fraud and abuse regarding elders which include the following:
    - Not providing healthcare, but charging for it.
    - Overcharging or double-billing for medical care or services.
    - Getting kickbacks for referrals to other providers or for prescribing certain drugs.
    - Overmedicating or under medicating.
    - Recommending fraudulent remedies for illnesses or other medical conditions.
    - Medicaid fraud.

HEALTH CONSEQUENCES

The health consequences of elder abuse are very serious. Elder abuse can destroy an elderly person's quality of life. American Medical Association White Paper on Elderly Health (1990) listed the following health consequences associated with elder abuse.

- Declining functional abilities
- Increased dependency
- Increased sense of helplessness
- Increased stress
- Worsening psychological decline

- Premature mortality and morbidity
- Depression and dementia
- Malnutrition
- Bed sores
- Death

The risks of death for elder abuse victims are three times higher than for non-victims (Hildreth, 2011).

RISK FACTORS

An exploratory attempt was made to examine a sample population of six elders' focus groups and two focus groups of health professionals working with the elderly, and their perception of elder abuse, during the year 2001 in five developing countries (Argentina, Brazil, Kenya, Lebanon and India) as well as in Sweden, Canada and Austria. The majority of elderly people that had been interviewed affirm that societal or as we also define it structural abuse' is the most frequent type of abuse, at least in most Latin American countries (WHO/INPEA, 2001a, 2001b).

The elders' focus groups which were part of the research identified other risk factors as:

- Being old
- Being ill
- Living alone
- Isolation
- Family history of mistreatment
- Lack of social network
- Lack of information about available resources
- Poor contact with peers
- Intergenerational Conflict (WHO/INPEA, 2002b)

The final analysis of the major themes which arose in the different countries revealed remarkable similarities and indeed was virtually universal across the participating nations, with older people perceiving abuse under three broad headings:

- **Neglect:** Isolation, abandonment and social exclusion
- **Violation:** Of human, legal and medical rights
- **Deprivation:** Of choices, decisions, status, finances and respect (WHO/INPEA, 2002b)

There are several risk factors, which increase the likelihood that an elderly person will become a victim of elder abuse (Cooper, Selwood, & Livingston, 2008). Such risk factors for elder abuse include an elderly person who:

- Has memory problems (such as dementia).
- Has physical disabilities.
- Has depression, loneliness, or lack of social support.

- Abuses alcohol or other substances.
- Is verbally or physically combative with the caregiver.
- Has a shared living situation.

There are also several risk factors, which increase the likelihood that a caregiver will participate in elder abuse (Cooper, Selwood., & Livingston, 2008). Such risk factors for elder abuse include a caregiver who:

- Feels overwhelmed or resentful.
- Has a history of substance abuse or a history of abusing others.
- Is dependent on the older person for housing, finances, or other needs.
- Has mental health problems.
- Is unemployed.
- Has a criminal history.
- Has a shared living situation.

Social Support

Social support refers to the physical and psychological comfort provided by other people (Sarason, Sarason, & Pierce, 1994). Social support consists of the tangible and intangible rewards and assistance provided by significant others. Social support is multidimensional. Social support can be viewed as a component of coping. It is effective regardless of the kind of coping strategies that are used (Frazier, Tix, Klein, &Arikian, 2000). It can also be beneficial in case of management of elder abuse. An elderly person facing abuse may need support. Social support can provide them comfort and minimize their problems. Social support is relevant to health in the case of elder abuse. Perceptions of the availability and quality of social support differ from the so called normal older people and elder abuse. Thirteen types of social support are considered here which are based on the acronym SOCIAL SUPPORT.

The spousal support is very much needed to eradicate the abuse of older women. It is often noticed the long-term spousal abuse against women. In some situations, the abuse is "domestic violence grown old," a situation in which the abusive behaviour of a spouse or partner continues into old age. This is an important type of support because the domestic violence of older people is often not reported and consequently strategies, which have proved effective within the domestic violence arena, have not been effectively utilized into circumstances involving the abuse of older people by the family members. In some situations, an older couple may be attempting to care and support each other and failing, in the absence of external support. Support your loved ones as much as you can in everything they do, no matter what their choices are.

Others Support

An abuser can be a partner, relative, a friend or neighbor, a volunteer worker, a maid servant, practitioner, solicitor, or any other individual with the intent to deprive a vulnerable person of their resources. Others support can prevent the elder abuse. Friends and family support may help in solving problems. If the elder abuse people want to receive support from significant others, then give them support in your relationships.

Community Support

Traditional forms of family and community support are being weakened as a consequence of the global modernization process. As a result, older people become at risk. Community support in responding to elder abuse can contribute to elderly persons' safety. Communities can develop programs that are structured around meeting the needs of elderly persons.

Institutional Support

Institutional support is very much needed in the caring process of the elderly. Providing services to the elderly reflects the motive of the institution rather than the impact upon the older persons. With the aging of today's population, there is the potential that elder abuse will increase unless it is more comprehensively supported by institutions.

Affective Support

Elderly people who received affective social support from significant others may benefit more in managing elder abuse. Affective support is most appropriate when the elderly people suffer from chronic illnesses. This type of support is beneficial to emotional and mental health.

Legal Support

The National Policy on Older Persons 1999, as a logical sequence to the constitutional directive, under the chapter on "Directive Principles of State Policy". A National Council for Older Persons (NCOP) was constituted by the Ministry of Social Justice and Empowerment to operationalize the National Policy on Older Persons. The legal support to protect elders will also help to minimize elder abuse and will provide improved assistance to victims of elder abuse. The Maintenance and Welfare of Parents and Senior Citizens Bill, 2007 seeks to make it a legal obligation for children and heirs to provide maintenance to senior citizens (Parker, 2007).

State Government Support

In India the state government establishes old age home per district with a minimum capacity of 150 senior citizens per home. The state government may also prescribe a scheme for the management of such homes. The scheme shall specify standards and services to be provided including those required for medical care and entertainment of residents of these old age homes.The state government shall ensure that government hospitals and those funded by the government provide beds for all senior citizens as far as possible. It shall ensure separate queues for senior citizens, expand facilities for treatment of diseases and expand research for chronic elderly diseases and aging. Every district hospital shall also earmark facilities for geriatric patients. The state government should be responsible for the management of the elder abuse and publicizing the provisions available in the Bill. The District Magistrate should take the responsibility for implementing the provisions of the Maintenance and Welfare of Parents and Senior Citizens Bill, 2007.

Unconditional Support

The support provided unconditional possibly may response more effectively how to live and combat the problem of older abuse. This kind of support is invisible. Elderly person can get unconditional support from the people in their life. Elderly people who are abused can create relationships of their choices they make, they are always safe, accepted and supported in every possible way. Receiving this kind of support means allowing the people in old age life to accept and support the choices. To begin with, elderly people need to have people in their life who are willing and able to support you unconditionally. If abused people are in relationships with meaningful people, and allow themselves to receive support from them, they can manage the problems easily.

Police Support

The majority of abusers are relatives, typically the older adult's spouse or sons and daughters, although the type of abuse differs according to the relationship. In some situations, the abuse is "domestic violence grown old," a situation in which the abusive behaviour of a spouse or partner continues into old age. Police support is required in such cases to prevent the deviant behavior of the perpetrator and for personal safety.

Physicians Support

Physicians and other medical personnel can play a vital role in assisting elder abuse victims. Although there has been an increase in awareness of elder abuse over the years, physicians tend to only report 2% of elder abuse cases. Reasons for lack of reporting by physicians include a lack of current knowledge concerning state laws on elder abuse, concern about angering the abuser and ruining the relationship with the elderly patient, possible court appearances, lack of cooperation from elderly patients or families, and lack of time and reimbursement (American Medical Association White Paper on Elderly Health, 1990). Through education and training on elder abuse, health care professionals can better assist elder abuse victims. This type of support is helpful, even if the communication between the physician and the client is online. There are some diseases of the geriatric patients which are more likely to motivate this kind of support than others.

Old Age Home Support

The older adult may lack the needed resources, as a result of poverty, or other situation in the family. In this context, Old Age Home support can be very helpful for managing elder abuse. This type of support is very essential in terms of caring about elderly health and well-being. Older people because of illness or any other reason generally ignore the consumption of food or water; cleanliness (bathing and personal hygiene); adequate clothing for climate protection; adequate safety; clean and healthy surroundings; medical attention for serious illness; essential medications. These provisions they may get in old age homes. Caregivers and other individuals working in old age homes should take the responsibility of managing elder abuse. Older people living in old age homes would hope to gain meaningful existence. The Maintenance and Welfare of Parents and Senior Citizens Bill, 2007 permits state governments to establish old age homes in every district. As of 2005, there were 1,018 Old Age Homes in India. Of the

739 homes for which detailed information is available, 427 homes are free of cost, 153 old age homes are on a pay and stay basis, and 146 homes have both free as well as pay and stay facilities. The Bill grants state governments permission to establish and maintain old age homes 'as it may deem necessary, in a phased manner,' beginning with 'at least one in each district.' There is no obligation on state governments to establish these homes. The Bill specifies that each old age home should accommodate at least 150 senior citizens. Specifying such details in the Bill reduces the flexibility to cater to differing local conditions and needs (Parker, 2007). The Bill grants state governments permission to establish and maintain old age homes 'as it may deem necessary, in a phased manner,' beginning with 'at least one in each district.' There is no obligation on state governments to establish these homes. The Bill specifies that each old age home should accommodate at least 150 senior citizens. Specifying such details in the Bill reduces the flexibility to cater to differing local conditions and needs (Parker, 2007).

Relatives Support

The majority of abusers are relatives, typically the older adult's spouse/partner or sons and daughters, although the type of abuse differs according to the relationship. Hence relatives support includes adult children and their spouses or partners, their offspring and other extended family members. Family relationships, neighbors and friends, are all socially considered as relationships of trust, whether or not the older adult actually thinks of the people as "trustworthy". In order to alleviate the problem of elder abuse, establishment of relationship is of paramount importance. In some situations, an older couple may be attempting to care and support each other and failing, in the absence of external support. With sons and daughters, it tends to be financial abuse, justified by a belief that it is nothing more than the "advance inheritance" of property, valuables and money.

Talking Support

The act of talking is to someone is another type of support. When the elderly faces the problem of elder abuse, telling others about their difficulties not only will reduce negative feelings but also reduces the incidences of health problems. Talking will help whether it is to a relative, friend, or therapist. Talking may involve a story telling that ties together experiences.

CONCLUSION

It is necessary to examine elder abuse from psychological, sociological, gender, legal, socio-economic and community perspectives in order to understand the meaning of this phenomenon. Policies and programmes should address the issues linked with the prevention of elder abuse. Developing countries should try to design public policies to prevent abuse by meeting basic needs, health care, initiating community programmes to stimulate social interaction; creating social support networks; and working with older people to create 'self-help' programmes.

Since abuse of elder people is a complex phenomenon, it therefore requires effective prevention and management strategies. Strategies should address to meet the basic needs (e.g. food, shelter), psychological needs (e.g. safety and security) and health care of elder abuse persons. Moreover, there is also need to examine the roles of elderly people beneficial to society, communities and family relationships.

Elder abuse prevention can only be successful in a culture that has value systems such as compassion and respect, and provides social support to the elderly people.

Expanding social support provides elderly to hear problems and offer a more objective perspective on the situation than their own. Therefore, to strengthen support system, elderly people need to be optimistic and maintain patience even in the face of life's toughest challenges. Receiving and providing support is one of the most important weapons to cope with elder abuse.

All dimensions of social support suggested in this article may not be equally responsive in managing the problem of elder abuse. Subjective perceptions of social support are more strongly associated with health outcomes than other dimensions (Wethington & Kessler, 1986). Research is needed to explore the role of various types of social support over significant periods of time to manage the problem of elder abuse.

We strongly recommend that the problem of elder abuse can be managed through health and social education. Education can be considered as the most effective method of preventing elder abuse. Education can be imparted through reading books and booklets on elder abuse prevention, by regular publicity in the media, and by providing information to older people. Through education we can raise awareness among older people about the type of abuse, the setting where they occur, health consequences and the risk factors associated with elder abuse.

Legal support to the cases of elder abuse is inadequate because the agencies do not take personal abuse into account or just ignoring the older people problems. Alleviating the problem of elder abuse requires proper legal remedies to respond to them and how to implement the remedies available. Governmental and non-governmental organizations need to form relationships with older people and provide the adequate services to face and deal with elder abuse.

Living with dignity should be enhanced in elderly people. To meet this objective, society should recognize the contribution and strengths of older people and address the violation of their rights including abuse either in the homes, hospital or old age homes. Daichman (2005) advocated that, "in the developing world, elder abuse will also be recognized not only as a social but also as a health problem by both governments and society" (p. 330).

Rehabilitation Counselling can be considered as one of the supportive intervention in solving the problem of elder abuse. Counselling of older people as well as the younger generation needs to be prioritizing to adjust to the needs and circumstances. Family counselling may also be an important component of management of elder abuse for both the younger as well as the older generation.

REFERENCES

Action on Elder Abuse. (1995). *Action on elder abuse's definition of elder abuse*. London: Bulletin, May/June.

Action on elder abuse. (n. d.) Retrieved October 12, 2007 from elderabuse.org.uk

Advocare Incorporated. (2017). Signs and symptoms of elder abuse and neglect in care. Advocare Incorporated. Retrieved 16 December 2012 from http://www.advocare.org.au/help-with-aged-care-complaints/signs-and-symptoms-of-eld/

American Medical Association White Paper on Elderly Health. (1990). Report on the Council on Scientific Affairs. *Archives of Internal Medicine, 150*, 2459–2472. doi:10.1001/archinte.1990.00390230019004 PMID:2288622

Bhatia, M. S., Srivastava, S., & Bansal, S. (2008). Elder abuse. *Delhi Psychiatry Journal, 11*(2), 150–154.

Cook-Daniels, L. (2003b). 2003 is the year elder abuse hits the international state. *Victimization of the Elderly and Disabled, 5*, 65-66, 76.

Cooper, C., Selwood, A., & Livingston, G. (2008). The prevalence of elder abuse and neglect: A systematic review. *Age and Ageing, 37*(2), 151–160. doi:10.1093/ageing/afm194 PMID:18349012

Daichman, L. S. (2005). Elder abuse in developing nations. In M. L. Johnson, V. L. Bengston, P. G. Coleman, & T. B. L. Kirkwood (Eds.), *The Cambridge handbook of age and ageing* (pp. 323–331). Cambridge: Cambridge University Press. doi:10.1017/CBO9780511610714.032

Dong, X. (2005). Medical implications of elder abuse and neglect. *Clinics in Geriatric Medicine, 21*(2), 293–313. doi:10.1016/j.cger.2004.10.006 PMID:15804552

Frazier, P. A., Tix, A. P., Klein, C. D., & Arikian, N. J. (2000). Testing theoretical models of the relations between social support, coping, and adjustment to stressful life events. *Journal of Social and Clinical Psychology, 19*(3), 314–335. doi:10.1521/jscp.2000.19.3.314

Hildreth, C. J. (2011). *Elder Abuse. Jama, 306*(5), 568. doi:10.1001/jama.306.5.568

Jackson, S., & Hafemeister, T. (2012). Pure financial exploitation vs. Hybrid financial exploitation co-occurring with physical abuse and/or neglect of elderly persons. *Psychology of Violence, 2*(3), 285–296. doi:10.1037/a0027273

Nursing Home Abuse Laws (NHAL). USA. (2017). Retrieved from https://www.hg.org/nursing-home-abuse.html

Parker, P. N. (2007, July 6). The maintenance and welfare of parents and senior citizens bill.

Robinson, L., Benedictis, T. D., & Segal, J. (2012). Elder abuse and neglect: Warning signs, risk factors, prevention, and help.

Sarason, I. G., Sarason, B. R., & Pierce, G. (1994). Social support: Global and relationship-based levels of analysis. *Journal of Social and Personal Relationships, 11*(2), 295–312. doi:10.1177/0265407594112008

Shilling, D. (2008). Improving the court system's response to elder abuse. *Victimization of the Elderly and Disabled, 11*, 49, 51-52, 59, 62-63.

Wethington, E., & Kessler, R. C. (1986). Perceived support, received support, and adjustment to stressful life events. *Journal of Health and Social Behavior, 27*(1), 78–89. doi:10.2307/2136504 PMID:3711634

WHO. (n.d.). WHO/NMH/NPH/02.2.

WHO/INPEA. (2001a). *Daichman, L., Guido, O., Aguas, S., &Bertone, M. National report on elder abuse in Argentina*. Geneva: WHO.

WHO/INPEA. (2001b). *L. Machado, National report on elder abuse in Brazil*. Geneva: WHO.

WHO/INPEA (2002b).*Missing voices: views of older persons on elder abuse.*

KEY TERMS AND DEFINITIONS

Elder Abuse: Elder abuse is a single, or repeated act, or lack of appropriate action, occurring within any relationship where there is an expectation of trust, which causes harm of distress to an older person".

Old Age Homes: Homes for the aged are ideal for elderly people who are alone, face health problems, depression and loneliness.

Social Support: Social support is the feeling or experience of having others who love and care for an individual.

Section 2

Cognition and Cognitive Impairment in Ageing and Clinical Outcome

Chapter 6
Cognitive Functions in the Geriatric Population

Shivani Sharma
All India Institute of Medical Sciences, India

Ashima Nehra
All India Institute of Medical Sciences, India

ABSTRACT

This chapter describes how one of the challenging issues of clinical diagnosis is distinguishing between the cognitive deficits manifested in normal aging, depression, mild cognitive impairment (MCI) and dementia. The diagnostic challenge is that there is a great deal of overlap in the symptom constellations of these conditions. It is thus important to establish conceptual and clinical criteria with sufficient predictive validity to accurately identify differences and similarities in cognitive states to justify initiation of appropriate treatments.

INTRODUCTION

The world population continues to grow older rapidly as fertility rates have fallen to very low levels in most world regions and people tend to live longer. When the global population reached 7 billion in 2012, 8% were aged 65 and over. In 2015, 3 years later, the older population rose by 55 million and the proportion of the older population reached 8.5 percent of the total population (He, Goodkind & Kowal, 2016). Old age makes one susceptible to a gamut of diseases and disorders. While some of them affect the physical functioning, others affect mood and cognitive functioning, casting a serious impact on quality of life, daily functioning and independence. Changes in cognition with aging are not universal and there is considerable variability. With increase in age, decline in cognitive ability becomes more and more pronounced. Age related decline of abilities of memory, attention and executive function have been most widely investigated. More pronounced deficits in these and other cognitive domains have been reported in mild cognitive impairment, depression and dementia. However, there is a great deal of overlap in the symptoms of the stated conditions, making it difficult to differentiate between them (see Table 1).

DOI: 10.4018/978-1-5225-3480-8.ch006

Further, these cognitive abilities (especially executive functioning) are directly related to independence of performing activities of daily living. Thus, reiterating the need to maintain proficiency of the same. However, literature has revealed impairment in the same, thus pointing to dependence on others. However, a common misconception is that loss of abilities like memory, attention, and other mental facilities that help us to think clearly and maintain social relationships, decline inevitably, and become untreatable as we age. Increasing number of studies suggest that the brain is malleable even in later life (Kueider & Rebok, 2014). Thus, the authors propose to write a chapter on the similarities and differences in cognitive functioning of the geriatric population with respect to normal aging, mild cognitive impairment, depression, and dementia. A clear distinction between these is pivotal not only in terms of creating awareness but also from the perspective of diagnosis and rehabilitation.

BACKGROUND

Cognitive change as a normal process of aging has been well documented in the scientific literature. Mental abilities change throughout life, first as a result of brain maturation and later with aging of brain cells. Some cognitive abilities, such as vocabulary, are resilient to brain aging and may even improve with age. Other abilities, such as conceptual reasoning, memory, and processing speed, decline gradually over time. There is also significant variation among older adults in the rate of decline in some of these abilities, such as measures of perceptual reasoning and processing speed (Harada, Love & Triebel, 2013). Although differences between the young and elderly can be shown in some cognitive areas, declining ability does not translate into impairment of daily activities. These changes are subtle. However, these changes can be noted on cognitive testing in terms of severity of impairment (Example: On cognitive testing, when scored based on age and education matched norms, an individual with MCI is more likely to score below the normal performance of ± 1 standard deviation. Further, the differences are sometimes so subtle that that some MCI patients may reveal an overall 'normal' score, however, reflecting certain affected sub domains of cognitive functioning). MCI definitions can be broadly classified as amnestic and non-amnestic. Amnestic MCI is characterized by a primary memory disorder with less-impaired function in other neurocognitive domains (Lopez et al., 2003). Non-amnestic MCI, on the other hand, is characterized by impairment in 1 or more neurocognitive domains other than memory, including

Table 1. Comparison of cognitive deficits in normal aging, mild cognitive impairment, depression and dementia

Cognitive Domain	Normal Aging	Mild Cognitive Impairment	Depression	Dementia
Memory	x	x	x	x
Attention	x	x	x	x
Language		x	x	x
Executive Function	x	x	x	x
Visuospatial Ability	x	x	x	x
Psychomotor Ability		x	x	x

language, executive function, and visuospatial skills (Petersen, 2004). While most studies indicate that amnestic MCI progresses to Alzheimer disease (AD), non-amnestic MCI is more likely to progress to dementias other than AD (Steffens et al., 2008).

Depression is a disorder of mood that produces sad feelings, negative thoughts, and disruptions of sleep, appetite, thinking, and energy level. Although most clinicians diagnose depression based on a categorical approach like that in the Diagnostic and Statistical Manual of Mental Disorders, Fifth Revision (DSM-V) (APA, 2013), it is important to recognize that any depressive symptoms that impair cognition or activities of daily living (ADLs) are clinically significant (Potter & Steffens, 2007).One problem with understanding the relationship of depression to MCI is that depression has often been excluded from the definition of this condition. Although this exclusion initially occurred because depression was viewed as a "pseudo-dementia" that confounds the detection of "true" impairment, research now indicates a high rate of co-occurrence between depression and MCI that raises the risk for persistent cognitive impairment and dementia (Potter & Steffens, 2007). Dementia refers to an outcome of changes in the brain that produce dysfunction in memory, thinking, communication, and praxis that impairs an individual's ability to function in daily life. Different types of Dementia are characterized by cognitive impairment in different domains (Table 1). Although research has not yet resolved whether depression is more accurately characterized as a risk or prodrome of dementia, the important clinical issue is that the 2 conditions are frequently linked; thus, the presence of depression, particularly of late onset, raises attention to screening for cognitive impairment as part of a long-term approach to care. One of the challenging issues of clinical diagnosis is distinguishing between individuals with normal aging, depression, MCI and dementia. The diagnostic challenge is that there is a great deal of symptom overlap between these conditions. For instance, the symptom constellation of decreased concentration and processing speed, irritability, sleep loss, fatigue, and anhedonia that occur in depression are similar to the constellation of memory loss, agitation, sleep-wake disturbance, and apathy that often occur in dementia (Potter & Steffens, 2007). Despite similarities between these conditions, careful attention to clinical history and presentation can help distinguish between them.

In the sections to follow, the authors attempt to provide an outline of the neuropsychological functioning (definitions in Table 2) and impairment as a result of normal aging, mild cognitive impairment, depression and dementia.

NORMAL AGING

Intelligence

Crystallized intelligence is less subject to decay as a result of rehearsal, practice and use of knowledge. These abilities remain relatively stable and may even gradually improve in the later decades of life as they are a product of the accumulated knowledge (Zillmer, Spiers & Culbertson, 2007). In contrast, fluid abilities (table) which involve novel reasoning and efficiency in solving new problems have been found to peak around the third decade of life and decline thereafter (Harada et al., 2013). It has been found that executive function, processing speed, memory and psychomotor ability fall under this broad domain (Harada et al., 2013).

Language

It is a complex cognitive domain composed of crystallized and fluid cognitive abilities. This ability remains stable over time with even an increase in vocabulary with age (Hayden & Welsh-Bohmer, 2011; Singh-Manoux et al., 2012). However, an exception to this general trend of stability is naming (ability to see a common object and name it) and verbal fluency (ability to generate or perform words for a certain category) (Singh-Manouxet al., 2012; Salthouse, 2010).

Memory

The most common complaint among older adults is that of change in memory. Like attention, memory is not a unitary construct; some kinds of memory remain relatively intact with age while others show significant declines (Glisky, 2007). Age related decline in this domain may also be a function of decline in processing speed, cognitive control or use of mnemonic devices. Unlike declarative memory, non-declarative memory remains unchanged in the later decades of life (Harada et al., 2013). Episodic memory has been found to be the most susceptible to the aging brain and most affected my normal aging (Glisky, 2007). Although many older adults believe that their memories for remote events are better than their memories for recent events, it is likely that older memories have become more gist like, retaining the general core information but lacking other details. More problematic for older adults is remembering context or source information: where or when something was heard or read, or even whether something actually happened or was just thought about. Semantic memory however, has been found be intact and even enhanced in older adults. Autobiographical memory which involves memory of one's past personal experiences is both episodic and semantic in nature. Literature revels that this ability is largely preserved in older adults (Rubin, 2000).

In general, older adults show normal acquisition of procedural skills in both motor and cognitive domains and retain them across the lifespan. With high levels of expertise, there is often little slowing of skilled performance with age, although some individual components of the skill may decline (Salthouse, 1984). Older adults do quite well on Prospective memory daily tasks, using a variety of external aids such as calendars and appointment books to remind themselves of these activities (West, Herndon, & Covell, 2003).Prospective memory may also rely on some aspect of working memory to maintain future intentions over time and likely also involves divided attention, both functions that show age-related deficits (Glisky, 2007).Memory can also be understood through the stages of encoding, storage and retrieval. While encoding (rate of acquisition of new information) and retrieval (ability to recall learnt information) declines with age, retention of information that is successfully encoded (storage), remains relatively stable in older adults.

Executive Functions

Executive Functions are an umbrella term for the three core EFs as agreed upon by different researchers: Inhibition (inhibitory control, which includes self-control (behavioural inhibition) and interference control (selective attention and cognitive inhibition)), working memory (WM), and cognitive flexibility (also called set shifting, mental flexibility, or mental set shifting) (Diamond, 2012). From these, higher

Table 2. Definitions and examples of cognitive domains

Cognitive Domain	Sub Domain/ Ability	Definition	Example
Intelligence	Fluid Intelligence	Novel reasoning and efficiency of problem solving or responding to abstract ideas	Coming up with a new approach to solve a problem at hand
	Crystallized Intelligence	Stored knowledge and habitual ways of acting or solving problems built up over a lifetime	Knowing the answer to the first prime minister of India
Language	Expressive Language	Ability to produce language	Giving a string of comprehendible instructions
	Receptive Language	Understanding or recognition of linguistic information	Understanding a string of instructions
Memory	Declarative (explicit) • Semantic • Episodic (Autobiographical)	Conscious recollection of facts and events • General world knowledge accumulated throughout life • Memory for personally experienced events that occurred in a particular place and time	• Knowing the year in which India got Independence • Remembering how one celebrated their 18th birthday
	Non- Declarative (implicit) • Procedural • Prospective	Memory for how to do things • Knowledge of skills and procedures • Remembering to perform intended actions in the future	• Remembering how to ride a bicycle • Remembering to take medicine after meals
Executive Functions		Group of highly interrelated functions that include planning, initiation, and regulation of behavior, working memory, response inhibition, and task switching	Planning a complex multi staged activity and carrying it out successfully
Working Memory		Active memory system on which information is manipulated and assembled to help us comprehend language, make decisions and solve problems	Spelling a word backwards
Visouspatial abilities/ Construction		Object perception, the ability to recognize familiar objects and spatial perception, the ability to appreciate the physical location of objects either alone or in relation to other objects/ ability to put together individual parts to make a coherent whole	Navigating through a map in an unfamiliar location
Attention	Selective Attention	Ability to attend to some stimuli while disregarding others that are irrelevant to the task at hand	Focusing on reading a book in a noisy coffee house
	Divided Attention	Processing of two or more sources of information at the same time	Talking on the phone while driving
	Sustained Attention	Ability to maintain concentration on a task over an extended period of time	Concentrating throughout a 3 hour lecture

order EFs of reasoning, problem-solving and planning are built (Collins & Koechlin, 2012; Lunt et al., 2012). These functions make it possible to play with mentally with ideas, take time to think and act, meet unanticipated and novel challenges, resist temptations and stay focused. These skills are essential for our mental and physical health, success in life and in our social, cognitive and psychological aspects of development. Numerous studies have implied a decline in these abilities as a result of aging (Apfelbaum, Krendl & Ambady, 2010).

Working Memory

Working memory is a multidimensional cognitive construct which is an active memory system on which information is manipulated and assembled to help us comprehend language, make decisions and solve problems. This has been hypothesized as the fundamental source of age-related deficits in a variety of cognitive tasks, including long-term memory, language, problem solving, and decision making. In fact, the majority of theories of cognitive aging seem to implicate working memory (Baddeley, 2000). Older adults exhibit significant deficits in tasks that involve active manipulation, reorganization, or integration of the contents of working memory. Although the mechanisms underlying these age-related deficits are as yet poorly understood, the effects of such deficits are far-reaching.

Attention and Processing Speed

Processing speed is the speed with which cognitive activities are performed. Decline in this ability in the later years of life affects the above stated cognitive functions as well (Salthouse, 2010; Salthouse, Fristoe, Lineweaver, & Coon, 1995; Carlson, Hasher, Connelly & Zacks, 1995). Some form of attention is involved in virtually all other cognitive domains, except when task is habitual. Declines in attention can therefore have broad-reaching effects on one's ability to function adequately and efficiently in everyday life. Selective attention refers to the ability to attend to some stimuli while disregarding others that are irrelevant to the task at hand. Deficits found in many of selective attention tasks can be largely attributed to a general slowing of information processing in older adults rather than to selective attention deficits per se (Glisky, 2007). Divided attention tasks require the processing of two or more sources of information or the performance of two or more tasks at the same time. It has usually been associated with significant age-related declines in performance, particularly when tasks are complex.

Visuospatial Ability/ Construction

This group of cognitive functions involves the ability to understand space in two and three dimensions. Literature reveals impairment in tasks that require visual construction abilities. However, visuospatial abilities are believed to remain intact (Howieson, Holm, Kaye, Oken & Howieson, 1993).

MILD COGNITIVE IMPAIRMENT

MCI has been described as a cognitive disturbance representing the transitional or prodromal phase between normal aging and Dementia (Rivas-Vazquez, Mendez, Rey & Carrazana, 2004). Based on criteria by Petersen et al. (1999), Rivas-Vazquez et al. (2004) have devised a mnemonic device (SOUND) for the same:

- **S**ubjective memory complaints.
- **O**bjective memory deficit.
- **U**naffected overall cognition.
- **N**ormal capacity to perform Activities of Daily Living.
- **D**ementia criteria not met.

With the above-mentioned factors adjusted for age and education (Diniz, Pinto & Forlenza, 2008). A Meta-analysis carried out recently reported that, patients with MCI evolve to Dementia at approximately 10% per year (Bruscoli & Lovestone, 2004). Petersen reported that, after approximately 6 years, 80% of the MCI progress to dementia (Peterson et al., 2001). Although the original criteria of MCI focussed on memory complaints the recent classification has been expanded to encompass other cognitive domains like executive function, attention, language etc. Resulting in the following sub-types of MCI: MCI single domain- memory type, MCI single domain – non-memory type, multi domain including memory impairment and multi domain without memory impairment (Winbald et al., 2004). Due to the variation in neuropsychological profiles and aetiology of the stated sub types, it is believed that their progression over time can result in different outcomes (Petersen et al., 2001). For example: Single domain amnestic MCI may be a pre-dementia stage for AD however, single domain non-amnestic MCI may be a found in transitional phases to frontotemporal dementia, dementia with lewy bodies, vascular dementia or depressive disorders (Bennett et al., 2002). The following section delineates the neuropsychological functioning in MCI.

Memory

Memory deficits form the core problem in MCI. It is however difficult to derive a standard equation of these memory problems given the diversity in memory-related functions. Conceptually, for encoding of any form of memory, attention is the most important prerequisite. It is being increasingly recognized that attention deficits are prevalent in MCI (Yanhong, Chandra &Venkatesh, 2013). Studies have reported reduction in episodic memory as the most prevalent in MCI (Petersen, 2004). Decline in prospective memory (ability to remember and perform an intended action at an appropriate point in the future) can also serve as an early sign in of memory failure (Spíndola & Brucki, 2011). This type of memory is relevant for social functioning, adherence to treatment, and carrying out instrumental activities of daily living (Chasteen Park & Schwarz, 2001; Smith, Del Sala, Logie & Maylor, 2000). Additionally, both familiarity based memory and recollection have been found to be impaired in MCI (Wolk, Mancuso, Kliot, Arnold & Dickerson, 2013; Algarabel González et al., 2012). Studies have also shown that MCI patients have difficulties in all the stages of verbal memory processing including acquisition, consolidation, and recall stages (Hutchens et al., 2013). These memory deficits are not limited to the amnestic MCI, but are also present in non-amnestic MCI, albeit at lower intensities (Yanhong et al., 2013). However, subjects with MCI are often aware of their memory deficits (Seelye, Schmitter-Edgecombe & Flores, 2010). Thus, this meta-memory skill can be utilized to design interventions involving compensatory strategies for daily issues related to memory deficits.

Executive Functions

Executive functions are a group of highly interrelated functions that include planning, initiation, and regulation of behaviour, working memory, response inhibition, and task switching (Miyake et al., 2000). In contrast to the well-established finding of memory deficits in MCI, the executive function tests have revealed no-deficits on some studies to global impairments of EFs in others (Zheng et al., 2012). Analysis of day-to-day application of executive functions in MCI patients revealed impairments in episodic memory, executive function, semantic knowledge and arithmetic. At the same time, control and MCI groups performed significantly better than patients with AD on financial capacity and cognitive measures (Griffith et al., 2003).

Other Impairments

Other amnestic cognitive deficits in MCI include impairment in fluid intelligence, working memory and attention processing (Saunders & Summers, 2010, Kramer et al., 2006). Further subjects with MCI also exhibit deficits in visual personal familiarity and recognition of facial emotional expression (Jurjanzet al., 2011; Varjassyovaet al., 2013). Such deficits lead to impaired social cognition and may adversely impact the patients' efficacy in handling complex situations and tasks.

DEPRESSION

Depression is not a normal part of aging (Flint, 1994). It is a medical condition that affects many older adults and can often be successfully treated. Symptoms of depression include: low mood, loss of interest or pleasure in activities, disturbed sleep, fluctuation in weight, lack of energy, feeling of worthlessness, difficulty with concentration or decision making, noticeable restlessness or slow movement and frequent thoughts of suicide or an attempt of suicide (Palazzolo, 2015).The World Health Organization Global Burden of Disease Study ranked depression as the most burdensome disease in the world in terms of total disability-adjusted years among people in the middle years of life (Murray & Lopez 1996).It has been found that the combination of depression and cognitive impairment is present in roughly 25% of older adults and this is expected to double every 5 years after the age of 70 (Arve, Tilvis, Lehtonen, Valvanne & Sairanen, 1999). In some cases, these conditions may be related to the same underlying disorder while in others they may be relatively independent (Morimoto, Kanellopoulos & Alexopoulos, 2014). Results of a meta-analysis reveal that a history of depression doubles the risk of developing dementia later on in life (Ownby, Crocco, Acevedo, John & Loewenstein, 2006). Depression has been found to be highly prevalent in MCI and most dementias. It may be a risk factor for the subsequent development of Dementia or in some conditions, a prodromal symptom (Potter & Steffens, 2007). Some studies have shown that these patients report depression well before they report cognitive difficulties, raising the possibility that depression was a risk factor for dementia. Meta-analyses of the world literature suggested that history of depression was a risk factor for dementia (Jorm, 2001). However, studies that examine the temporal sequence reveal that although depressive symptoms preceded the onset of dementia, depression appear to be a prodrome rather than an independent predictor of dementia (Chen, Ganguli, Mulsant & DeKosky, 1999). Thus, depression might be a prodromal or early sign of dementia rather than a separate condition or risk factor for dementia. Impairment in attention, concentration and thinking ability are one of the key diagnostic criteria of depression. Meta-analysis on the neurocognitive deficits in depression has found impairment in domains in executive function, memory, processing speed to name a few (Veiel, 1997, Zakzanis, Leach & Kaplan, 1998). Studies reveal 33-50% of depressed individuals have cognitive impairment (Butters et al., 2004; Reischies & Neu, 2000).

Memory

Memory has been the most assessed function for evaluation of cognitive differences between depression and dementia. Evidence suggests deficits in episodic memory, learning and explicit verbal and visual memory in depression patients. However, other memory functions appear to be spared (Danion, Kauffmann-Muller, Grange, Zimmermann & Greth, 1995; Bazin, Perruchet, De Bonis & Feline, 1994). It is imperative to note here that these memory deficits are significantly mild when compared with dementia (Kang et al., 2014). Taking this comparison forward depressed patients show relatively mild impairment on recognition memory, encoding, forgetting and psychomotor speed (Hart & Kwentus, 1987; Miller & Lewis, 1977). Literature reveals that most common memory deficits being those related to tasks of recall or remembering. However, the sample sizes of these studies have been relatively small and the methodologies varied. Additionally, these memory deficits in spite of being significantly worse than normal individuals are comparably better than those associated with dementia. Most researchers have suggested that such differences represent general cognitive inefficiency and attention problems rather than a fundamental lack of ability. This can be seen in the differences between depression and dementia patients as well as in the temporariness of these deficits in the clinical picture of depression (Kang et al., 2014).

Executive Functions

Executive function impairment in depression have been studied widely. It has been found that deficits in planning, organizing, set shifting etc. have predicted low antidepressant response and functional disability. Further, such deficits occur at a rate of 20-30% in such patients (McIntyreet al., 2013). In general, significant EF impairments have been observed in subjects with more severe depression (Raskin, Friedman & DiMascio, 1982; Friedman, 1964). Processing speed impairment is another important executive function deficit observed in depression. It has been found that such impairments partially mediate the effect of depression on functioning. A more clinical outcome of this processing speed impairment is psychomotor slowing, which is almost universally found in the depressed patients, irrespective of the number of episodes (Brown et al., 2013). However, differences between normal and depressed patients on executive functioning are sufficiently subtle to not significantly influence scores on standard cognitive screening instruments (Bieliauskas, Costello & Terpenning, 1991; Bieliauskas, Boczar & Lamberty, 1991).

Speech and Language

Small numbers of studies have specifically examined speech-language function in elderly depressed patients. While most of the tasks used to measure cognitive abilities in above-mentioned studies have obvious receptive and expressive language components, it has been found that depressed patients perform better than patients with dementia on naming, repetition, general reading skill, syntax, and auditory verbal comprehension. At the same time, normal individuals tend to show better language performance than depressed patients overall, though these differences were considerably less obvious than those noted between depressed and AD patients (Gray, Rattan & Dean, 1986).

PSEUDO-DEMENTIA AND DELIRIUM

Pseudo-dementia is defined as cognitive impairment that mimics dementia however diminishes upon remission of depression (Morimoto et al., 2014). These patients have been found to have severe, however late onset of depression but mild dementia. Over decades of practice, clinicians have observed that findings of neuropsychological tests may not precisely match subjective complaints in MCI. In contrast, dementia patients are unconcerned about memory problems but reflect poor performance on testing. More differences between these patients have been recorded in order to aid the process the diagnosis (Table 3). Further, studies that examined depressed cognitively impaired patients over time, found that a significant proportion continued to experience progressive cognitive decline even after remission of depression (Reifler, 2000). Thus suggesting that the impairment recorded during depression was not 'pseudo' but a warning signal for more permanent cognitive decline in the future. Another condition that if often confused in dementia is *delirium* which is a state of severe confusion and rapid changes in brain function. However, it is important to differentiate between their key characteristics (Table 4).

DEMENTIA

Dementia does not describe a specific disease, but rather describes a clinical syndrome characterized by a loss of previously acquired cognitive functions that adversely affect an individual's ability to complete day to day activities (Schoenberg & Scott, 2011). The decline in cognitive functioning is greater than what occurs during the normal aging, depression and mild cognitive impairment. The most common types of dementia are: Alzheimer's disease, vascular dementia, Dementia with Lewy Bodies, fronto

Table 3. Difference between Dementia and Pseudo- dementia

No.	Dementia	Pseudodementia
1.	Forgetful behavior usually reported by family member	Detailed account of cognitive impairment provided
	Unconcerned about memory problems	Prominent subjective memory loss
2.	Emphasis on achievements	Emphasis on disability
3.	Unconcerned appearance	Communication of distress
4.	Usually liable affect	Severe depression
5.	Errors on examination after genuine attempts	Frequent "don't know" answers
6.	Recent memory impaired	Recent memory not impaired
7.	Confabulation may be present	Confabulation is rare
8.	Consistently poor performance on cognitive testing	Variability in performance on cognitive testing
9.	History of depression uncommon	History of manic/ depressive episodes may be present
10.	Aphasia, apraxia, agnosia are common	Language, recognition and motor skills are intact however, reduced psychomotor speed, sustained attention and executive function deficits are noted on neuropsychological testing

(Tripathi, 2014, Used with permission)

Table 4. Difference between Dementia and Delirium

No.	Dementia	Delirium
1.	Gradual onset (months to years)	Acute onset (hours to days)
2.	Chronic progression	Fluctuating course
3.	Clear consciousness	Impaired consciousness
4.	Impaired attention	Fluctuating impairment in attention
5.	Recent and remote memory impaired	Recent and immediate memory impaired
6.	Depressed mood, apathy	Fluctuating moods- anger, fear
7.	Difficulty in abstraction, judgment impaired	Fragmented and disorganized thinking
8.	Misperceptions present	More misperceptions, illusions, delusions and hallucinations than Dementia
9.	Withdrawn, agitated psychomotor activity	Hypo or hyper kinetic psychomotor activity

(Tripathi, 2014, Used with permission)

temporal dementia and Parkinson's disease with dementia. Some of these degenerative conditions have neuropathological signs that differentiate them from other conditions (e.g., tau mutations in AD), while others are a secondary result of multiple illnesses that have a primary central nervous system deterioration (e.g., hypertension and diabetes in vascular dementia). Dementias can be caused by a variety of medical (e.g., cerebrovascular, metabolic) and psychiatric illnesses (e.g., substance abuse) (Schoenberg &Scott, 2011). The cognitive deficits in dementia are not confined to memory and may include impairment in language, praxis, organisational skills, attention and judgement. Significant cognitive impairment results in loss of social functioning. Behavioural changes also occur that can be particularly troublesome to the family (Gifford & Jones, 2009). Different forms of dementia have characteristic presentations and patterns of cognitive change (Table 5).

A detailed history of symptom onset and the course of its progression can be very valuable in the differential diagnosis of dementia.

ISSUES, CONTROVERSIES, AND PROBLEMS

Thus, there is little knowledge and awareness about the subtle differences between normal aging and mild cognitive impairment as most elderly give into their fate of old age and believe the experienced level of decline and impairment is inevitable. Further, there is ongoing debate about whether depression is a risk factor for dementia or a prodrome of this condition. Additional uncertainty exists as depression in elderly causes cognitive impairment in its own right (Butters et al., 2000). Depression could result from a number of factors. It could be a psychological response to an individual self-awareness of cognitive deficits,

misinterpretation by others of a natural response to withdraw from previously enjoyed activities of dementia patients who find them hard and effortful, response to a prospect of having an incurable progressive disease (Ganguli, 2009). Thus, pointing to the need to draw up a detailed medical, psychiatric and psycho-social history of patients.

Table 5. Cognitive deficits in sub types of Dementia

Domains	Dementia				
	Alzheimer's Disease	**Vascular Dementia**	**Dementia With Lewy Bodies**	**Fronto-Temporal Dementia**	**Parkinson's Disease With Dementia**
Behavioral Observations	Irritability, social withdrawal	Symptoms of depression and apathy are common	Visual hallucinations and other psychiatric symptoms may be present	Prominent personality changes	Apathy and depression are common
Attention	Simple Attention intact Complex Attention Impaired	Often both impaired	Gross Impairment	Simple Attention intact Complex Attention Impaired	Simple Attention intact Complex Attention Impaired
Learning/ Memory	Prominent and progressive impairment especially for recent events	Severe impairment. Consolidation, free recall impaired Recognition intact	Learning impaired Visual, immediate and delayed memory impaired	Late impairment in immediate free recall	Slowed learning Encoding impaired
Language	Impaired fluency, naming, reading, comprehension Vocabulary intact	Variable degree of impairment	Verbal fluency and naming impaired	Varied impairment Fluency, naming, comprehension impaired	Impaired with dysarthria, hypophonia and micrographia Verbal fluency and naming impaired Repetition and comprehension intact
Visuo-perpectual/ visuo-constructional Ability	Impaired and worsens as disease progresses	Variable degree of impairment, if at all present	Severe impairment as disease progresses	Late impairment	Impairment worsened by motor deficits
Executive Function	Progressive difficulty in handling complex reasoning based tasks	Varied severity of impairment	Moderate to severe impairment may be present	Severe perseveration	Mild to moderate impairment present
Sensory/ Motor Ability	Olfaction may be impaired Dyspraxia common	Gait instability and rigidity	Simultaneous or late development of parkinsonian features	Poor motor programming may be present	Parkinsonian features before development of Dementia

Dysarthria: Slurred or slow speech which can be difficult to understand; Hypophonia: Soft speech, especially resulting from a lack of coordination in the vocal musculature.

Micrographia: Abnormally small, cramped handwriting, or the progression to continually smaller handwriting.

Dyspraxia: Difficulty in activities requiring coordination and movement.

(Adapted from Schoenberg and Scott, 2011 (Permission Pending); Gifford & Jones, 2009)

SOLUTIONS AND RECOMMENDATIONS

Due to lack of insight in patients, patients and informants (such as family members) may report conflicting views regarding the presence and severity of symptoms (thus implying the importance of being cognizant of early signs, Table 6) (Nehra & Bajpai, 2015). A history of cognitive changes over time, validated by knowledgeable informants, is therefore important for identifying the first diagnostic criterion. Critical features that may clarify a cause are onset, trajectory, time-course, and nature of the

Table 6. Strub and black Neuropsychological test battery components and corresponding neuropsychological tests

S.No.	Component	Description	Most Popular Tests
1.	History	Developmental, educational, social and vocational	Proforma based on clinical condition
2.	Behaviour	Attention, cooperation, level of effort, mood, rapport	Digit Symbol Substitution Test (DSST), Digit Span Test, Brief Test of Attention (BTA)
3.	Intelligence	General, verbal and non- verbal	Ravens Progressive Matrices (RPM) and Wechsler Adult Intelligence Scale (WAIS)
4.	Language	Auditory discrimination, single word and sentence comprehension, repetition	Boston Naming Test (BNT), Controlled Oral Word Association Test (COWA), Indian Aphasia Battery (IAB) and Verbal Adult Intelligence Scale (VAIS)
5.	Memory	Verbal and non- verbal memory, acquisition, immediate recall, recent and remote memory, incidental memory and recognition	California Verbal Learning Test (CVLT), PGI Memory Scale (PGIMS) and Wechsler Memory Scale (WMS)
6.	Abstract reasoning and Executive Functions	Verbal and non- verbal reasoning, problem solving, conceptual shifting	Trail Making Test (TMT), Stroop Test, Wisconsin Card Sorting Test (WCST), Iowa Gambling Test (IGT), Tower of London Test (TOL)
7.	Spatial Analysis and Constructional Ability	Paper and pencil reproduction, three dimensional constructions, reproduction from memory, visual analysis	Bender Visual Motor Gestalt Test (BVMGT), Rey Osterrieth Complex Figure Test (ROCF)
8.	Sensory Perceptual Ability	Visual, auditory and tactile perception	Same as above
9.	Geographic Orientation	Awareness of place and person	Mini Mental Status Examination (MMSE), Galveston Orientation and Amnesia Test (GOAT)
10.	Time Orientation	Awareness of time	Same as above
11.	Reading and Writing	Achievement in reading, spelling and calculation	Same as Language Tests
12.	Perceptual Motor Speed	Planning ability and concept manipulation	Finger Tapping Test (FTT), Digit Symbol Substitution Test (DSST), Bender Visual Motor Gestalt Test (BVMGT), Grooved Pegboard Test
13.	Strength	Motor strength and coordination	Same as above
14.	Personality	Focal signs	Rorschach Inkblot Test, 16 Personality Factor Questionnaire (16PF), Thematic Apperception Test (TAT), Myers-Briggs Type Indicator (MBTI)
15.	Social Functioning	Social adaptive functioning	Disease specific

Adapted from Tripathi, 2014 (Used with permission)

cognitive symptoms. Very rapid cognitive decline (e.g., weeks to months) is not typical of MCI due to AD, and should raise concerns for other causes, such metabolic disorders (McCarten, 2013; Holsinger, Deveau, Boustani & Williams, 2007). Thus, as mentioned above, cognitive impairment as a result of MCI can affect virtually all cognitive domains (Table 5). Estimated conversion rates from MCI to dementia range from 2-31%, with a mean annual conversion of 10.2% (Bruscoli & Lovestone, 2004) with some individuals also displaying persistent MCI without converting to dementia (Schonknecht, 2011). Although, cognitive impairment associated with MCI does not hamper independent functioning in activities of daily living, research suggests that it has a significant impact on psychological wellbeing and Quality of Life (Teng, Tassniyom & Lu, 2012). Reviews also reveal the presence of neuropsychiatric symptoms (such as depression, anxiety, agitation, irritability, sleep disturbance, fatigue) in such patients (Bombois, Derambure, Pasquier & Monaca, 2010). Thus, overall impacting daily functioning in terms of financial management, driving and scheduling to name a few (Gold, 2012) more debilitating results have been found in patients with dementia. Further, as mentioned above, depression can impair an older adult's ability to function and enjoy life and can contribute to poor health outcomes. Compared to older adults without depression, those with depression often need greater assistance with self-care and daily living activities and often recover more slowly from physical disorders. Without appropriate treatment, symptoms of depression can limit an older adult's ability to achieve successful aging (Palazzolo, 2015). Thus, detection of cognitive impairment is critical and deficits that are validated by neuropsychological testing should not be ignored or considered normal manifestation of aging (Ritchie, Artero & Touchon, 2001). In order to combat these issues, cognitive rehabilitation interventions along with cognitive behavior therapy can be used increase to frequency of engaging in positive lifestyle behaviors which can be thought of as protective factors which contribute to reduced risk of impairment.

Evidence from RCTs and clinical trials suggest that aerobic exercises, mental activities and social engagement have beneficial effects on cognitive functioning (Lin, O'Connor, Rossom, Perdue & Eckstrom, 2013). These factors contribute to the 'cognitive reserve capacity' of individuals. It is a hypothetical construct used to explain how individuals vary in severity of cognitive decline when neurodegenerative changes occur (Whalley, Deary, Appleton & Starr, 2004). Further, since it is not fixed, there are opportunities for modification and enhancement of the same through above stated factors and those of education and occupational achievement. Cognitive retraining activities can be of two types: (a) Restorative cognitive retraining activities directly target cognitive compromise by restoring abilities through neuroplasticity mechanisms like repeated practice on structured tasks of specific cognitive domains (Huckans et al., 2013; Bajpai, Tripathi, Dey & Nehra, In Press) and (b) Compensatory cognitive retraining activities directly target functional deficits by teaching skills and strategies to compensate for cognitive impairments so that the impact of these deficits on daily function and QOL can be reduced. Compensatory strategies can include internal strategies (e.g., using mnemonic devices compensate for memory difficulties), external strategies (e.g., time tables and navigation devices), or environmental strategies (e.g., eliminating distracting stimuli at work) (Huckans et al., 2013; Bajpai, Tripathi & Nehra, 2015).

The efficacy of these activities in rehabilitating cognitive functions has been seen in older adults, patients with MCI and Dementia. However, another set of mentally stimulating activities (such as reading, playing music) that increase an individual's active participation in their day to day life and draw from their hobbies and interests have also shown promising results (Kelly et al., 2014). The importance of and encouragement to engage in these types of activities communicated is through psycho-education programs. These interventions come under the umbrella of lifestyle interventions that target modifiable risk and protective factors by directly engaging individuals in healthy lifestyle practices (such as regular exercise, nutrition) (Huckans et al., 2013).Another set on interventions known as psychotherapeutic interventions directly target neuropsychiatric symptoms like depression and anxiety through techniques like Cognitive Behavior Therapy (CBT) and traditional relaxation and mindfulness (Huckans et al., 2013) Cognitive Behavior Therapy (CBT) is a structured, short term collaborative process between the client and therapist which is directed towards solving current problems and modifying dysfunctional (problematic) thinking and behavior. The therapist adopts a variety of methods of bring about a change in the clients thought process and belief system. However, the client is not passive in this process, the interaction is structured yet collaborative. The basic idea behind CBT is that when an individual realizes that there is a more productive and adaptive way of thinking, they change their thinking which further leads to improvement in their emotional states and behavior. Vast number of studies supports the effectiveness of CBT in treating depression symptoms in elderly. Studies have also shown continued effect of the same even after 1 year of follow up (Laidlaw et al., 2008). Further, aside from counselling patients on how to deal with their symptoms, dissemination of facts and statistics can also be comforting. For example, it can be revealed that only a minority of patients will progress to dementia annually. Further, many patients with MCI (40-70%) may not even progress to dementia even after 10 years.74 Importantly, some MCI patients (15-20%) have been found to have improved cognition1-2 years later, although the latter group may still remain at increased risk of future cognitive decline (Koepsell & Monsell, 2012; Plassman et al., 2008).

Thus, holistic history taking, longitudinal follow-up and serial cognitive assessments are useful since they allow a clearer assessment of patient's true baseline and trajectory of cognitive function over time, and decrease the risk that poor performance on a single assessment due to anxiety, fatigue, or acute illness leading to a false positive diagnosis (Langa & Levine, 2014).

FUTURE RESEARCH DIRECTIONS

Limited studies are available that point to the subtle differences between the overlapping cognitive deficits in the stated conditions. For instance, consistent findings have shown that episodic memory and executive functioning are the most sensitive measures in detecting individuals who may eventually develop Dementia (Chen et al., 2001). Further, investigators have also concluded that performance on fine and complex measures of psychomotor functioning may be as useful as traditional cognitive tests for detecting MCI, and should be incorporated in screening batteries (Rivas-Vazquez et al., 2004). However, there is still a dearth of such studies that can aid the process of differentiating between these conditions from a neuropsychological perspective (Nehra & Bajpai, 2013). Additionally, there is a dire need to investigate and standardize protocols for assessment with exhaustive history taking. Although it is not always necessary to evaluate exhaustively every aspect of mental functioning, certain critical functions should be assessed in every patient. These include level of consciousness, physical appearance, emotional status, attention, expressive and receptive language, memory, constructional ability and executive function.

History taking (Table 7) should be directed towards 4 major areas of clinical concern

- The presence or absence of the classic behavioural changes indicative of organic dysfunction (memory impairment or language disorder) must be established
- The possibility of functional psychiatric disorders must be considered
- Establish patients pre-morbid behaviour and level of functioning
- Evaluation of general medical status

Table 7. Signs to look out for

Cognitive Domain	Early Signs
Attention	• Poor concentration • Easily distracted • Cannot hold phone number in mind • Taking too long to complete tasks
Memory	• Poor recall of recent events • Repeating self • Needs reminders
Language	• Difficulty in keeping up with conversations • Word finding difficulty • Use of vague generic terms • Comprehension difficulty
Praxis, Somatosensory and Motor Functions	• Difficulty in use of familiar tools • Difficulty with sequencing of actions
Visuospatial Functions	Difficulty navigating familiar environment
Executive Functions	• Poor task persistence • Avoidance of multi stage activities

(Morimoto, Kanellopoulos & Alexopoulos, 2014)

CONCLUSION

Thus, the above stated conditions, namely, normal aging, mild cognitive impairment, depression, and dementia are linked closely to one another. As explained, the differences between normal aging and MCI are very subtle. Thus, in order to make the correct diagnosis, it is important to divulge more into these surface level differences and explore and evaluate sub domain differences through detailed neuropsychological assessment. However, there is a clear contrast between the cognitive functioning seen in MCI and Dementia which can most-importantly be differentiated through independence in performing activities of daily living. Further, depression is related to dementia and cognitive impairment in several ways (Ganguli, 2009):

- Both can occur together, independent from each other.
- Both can be manifestations of the same brain disease.
- Knowledge of presence of cognitive impairment can led to depression.
- Early onset of depression can be increase the probability for future development of dementia.

Although antidepressant medication is an important approach to treating depression, not all individuals respond to pharmacologic therapy, and some may experience adverse effects (Lyketsos et al., 2002). One useful approach in the context of cognitive impairment is to apply interventions that compensate for the compromised abilities. These interventions aim to reduce the symptoms, delay or prevent progression to dementia or increase the rate of conversion to normal cognition (Huckans et al., 2013).Similar approaches to cognitive-behavioural therapy and support groups have been helpful in facilitating problem solving and reducing negative affect among individuals with early dementia (Kasl-Godley &Gatz, 2000). Thus, developing guidelines for specific type of activities, defining degree of ability reflective of intact functioning would enhance sensitivity and specificity to diagnosis and holistic assessment.

REFERENCES

Algarabel González, S., Fuentes, M., Escudero, J., Pitarque, A., Peset, V., Mazón, J. F., & Meléndez Moral, J. C. (2012). Recognition memory deficits in mild cognitive impairment. *Neuropsychology, Development, and Cognition. Section B, Aging, Neuropsychology and Cognition*, *19*(5), 608–619. doi: 10.1080/13825585.2011.640657 PMID:22247955

Apfelbaum, E. P., Krendl, A. C., & Ambady, N. (2010). Age-related decline in executive function predicts better advice-giving in uncomfortable social contexts. *Journal of Experimental Social Psychology*, *46*(6), 1074–1077. doi:10.1016/j.jesp.2010.07.017

Arve, S., Tilvis, R. S., Lehtonen, A., Valvanne, J., & Sairanen, S. (1999). Coexistence of lowered mood and cognitive impairment of elderly people in five birth cohorts. *Aging (Milan, Italy)*, *11*(2), 90–95. PMID:10386168

Baddeley, A. (2000). The episodic buffer: A new component of working memory? *Trends in Cognitive Sciences*, *4*(11), 417–423. doi:10.1016/S1364-6613(00)01538-2 PMID:11058819

Bajpai, S., Tripathi, M., & Nehra, A. (2015). Cognitive Rehabilitation: A State Of The Art For Long Term Management Of Alzheimer Disease For Indian Population. In *Proceedings of 12th International Conference on Alzheimer's and Parkinson's Disease*. Nice, France.

Bajpai, S., Tripathi, M., Dey, A. B., & Nehra, A. (in press). Enhancing Memory & Activities of Daily Living (ADLs) In Patients with Early Alzheimer's disease using Memory Stimulation Intervention: A Randomized Controlled Trial. *International Journal of Advanced Medical and Health Research.*

Bazin, N., Perruchet, P., De Bonis, M., & Feline, A. (1994). The dissociation of explicit and implicit memory in depressed patients. *Psychological Medicine*, *24*(01), 239–245. doi:10.1017/S0033291700027008 PMID:8208889

Bennett, D. A., Wilson, R. S., Schneider, J. A., Evans, D. A., Beckett, L. A., Aggarwal, N. T., ... Bach, J. (2002). Natural history of mild cognitive impairment in older persons. *Neurology*, *59*(2), 198–205. doi:10.1212/WNL.59.2.198 PMID:12136057

Bieliauskas, L. A., Boczar, J., & Lamberty, G. (1991). Lack of depression effects on cognitive functions in the elderly. Journal of Clinical and Experimental Neuropsychology, 13(3), 433-433).

Bieliauskas, L. A., Costello, S., & Terpenning, M. (1991). Depression and screening for cognitive deficit in elderly patients. Journal of Clinical and Experimental Neuropsychology, 13(1), 101-101).

Bombois, S., Derambure, P., Pasquier, F., & Monaca, C. (2010). Sleep disorders in aging and dementia. *The Journal of Nutrition, Health & Aging*, *14*(3), 212–217. doi:10.1007/s12603-010-0052-7 PMID:20191256

Brown, P. J., Liu, X., Sneed, J. R., Pimontel, M. A., Devanand, D. P., & Roose, S. P. (2013). Speed of processing and depression affect function in older adults with mild cognitive impairment. *The American Journal of Geriatric Psychiatry*, *21*(7), 675–684. doi:10.1016/j.jagp.2013.01.005 PMID:23567401

Bruscoli, M., & Lovestone, S. (2004). Is MCI really just early dementia? A systematic review of conversion studies. *International Psychogeriatrics*, *16*(02), 129–140. doi:10.1017/S1041610204000092 PMID:15318760

Butters, M. A., Becker, J. T., Nebes, R. D., Zmuda, M. D., Mulsant, B. H., Pollock, B. G., & Reynolds, C. F. III. (2000). Changes in cognitive functioning following treatment of late-life depression. *The American Journal of Psychiatry*, *157*(12), 1949–1954. doi:10.1176/appi.ajp.157.12.1949 PMID:11097959

Butters, M. A., Whyte, E. M., Nebes, R. D., Begley, A. E., Dew, M. A., Mulsant, B. H., ... Reynolds, C. F. (2004). The nature and determinants of neuropsychological functioning in late-life depression. *Archives of General Psychiatry*, *61*(6), 587–595. doi:10.1001/archpsyc.61.6.587 PMID:15184238

Carlson, M. C., Hasher, L., Connelly, S. L., & Zacks, R. T. (1995). Aging, distraction, and the benefits of predictable location. *Psychology and Aging*, *10*(3), 427–436. doi:10.1037/0882-7974.10.3.427 PMID:8527063

Chasteen, A. L., Park, D. C., & Schwarz, N. (2001). Implementation intentions and facilitation of prospective memory. *Psychological Science*, *12*(6), 457–461. doi:10.1111/1467-9280.00385 PMID:11760131

Chen, P., Ganguli, M., Mulsant, B. H., & DeKosky, S. T. (1999). The temporal relationship between depressive symptoms and dementia: A community-based prospective study. *Archives of General Psychiatry*, *56*(3), 261–266. doi:10.1001/archpsyc.56.3.261 PMID:10078504

Chen, P., Ratcliff, G., Belle, S. H., Cauley, J. A., DeKosky, S. T., & Ganguli, M. (2001). Patterns of cognitive decline in presymptomatic Alzheimer disease: A prospective community study. *Archives of General Psychiatry*, *58*(9), 853–858. doi:10.1001/archpsyc.58.9.853 PMID:11545668

Collins, A., & Koechlin, E. (2012). Reasoning, learning, and creativity: Frontal lobe function and human decision-making. *PLoS Biology*, *10*(3), e1001293. doi:10.1371/journal.pbio.1001293 PMID:22479152

Danion, J. M., Kauffmann-Muller, F., Grangé, D., Zimmermann, M. A., & Greth, P. (1995). Affective valence of words, explicit and implicit memory in clinical depression. *Journal of Affective Disorders*, *34*(3), 227–234. doi:10.1016/0165-0327(95)00021-E PMID:7560551

Diamond, A. (2013). Executive functions. *Annual Review of Psychology*, *64*(1), 135–168. doi:10.1146/annurev-psych-113011-143750 PMID:23020641

Diniz, B. S., Pinto, J. A. Jr, & Forlenza, O. V. (2008). Do CSF total tau, phosphorylated tau, and β-amyloid 42 help to predict progression of mild cognitive impairment to Alzheimer's disease? A systematic review and meta-analysis of the literature. *The World Journal of Biological Psychiatry*, *9*(3), 172–182. doi:10.1080/15622970701535502 PMID:17886169

Flint, Alastair J. "Epidemiology and comorbidity of anxiety disorders in the elderly." *The American Journal of Psychiatry* 151.5 (1994): 640.

Friedman, A. S. (1964). Minimal effects of severe depression on cognitive functioning. *Journal of Abnormal and Social Psychology*, *69*(3), 237–243. doi:10.1037/h0048608 PMID:14210773

Ganguli, M. (2009). Depression, cognitive impairment and dementia: Why should clinicians care about the web of causation? *Indian Journal of Psychiatry*, *51*(5), 29. PMID:21416013

Gifford, J., & Jones, R. (2009). Assessment and treatment of cognitive deficits in dementia. *The Prescriber*, *20*(6), 45–49. doi:10.1002/psb.490

Glisky, E. L. (2007). Changes in cognitive function in human aging. In *Brain aging: Models, methods, and mechanisms* (pp. 3-20).

Gold, D. A. (2012). An examination of instrumental activities of daily living assessment in older adults and mild cognitive impairment. *Journal of Clinical and Experimental Neuropsychology*, *34*(1), 11–34. doi:10.1080/13803395.2011.614598 PMID:22053873

Gray, J. W., Rattan, A. I., & Dean, R. S. (1986). Differential diagnosis of dementia and depression in the elderly using neuropsychological methods. *Archives of Clinical Neuropsychology*, *1*(4), 341–349. doi:10.1093/arclin/1.4.341 PMID:14591414

Griffith, H. R., Belue, K., Sicola, A., Krzywanski, S., Zamrini, E., Harrell, L., & Marson, D. C. (2003). Impaired financial abilities in mild cognitive impairment A direct assessment approach. *Neurology*, *60*(3), 449–457. doi:10.1212/WNL.60.3.449 PMID:12578926

Harada, C. N., Love, M. C. N., & Triebel, K. L. (2013). Normal cognitive aging. *Clinics in Geriatric Medicine*, *29*(4), 737–752. doi:10.1016/j.cger.2013.07.002 PMID:24094294

Hart, R. P., & Kwentus, J. A. (1987). Psychomotor slowing and subcortical-type dysfunction in depression. *Journal of Neurology, Neurosurgery, and Psychiatry*, *50*(10), 1263–1266. doi:10.1136/jnnp.50.10.1263 PMID:3681304

Hayden, K. M., & Welsh-Bohmer, K. A. (2011). Epidemiology of cognitive aging and Alzheimer's disease: contributions of the cache county utah study of memory, health and aging. In *Behavioral Neurobiology of Aging* (pp. 3–31). Springer Berlin Heidelberg. doi:10.1007/7854_2011_152

He, W., Goodkind, D., &Kowal, P. (2016). An aging world: 2015. International population reports.

Holsinger, T., Deveau, J., Boustani, M., & Williams, J. W. (2007). Does this patient have dementia? *Journal of the American Medical Association*, *297*(21), 2391–2404. doi:10.1001/jama.297.21.2391 PMID:17551132

Howieson, D. B., Holm, L. A., Kaye, J. A., Oken, B. S., & Howieson, J. (1993). Neurologic function in the optimally healthy oldest old Neuropsychological evaluation. *Neurology*, *43*(10), 1882–1882. doi:10.1212/WNL.43.10.1882 PMID:8413942

Huckans, M., Hutson, L., Twamley, E., Jak, A., Kaye, J., & Storzbach, D. (2013). Efficacy of cognitive rehabilitation therapies for mild cognitive impairment (MCI) in older adults: Working toward a theoretical model and evidence-based interventions. *Neuropsychology Review*, *23*(1), 63–80. doi:10.1007/s11065-013-9230-9 PMID:23471631

Hutchens, R. L., Kinsella, G. J., Ong, B., Pike, K. E., Clare, L., Ames, D., ... Parsons, S. (2013). Relationship between control beliefs, strategy use, and memory performance in amnestic mild cognitive impairment and healthy aging. *The Journals of Gerontology. Series B, Psychological Sciences and Social Sciences*, *68*(6), 862–871. doi:10.1093/geronb/gbt016 PMID:23550087

Jorm, A. F. (2001). History of depression as a risk factor for dementia: An updated review. *The Australian and New Zealand Journal of Psychiatry*, *35*(6), 776–781. doi:10.1046/j.1440-1614.2001.00967.x PMID:11990888

Jurjanz, L., Donix, M., Amanatidis, E. C., Meyer, S., Poettrich, K., Huebner, T., ... Holthoff, V. A. (2011). Visual personal familiarity in amnestic mild cognitive impairment. *PLoS One*, *6*(5), e20030. doi:10.1371/journal.pone.0020030 PMID:21625502

Kang, H., Zhao, F., You, L., Giorgetta, C., Venkatesh, D., Sarkhel, S., & Prakash, R. (2014). Pseudo-dementia: A neuropsychological review. *Annals of Indian Academy of Neurology*, *17*(2), 147. doi:10.4103/0972-2327.132613 PMID:25024563

Kasl-Godley, J., & Gatz, M. (2000). Psychosocial interventions for individuals with dementia: An integration of theory, therapy, and a clinical understanding of dementia. *Clinical Psychology Review*, *20*(6), 755–782. doi:10.1016/S0272-7358(99)00062-8 PMID:10983267

Kelly, M. E., Loughrey, D., Lawlor, B. A., Robertson, I. H., Walsh, C., & Brennan, S. (2014). The impact of cognitive training and mental stimulation on cognitive and everyday functioning of healthy older adults: A systematic review and meta-analysis. *Ageing Research Reviews*, *15*, 28–43. doi:10.1016/j.arr.2014.02.004 PMID:24607830

Koepsell, T. D., & Monsell, S. E. (2012). Reversion from mild cognitive impairment to normal or near-normal cognition Risk factors and prognosis. *Neurology*, *79*(15), 1591–1598. doi:10.1212/WNL.0b013e31826e26b7 PMID:23019264

Kramer, J. H., Nelson, A., Johnson, J. K., Yaffe, K., Glenn, S., Rosen, H. J., & Miller, B. L. (2006). Multiple cognitive deficits in amnestic mild cognitive impairment. *Dementia and Geriatric Cognitive Disorders*, *22*(4), 306–311. doi:10.1159/000095303 PMID:16931884

Kueider, A., & Rebok, G. (2014). Cognitive Training for Older Adults: What Is It and Does It Work? Center on Ageing, American Institutes for Research.

Laidlaw, K., Davidson, K., Toner, H., Jackson, G., Clark, S., Law, J., ... Cross, S. (2008). A randomised controlled trial of cognitive behaviour therapy vs treatment as usual in the treatment of mild to moderate late life depression. *International Journal of Geriatric Psychiatry*, *23*(8), 843–850. doi:10.1002/gps.1993 PMID:18311844

Langa, K. M., & Levine, D. A. (2014). The diagnosis and management of mild cognitive impairment: A clinical review. *Journal of the American Medical Association*, *312*(23), 2551–2561. doi:10.1001/jama.2014.13806 PMID:25514304

Lin, J. S., O'Connor, E., Rossom, R. C., Perdue, L. A., & Eckstrom, E. (2013). Screening for cognitive impairment in older adults: A systematic review for the US Preventive Services Task Force. *Annals of Internal Medicine*, *159*(9), 601–612. PMID:24145578

Lopez, O. L., Jagust, W. J., DeKosky, S. T., Becker, J. T., Fitzpatrick, A., Dulberg, C., ... Carlson, M. (2003). Prevalence and classification of mild cognitive impairment in the Cardiovascular Health Study Cognition Study: Part 1. *Archives of Neurology*, *60*(10), 1385–1389. doi:10.1001/archneur.60.10.1385 PMID:14568808

Lunt, L., Bramham, J., Morris, R. G., Bullock, P. R., Selway, R. P., Xenitidis, K., & David, A. S. (2012). Prefrontal cortex dysfunction and 'Jumping to Conclusions': Bias or deficit? *Journal of Neuropsychology*, *6*(1), 65–78. doi:10.1111/j.1748-6653.2011.02005.x PMID:22257612

Lyketsos, C. G., Lopez, O., Jones, B., Fitzpatrick, A. L., Breitner, J., & DeKosky, S. (2002). Prevalence of neuropsychiatric symptoms in dementia and mild cognitive impairment: Results from the cardiovascular health study. *Journal of the American Medical Association*, *288*(12), 1475–1483. doi:10.1001/jama.288.12.1475 PMID:12243634

McCarten, J. R. (2013). Clinical evaluation of early cognitive symptoms. *Clinics in Geriatric Medicine*, *29*(4), 791–807. doi:10.1016/j.cger.2013.07.005 PMID:24094297

McIntyre, R. S., Cha, D. S., Soczynska, J. K., Woldeyohannes, H. O., Gallaugher, L. A., Kudlow, P., ... Baskaran, A. (2013). Cognitive deficits and functional outcomes in major depressive disorder: Determinants, substrates, and treatment interventions. *Depression and Anxiety*, *30*(6), 515–527. doi:10.1002/da.22063 PMID:23468126

Miller, E., & Lewis, P. (1977). Recognition memory in elderly patients with depression and dementia: A signal detection analysis. *Journal of Abnormal Psychology*, *86*(1), 84–86. doi:10.1037/0021-843X.86.1.84 PMID:838953

Miyake, A., Friedman, N. P., Emerson, M. J., Witzki, A. H., Howerter, A., & Wager, T. D. (2000). The unity and diversity of executive functions and their contributions to complex "frontal lobe" tasks: A latent variable analysis. *Cognitive Psychology*, *41*(1), 49–100. doi:10.1006/cogp.1999.0734 PMID:10945922

Morimoto, S. S., Kanellopoulos, T., & Alexopoulos, G. S. (2014). Cognitive Impairment in Depressed Older Adults: Implications for Prognosis and Treatment. *Psychiatric Annals*, *44*(3), 138–142. doi:10.3928/00485713-20140306-05 PMID:25821256

Murray, C. J., & Lopez, A. D. (1996). Evidence-based health policy--lessons from the Global Burden of Disease Study. *Science*, *274*(5288), 740–743. doi:10.1126/science.274.5288.740 PMID:8966556

Nehra, A., & Bajpai, S. (2013). *The Importance of Diagnosis & Assessment of Dementia: From a Neuropsychological Perspective. Alzheimer's & related Disorders Society of India (ARSDI)* (pp. 43–46). Delhi Chapter.

Nehra, A., & Bajpai, S. (2015). *Normal Aging Versus Dementia: Which signs to look for? Alzheimer's & Related Disorders Society of India (ARSDI)*. Delhi Chapter.

Ownby, R. L., Crocco, E., Acevedo, A., John, V., & Loewenstein, D. (2006). Depression and risk for Alzheimer disease: Systematic review, meta-analysis, and metaregression analysis. *Archives of General Psychiatry*, *63*(5), 530–538. doi:10.1001/archpsyc.63.5.530 PMID:16651510

Palazzolo, J. (2015). Cognitive Behavioral Therapy for Depression and Anxiety in the Elderly. *Ann Depress and Anxiety*, *2*(6), 1063.

Petersen, R. C. (2004). Mild cognitive impairment as a diagnostic entity. *Journal of Internal Medicine*, *256*(3), 183–194. doi:10.1111/j.1365-2796.2004.01388.x PMID:15324362

Petersen, R. C., Doody, R., Kurz, A., Mohs, R. C., Morris, J. C., Rabins, P. V., ... Winblad, B. (2001). Current concepts in mild cognitive impairment. *Archives of Neurology*, *58*(12), 1985–1992. doi:10.1001/archneur.58.12.1985 PMID:11735772

Petersen, R. C., Smith, G. E., Waring, S. C., Ivnik, R. J., Tangalos, E. G., & Kokmen, E. (1999). Mild cognitive impairment: Clinical characterization and outcome. *Archives of Neurology*, *56*(3), 303–308. doi:10.1001/archneur.56.3.303 PMID:10190820

Plassman, B. L., Langa, K. M., Fisher, G. G., Heeringa, S. G., Weir, D. R., Ofstedal, M. B., ... Steffens, D. C. (2008). Prevalence of cognitive impairment without dementia in the United States. *Annals of Internal Medicine*, *148*(6), 427–434. doi:10.7326/0003-4819-148-6-200803180-00005 PMID:18347351

Potter, G. G., & Steffens, D. C. (2007). Contribution of depression to cognitive impairment and dementia in older adults. *The Neurologist*, *13*(3), 105–117. doi:10.1097/01.nrl.0000252947.15389.a9 PMID:17495754

Raskin, A., Friedman, A. S., & DiMascio, A. (1982). Cognitive and performance deficits in depression. *Psychopharmacology Bulletin*, *18*(4), 196–202. PMID:7156290

Reifler, B. V. (2000). A case of mistaken identity: Pseudodementia is really predementia. *Journal of the American Geriatrics Society*, *48*(5), 593–594. doi:10.1111/j.1532-5415.2000.tb05010.x PMID:10811557

Reischies, F. M., & Neu, P. (2000). Comorbidity of mild cognitive disorder and depression–a neuropsychological analysis. *European Archives of Psychiatry and Clinical Neuroscience*, *250*(4), 186–193. doi:10.1007/s004060070023 PMID:11009071

Ritchie, K., Artero, S., & Touchon, J. (2001). Classification criteria for mild cognitive impairment A population-based validation study. *Neurology*, *56*(1), 37–42. doi:10.1212/WNL.56.1.37 PMID:11148233

Rivas-Vazquez, R. A., Mendez, C., Rey, G. J., & Carrazana, E. J. (2004). Mild cognitive impairment: New neuropsychological and pharmacological target. *Archives of Clinical Neuropsychology*, *19*(1), 11–27. doi:10.1093/arclin/19.1.11 PMID:14670376

Rubin, D. C. (2000). Autobiographical memory and aging.

Salthouse, T. A. (1984). Effects of age and skill in typing. *Journal of Experimental Psychology. General*, *113*(3), 345.

Salthouse, T. A. (2010). Selective review of cognitive aging. *Journal of the International Neuropsychological Society: JINS*, *16*(5), 754–760. doi:10.1017/S1355617710000706 PMID:20673381

Salthouse, T. A., Fristoe, N. M., Lineweaver, T. T., & Coon, V. E. (1995). Aging of attention: Does the ability to divide decline? *Memory & Cognition*, *23*(1), 59–71. doi:10.3758/BF03210557 PMID:7885266

Saunders, N. L., & Summers, M. J. (2010). Attention and working memory deficits in mild cognitive impairment. *Journal of Clinical and Experimental Neuropsychology*, *32*(4), 350–357. doi:10.1080/13803390903042379 PMID:19787522

Schoenberg, M. R., & Scott, J. G. (2011). *The little black book of neuropsychology: A syndrome-based approach*.

Schönknecht, P. (2011). Neurobiological and psychological aspects of mild cognitive impairment Bridging the gap.

Seelye, A. M., Schmitter-Edgecombe, M., & Flores, J. (2010). Episodic memory predictions in persons with amnestic and nonamnestic mild cognitive impairment. *Journal of Clinical and Experimental Neuropsychology*, *32*(4), 433–441. doi:10.1080/13803390903201751 PMID:20397298

Singh-Manoux, A., Kivimaki, M., Glymour, M. M., Elbaz, A., Berr, C., Ebmeier, K. P., ... Dugravot, A. (2012). Timing of onset of cognitive decline: Results from Whitehall II prospective cohort study. *BMJ (Clinical Research Ed.)*, *344*, d7622. doi:10.1136/bmj.d7622 PMID:22223828

Smith, G., Del Sala, S., Logie, R. H., & Maylor, E. A. (2000). Prospective and retrospective memory in normal ageing and dementia: A questionnaire study. *Memory (Hove, England)*, *8*(5), 311–321. doi:10.1080/09658210050117735 PMID:11045239

Teng, E., Tassniyom, K., & Lu, P. H. (2012). Reduced quality-of-life ratings in mild cognitive impairment: Analyses of subject and informant responses. *The American Journal of Geriatric Psychiatry*, *20*(12), 1016–1025. doi:10.1097/JGP.0b013e31826ce640 PMID:23018474

Varjassyová, A., Hořínek, D., Andel, R., Amlerova, J., Laczó, J., Sheardová, K., ... Geda, Y. E. (2013). Recognition of facial emotional expression in amnestic mild cognitive impairment. *Journal of Alzheimer's Disease*, *33*(1), 273–280. PMID:22954669

Veiel, H. O. (1997). A preliminary profile of neuropsychological deficits associated with major depression. *Journal of Clinical and Experimental Neuropsychology*, *19*(4), 587–603. doi:10.1080/01688639708403745 PMID:9342691

West, R., Herndon, R. W., & Covell, E. (2003). Neural correlates of age-related declines in the formation and realization of delayed intentions. *Psychology and Aging*, *18*(3), 461–473. doi:10.1037/0882-7974.18.3.461 PMID:14518808

Whalley, L. J., Deary, I. J., Appleton, C. L., & Starr, J. M. (2004). Cognitive reserve and the neurobiology of cognitive aging. *Ageing Research Reviews*, *3*(4), 369–382. doi:10.1016/j.arr.2004.05.001 PMID:15541707

Wolk, D. A., Mancuso, L., Kliot, D., Arnold, S. E., & Dickerson, B. C. (2013). Familiarity-based memory as an early cognitive marker of preclinical and prodromal AD. *Neuropsychologia*, *51*(6), 1094–1102. doi:10.1016/j.neuropsychologia.2013.02.014 PMID:23474075

Yanhong, O., Chandra, M., & Venkatesh, D. (2013). Mild cognitive impairment in adult: A neuropsychological review. *Annals of Indian Academy of Neurology*, *16*(3), 310. doi:10.4103/0972-2327.116907 PMID:24101808

Zakzanis, K., Leach, L., & Kaplan, E. (1998). On the nature and pattern of neurocognitive function in major depressive disorder. *Cognitive and Behavioral Neurology*, *11*(3), 111–119. PMID:9742509

Zheng, D., Dong, X., Sun, H., Xu, Y., Ma, Y., & Wang, X. (2012). The overall impairment of core executive function components in patients with amnestic mild cognitive impairment: A cross-sectional study. *BMC Neurology*, *12*(1), 138. doi:10.1186/1471-2377-12-138 PMID:23164134

Zillmer, E. A., Spiers, M. V., & Culbertson, W. (2007). *Principles of neuropsychology*. Nelson Education.

KEY TERMS AND DEFINITIONS

Attention: It is the concentration of awareness on some phenomenon to the exclusion of other stimuli in the environment.

Cognition: Cognition is a term referring to the mental processes involved in gaining knowledge and comprehension. These processes include thinking, knowing, remembering, judging and problem-solving.

Delirium: It is a state of severe confusion and rapid changes in brain function. However, it is differentiated from Dementia by acute onset, fluctuating course and impaired consciousness.

Executive Function: Executive functions are a set of cognitive processes that are necessary for the cognitive control of behavior: selecting and successfully monitoring behaviors that facilitate the attainment of chosen goals. Executive functions include basic cognitive processes such as attentional control, cognitive inhibition, inhibitory control, working memory, and cognitive flexibility. Higher order executive functions require the simultaneous use of multiple basic executive functions and include planning and fluid intelligence.

Impairment: A state of diminished or weakened ability especially in a specified faculty/ domain

Language: Language is a formal system of communication which involves the combination of words and/or symbols, whether written or spoken, as well as some rules that govern them.

Memory: Memory is the faculty of the mind by which information is encoded, stored and retrieved.

Neuropsychological Rehabilitation: Neuropsychological rehabilitation can be defined as teaching or retraining activities aimed at improving and alleviating symptoms associated with brain damage or brain dysfunction

Processing Speed: It is the speed with which various cognitive activities are performed.

Pseudo-Dementia: It is defined as cognitive impairment that mimics dementia however diminishes upon remission of depression. Further, it is marked by detailed account of cognitive impairment, subjective memory loss and frequent "don't know" answers.

Visuospatial Ability: It is the capacity to identify visual and spatial relationships among objects. Visuospatial ability is measured in terms of the ability to imagine objects, to make global shapes by locating small components.

Chapter 7
Cognition in Ageing:
Implications for Assessment and Intervention

Susmita Halder
Institute of Psychiatry, India

Akash Kumar Mahato
Amity University, India

ABSTRACT

This chapter focuses on cognitive functions and impairment in the elderly; its implications in daily functioning with inputs on differences in the existing literature. The chapter further focuses on the diagnostic and assessment issues and intervention strategies. Ageing is an inevitable phase of life and encompasses changes in physical, psychological and social realms of an individual. Concern with the dwindling health and presence of any medical issues make the geriatric population prone to develop mental health conditions. Poor memory and reduced functional ability is one of the common complaints from older adults coming to psychiatric or neurology clinics. Cognitive functions have been well documented regarding their role in daily functioning of an individual. With growing age of the brain; while some cognitive functions do slow down; some of the functions do evolve better with experience. In this context, it is important to differentiate between normal age related cognitive changes and symptoms of any degenerative disease.

INTRODUCTION

Weakening of bodily and mental functions with age is an inevitable phase of human life. Advances in medicine have enhanced the life span of humans across the globe. As per United Nations World population ageing report (2015), the elderly population across the world is growing with steady acceleration; and by year 2030, the number of people aged 60 years or above is projected to reach 1.4 billion, a growth of 56 percent. And by 2050, the global population of older persons is projected to more than double its

DOI: 10.4018/978-1-5225-3480-8.ch007

size in 2015, reaching nearly 2.1 billion. It is imperative that with this enormous number of people, the ratio of those seeking medical attention will also be very high. As per an estimate, in year 2015, 46.8 million people across the world suffered from dementia and this number is projected to reach 131.5 million by year 2050 (ADI, 2015). The cumulative incidence of Alzheimer dementia has been estimated to rise from about 5% by age 70 to 50% by age 90, making it a very common disease (Hebert et al., 1995). Increasing longevity and demographic shifts in many societies will stress the health systems unless a cure for AD is found or at least any therapy that postpones the onset of the dementia by 5 to 10 years for the time being (Wimo, Jonsson & Winblad, 2006).

The chapter focuses on how cognition changes over age and whether all aged do have cognitive impairment. And if cognitive impairment does happen, what is its impact on daily functioning of the individual and the intervention strategies. Existing literature support that with age cognitive functions do get lowered, however this is not uniform. Cognitive ageing can be seen as decline in mental functions of an individual with increasing age. This decline in mental functions is more pronounced in fluid mental abilities (Deary et al., 2009) which include memory functions, processing speed, executive functions and reasoning. Compared to this, the crystallized mental capabilities like verbal abilities, general knowledge are less affected. While all mental functions are required for optimum functioning in daily life, the lowering of these functions brings down the fluency and independence in daily living. Attempts to classify cognitive decline dates back several decades, as Kral (1962) introduced the term 'benign senescent forgetfulness' to differentiate between normal memory function, pathological memory processes and mild form of memory loss. Well established longitudinal studies, like Schaie and Hofer (2001) suggested categories of aged people depending on type of cognitive deterioration they have and could be put as:

- Those who age normally,
- The super normal,
- Those who have mild cognitive impairment, and
- Those who develop dementia.

It is imperative from this type of classification that cognitive ageing is not uniform and some individuals can have healthy cognitive functions and function very independently till their death. However, the number of such super normals is comparatively much less than the more frequent group of normal ageing. The normal ageing group characteristically reach an asymptote in their 30's or early 40's, maintain a plateau until late 50's or early 60's followed by a modest decline on most abilities through the early 80's (Schaie, 2008). From a clinical perspective, this becomes obvious that consultation with medical experts for complaints relating to cognitive ageing is proportional to the severity of the impairment. However, severity of symptoms itself may not warrant the person to seek medical assistance, and family members wait until severe medical conditions or behavioural problems.

CHARACTERISTICS OF COGNITIVE AGEING

The profile of people coming to clinics with complain related to cognitive ageing range from forgetfulness, repeating task already done or insisting on having done the task not done in actual, asking same question again and again, forgetting name of people, difficulty in recalling address, travel independently, forgetting route to home and so on. Associated features of irritability, low mood, agitation, stubbornness, increased or decreased speech productions are often reported. The impact of reported symptoms varies from person to person depending on premorbid functioning, occupational engagement as well as familial engagements and support. It is important to assess and see the level of cognitive functions of ageing people reporting with related problems, so that appropriate management plans are drawn and non-significant symptoms are addressed accordingly.

CONCEPT OF MILD COGNITIVE IMPAIRMENT (MCI)

Mild cognitive impairment can be best understood as an intermediate or transitional stage between age appropriate normal cognitive aging and dementia. That is, the syndrome is higher in severity of age related cognitive decline but not severe enough to cause major dysfunction and diagnosed as dementia. The term Mild cognitive impairment was introduced by Reisberg (1988) as he described the stages of cognitive decline in dementia. The concept of Mild cognitive impairment may not be very new but its relative use in clinical practice could be dubious, as clinician may tend to diagnose cases only as dementia or not dementia. Peterson and colleagues (1999) defined the core diagnostic criteria of Mild Cognitive Impairment as follows;

- Memory complaint
- Objective memory impairment for age
- Normal general cognitive function
- Normal activities of daily living and
- No dementia

The syndrome of MCI is suggested to be heterogeneous with four subtypes:

1. Amnestic MCI, single domain
2. Amnestic MCI, multiple domain
3. Non- Amnestic MCI, single domain
4. Non- Amnestic MCI, multiple domain

The amnestic MCI primarily involves only memory impairment in single or multiple domains; while the non- amnestic type includes discrete cognitive impairments other than memory functions, that can be in single or multiple domains.

It is pretty obvious that the more severe form of cognitive impairment or dementia is easy to diagnose, but mild cognitive impairment pose some challenge in assessment and diagnosis. Much of this challenge comes from lack of normative data for age appropriate cognitive decline. As MCI is an intermediate stage between age appropriate cognitive decline and dementia; the boundary between the categories may appear diffuse making it difficult to differentiate between MCI with age related cognitive decline.

COMPARATIVE PRESENTATION OF NORMAL AGING WITH MCI AND ALZHEIMER'S

The following Table 1 is a description of cognitive decline and complaints in normal aging group compared with actual individual cases with mild cognitive impairment and Alzheimer's disease. The profile of normal aged in the Table 1 is taken from study on 50 healthy subjects aged 60-70 years, selected through purposive sampling (Thapliyal, Halder & Mahato, 2016). The findings are interesting, considering the mean MMSE score of the normal ageing sample was 26 which suggest no gross cognitive impairment. Despite this there were several domains of memory, where impairment was noticed. Verbal fluency and response inhibition of this group was impaired compared to available comparable normative data. Most importantly, the group had no dysfunction in activities of daily living and did not consult anybody for the subtle impairments in the cognitive functions. This also brings into light, the orientation of family members and their acceptance of age related changes in functionality and memory issues. Probably it would be easy to differentiate a person with mild cognitive impairment with that of dementia, but could be difficult to differentiate with normal age-related impairment. There could be dearth of global data over how much of a population slides down from normal age-related decline to mild cognitive impairment and further into dementia; but here lies the importance of early identification and early intervention to retard this progression. The comparative profile of normal aging, MCI and Alzheimer's disease, suggests

Table 1. Comparative presentation of normal aging with mci and Alzheimer's

	Normal Aging	MCI	Alzheimer's Disease
Age	60-70 years. Mean age 63.6 years	60 years, Male educated upto10th	62 years, Male
Reported complaints	None reported	Memory problems,forgetfulness, difficulty remembering things	Difficulty in remembering information, parts of conversation, date and time; inability to perform role at workplace and home with responsibility
Memory functions	Mean MMSE- 26.62 Intact recent and remote memory. Reduced verbal working memory. Deficits in visual–spatial memory.	Nothing significant on dementia rating scale, or not demented But impairment in recent memory, delayed recall, verbal retention for dissimilar pairs, visual retention and recognition	MMSE score- 16. significant impairment in all domains, recall, retention, recognition
Problem solving	-	-	Poor problem-solving skill, poor comprehension
Attention	Reduced temporal sequencing. Poor attention and concentration	Poor attention and concentration	Significantly impaired
Visuo- Motor Visuo spatial	None	Mild level	Difficulty in reception of stimuli, consolidated execution of tasks
Language	Lowered verbal fluency and semantic processing ability or word knowledge.	Mild level of impairment	Grossly impaired
Activities of daily living	No impairment reported	None	IDEAS 6 (global score) Gross difficulties
Mood symptoms	None reported	None	High Irritability

that the distinction between normal aging and mild cognitive impairment are very subtle and could be difficult to differentiate unless assessed on formal assessment tools. Considering that MCI is a gradual progression from stage of normal ageing towards Alzheimer's, this becomes a vital stage for intervention.

IMPACT OF COGNITIVE DECLINE ON DAILY LIFE

The impact of cognitive decline could be grave and different people react and cope differently with the changes. As described earlier, forgetfulness could be the most common complaint. The severity can range from forgetting simple instruction, forgetting items or locating items at home, to forgetting names of acquaint people family members, addresses. Individuals can repeat doing the same task or be convinced of doing the task without doing it. Memory impairment can have an impact on communication with others as individual fail to relate or recollect events. They have difficulty in understanding multiple instructions and taking complex decisions. People with cognitive impairment are also at risk of financial fraud and exploitation. The cognitive decline may impact an individual's capacity to travel independently and they may need an assistant when stepping outside home. Individuals react to these changes in different ways. Some may withdraw and confine themselves at home. Some may be more rigid recognising the symptoms but unwilling to take assistance of other, putting themselves at risk. Symptoms of low mood, irritability and agitation are often reported by family members of clients with cognitive decline.

FRAMEWORK OF COGNITIVE ASSESSMENT IN ELDERLY

When talking about cognitive decline in elderly one may not be at fault of thinking about memory impairment only. However, cognitive decline could manifest in different domains starting from memory, to language, visuo-spatial skills, executive functions, attention, psychomotor speed, and information processing. It is advised to go for a thorough neuro-cognitive evaluation, so that functioning level of each domain is clear to the client as well as therapist. However, this may not be possible always to go for detail evaluation and subsequently domain specific assessment could be done. The following domains after initial screening need to be carefully examined and cross checked with caregivers to correlate.

- Memory
- Language and Speech
- Attention
- Visuo spatial
- Motor functions
- Executive functions
- Family Rating

The assessment tools mentioned along are general reference and not exhaustive. There could be several other assessment tools which could be more suitable for individual assessment of elderly people with cognitive decline.

Initial Screening

The mini mental status examination (MMSE) developed by Folstein and Folstein (1975) over the years has established itself as a gold standard in screening for cognitive impairment. The tool is probably one of the most widely used screening tools across the world. While there are minor variations over the cut-off score for different people depending on years of schooling or age; the tool is a highly reliable and valid instrument for screening cognitive impairment. However, certain limitations erupt when the client taking the assessment is either illiterate or is unable to respond due to some other comorbid condition. The tool also has limitation in detecting cognitive impairment in highly educated. To counter this, higher cut-offs have been suggested (O'Bryantt et al., 2008). The tool is available in English and translated into local vernacular; but many clinicians may end up using the tool with clients not familiar with the language, making the finding invalid. While MMSE has a strong literature to support its screening capability, the tool does not give impression regarding finer cognitive domains, neither it claims so. As mentioned in the study quoted above (Thapliyal et al., 2016), the study samples had subtle cognitive impairment, despite having scores above cut-off on the MMSE. Some other screening tools that can be used for detection of Mild Cognitive Impairment, are the Montreal Cognitive Assessment (Nasreddine et al., 2005), which has a sensitivity of 80 to 100% and specificity of 50 to 76% for detecting MCI (Langa & Levine, 2014).

Memory

Memory is one of the most important cognitive functions. It is a complex process that includes encoding, storage, and retrieval of information. The process while may sound simple, is not that simple and helpful only when the person is able to retrieve the desired information. While family and care givers of ageing clients may complain of 'poor and weakened memory'; memory itself is not a single entity and have different forms or levels. Each form of memory has different impact on overall functioning of ageing people and widely documented in literature. Thus, it is important to assess different domains of memory in ageing population, as not all domains of memory will get impaired and some remain intact despite ageing.

Among all the domains of memory, the working memory or the short-term memory appears to have relatively higher importance. Working memory is vital for performing mental operations that helps in communicating with others, calculation, relating our ideas to behaviour and meaningful analysis of consistent inflow of information. Impairment in working memory translates into difficulty in maintaining conversation, forgetting instruction or tasks, repeating question. The capacity as well as duration for which information can be held in working memory is limited, thus any decline in working memory will have its impact on daily functioning.

There are a host of assessment tools for assessing memory functions, like the Wechsler Memory Scale (WMS): The WMS is one of the most widely used tools to assess memory functions. Currently in its fourth edition, the Wechsler Memory Scale IV (WMS IV) is suitable for age ranges 16 to 90 years. The scale has good psychometric properties and scores are summarized into five indexes, namely auditory memory, visual memory, visual working memory, immediate memory and delayed memory. The scale is known to differentiate clinical groups such as dementia or neurological disorders (Hunsley & Lee, 2010; Kessels, Overbeek & Bouman, 2015); however certain subcomponents of the scale are doubted of its efficacy in detecting subtle impairment in the mild cognitive impairment population (Pike et al., 2013)

Rey Auditory Verbal Learning Test (RAVLT): The RAVLT is a brief pencil-and-paper measure that assesses immediate memory span, new learning, susceptibility to interference, and recognition memory (Strauss & Spreen, 2006). It is an established tool to measure verbal memory in people aged 16 years and older. Literatures suggests its utility in differentiating memory functions in healthy controls, mild cognitive impairment and dementia (Ramlall, Chipps, Bhigiee, & Pillay, 2014)

Language and Speech

With growing age and reducing command over linguistic complexity, older adults tend to use short sentences for communication. While language deficits are very clear in dementia, there may not be gross deficits or observable difficulties in age associated cognitive decline. However, studies do suggest a parallel between linguistic deficits in mild cognitive impairment and dementia (Taler & Phillips, 2008). It is vital to assess certain aspects of language and speech like verbal fluency, naming capacity, syntactic processing as well as receptive language. The Controlled Oral Word Association Test (COWA) is an easy measure of phonemic verbal fluency with simple construct where participant is asked to name words beginning with specific letters excluding proper noun. Phonemic verbal fluency is a valuable approach for detecting cognitive alterations in the aged, given its stability throughout the ageing process (Steiner et al., 2008).

The other component of verbal fluency is semantic, also referred to as category fluency and assessed by different versions of naming tests like the Boston Naming Test, Category Fluency test, Animal Naming test to a name a few. Review suggests that when the specificities of the various verbal fluency test measures are equated, the animal naming verbal fluency test score is most sensitive measure to distinguish normal aging from dementia (Diesfeldt, Vander Elst, & Jolles, 2009). Longitudinal studies representing repeated evaluations of letter and category fluency over a group average of 2.3 to 5.9 years also confirm greater longitudinal declines in category compared to letter fluency. Longitudinal declines in fluency also differentiate unimpaired participants from those who will develop Alzheimer's disease (Clark et al., 2009). Thus, verbal fluency is an important component for assessment.

Attention

One of the most vital cognitive functions, attention is integral in processing the information human brain is presented with. It has been conceptualized as the gateway for information inflow to the brain (Cohen, 1993) and allows the individual to filter relevant and irrelevant information as per the individual and monitor appropriate response to the stimuli. Attention functions decline with age and the function is affected in majority of patients of neurological disorders. Thus, it needs to be assessed in elderly people brought for consultation. A host of measures for assessing attention are available. While the Digit span test and digit symbol tests are simple in construct; tests like the Trail Making Test (TMT) assess visual search, scanning, sequencing, switching and speed aspects (Spreen & Strauss, 2006).

Visuo-Spatial

This involves the ability to understand space in two and three dimensions. One component of it is construction skills that involves the ability to put together individual parts to make a coherent whole and is subject to decline over time (Howieson, Holm, Kaye,Oken, & Howieson,1993).The other component is visuo-spatial abilities that includes object perception, the ability to recognize familiar objects such as household items or faces, and spatial perception, the ability to appreciate the physical location of objects either alone or in relation to other objects remain intact (Harada, Natelson Love, & Triebel, 2013). Research has shown that spatial-sequential working memory is subject to age-related decline (Brown, 2016).

Several other studies also suggest that spatial working memory decline across aging that could contribute to age-dependent deterioration in both visuo-motor learning processes. However, spatial working memory integrity seems to affect strategic learning decline even after controlling for aging (Luis A, Rosalinda, Israel, & Juan, 2015). The clock drawing test is a popular measure of visual perception and can be administered on both children as well as adults. It assesses visual spatial abilities, executive control and visual inattention processes of the individual and has adequate test retest reliability (Spreen & Strauss, 2006).

Motor Functions

Motor functions are apparently the most observable because of gait, hand movements of the individual and decline in motor functions could be quite intriguing. Review suggests motor functions are not significantly impaired in normal aging but could be in very mild Alzheimer's (Pettersson, Olsson, & Wahlund, 2005). Motor functions thus need to be assessed in elderly clients reporting with cognitive problems. The Grooved pegboard can be used to assess motor function reliably in person 6-85 years of age. Another common assessment is the Finger tapping or the Finger oscillation test.

Executive Functions

Executive functions are central for self -regulation. Seen as regulated by the frontal region of the brain, the functions help us in selecting and monitoring our behaviour. Defined as collection of processes that are responsible for guiding, directing, and managing cognitive, emotional, and behavioural functions, particularly during active, novel problem solving (Gioia, Isquith, Guy, & Kenworthy, 2000). Lezak described four components of executive functions that are volition; planning; purposive action; and effective performance (Lezak et al., 2004). The stroop test, Category test, Wisconsin card sorting test are some of the reliable and popular measures of executive functions in use.

Family Rating

Although not exactly an assessment of cognitive domains, it is vital to take a view point of family members and caregivers about the functioning of their ward. Family can provide vital information regarding activities of daily living, behavioural, and mood issues regarding the client.

INTERVENTIONS

Intervention for age related cognitive decline may appear like delaying the inevitable. Much of the management for advanced stages of cognitive decline i.e. dementia relies on pharmacological treatment, dietary supplements, and physical exercise. Cognitive retraining, life style management and family support are other psychosocial methods of intervention used in cognitive decline. It is important to remind that there is not much of functional impairment in normal ageing as well as mild cognitive impairment. It is only in advanced stage that functional impairments are apparent. This stresses the importance of early identification and customized treatment plan for the elderly. Early identification can help in smooth progression and easy adaptability of the family members as well as the client for the expected emotional and behavioural changes. Appropriate measures can at least delay the process if not prevent the condition from worsening. Following intervention strategies can be adopted in clients with cognitive decline. This is a general frame and could be customised as per the needs of the client and feasibilities.

1. Early identification.
2. Psychoeducation and counselling to family and caregivers.
3. Addressing risk factors and other medical conditions.
4. Management of mood symptoms.
5. Daily activity scheduling (guided/ independent).
6. Involvement in physical activity and leisure activity.
7. Cognitive retraining.
8. Behavioural management.
9. Environmental Restructuring.

Early Identification

Early identification of cognitive decline in elderly could be a debatable issue for a practical reason. First, families or client themselves are aware of the certain decline in cognitive capabilities of their elderly member and take it as a natural process. Consultation with professionals happens mostly when there is gross problem in daily functioning or development of other behavioural issue. By then the decline already becomes apparent. In such condition, how much the cognitive decline can be slowed or reversed, if possible depends on the type and severity of decline itself (Katona, Cooper & Robertson, 2016). It is very important to assess onset, whether fast or slow as well as severity using appropriate rating scales when discussing cognitive decline and memory loss.

From research perspective, literature do suggest that cognitive decline can be predicted, but from therapeutic perspective, it could be difficult to practice, unless family members get their elderly member screened before onset of obvious symptoms. But this does not limit the importance of early identification. There are obvious benefits of early screening that can help planning management of the client. It also allows caregivers to plan for future (Scott & Donnelly, 2005).

First and foremost, it allows the clinician to rule out conditions that are not true cognitive decline e.g., vitamin B12 deficiency, hypothyroidism, depression to name a few, in which client may complain about forgetfulness. Many of the conditions that appear similar like cognitive decline or dementia could be reversible, and have different management plan, thus early identification has an important role. As clients at this stage often develop several other comorbid medical conditions like cardiovascular disease; early identification helps in better pharmacological management, diet management and lifestyle measures.

Early identification gives valuable insight to family and care givers about the nature of the condition helping them plan and prepare for it. The client can also take decisions regarding financial and property inheritance related matters. While family members are aware of the clinical condition of their client, care giving can often become strenuous leading to critical comment, ignorance or even ill treatment to clients. Early identification can help prepare family and care givers to cope with the situation and provide better care giving to their elderly member.

Psychoeducation to Family and Caregivers

Psychoeducation in itself is not a treatment method, rather an educative module aimed to improve insight and awareness of client as well as caregivers regarding the illness condition. Psychoeducation has been indicated mostly in psychotic conditions and established itself as an evidenced based practise in schizophrenia, but it is equally beneficial in non-psychotic conditions, where treatment requires an insight into altered behaviour of the client. Several models of Psychoeducation have been proposed, that target patient with psychosis and their family members (Bhattacharjee et al., 2011). The theme of these models can be borrowed effectively for caregivers of clients with cognitive decline. The Psychoeducation model that can be best incorporated is the comprehensive model, which includes informative, supportive and family oriented approach. The family members especially the direct caregivers need to be explained about the declining cognitive status of their member, and how it translates into impairment in daily activities and changes in behaviour and emotions. The aim of gaining this insight is also on generalization of the information in relation to client's behaviour across different settings. Risk of increased stress is an issue, when family members come to know about this relatively unknown aspect. However there lies a general acceptance of decline of functions in ageing people, and any increased concerns are temporary only. Psychoeducation helps in reducing the care burden and also improving coping of the care givers. The family centred component of psychoeducation let the caregivers vent out their feelings and realise that their feeling of burnout and any subsequent guilt is normal and help them cope better with the situation.

Addressing Risk Factors and Management of Other Medical Conditions

It is very vital to address risk factors while interviewing the elderly clients. A positive family history of dementia may increase the probability of the person developing cognitive decline (Wolters et al., 2017). Similarly, a positive history of medical conditions like heart disease, stroke, obesity or increased cholesterol levels, diabetes mellitus is reported to be linked and increases the risk of cognitive decline, thus need to be checked. Medical conditions like hearing impairment though may not be directly linked with cognitive decline, it can make the person confined to himself or hesitant to engage in social interaction leading to other emotional manifestations and thus need to be checked. A personal history of smoking or tobacco use, and other drug use needs to be explored and the client need to be counselled regarding this. Habit of not indulging in any physical exercise in past and present can also have an impact and need to be incorporated. While the available literature may suggest a long list of risk factors, they do not guarantee cognitive decline and thus individual cases should be assessed as per the more dominant risk factors apparent from history and family members reporting.

Management of Mood Symptoms

Caregivers often complain of development of grumpiness, irritability, withdrawnness, rigidity or stubbornness in their elderly wards. While this can be because of the ageing, which makes them more sensitive and less tolerant to environmental changes and situations; there could be underlying depression that needs to be screened. Any significant and persistent change in sleep and appetite patterns increased or decreased socialization need to be explored for underlying mood symptoms and addressed with pharmacotherapy if required.

Daily Activity Scheduling (Guided/ Independent)

A structured daily routine is an important component in management of elderly, as lack of engagement could be a big contributor to loneliness and subsequent feelings of irritation, reduced feeling of self-competency. Normal aged people in absence of apparent decline in functioning may prefer on their own to engage in some activity which could be unstructured or sitting idle watching television or sleeping at odd hours. But it is beneficial to frame a daily routine for aged people at risk. This could be independent for better functioning people, and guided if the person appears to be slack. The routine may specify timeline for activities of daily living along with specification on sleeping hours if any in afternoon, involvement in appropriate physical activity and exercises, leisure activities as well as involvement in brain stimulating activities like reading newspapers & magazines, solving puzzles and crosswords. Elderly people often have a tendency to stop writing, as they are no more in active occupation, and engage in any writing only when having some financial dealing at banks or writing any letter to authority. They may be motivated to engage in writing a daily diary, old experiences to share or even religious text content.

COGNITIVE RETRAINING

Cognitive retraining is a promising non-pharmacological intervention for cognitive impairment and indicated in host of clinical populations including schizophrenia, traumatic brain injury, ADHD as well as mild cognitive impairment. Prospective and controlled studies have demonstrated certain indication of cognitive training in elderly. Cognitive retraining works on the principle of neuroplasticity of the brain (Leung et al, 2015) and takes either remediating approach, compensatory or adaptive approach to improve on neurocognitive abilities of the client. Cognitive remediation programmes are highly customized depending on the clinical diagnosis and severity of the symptoms.

A question arises whether cognitive remediation techniques can be used for age related cognitive decline in absence of significant cognitive impairment. Although there is no significant impairment, the profile of normal aged population is different than that of younger population. Thus, cognitive remediation techniques can be employed for age related cognitive decline, albeit to reduce the risk of further decline into mild cognitive impairment and further into dementia. The techniques can be customized as per the identified decline in cognitive functions of the individual and may not be as rigid compared to programmes for mild cognitive impairment or dementia group. It could have a major component of brain stimulating tasks that are challenging as well as interesting for the individual. Normal elderly people usually have plenty of free time that can be used for learning new skills such as computer, email and use of internet for those who did not had previous exposure. Playing and solving crosswords or puzzles can also be used.

BEHAVIOURAL MANAGEMENT

As mentioned earlier, older people can present with a host of behavioural changes. Some of these behaviours may be temporary and reactive in nature while some may be unprovoked and a regular feature. Family and care givers do ignore minor issues initially but find themselves in a fix when their older wards have repeated and severe behavioural issues like aggression leading to verbal or physical abuse, wandering behaviour, stubborn, uncooperative, and rigid behaviour like not sticking to specified diet and bowel routines risking own health, disinhibited behaviour etc. While much of the severe behavioural issues are seen in advanced stages as in dementia, certain features may be evident at early stages too. It is vital to understand whether the behaviour is a manifestation of dysfunction or secondary to stress, difficulty in coping with demanding situations or attention seeking behaviour. It helps to establish a clear communication with such clients and understand if they want to express something. While pharmacological interventions help in reducing symptoms, behavioural strategies too can be employed to reduce the frequency and re-occurrence of the behaviour. A simple ABC approach can be used to assess why the person is engaging in a particular behaviour. Elderly wards at times need clear and stern guidelines to maintain diet, timely compliance of medicine, toilet use as well. Behavioural management does not mean to give punishment or verbally harsh, but to understand the underlying reasons and adopt appropriate strategies.

ENVIRONMENTAL RESTRUCTURING

Environmental restructuring while have been suggested as one of the non-pharmacological interventions in Alzheimer's disease; restructuring the home environment and surrounding can have good effect in age related cognitive decline too. While the original concept is to provide a safe and structured atmosphere at home to clients where they do not get confused with too many choices to do and are supported by signage; environmental restructuring can be customised for normal aged population too.

CONCLUSION

Decline in cognitive ability with age does have its impact on the greying person in varying severity. While the process is inevitable, not all elderly people develop dementia. With ever increasing population of elder people across the world; managing this population which is on threshold of developing behavioural and emotional dysfunctional behaviour secondary to cognitive decline would be a challenging task. There are no definite probabilities of what percentage of people with mild cognitive impairment will deteriorate further into dementia, and the MCI group somehow appears to be focus of research than clinical practice. The lack of data on cognitive functions of normal ageing people to be compared with MCI also add into this. There could be certain markers that differentiate the normal ageing and MCI from each other. A thorough assessment of individuals brought into consultation to check these markers as well as early intervention could be the key for optimum functioning of the elderly individual.

REFERENCES

Bhattacharjee, D., Rai, A. K., Singh, N. K., Kumar, P., Munda, S. K., & Das, B. (2011). Psychoeducation: A measure to strengthen psychiatric treatment. *Delhi Psychiatric Journal, 14*(1), 33–39.

Brown, L. A. (2016). Spatial-Sequential Working Memory in Younger and Older Adults: Age Predicts Backward Recall Performance within Both Age Groups. *Frontiers in Psychology, 7*, 1514. doi:10.3389/fpsyg.2016.01514 PMID:27757096

Clark, L. J., Gatz, M., Zheng, L., Chen, Y. L., McCleary, C., & Mack, W. J. (2009). Longitudinal verbal fluency in normal aging, preclinical and prevalent Alzheimer disease. *American Journal of Alzheimer's Disease and Other Dementias, 24*(6), 461–468. doi:10.1177/1533317509345154 PMID:19759254

Cohen, R. A. (1993). *The Neuropsychology of Attention*. New York: Plenum Press. doi:10.1007/978-1-4419-7463-1

Deary, I. J., Corley, J., Gow, A. J., Harris, S. E., Houlihan, L. M., Marioni, R. E., ... Starr, J. M. (2009). Age associated cognitive decline. *British Medical Bulletin, 92*(1), 135–152. doi:10.1093/bmb/ldp033 PMID:19776035

Diesfeldt, H. F., Vander Elst, W., & Jolles, J. (2009). Category fluency (animals, professions) in normal cognitive ageing and dementia. *Tijdschriftvoor Gerontologie en Geriatrie., 40*(2), 54-71. Retrieved from https://www.ncbi.nlm.nih.gov/pubmed/19472572

Folstein, M. F., Folstein, S. E., & McHugh, P. R. (1975). Mini-mental state: A practical method for grading the cognitive state of patients for the clinician. *Journal of Psychiatric Research, 12*(3), 189–198. doi:10.1016/0022-3956(75)90026-6 PMID:1202204

Gioia, G. A., Isquith, P. K., Guy, S. C., & Kenworthy, L. (2000). *BRIEF: Behavior Rating Inventory of Executive Function Professional Manual*. Lutz, FL: PAR.

Harada, C. N., Natelson Love, M. C., & Triebel, K. (2013). Normal Cognitive Aging. *Clinics in Geriatric Medicine, 29*(4), 737–752. doi:10.1016/j.cger.2013.07.002 PMID:24094294

Hebert, L. E., Scherr, P. A., Beckett, L. A., Albert, M. S., Pilgrim, D. M., Chown, M. J., ... Evans, D. A. (1995). Age-specific incidence of Alzheimer's disease in a community population. *Journal of the American Medical Association, 273*(17), 1354–1359. doi:10.1001/jama.1995.03520410048025 PMID:7715060

Howieson, D. B., Holm, L. A., Kaye, J. A., Oken, B. S., & Howieson, J. (1993). Neurologic function in the optimally healthy oldest old. Neuropsychological evaluation. *Neurology, 43*(10), 1882–1886. doi:10.1212/WNL.43.10.1882 PMID:8413942

Hunsley, J., & Lee, C. M. (2010). *Introduction to clinical psychology: An evidence-based approach*. New York: John Wiley & Sons, Inc.

Katona, C., Cooper, C., & Robertson, M. (2016). *Psychiatry at a glance*. New Delhi: Wiley Blackwell.

Kessels, P. C., Overbeek, A., & Bouman, Z. (2015). Assessment of verbal and visuospatial working memory in mild cognitive impairment and Alzheimer's dementia. *Dementia &Neuropsycholgia, 9*(3), 301-305. Retrieved http://www.scielo.br/pdf/dn/v9n3/1980-5764-dn-9-03-00301.pdf

Kral, V. A. (1962). Senescent forgetfulness: Benign and malignant. *Canadian Medical Association Journal*, *86*(6), 257–260. PMID:14459267

Langa, K. M., & Levine, D. A. (2014). The Diagnosis and Management of Mild Cognitive Impairment: A Clinical Review. *Journal of the American Medical Association*, *312*(23), 2551–2561. doi:10.1001/jama.2014.13806 PMID:25514304

Leung, N. T. Y., Tam, H. M. K., Chu, L. W., Kwok, T. C. Y., Chan, F., Lam, L. C. W., ... Lee, T. M. C. (2015). Neural Plastic Effects of Cognitive Training on Aging Brain. *Neural Plasticity*, *2015*, 1–9. doi:10.1155/2015/535618 PMID:26417460

Lezak, M. D., Howieson, D. B., & Loring, D. W. (2004). *Neuropsychological assessment* (4th ed.). New York: Oxford UniversityPress.

Luis, A. U. C., Rosalinda, D., Israel, V. P., & Juan, F. R. (2015). The Effect of Spatial Working Memory Deterioration on Strategic Visuomotor Learning across Aging. *Behavioural Neurology*. Retrieved from https://www.hindawi.com/journals/bn/2015/512617/

Nasreddine, Z. S., Phillips, N. A., Bedirian, V., Charbonneau, S., Whitehead, V., Collin, I., ... Chertkow, H. (2005). The Montreal Cognitive Assessment, MoCA: A brief screening tool for mild cognitive impairment. *Journal of the American Geriatrics Society*, *53*(4), 695–699. doi:10.1111/j.1532-5415.2005.53221.x PMID:15817019

O'Bryant, S. E., Humphreys, J. D., Smith, G. E., Ivnik, R. J., Graff-Radford, N. R., ... Lucas, J. A. (2008). Detecting Dementia with the Mini-Mental State Examination (MMSE) in Highly Educated Individuals. *Archives of Neurology*, *65*(7), 963–967. PMID:18625866

Petersen, R. C., Smith, G. E., Waring, S. C., Ivnik, R. J., Tangalos, E. G., & Kokmen, E. (1999). Mild cognitive impairment: Clinical characterization and outcome. *Archives of Neurology*, *5*(3), 303–308. doi:10.1001/archneur.56.3.303 PMID:10190820

Pettersson, A. F., Olsson, E., & Wahlund, L. O. (2005). Motor function in subjects with mild cognitive impairment and early Alzheimer's disease. *Dementia and Geriatric Cognitive Disorders*, *19*(56), 299–304. doi:10.1159/000084555 PMID:15785030

Pike, K. E., Kinsella, G. J., Ong, B., Mullaly, E., Rand, E., Storey, E., ... Parsons, S. (2013). Is the WMS-IV verbal paired associates as effective as other memory tasks in discriminating amnestic mild cognitive impairment from normal aging? *The Clinical Neuropsychologist*, *27*(6), 908–923. Retrieved https://www.ncbi.nlm.nih.gov/pubmed/23767765 doi:10.1080/13854046.2013.809149 PMID:23767765

Ramlall, S., Chipps, J., Bhigjee, A. I., & Pillay, B. J. (2014). Sensitivity and specificity of neuropsychological tests for dementia and mild cognitive impairment in a sample of residential elderly in South Africa. *South African Journal of Psychiatry*, *20*(4), 153–159. doi:10.4102/sajpsychiatry.v20i4.558

Reisberg, B., Ferris, S., de Leon, M. J., Franssen, E. S. E., Kluger, A., Mir, P., ... Cohen, J. (1988). Stage-specific behavioral, cognitive, and in vivo changes in community residing subjects with age-associated memory impairment and primary degenerative dementia of the Alzheimer type. *Drug Development Research*, *15*(2-3), 101–114. doi:10.1002/ddr.430150203

Schaie, K. W. (2008). Historical processes and patterns of cognitive ageing. In S. M. Hofer & D. F. Alwin (Eds.), *Handbook of Cognitive Aging: Interdisciplinary Perspectives* (pp. 368–383). Thousand Oaks, CA: Sage Pub. Inc. doi:10.4135/9781412976589.n23

Schaie, K. W., & Hofer, S. M. (2001). Longitudinal studies in research of ageing. In J. E. Birren & K. W. Schaie (Eds.), *Handbook of the Psychology of ageing* (5th ed., pp. 55–77). San Diego, CA: Academic Press.

Scott, D., & Donnelly, M. (2005). The early identification of cognitive impairment. A stakeholder evaluation of a 'Dementia Awareness Service' in Belfast. *Dementia (London)*, *4*(2), 207–232. doi:10.1177/1471301205051093

Steiner, V. A. G., Mansur, L. L., Brucki, S. M., & Nitrini, R. (2008). Phonemic verbal fluency and age: A preliminary study. *Dementia & Neuropsychologia*, *2*(4), 328–332. doi:10.1590/S1980-57642009DN20400017

Strauss, E., Sherman, E. M. S., & Spreen, O. A. (2006). *Compendium of Neuropsychological Tests: Administration, norms, and commentary* (3rd ed.). Oxford: Oxford University Press.

Taler, V., & Phillips, N. A. (2008). Language performance in Alzheimer's disease and mild cognitive impairment: A comparative review. *Journal of Clinical and Experimental Neuropsychology*, *30*(5), 501–556. doi:10.1080/13803390701550128 PMID:18569251

Thapliyal, G., Halder, S., & Mahato, A. (2016). Memory, verbal fluency and response inhibition in normal aging. *Journal of Geriatric Mental Health*, *3*(2), 145–149. doi:10.4103/2348-9995.195636

United Nations, Department of Economic and Social Affairs, Population Division. (2015). *World Population Ageing 2015* (ST/ESA/SER.A/390).

Wimo, A., Jonsson, L., & Winblad, B. (2006). An estimate of the worldwide prevalence and direct costs of dementia in 2003. *Dementia and Geriatric Cognitive Disorders*, *21*(3), 175–181. doi:10.1159/000090733 PMID:16401889

Wolters, F. J., Van der Lee, S. J., Koudstaal, P. J., Van Duijn, C. M., Hofman, A., & Ikram, M. K. … Ikram, M. A. (2017). Parental family history of dementia in relation to subclinical brain disease and dementia risk [Abstract]. *Neurology*. Retrieved from http://www.neurology.org/content/early/2017/03/29/WNL.0000000000003871.abstract

KEY TERMS AND DEFINITIONS

Assessment: Assessment is a consideration of someone or something and a judgment about them. In reference to cognition, it is the assessment of different cognitive capabilities of an individual for diagnostic, therapeutic and research purpose.

Cognitive Ageing: Cognitive ageing is the change in cognitive abilities due to increasing age. It is a normal phenomenon and certain functions like memory, processing speed and reasoning are more prone to decline with age.

Impairment: Impairment in reference to cognition is marked decline in cognitive functions that is significantly lower than the age appropriate standards.

Intervention: Interventions are actions taken to improve an existing condition. It is multi pronged in cognitive aging and may include early identification, psycho-education, reducing risks, addressing co morbidity and cognitive retraining.

Chapter 8
Mild Cognitive Impairment:
Evolution of the Clinical Diagnosis

Pallavi Sinha
North Delhi Municipal Corporation Medical College, India & Hindu Rao Hospital, India

Amit Garg
Felicity Mindcare Clinic, India

ABSTRACT

This chapter describes how the world population is ageing with the advances in medical health technology. Longevity allows many humans to live beyond the sixth and seventh decade. With this comes the added medical co-morbidity that one sees with healthy ageing. Mild cognitive impairment (MCI) includes a heterogeneous group of persons who have declining deficits in cognitions with minimal impairment in doing complex activities with no deficits in daily activities and in the absence of dementia. The purpose of this chapter is to acquaint the readers with the concept of Mild Cognitive Impairment and the evolution of the diagnosis to its current nosological status. It will further elaborate on the assessment and management of patients with MCI.

INTRODUCTION

Ageing is a worldwide phenomenon. Demographically, nations across both developed and developing world are seeing a boom in the number of individuals in the elderly age group. While some degree of memory impairment is considered normal as the human brain ages, a sub-category of persons develops significant problems in cognition. It is postulated that only about 1% of individuals go through life without any cognitive impairment (Petersen, 2011). However, the vast majority develops cognitive impairments that can be put on a continuum from normal ageing to dementia. The cognitive impairment present in normal ageing is subtle and minimal without causing any dysfunction in the patient's day-to-day living. On the other end of the spectrum is dementia, which carries significant impairment in memory along with other cognitive domains causing an impact on the person's ability to live independently and manage activities of daily living. In between lies the concept of mild cognitive impairment (MCI), which

DOI: 10.4018/978-1-5225-3480-8.ch008

represents an intermediate state of cognitive impairment. This intermediate state of cognitive impairment has received many definitions and labels but the one that has persevered and used maximally is Mild Cognitive Impairment.

The concept of mild cognitive impairment was first introduced by Resiberg et al. in 1988 as a descriptive term referring to the stage 3 of Global Deterioration Scale which was considered to be an intermediate stage (Reisberg, Ferris, & de Leon, 1988). Less than a decade later, Peterson et al used MCI as a separate diagnostic entity not linked to predefined rating scale (Petersen et al., 1995). They developed their conceptualization from an observation of clinical signs and cognitive performance in a longitudinal community based study of ageing and dementia. This development was stimulated by the fact that a transitional zone lay between normal ageing and dementia, and that the latter was not necessarily a binary diagnosis of being present or absent. Over the years, the concept was redefined and re-evaluated by multiple researchers as a possible condition where preventive measures could be utilized. Over the past 25 years, patients with MCI have undergone extensive research from the clinical, imaging, genetic, pathological and epidemiological perspective (Petersen et al., 2014). MCI received this additional attention as a potential syndrome to develop interventions to prevent dementia, something that has still not been clearly established despite two decades of clinical research.

EVOLUTION OF CRITERIA FOR MILD COGNITIVE IMPAIRMENT

It would be simplistic to assume MCI as a transitional state between normal ageing and dementia. However there appears some overlap between both MCI with normal ageing and MCI with dementia. The original 1999 Mayo criteria assumed MCI to be a precursor state for Alzheimer's Dementia and emphasized on episodic memory impairment. These were (Petersen et al., 1999):

1. Memory complaint, preferably corroborated by informant
2. Memory impairment documented according to appropriate reference values
3. Essentially normal performance in non-memory cognitive domains
4. Generally reserved activities of daily living
5. Absence of dementia

However, since not all MCI progressed to Alzheimer's dementia, a broader conceptualization of the diagnostic criteria were required. A neuropsychological assessment of a subset of patients with MCI revealed subtle deficits in other cognitive domains like executive functioning, language and visuo-spatial skills (Molano et al., 2010). These patients were at higher risk of converting to Lewy body dementia or fronto-temporal dementia. With the expanding literature on MCI suggesting that it is a heterogenous group and not just a precursor of Alzheimer's dementia, the revised Mayo criteria were published in 2003 (Petersen, 2004) which expanded to include cognitive deficits in domains other than memory. They divided MCI into amnestic MCI (aMCI) and Non-amnestic MCI (naMCI) based on the type of cognitive deficits present.

Amnestic MCI is characterized by episodic memory impairment, which is not severe enough to classify as dementia. The person is able to carry out his activities of daily living independently with only minor difficulties. aMCI is further sub-divided into deficits in memory alone and deficits in memory and other cognitive domains. Non-amnestic MCI is characterized by subtle deficits in other cognitive domain of attention, executive functions, language skills or visuo-spatial skills. Memory is relatively well preserved in naMCI. Non-amnestic MCI can have deficits in single or multiple non-memory domains. Essentially the revised Mayo criteria of 2003 now divided MCI into four possible clinical subtypes: (i) aMCI–single domain, (ii) aMCI–multiple domain, (iii) naMCI–single domain and (iv) naMCI–multiple domain.

In 2011, the National Institute on Aging-Alzheimer's Association (NIA-AA) work group proposed a set of research criteria for MCI specifically due to Alzheimer's disease. While the core clinical criteria are similar to those of the revised 2003 Mayo criteria, they in addition proposed the use of biomarkers and provide a guideline for predicting the progression of MCI to Alzheimer's Dementia (Albert et al., 2011). The group however specified that the biomarkers remained uninformative for the definition of MCI. The use of biomarkers has been proposed for research and clinical trials to ascertain the aetiology of MCI and currently two set of biomarkers are used to predict conversion of MCI into Alzheimer's dementia. These are a) biomarkers of amyloid beta deposition and b) biomarkers of neuronal injury. According to the NIA- AA workgroup (Albert et al., 2011), valid indicators of amyloid beta (Aβ) deposition are: (i) cerebrospinal fluid concentrations of Aβ42 (CSF Aβ42) and (ii) positron emission tomography (PET) amyloid imaging; valid indicators of neuronal injury are: (i) CSF tau/phosphorylated tau, (ii) hippocampal volume or medial temporal atrophy by volumetric measures or visual rating, (iii) rate of brain atrophy, (iv) fluoro-deoxyglucose (FDG) PET imaging and (v) SPECT perfusion imaging.

The Diagnostic and Statistical Manual for Mental Disorders (DSM-5) published by the American Psychiatric Association was revised in 2103 and formally acknowledged mild cognitive impairment as a diagnostic entity (American Psychiatric Association, 2013). It changed the nomenclature to neurocognitive disorders with major neurocognitive disorder replacing dementia and mild neurocognitive disorder used for mild cognitive impairment. The DSM 5 devised a two-step aetiology based criteria. The first step was for defining the mild neurocognitive disorder and second step was ascertaining its aetiology. The criteria for mild neurocognitive disorder includes (i) clinical concern raised by the patient or an informant, or observations made by the clinician, (ii) cognitive impairment in one or more cognitive domains preferably relative to appropriate normative data for that individual, (iii) preservation of functional independence and (iv) no dementia (American Psychiatric Association, 2013). These criteria were similar to the revised Mayo criteria and though the nomenclature of the disorder may be different, the basis for diagnosis remained similar.

EPIDEMIOLOGY

A vast pool of data exists on the epidemiology of MCI. However there exist also significant variations in these data owing to the heterogeneity that the MCI syndrome holds. Petersen and Morris outlined the main sources of variability in research on MCI (Petersen & Morris, 2005): (1) criteria for MCI, (2) implementation of the criteria, (3) source of subjects, and (4) reference standards for normal performance. Thus, keeping these limitations in mind, the overall prevalence of MCI in the elderly populations ranges between 2% to 20%(Ganguli, Dodge, Shen, & DeKosky, 2004; Lopez et al., 2012). The Mayo Clinic Study of Ageing, a prospective study found the prevalence of MCI in the community at 16%, with aMCI at 11.1% and naMCI at 4.9% (Petersen et al., 2010). They also reported that the prevalence increased with age and was found to be more common in males and those carrying APOEe3e4 0r e4e4 genotype.

Longitudinal studies observing the outcome of MCI have reported a greater conversion to dementia as compared to the normal population (Busse, Hensel, Gühne, Angermeyer, & Riedel-Heller, 2006; Lopez et al., 2012). The annual rate of conversion of MCI to dementia is 5-10% in community-based studies and 10-15% in specialty clinics. The higher rates in specialty clinics may reflect the greater cognitive impairment that may be present in those seeking evaluation in clinic setting. It is pertinent to note that the annual incidence of dementia in the general population has been observed to be 1-2% per year, which is significantly lower than the conversion rates seen in MCI patients. This reflects that a major proportion of patients with MCI are at high risk of developing dementia. However, all patients who are diagnosed with MCI do not eventually develop dementia in the long term. Around 25-30% of patients with MCI have been seen to return to normal cognition in follow up studies (Manly et al., 2008) though this does not preclude conversion to dementia over longer follow-up. Indeed, the conversion to dementia can be as high as 80% after 6 years of diagnosis of MCI (Busse et al., 2006).

RISK FACTORS FOR MILD COGNITIVE IMPAIRMENT

Despite the heterogeneity that MCI holds, it provides an opportunity for prompt identification of patients at risk of evolving into dementia and development of pharmacological and non-pharmacological therapy as preventive measures. It is therefore prudent to identify risk factors especially those that can be modified to prevent this morbidity. As is expected, older age and lower education status is a major risk factor for development of MCI (Ward, Arrighi, Michels, & Cedarbaum, 2012). Cardiovascular risk factors have been evaluated in multiple studies to see their relation with cognitive decline. Though cross-sectional studies gave divergent views, longitudinal studies have demonstrated hypertension to be associated with cognitive decline (Birns & Kalra, 2009). The causal link between diabetes mellitus and cognitive deficits is supported by numerous biochemical (Brownlee, 2001), imaging-related (Biessels, Koffeman, & Scheltens, 2006), and histo-pathological findings (Sonnen et al., 2009).Prospective studies that have analysed the data after correcting for the effect of confounding variables like hypertension, stroke have also emphasized on diabetes mellitus as an independent risk factor for cognitive impairment(Luchsinger et al., 2007; Yaffe et al., 2004). In the study by Luchsinger et al (2007), the risk of MCI attributable to diabetes was found to be 8.8% and that diabetes was linked to higher rates of amnestic MCI. The longer duration of diabetes, lack of anti-diabetic medication, and greater number of hypoglycemic episodes were associated with an increased risk of cognitive impairment (Logroscino, Kang, & Grodstein, 2004; Okereke et al., 2008; Whitmer, Karter, Yaffe, Quesenberry, & Selby, 2009). Similarly, a large population based study has found hypercholesterolemina to be associated with development of MCI in later life (Kivipelto et al., 2001) and some evidence suggests that statins can lower the risk of cognitive decline (Haag, Hofman, Koudstaal, Stricker, & Breteler, 2009). Newer research has found chronic renal failure to be an independent risk factor for development of MCI (Etgen, Bickel, & Forstl, 2010). The metabolic changes present in chronic renal failure like hyperhomocystinemia, coagulation disorders, anemia and inflammation may have contributory role in the development of cognitive impairment. Most longitudinal studies have also found a significant association between chronic renal failure and MCI even with mild to moderate restriction in renal functioning (Buchman et al., 2009; Etgen et al., 2009; Kurella et al., 2005). Nutritional and metabolic factors have also been studied as risk factors for MCI. Both cross-sectional and longitudinal studies have shown an association between vitamin B12 deficiency and the development of MCI (Clarke et al., 2007; Hin et al., 2006) but none of the randomized controlled trials conducted to date have shown any significant improvement in cognitive functioning with vitamin B12 substitution (Seal, Metz, Flicker, & Melny, 2002; van Uffelen, Chinapaw, van Mechelen, & Hopman-

Rock, 2008). Similarly, though vitamin D is used in the synthesis of neurotrophic factors and regulation of receptors in the memory relevant regions of the brain namely hippocampus (Brewer et al., 2001), prospective cohort studies have failed to find any association between cognitive impairment and 25-hydroxyvitamin D levels (Slinin et al., 2010). Homocysteine levels have also been studied in the context of ageing as its level is seen to rise as age increases. Though cross-sectional studies reported a relation between hyperhomocysteinemia and cognitive impairment, this has largely been disproved by longitudinal studies (Etgen et al., 2010).

The available research on subclinical hypothyroidism, testosterone and oestrogen also largely finds no significant association with MCI (Ceresini et al., 2009; Lethaby, Hogervorst, Richards, Yesufu, & Yaffe, 2008; Roberts et al., 2006; Warren, Serby, & Roane, 2008). In contrast to the hormonal risk factors, there is strong evidence for risk factors pertaining to lifestyle and MCI. Specific regional diet like the Mediterranean diet has been found to have protective effect on cognitive decline via improved carbohydrate metabolism coupled with antioxidative and anti-inflammatory mechanisms (Solfrizzi et al., 2008). Mediterranean diet consists of a diet rich in fruits, vegetable, fish and unsaturated fats and is largely void of meat. It has been seen to have a dose dependent protective effect with longitudinal studies reporting a 28% reduction in risk of MCI after sustained use of high proportion of Mediterranean diet (Féart, Samieri, & Barberger-Gateau, 2010; Scarmeas et al., 2009). In addition to diet, physical exercise has also been extensively studied with a recent meta-analysis of 15 prospective cohort studies showing that both intense and moderate exercise reduces the risk of occurrence of MCI by atleast 35% (Sofi et al., 2011).

PREDICTORS OF DEVELOPMENT OF DEMENTIA

It is clear from longitudinal studies that the risk of developing dementia in patients with MCI is much more than that seen in the normal population. But there is also a subset of patients with MCI who remain cognitively stable or may even revert back to normal cognition. What separates this subset of patients with a good prognosis? Over the years, researchers have evaluated clinical, neurochemical, genetic and radiographic factors leading to conversion of MCI into dementia. While no single factor can predict development of dementia, a few biomarkers have been identified that can predict this conversion to some extent.

These potential biomarkers can be divided into:

1. **Clinical Biomarker:** The degree of cognitive impairment at the time presentation can predict the risk of developing dementia. Greater the impairment, higher is the risk (Dickerson, Sperling, Hyman, Albert, & Blacker, 2007; Visser et al., 2009). This factor has been replicated in many clinical trials and reflects the underlying severity and extent of neuro-pathological involvement. In addition, baseline deficits in episodic memory i.e. Amnestic MCI predicts conversion to Alzheimer's dementia (Landau et al., 2010).
2. **Genetic Biomarker:** Longitudinal data have shown that progression to dementia is more rapid among carriers of the apolipoprotein (APOE) ε4 allele than among non-carriers (Bonham et al., 2016; Petersen et al., 1995; Viticchi et al., 2017). APOE ε4 is considered to be one of the strongest genetic risk factors for development of Alzheimer's dementia. Corollary to this, the absence APOE ε4 polymorphism suggests stability of MCI diagnosis (Clem et al., 2017). However, a strong genetic

base of MCI is not supported by concordance studies among twins, which showed no difference in level of concordance between monozygotic and dizygotic twins (Caracciolo, Gatz, Xu, Pedersen, & Fratiglioni, 2012).

3. **Neuroimaging Biomarker:** Quantitative magnetic resonance imaging has been extensively studied in the context of MCI. Studies have noted that patients whose volumetric assessment of the hippocampus fell at or below the 25th percentile for age and sex had2-3 times higher risk of progression of amnestic MCI to dementia as compared to those patients whose hippocampal measure was at or above the 75th percentile (Jack et al., 2010). While amnestic MCI has greater volume loss in the hippocampus and amygdala compared to normal subjects, the multi domain MCI is shown to have greater volume loss in the parietal, superior temporal, and frontal regions, with less involvement of the hippocampus (Bell-McGinty et al., 2005).

Functional imaging techniques, such as 18-fluorodeoxyglucose positron-emission tomography (FDG-PET) have also been used in experimental studies. Available data suggests that MCI syndrome that has a pattern of temporo-parietal hypometabolism, which is seen in Alzheimer's disease, carries a greater progression to dementia (Drzezga et al., 2005; Landau et al., 2010). The FDG-PET scan has also shown to have a good correlation with cognitive measures in patients with MCI, with a sensitivity of 92% and a specificity of 89% to predict conversion to Alzheimer's dementia (Drzezga et al., 2005). Functional MRI studies are usually conducted in research settings and have found that subjects with MCI have a greater activation of the hippocampus compared to normal controls and subjects with AD in memory tasks (Dickerson et al., 2007). A combination of multiple neuroimaging techniques has allowed researchers to examine the pathophysiology of transition from MCI to dementia.

Both MRI and FDG PET are considered as surrogate markers of neuronal degeneration in a model of temporal evolution of disease-specific pathology as proposed by Jack et al (Jack et al., 2010). According to this hypothesis, amyloid biomarkers appear before markers of neuronal injury; possibly 10-20 years before symptoms appear. Amyloid labeled ligands like carbon-11 Pittsburgh Compound B (PiB) can be used to localize regional cerebral patterns of amyloid deposition. PET molecular imaging has shown increased amyloid β burden in progressive MCI, particularly in the lateral frontal cortex, posterior cingulate cortex, regions of the medial and lateral parietal lobe, and the lateral temporal lobe (Forsberg et al., 2008; Koivunen et al., 2008).

4. **CSF Biomarker:** The altered pattern of CSF proteins seen in patients of Alzheimer's dementia is also seen in MCI patients specially those at higher risk of conversion to dementia. This is shown in CSF studies as high tau or phosphorylated tau proteins with decreased amyloid-β42 (Aβ42) proteins (Clark et al., 2003). Hansson et al further reported that abnormal concentration of T-tau, P-tau 181 and Aβ42 in CSF are strongly associated with further development of Alzheimer's dementia in patients with MCI (Hansson et al., 2006). Though these finding may appear appealing, there is a great variability in the tau and Aβ42 levels in patients with Alzheimer's dementia and a negative CSF result may not conclusively rule out the presence of Alzheimer's pathology in MCI patients (Clark et al., 2003).

It appears that the best prediction model for conversion of MCI to dementia will come from a combination of neuroimaging and neurochemical biomarkers. The National Institute on Aging-Alzheimer's Association (Albert et al., 2011) has also therefore incorporated these biomarkers of amyloid deposition and neuronal injury into their criteria to grade the certainty that the MCI syndrome was due to Alzheimer's aetiology (Table 1). However, at present, these biomarkers are not routinely used in clinical practice but are reserved for primarily clinical research. The lack of established standardized cut off points in neuroimaging studies makes it difficult to incorporate it into routine clinical practice. There is also a need to reach a consensus on the application of CSF biomarkers in clinical practice because it currently varies from country to country, and even from site to site (Herukka et al., 2017). The application of biomarkers in routine clinical practice is also hampered by the lack of access and high cost of utilization. Despite the caveats, a combination of biomarkers can be used at individual patient level when done in the context of the patient's presenting symptoms.

On the other end of the cognitive continuum, studies have also been conducted to see predictors of reversion of MCI into normal cognition. Pandya et al undertook a prospective cohort study and reported that at 2 years, 14% of patients with MCI reverted to normal cognition, 51% remained MCI, and 35% progressed to dementia. Significant variables found to be associated with MCI reversion were younger age, being unmarried, absence of APOE ε4 allele, lower severity score, and higher memory/language test scores (Pandya, Lacritz, Weiner, Deschner, & Woon, 2017). A similar case-control study by Sachdeva et al. (2013) suggested that reversion to baseline normal cognition was more likely if patients had greater level of mental activity, better control over blood pressure, greater openness to experience, a larger left hippocampus/amygdala, better visual acuity, or better smelling ability (Sachdev et al., 2013).

ASSESSMENT FOR MILD COGNITIVE IMPAIRMENT

The distinction between mild cognitive impairment and normal ageing can be a challenging process for a clinician. The first and foremost complaint that brings patients to the clinic is problems in memory. The memory loss usually involves episodic memory in amnestic MCI and patients often report about forgetting appointments, conversations. It is usually noted by the patient himself or by a close informant. A neuropsychological evaluation will help in differencing mild cognitive impairment from normal ageing but is routinely not done at first contact. Instead tests like Montreal Cognitive Assessment or the Short test of mental status can be used in the clinic to screen for cognitive impairment. In comparison to the Mini Mental Status Examination, the above two tests are more sensitive and specific at detecting MCI (Nasreddine et al., 2005; Tang-Wai et al., 2003). It is also important to rule out reversible cause of mild cognitive impairment like depression or anticholinergic side effects of medications.

Table 1. The National Institute on Aging and Alzheimer's Association Criteria for Biomarker Certainty That the Mild Cognitive Impairment Syndrome is Caused by Alzheimer Disease

High Likelihood: The core clinical symptoms and both amyloid β and neuronal damage biomarkers are present
Intermediate Likelihood: The core clinical symptoms and a single positive biomarker (either amyloidβ deposition or neuronal damage) are present
Unlikely to Be Due to Alzheimer Disease: The core clinical symptoms are present and neither types of biomarkers are positive
Amyloid markers identified by CSF or amyloid ligand scans Neuronal damage identified by CSF, MRI, or FDG-PET scans

(Albert et al., 2011)

The detailed neuropsychological assessment of patients with MCI will show objective deficits in memory and other cognitive domains. Scores on these tests in patients with MCI will usually be 1 to 1.5 standard deviations below the mean values seen for the age and education matched controls on culturally appropriate normative data (Albert et al., 2011). However, it should be noted that these ranges are guidelines and not cut off scores.

The deficits in episodic memory (ability to learn and retain new information) is usually seen in amnestic MCI and can be tested by the Rey Auditory Verbal Learning Test (Vakil, Greenstein, & Blachstein, 2010) or the California Verbal Learning Test (Paolo, Troster, & Ryan, 1997). Other cognitive domains like executive functions (e.g., set-shifting, reasoning, problem-solving, planning), language (e.g., naming, fluency, expressive speech, and comprehension), visuo-spatial skills, and attentional control (e.g., simple and divided attention) should also be evaluated using appropriate tests (Albert et al., 2011). Validated tools that can be used are: the Trail making test for executive function (Tombaugh, 2004), Boston naming test for language functions (Williams, Mack, & Henderson, 1989), figure copying for spatial skills and digit span forward for testing attention. The impairment in patients with MCI can be memory only or in more than one cognitive domain. Patients with MCI are able to carry out their daily activities independently. Their activities of daily living like eating, dressing is usually normal though they might have mild impairment in instrumental activities of daily living like problems at job, paying bills. The Functional activities questionnaire (Pfeffer, Kurosaki, Harrah, Chance, & Filos, 1982) can be used to evaluate daily functioning though a careful and detailed history will be sufficient to determine functioning. It is important to note that daily functional activities will be impaired in dementia and not MCI.

Studies have also reported the presence of neuropsychiatric symptoms in 35-75% of patients with MCI with the most common behavioral abnormalities being depression, apathy, anxiety and irritability (Apostolova & Cummings, 2008). They can be evaluated using clinical interview or appropriate rating scales. These behavioral abnormalities are similar to those seen in Alzheimer's dementia. The occurrence of neuropsychiatric symptoms for the first time in the elderly population should also raise the suspicion for an underlying mild cognitive impairment (Gallagher, Fischer, & Iaboni, 2017).

MANAGEMENT OF MILD COGNITIVE IMPAIRMENT

From a clinical view, patients with mild cognitive impairment should not be labeled as prodromal Alzheimer's dementia. As has been previously noted, the MCI syndrome is a dynamic and heterogeneous condition and a proportion of patients either stabilize their cognitive impairment or even return to baseline cognition. Therefore, it would be hasty to label as a pre-dementia state since the outcome is uncertain. There is however a subset of patients with amnestic MCI who are positive for biomarkers of amyloid deposition and/or neuronal injury who stand at high risk of converting to Alzheimer's dementia. Identification of this subset can allow better monitoring and early identification of Alzheimer's dementia. The National Institute for Health and Care Excellence (NICE) guidelines also recommend follow-up to ensure dementia is diagnosed timely and care planned at an early stage (National Collaborating Centre for Mental Health (UK), 2007). Since currently there is no available treatment for MCI, efforts are needed to delay the development of dementia if possible. Jorm et al. (1987) had calculated that dementia prevalence could be halved if its onset were to be delayed by 5 years (Jorm, Korten, & Henderson, 1987). Therefor intervention aimed at modifying risk factors, neuro-protection and increasing cognitive reserve could be used in those patients at high risk of converting to dementia.

PHARMACOLOGICAL TREATMENT

Currently there is no drug approved for the use in mild cognitive impairment by the Food and Drug Administration (FDA). Acetyl cholinesterase inhibitors like rivastigmine, galantamine and donepezil used in Alzheimer's dementia have not been seen to be of any benefit in MCI. A systematic review of randomized controlled trials of acetyl cholinesterase inhibitors have shown that the marginal beneficial effects they provided were outweighed by the adverse effects including an unexplained increased risk of mortality with galantamine (Raschetti, Albanese, Vanacore, & Maggini, 2007). The effectiveness of donepezil in delaying dementia in amnestic MCI was evaluated by the Alzheimer's Disease Cooperative Study in a placebo controlled RCT. They reported a lower rate of progression to Alzheimer's disease during the first 12 months of treatment, but the rate of progression to Alzheimer's disease after three years was similar to the placebo group (Petersen et al., 2005). Subsequent analyses of the results showed that the treatment effect was more prominent among ApoE4 carriers, with a reduction in risk apparent throughout the 36-month study (Petersen & Negash, 2008). Thus, till date, acetyl cholinesterase inhibitors are not to be routinely used in patients with MCI. Amongst the acetyl cholinesterase inhibitors, Donepezil is the only agent, which has shown some effect in delaying progression in ApoE4 positive amnestic MCI patients (Petersen et al., 2005).

In an attempt to limit the neuro-inflammation hypothesized in dementia, Thal and colleagues studied the COX 2 inhibitor, Rofecoxib in a placebo controlled RCT in patients with amnestic MCI and found no beneficial effect with this anti-inflammatory agent (Thal et al., 2005). Other pharmacological agents like vitamin E& B, oestrogen and testosterone replacement therapy, gingko biloba and omega 3 fatty acids have also not found to be useful in preventing conversion of MCI to dementia (Chertkow et al., 2008). There is encouraging evidence for Piribedil, a dopamine agonist which was found to be effective in improving the global cognitive functions in MCI patients (Nagaraja & Jayashree, 2001). Other classes of drugs currently being studied include statins, nicotine patch, anti-amyloid drugs (e.g., β-secretase inhibitors, gamma-secretase inhibitors, glycosaminoglycan mimetics, amyloid immunotherapy) and ampakines (Chertkow et al., 2008). These are however far from getting approval for routine clinical practice.

Treatment of vascular risk factors like hypertension has some moderate evidence in delaying the progression of dementia (Forette et al., 2002). Evidence for other vascular risk factors, like dyslipidemia and hypercholesterolemia id meager. It also important to identify and treat comorbid psychiatric conditions like depression as the latter may further increase the risk of developing dementia (Alexopoulos, Meyers, Young, Mattis, & Kakuma, 1993; Palmer et al., 2007).

NON-PHARMACOLOGICAL TREATMENT

There is some evidence for non-pharmacological interventions, such as cognitive training and physical exercise, which may be neuro-protective or compensatory. There is some evidence of a potential benefit from cognitive rehabilitation, including the use of mnemonics, association strategies, and computer- assisted training programs (Jean, Bergeron, Thivierge, & Simard, 2010; Massoud et al., 2007). A systematic review by Gates et also found cognitive exercises to produce moderate-to-large beneficial effects on memory-related outcomes (Gates, Sachdev, Fiatarone Singh, & Valenzuela, 2011). The data to date suggest that cognitive intervention is more efficient in people with relatively mild cognitive deficits (healthy older adults and people with mild cognitive impairment) than in people with mild dementia (Chertkow et al., 2008). Exercise especially aerobic exercise has also shown promising results in delaying the progression to dementia (McDonnell, Smith, & Mackintosh, 2011; Miller, Taler, Davidson, & Messier, 2012). Other lifestyle modification like following a Mediterranean diet can also have a positive impact. A recent metanalysis of available trials showed that following a Mediterranean diet can help in not just preventing MCI but reducing the progression of MCI to dementia (Singh et al., 2014).

CONCLUSION

Though there is no established treatment for MCI yet there is moderate evidence for intervention that can prevent or delay the progression to dementia. What may be required will be a combination of medication, cognitive training and lifestyle modifications to provide maximum benefit to the patient with MCI. It is hoped that in the future the diagnostic power of this clinical syndrome would have improved and patients that are bound to develop dementia are identified early and treated. Just like other non-communicable diseases like diabetes, hypertension, which can be screened for early and managed without any major deterioration in quality of life, one hopes that dementia also reaches this fate. It is anticipated that in the years to come, biomarkers are understood better so that asymptomatic patients can be identified, and dementia may be prevented if possible. In the meantime, MCI will advance our understanding and help develop interventions with the goal of finding preventive therapies for these neurodegenerative disorders.

REFERENCES

Albert, M. S., DeKosy, S. T., Dickson, D., Dubois, B., Feldman, H. H., Fox, N. C., ... Phelps, C. H. (2011). The diagnosis of mild cognitive impairment due to Alzheimer's disease: Recommendations from the National Institute on Aging-Alzheimer's Association workgroups on diagnostic guidelines for Alzheimer's disease. *Alzheimer's & Dementia: The Journal of the Alzheimer's Association*, *7*(3), 270–279. doi:10.1016/j.jalz.2011.03.008 PMID:21514249

Alexopoulos, G. S., Meyers, B. S., Young, R. C., Mattis, S., & Kakuma, T. (1993). The course of geriatric depression with "reversible dementia": A controlled study. *The American Journal of Psychiatry*, *150*(11), 1693–1699. doi:10.1176/ajp.150.11.1693 PMID:8105707

American Psychiatric Association. (2013). *Diagnostic and Statistical Manual of Mental Disorders: DSM 5* (5th ed.). Washington, DC: American Psychiatric Association.

Apostolova, L. G., & Cummings, J. L. (2008). Neuropsychiatric manifestations in mild cognitive impairment: A systematic review of the literature. *Dementia and Geriatric Cognitive Disorders*, *25*(2), 115–126. doi:10.1159/000112509 PMID:18087152

Bell-McGinty, S., Lopez, O. L., Meltzer, C. C., Scanlon, J. M., Whyte, E. M., Dekosky, S. T., & Becker, J. T. (2005). Differential cortical atrophy in subgroups of mild cognitive impairment. *Archives of Neurology*, *62*(9), 1393–1397. doi:10.1001/archneur.62.9.1393 PMID:16157746

Biessels, G. J., Koffeman, A., & Scheltens, P. (2006). Diabetes and cognitive impairment. Clinical diagnosis and brain imaging in patients attending a memory clinic. *Journal of Neurology*, *253*(4), 477–482. doi:10.1007/s00415-005-0036-4 PMID:16283097

Birns, J., & Kalra, L. (2009). Cognitive function and hypertension. *Journal of Human Hypertension*, *23*(2), 86–96. doi:10.1038/jhh.2008.80 PMID:18650838

Bonham, L. W., Geier, E. G., Fan, C. C., Leong, J. K., Besser, L., Kukull, W. A., ... Yokoyama, J. S. (2016). Age-dependent effects of APOE ε4 in preclinical Alzheimer's disease. *Annals of Clinical and Translational Neurology*, *3*(9), 668–677. doi:10.1002/acn3.333 PMID:27648456

Brewer, L. D., Thibault, V., Chen, K. C., Langub, M. C., Landfield, P. W., & Porter, N. M. (2001). Vitamin D hormone confers neuroprotection in parallel with downregulation of L-type calcium channel expression in hippocampal neurons. *The Journal of Neuroscience*, *21*(1), 98–108. PMID:11150325

Brownlee, M. (2001). Biochemistry and molecular cell biology of diabetic complications. *Nature*, *414*(6865), 813–820. doi:10.1038/414813a PMID:11742414

Buchman, A. S., Tanne, D., Boyle, P. A., Shah, R. C., Leurgans, S. E., & Bennett, D. A. (2009). Kidney function is associated with the rate of cognitive decline in the elderly. *Neurology*, *73*(12), 920–927. doi:10.1212/WNL.0b013e3181b72629 PMID:19657107

Busse, A., Hensel, A., Gühne, U., Angermeyer, M. C., & Riedel-Heller, S. G. (2006). Mild cognitive impairment: Long-term course of four clinical subtypes. *Neurology*, *67*(12), 2176–2185. doi:10.1212/01.wnl.0000249117.23318.e1 PMID:17190940

Caracciolo, B., Gatz, M., Xu, W., Pedersen, N. L., & Fratiglioni, L. (2012). Differential distribution of subjective and objective cognitive impairment in the population: A nation-wide twin-study. *Journal of Alzheimer's Disease*, *29*(2), 393–403. PMID:22233768

Ceresini, G., Lauretani, F., Maggio, M., Ceda, G. P., Morganti, S., Usberti, E., ... Ferrucci, L. (2009). Thyroid function abnormalities and cognitive impairment in elderly people: Results of the Invecchiare in Chianti study. *Journal of the American Geriatrics Society*, *57*(1), 89–93. doi:10.1111/j.1532-5415.2008.02080.x PMID:19054181

Chertkow, H., Massoud, F., Nasreddine, Z., Belleville, S., Joanette, Y., Bocti, C., ... Bergman, H. (2008). Diagnosis and treatment of dementia: 3. Mild cognitive impairment and cognitive impairment without dementia. *Canadian Medical Association Journal*, *178*(10), 1273–1285. doi:10.1503/cmaj.070797 PMID:18458258

Clark, C. M., Xie, S., Chittams, J., Ewbank, D., Peskind, E., Galasko, D., ... Trojanowski, J. Q. (2003). Cerebrospinal fluid tau and beta-amyloid: How well do these biomarkers reflect autopsy-confirmed dementia diagnoses? *Archives of Neurology*, *60*(12), 1696–1702. doi:10.1001/archneur.60.12.1696 PMID:14676043

Clarke, R., Birks, J., Nexo, E., Ueland, P. M., Schneede, J., Scott, J., ... Evans, J. G. (2007). Low vitamin B-12 status and risk of cognitive decline in older adults. *The American Journal of Clinical Nutrition*, *86*(5), 1384–1391. PMID:17991650

Clem, M. A., Holliday, R. P., Pandya, S., Hynan, L. S., Lacritz, L. H., & Woon, F. L. (2017). Predictors That a Diagnosis of Mild Cognitive Impairment Will Remain Stable 3 Years Later. *Cognitive and Behavioral Neurology*, *30*(1), 8–15. doi:10.1097/WNN.0000000000000119 PMID:28323681

Dickerson, B. C., Sperling, R. A., Hyman, B. T., Albert, M. S., & Blacker, D. (2007). Clinical prediction of Alzheimer disease dementia across the spectrum of mild cognitive impairment. *Archives of General Psychiatry*, *64*(12), 1443–1450. doi:10.1001/archpsyc.64.12.1443 PMID:18056553

Drzezga, A., Grimmer, T., Riemenschneider, M., Lautenschlager, N., Siebner, H., Alexopoulus, P., ... Kurz, A. (2005). Prediction of individual clinical outcome in MCI by means of genetic assessment and (18)F-FDG PET. *Journal of Nuclear Medicine*, *46*(10), 1625–1632. PMID:16204712

Etgen, T., Bickel, H., & Förstl, H. (2010). Metabolic and endocrine factors in mild cognitive impairment. *Ageing Research Reviews*, *9*(3), 280–288. doi:10.1016/j.arr.2010.01.003 PMID:20109582

Etgen, T., Sander, D., Chonchol, M., Briesenick, C., Poppert, H., Förstl, H., & Bickel, H. (2009). Chronic kidney disease is associated with incident cognitive impairment in the elderly: The INVADE study. *Nephrology, Dialysis, Transplantation*, *24*(10), 3144–3150. doi:10.1093/ndt/gfp230 PMID:19461010

Féart, C., Samieri, C., & Barberger-Gateau, P. (2010). Mediterranean diet and cognitive function in older adults. *Current Opinion in Clinical Nutrition and Metabolic Care*, *13*(1), 14–18. doi:10.1097/MCO.0b013e3283331fe4 PMID:19834324

Forette, F., Seux, M. L., Staessen, J. A., Thijs, L., Babarskiene, M. R., & Babeanu, S., … Systolic Hypertension in Europe Investigators. (2002). The prevention of dementia with antihypertensive treatment: New evidence from the Systolic Hypertension in Europe (Syst-Eur) study. *Archives of Internal Medicine*, *162*(18), 2046–2052. doi:10.1001/archinte.162.18.2046 PMID:12374512

Forsberg, A., Engler, H., Almkvist, O., Blomquist, G., Hagman, G., Wall, A., ... Nordberg, A. (2008). PET imaging of amyloid deposition in patients with mild cognitive impairment. *Neurobiology of Aging*, *29*(10), 1456–1465. doi:10.1016/j.neurobiolaging.2007.03.029 PMID:17499392

Gallagher, D., Fischer, C. E., & Iaboni, A. (2017). Neuropsychiatric Symptoms in Mild Cognitive Impairment. *Canadian Journal of Psychiatry*, *62*(3), 161–169. doi:10.1177/0706743716648296 PMID:28212495

Ganguli, M., Dodge, H. H., Shen, C., & DeKosky, S. T. (2004). Mild cognitive impairment, amnestic type: An epidemiologic study. *Neurology*, *63*(1), 115–121. doi:10.1212/01.WNL.0000132523.27540.81 PMID:15249620

Gates, N. J., Sachdev, P. S., Fiatarone Singh, M. A., & Valenzuela, M. (2011). Cognitive and memory training in adults at risk of dementia: A systematic review. *BMC Geriatrics*, *11*(1), 55. doi:10.1186/1471-2318-11-55 PMID:21942932

Haag, M. D. M., Hofman, A., Koudstaal, P. J., Stricker, B. H. C., & Breteler, M. M. B. (2009). Statins are associated with a reduced risk of Alzheimer disease regardless of lipophilicity. The Rotterdam Study. *Journal of Neurology, Neurosurgery, and Psychiatry*, *80*(1), 13–17. doi:10.1136/jnnp.2008.150433 PMID:18931004

Hansson, O., Zetterberg, H., Buchhave, P., Londos, E., Blennow, K., & Minthon, L. (2006). Association between CSF biomarkers and incipient Alzheimer's disease in patients with mild cognitive impairment: A follow-up study. *Lancet Neurology*, *5*(3), 228–234. doi:10.1016/S1474-4422(06)70355-6 PMID:16488378

Herukka, S.-K., Simonsen, A. H., Andreasen, N., Baldeiras, I., Bjerke, M., Blennow, K., ... Waldemar, G. (2017). Recommendations for cerebrospinal fluid Alzheimer's disease biomarkers in the diagnostic evaluation of mild cognitive impairment. *Alzheimer's & Dementia. The Journal of the Alzheimer's Association*, *13*(3), 285–295. doi:10.1016/j.jalz.2016.09.009 PMID:28341066

Hin, H., Clarke, R., Sherliker, P., Atoyebi, W., Emmens, K., Birks, J., ... Evans, J. G. (2006). Clinical relevance of low serum vitamin B12 concentrations in older people: The Banbury B12 study. *Age and Ageing*, *35*(4), 416–422. doi:10.1093/ageing/afl033 PMID:16709605

Jack, C. R., Wiste, H. J., Vemuri, P., Weigand, S. D., Senjem, M. L., Zeng, G., ... Knopman, D. S. (2010). Brain beta-amyloid measures and magnetic resonance imaging atrophy both predict time-to-progression from mild cognitive impairment to Alzheimer's disease. *Brain*, *133*(11), 3336–3348. doi:10.1093/brain/awq277 PMID:20935035

Jean, L., Bergeron, M.-E., Thivierge, S., & Simard, M. (2010). Cognitive intervention programs for individuals with mild cognitive impairment: Systematic review of the literature. *The American Journal of Geriatric Psychiatry*, *18*(4), 281–296. doi:10.1097/JGP.0b013e3181c37ce9 PMID:20220584

Jorm, A. F., Korten, A. E., & Henderson, A. S. (1987). The prevalence of dementia: A quantitative integration of the literature. *Acta Psychiatrica Scandinavica*, *76*(5), 465–479. doi:10.1111/j.1600-0447.1987.tb02906.x PMID:3324647

Kivipelto, M., Helkala, E. L., Hänninen, T., Laakso, M. P., Hallikainen, M., Alhainen, K., ... Nissinen, A. (2001). Midlife vascular risk factors and late-life mild cognitive impairment: A population-based study. *Neurology*, *56*(12), 1683–1689. doi:10.1212/WNL.56.12.1683 PMID:11425934

Koivunen, J., Pirttilä, T., Kemppainen, N., Aalto, S., Herukka, S.-K., Jauhianen, A. M., ... Soininen, H. (2008). PET amyloid ligand [11C]PIB uptake and cerebrospinal fluid beta-amyloid in mild cognitive impairment. *Dementia and Geriatric Cognitive Disorders*, *26*(4), 378–383. doi:10.1159/000163927 PMID:18931497

Kurella, M., Chertow, G. M., Fried, L. F., Cummings, S. R., Harris, T., Simonsick, E., ... Yaffe, K. (2005). Chronic kidney disease and cognitive impairment in the elderly: The health, aging, and body composition study. *Journal of the American Society of Nephrology*, *16*(7), 2127–2133. doi:10.1681/ASN.2005010005 PMID:15888561

Landau, S. M., Harvey, D., Madison, C. M., Reiman, E. M., Foster, N. L., Aisen, P. S., ... Jagust, W. J. (2010). Comparing predictors of conversion and decline in mild cognitive impairment. *Neurology*, *75*(3), 230–238. doi:10.1212/WNL.0b013e3181e8e8b8 PMID:20592257

Lethaby, A., Hogervorst, E., Richards, M., Yesufu, A., & Yaffe, K. (2008). Hormone replacement therapy for cognitive function in postmenopausal women. *Cochrane Database of Systematic Reviews*, (1): CD003122. PMID:18254016

Logroscino, G., Kang, J. H., & Grodstein, F. (2004). Prospective study of type 2 diabetes and cognitive decline in women aged 70-81 years. *BMJ (Clinical Research Ed.)*, *328*(7439), 548. doi:10.1136/bmj.37977.495729.EE PMID:14980984

Lopez, O. L., Becker, J. T., Chang, Y. F., Sweet, R. A., DeKosky, S. T., Gach, M. H., ... Kuller, L. H. (2012). Incidence of mild cognitive impairment in the Pittsburgh Cardiovascular Health Study–Cognition Study. *Neurology*, *79*(15), 1599–1606. doi:10.1212/WNL.0b013e31826e25f0 PMID:23019262

Luchsinger, J. A., Reitz, C., Patel, B., Tang, M. X., Manly, J. J., & Mayeux, R. (2007). Relation of diabetes to mild cognitive impairment. *Archives of Neurology*, *64*(4), 570–575. doi:10.1001/archneur.64.4.570 PMID:17420320

Manly, J. J., Tang, M. X., Schupf, N., Stern, Y., Vonsattel, J.-P. G., & Mayeux, R. (2008). Frequency and course of mild cognitive impairment in a multiethnic community. *Annals of Neurology*, *63*(4), 494–506. doi:10.1002/ana.21326 PMID:18300306

Massoud, F., Belleville, S., Bergman, H., Kirk, J., Chertkow, H., Nasreddine, Z., ... Freedman, M. (2007). Mild cognitive impairment and cognitive impairment, no dementia: Part B, therapy. *Alzheimer's & Dementia*, *3*(4), 283–291. doi:10.1016/j.jalz.2007.07.002 PMID:19595949

McDonnell, M. N., Smith, A. E., & Mackintosh, S. F. (2011). Aerobic exercise to improve cognitive function in adults with neurological disorders: A systematic review. *Archives of Physical Medicine and Rehabilitation*, *92*(7), 1044–1052. doi:10.1016/j.apmr.2011.01.021 PMID:21704783

Miller, D. I., Taler, V., Davidson, P. S. R., & Messier, C. (2012). Measuring the impact of exercise on cognitive aging: Methodological issues. *Neurobiology of Aging*, *33*(3), 622.e29–622.e43. doi:10.1016/j.neurobiolaging.2011.02.020 PMID:21514694

Molano, J., Boeve, B., Ferman, T., Smith, G., Parisi, J., Dickson, D., ... Petersen, R. (2010). Mild cognitive impairment associated with limbic and neocortical Lewy body disease: A clinicopathological study. *Brain*, *133*(Pt 2), 540–556. doi:10.1093/brain/awp280 PMID:19889717

Nagaraja, D., & Jayashree, S. (2001). Randomized study of the dopamine receptor agonist piribedil in the treatment of mild cognitive impairment. *The American Journal of Psychiatry*, *158*(9), 1517–1519. doi:10.1176/appi.ajp.158.9.1517 PMID:11532743

Nasreddine, Z. S., Phillips, N. A., Bédirian, V., Charbonneau, S., Whitehead, V., Collin, I., ... Chertkow, H. (2005). The Montreal Cognitive Assessment, MoCA: A brief screening tool for mild cognitive impairment. *Journal of the American Geriatrics Society*, *53*(4), 695–699. doi:10.1111/j.1532-5415.2005.53221.x PMID:15817019

National Collaborating Centre for Mental Health (UK). (2007). *Dementia: A NICE-SCIE Guideline on Supporting People With Dementia and Their Carers in Health and Social Care*. Leicester, UK: British Psychological Society.

Okereke, O. I., Kang, J. H., Cook, N. R., Gaziano, J. M., Manson, J. E., Buring, J. E., & Grodstein, F. (2008). Type 2 diabetes mellitus and cognitive decline in two large cohorts of community-dwelling older adults. *Journal of the American Geriatrics Society*, *56*(6), 1028–1036. doi:10.1111/j.1532-5415.2008.01686.x PMID:18384580

Palmer, K., Berger, A. K., Monastero, R., Winblad, B., Bäckman, L., & Fratiglioni, L. (2007). Predictors of progression from mild cognitive impairment to Alzheimer disease. *Neurology*, *68*(19), 1596–1602. doi:10.1212/01.wnl.0000260968.92345.3f PMID:17485646

Pandya, S. Y., Lacritz, L. H., Weiner, M. F., Deschner, M., & Woon, F. L. (2017). Predictors of Reversion from Mild Cognitive Impairment to Normal Cognition. *Dementia and Geriatric Cognitive Disorders*, *43*(3-4), 204–214. doi:10.1159/000456070 PMID:28301848

Paolo, A. M., Troster, A. I., & Ryan, J. J. (1997). California Verbal Learning Test: Normative data for the elderly. *Journal of Clinical and Experimental Neuropsychology*, *19*(2), 220–234. doi:10.1080/01688639708403853 PMID:9240482

Petersen, R. C. (2004). Mild cognitive impairment as a diagnostic entity. *Journal of Internal Medicine*, *256*(3), 183–194. doi:10.1111/j.1365-2796.2004.01388.x PMID:15324362

Petersen, R. C. (2011). Clinical practice. Mild cognitive impairment. *The New England Journal of Medicine*, *364*(23), 2227–2234. doi:10.1056/NEJMcp0910237 PMID:21651394

Petersen, R. C., Caracciolo, B., Brayne, C., Gauthier, S., Jelic, V., & Fratiglioni, L. (2014). Mild cognitive impairment: A concept in evolution. *Journal of Internal Medicine*, *275*(3), 214–228. doi:10.1111/joim.12190 PMID:24605806

Petersen, R. C., & Morris, J. C. (2005). Mild cognitive impairment as a clinical entity and treatment target. *Archives of Neurology*, *62*(7), 1160–1163, discussion 1167. doi:10.1001/archneur.62.7.1160 PMID:16009779

Petersen, R. C., & Negash, S. (2008). Mild cognitive impairment: An overview. *CNS Spectrums*, *13*(1), 45–53. doi:10.1017/S1092852900016151 PMID:18204414

Petersen, R. C., Roberts, R. O., Knopman, D. S., Geda, Y. E., Cha, R. H., Pankratz, V. S., ... Rocca, W. A. (2010). Prevalence of mild cognitive impairment is higher in men. The Mayo Clinic Study of Aging. *Neurology*, *75*(10), 889–897. doi:10.1212/WNL.0b013e3181f11d85 PMID:20820000

Petersen, R. C., Smith, G. E., Ivnik, R. J., Tangalos, E. G., Schaid, D. J., Thibodeau, S. N., ... Kurland, L. T. (1995). Apolipoprotein E status as a predictor of the development of Alzheimer's disease in memory-impaired individuals. *Journal of the American Medical Association*, *273*(16), 1274–1278. doi:10.1001/jama.1995.03520400044042 PMID:7646655

Petersen, R. C., Smith, G. E., Waring, S. C., Ivnik, R. J., Tangalos, E. G., & Kokmen, E. (1999). Mild cognitive impairment: Clinical characterization and outcome. *Archives of Neurology*, *56*(3), 303–308. doi:10.1001/archneur.56.3.303 PMID:10190820

Petersen, R. C., Thomas, R. G., Grundman, M., Bennett, D., Doody, R., Ferris, S., ... Thal, L. J. (2005). Vitamin E and donepezil for the treatment of mild cognitive impairment. *The New England Journal of Medicine*, *352*(23), 2379–2388. doi:10.1056/NEJMoa050151 PMID:15829527

Pfeffer, R. I., Kurosaki, T. T., Harrah, C. H., Chance, J. M., & Filos, S. (1982). Measurement of Functional Activities in Older Adults in the Community. *Journal of Gerontology*, *37*(3), 323–329. doi:10.1093/geronj/37.3.323 PMID:7069156

Raschetti, R., Albanese, E., Vanacore, N., & Maggini, M. (2007). Cholinesterase inhibitors in mild cognitive impairment: A systematic review of randomised trials. *PLoS Medicine*, *4*(11), e338. doi:10.1371/journal.pmed.0040338 PMID:18044984

Reisberg, B., Ferris, S. H., de Leon, J., Franssen, E. S. E., Kluger, A., Mir, P., ... Cohen, J. (1988). Stage-specific behavioral, cognitive, and in vivo changes in community residing subjects with age-associated memory impairment (AAMI) and primary degenerative dementia of the Alzheimer type. *Drug Development Research*, *15*(2-3), 101–114. doi:10.1002/ddr.430150203

Roberts, L. M., Pattison, H., Roalfe, A., Franklyn, J., Wilson, S., Hobbs, F. D. R., & Parle, J. V. (2006). Is subclinical thyroid dysfunction in the elderly associated with depression or cognitive dysfunction? *Annals of Internal Medicine*, *145*(8), 573–581. doi:10.7326/0003-4819-145-8-200610170-00006 PMID:17043339

Sachdev, P. S., Lipnicki, D. M., Crawford, J., Reppermund, S., Kochan, N. A., Trollor, J. N., ... Team, A. S. (2013). Factors Predicting Reversion from Mild Cognitive Impairment to Normal Cognitive Functioning: A Population-Based Study. *PLoS One*, *8*(3), e59649. doi:10.1371/journal.pone.0059649 PMID:23544083

Scarmeas, N., Stern, Y., Mayeux, R., Manly, J. J., Schupf, N., & Luchsinger, J. A. (2009). Mediterranean diet and mild cognitive impairment. *Archives of Neurology*, *66*(2), 216–225. doi:10.1001/archneurol.2008.536 PMID:19204158

Seal, E. C., Metz, J., Flicker, L., & Melny, J. (2002). A randomized, double-blind, placebo-controlled study of oral vitamin B12 supplementation in older patients with subnormal or borderline serum vitamin B12 concentrations. *Journal of the American Geriatrics Society*, *50*(1), 146–151. doi:10.1046/j.1532-5415.2002.50020.x PMID:12028259

Singh, B., Parsaik, A. K., Mielke, M. M., Erwin, P. J., Knopman, D. S., Petersen, R. C., & Roberts, R. O. (2014). Association of Mediterranean diet with Mild Cognitive Impairment and Alzheimer's disease: A Systematic Review and Meta-Analysis. *Journal of Alzheimer's Disease*, *39*(2), 271–282. PMID:24164735

Slinin, Y., Paudel, M. L., Taylor, B. C., Fink, H. A., Ishani, A., Canales, M. T., ... Osteoporotic Fractures in Men (MrOS) Study Research Group. (2010). 25-Hydroxyvitamin D levels and cognitive performance and decline in elderly men. *Neurology, 74*(1), 33–41.

Sofi, F., Valecchi, D., Bacci, D., Abbate, R., Gensini, G. F., Casini, A., & Macchi, C. (2011). Physical activity and risk of cognitive decline: A meta-analysis of prospective studies. *Journal of Internal Medicine*, *269*(1), 107–117. doi:10.1111/j.1365-2796.2010.02281.x PMID:20831630

Solfrizzi, V., Capurso, C., Introno, A., D', , Colacicco, A. M., Santamato, A., & Ranieri, M. (2008). Lifestyle-related factors in predementia and dementia syndromes. *Expert Review of Neurotherapeutics*, *8*(1), 133–158. doi:10.1586/14737175.8.1.133 PMID:18088206

Sonnen, J. A., Larson, E. B., Brickell, K., Crane, P. K., Woltjer, R., Montine, T. J., & Craft, S. (2009). Different patterns of cerebral injury in dementia with or without diabetes. *Archives of Neurology*, *66*(3), 315–322. doi:10.1001/archneurol.2008.579 PMID:19139294

Tang-Wai, D. F., Knopman, D. S., Geda, Y. E., Edland, S. D., Smith, G. E., Ivnik, R. J., ... Petersen, R. C. (2003). Comparison of the short test of mental status and the mini-mental state examination in mild cognitive impairment. *Archives of Neurology*, *60*(12), 1777–1781. doi:10.1001/archneur.60.12.1777 PMID:14676056

Thal, L. J., Ferris, S. H., Kirby, L., Block, G. A., Lines, C. R., Yuen, E., ... Reines, S. A. (2005). A randomized, double-blind study of rofecoxib in patients with mild cognitive impairment. *Neuropsychopharmacology*, *30*(6), 1204–1215. doi:10.1038/sj.npp.1300690 PMID:15742005

Tombaugh, T. N. (2004). Trail Making Test A and B: Normative data stratified by age and education. *Archives of Clinical Neuropsychology*, *19*(2), 203–214. doi:10.1016/S0887-6177(03)00039-8 PMID:15010086

Vakil, E., Greenstein, Y., & Blachstein, H. (2010). Normative data for composite scores for children and adults derived from the Rey Auditory Verbal Learning Test. *The Clinical Neuropsychologist*, *24*(4), 662–677. doi:10.1080/13854040903493522 PMID:20155574

van Uffelen, J. G. Z., Chinapaw, M. J. M., van Mechelen, W., & Hopman-Rock, M. (2008). Walking or vitamin B for cognition in older adults with mild cognitive impairment? A randomised controlled trial. *British Journal of Sports Medicine*, *42*(5), 344–351. doi:10.1136/bjsm.2007.044735 PMID:18308888

Visser, P. J., Verhey, F., Knol, D. L., Scheltens, P., Wahlund, L.-O., Freund-Levi, Y., ... Blennow, K. (2009). Prevalence and prognostic value of CSF markers of Alzheimer's disease pathology in patients with subjective cognitive impairment or mild cognitive impairment in the DESCRIPA study: A prospective cohort study. *Lancet Neurology*, *8*(7), 619–627. doi:10.1016/S1474-4422(09)70139-5 PMID:19523877

Viticchi, G., Falsetti, L., Buratti, L., Sajeva, G., Luzzi, S., Bartolini, M., ... Silvestrini, M. (2017). Framingham Risk Score and the Risk of Progression from Mild Cognitive Impairment to Dementia. *Journal of Alzheimer's Disease*, *59*(1), 67–75. doi:10.3233/JAD-170160 PMID:28582863

Ward, A., Arrighi, H. M., Michels, S., & Cedarbaum, J. M. (2012). Mild cognitive impairment: Disparity of incidence and prevalence estimates. *Alzheimer's & Dementia*, *8*(1), 14–21. doi:10.1016/j.jalz.2011.01.002 PMID:22265588

Warren, M. F., Serby, M. J., & Roane, D. M. (2008). The effects of testosterone on cognition in elderly men: A review. *CNS Spectrums*, *13*(10), 887–897. doi:10.1017/S1092852900016990 PMID:18955944

Whitmer, R. A., Karter, A. J., Yaffe, K., Quesenberry, C. P., & Selby, J. V. (2009). Hypoglycemic episodes and risk of dementia in older patients with type 2 diabetes mellitus. *Journal of the American Medical Association*, *301*(15), 1565–1572. doi:10.1001/jama.2009.460 PMID:19366776

Williams, B. W., Mack, W., & Henderson, V. W. (1989). Boston naming test in Alzheimer's disease. *Neuropsychologia*, *27*(8), 1073–1079. doi:10.1016/0028-3932(89)90186-3 PMID:2797414

Yaffe, K., Blackwell, T., Kanaya, A. M., Davidowitz, N., Barrett-Connor, E., & Krueger, K. (2004). Diabetes, impaired fasting glucose, and development of cognitive impairment in older women. *Neurology*, *63*(4), 658–663. doi:10.1212/01.WNL.0000134666.64593.BA PMID:15326238

KEY TERMS AND DEFINITIONS

Amnesia: Loss of memory.

Activity of Daily Living: Basic self-care tasks like bathing, eating.

Cognitions: Mental process of acquiring information and understanding it through thought, experience and perception.

Dementia: Impairment in memory and/ or other cognitive domains with difficulty in carrying out activities of daily living.

Executive Functions: Mental process required for planning, organizing and completing tasks.

Mild Cognitive Impairment: Presence of clinically observed and significant impairment in cognitive functions without any deficits in day to day functioning.

Memory: Memory as a mental process of storing, encoding and retrieving information.

Chapter 9
Brain Ageing and Cognitive Impairment:
Implications, Treatment, and Care

Rajpal Kaushik
West Delhi Psychiatry Centre, India

Pratima Kaushik
Amity University, India

ABSTRACT

This chapter describes how an individual progresses towards aging, several age-related cognitive declines are becoming an ever-increasing problem. Ageing causes changes to brain size, vasculature, and cognition. Protective factors that reduce cardiovascular risk, namely regular exercise, a healthy diet, and low to moderate alcohol intake, seem to aid the ageing brain as does increase cognitive effort in the form of education or occupational attainment. A healthy life both physically and mentally may be the best defense against the changes of an ageing brain. This chapter aims to characterize changes in brain structure with aging, and to investigate relationships between brain aging and cognitive decline. Along with these it will make and attempt to identify possible management, treatment and preventive measures for managing cognitive impairment in brain ageing and promoting cognitive reserve for healthy brain ageing.

INTRODUCTION

With the world facing an aging demographic, strategies to preserve cognitive and physiological functions and prevent age-related diseases are of government priority in many countries (Kirkwood, 2008); early cognitive decline is a stage where intervention is most likely to be effective. The biological basis of cognitive ability and how it changes with age is therefore of enormous interest (Deary, Penke, & Johnson, 2010). In particular, the biological basis of cognitive reserve, of which childhood mental ability is a useful index (Whalley et al., 2004), is important in any life course approach to cognitive aging. Over the last few decades, a large body of research has been conducted to identify those changes in cognition

DOI: 10.4018/978-1-5225-3480-8.ch009

that represent the normally aging brain by contrast to those that may be evidence of brain pathology. The areas of cognition that are often examined in this context include memory, language, visuospatial ability, speed of information processing, attention and executive functioning.

The effects of ageing on the brain and cognition are widespread and have multiple etiologies. Ageing has its effects on the molecules, cells, vasculature, gross morphology, and cognition. Using National Institute of Mental Health criteria in an elderly population it was reported that a high (38.4%) prevalence of age-associated memory impairment (AAMI). In a study of the International Psychogeriatric Association proposed criteria for 'ageing-associated cognitive decline' (AACD). The prevalence was slightly related to age and education. The rate was lowest in the oldest age of 75 - 78 years (20.5%) and highest in the age of 71 -74 years (30%). Subjects with less than 4 years of education had the lowest (14.3%) and subjects with more than 6 years of education had the highest rate (29.4%) for AACD (Hanninen et al., 1996). Brain ageing has been reported due to several reasons. In this cohort, irrespective of the clinical symptoms, the frequency of Alzheimer's disease-related pathology is between 19 and 67%, of Lewy body pathology is between 6 and 39%, of vascular pathologies is between 28 and 70%, of TDP-43 proteinopathy is between 13 and 46%, of hippocampal sclerosis is between 3 and 13% and, finally, of mixed pathologies is between 10 and 74%. Some studies also mention tauopathies. White-matter pathologies are not discussed specifically in all studies, although these lesions may be present in more than 80% of the aging brains (Rahimi & Kovacs, 2014).

Age-associated cognitive decline is becoming more and more prevalent. There are many causes of dementia, but neurodegenerative diseases (NDDs) are thought to be one of the most prevalent in the aging population. Indeed, during the last century neuropathological examinations have demonstrated that the brains of the majority of the individuals with cognitive decline show Alzheimer's disease (AD)-related pathologies, including neurofibrillary tangles and senile plaques. This observation led to the concept that Alzheimer's' Disease is the most frequent neurodegenerative diseases and cause of cognitive decline in older people. Community-based neuropathology studies have shown that complex constellations of underlying pathologies may lead to cognitive decline, and that the number of possible combinations increases in the aging brain.

Structural alterations observed mostly in cross-sectional imaging studies may, however, be related to events much earlier in life, and not all attributable just to advancing age (Penke et al., 2010). For example, the size and function of the brain in old age is likely related to its size and functional ability in early life, and even to in utero factors (Shenkin et al., 2009). Resistance to vascular disease and its effects on the heart, brain and other organs may also be 'preset' in utero. Genetic, and early life social, environmental, educational and nutritional factors may, therefore, all interact and lead to events in adulthood that influence the state of the brain and its vulnerability to additional insults in old age (Deary et al., 2009; Deary & Johnson, 2010).

Mental abilities change throughout life, first as a result of brain maturation and later with aging of brain cells and their billions of complex interconnections. As people age, their movements and reflexes slow and their hearing and vision weaken. Ageing has its effects on the molecules, cells, vasculature, gross morphology, and cognition. With ageing, the brains shrink in volume, particularly in the frontal cortex. Vasculature ageing and rising of blood pressure increases the possibility of stroke and as a result ischaemia increases and white matter may develop lesions. Memory decline also occurs with ageing and brain activation becomes more bilateral for memory tasks. Genetics, neurotransmitters, hormones, and experience play important role in brain ageing. But, it is not all negative, higher levels of education or occupational attainment may act as a protective factor. Also protective are a healthy diet, low to moderate alcohol intake, and regular exercise. Biological ageing is not tied absolutely to chronological ageing and it may be possible to slow biological ageing and even reduce the possibility of suffering from age related diseases such as dementia.

In the living human brain, changes in structural and functional brain imaging are interpreted to reflect neuroplasticity. There are numerous examples in the literature of neuroimaging data interpreted as evidence of neuroplasticity across a range of behavioral or environmental manipulations or interventions, including increased gray matter volumes (volumetric magnetic resonance imaging), increased white matter functional integrity (diffusion tensor imaging), and increased cerebral blood flow or glucose metabolism, particularly increased functional connectivity (positron emission tomography, single photon emission computerized tomography). Neuroplasticity can be defined as a final common pathway of neurobiological processes, including structural, functional, or molecular mechanisms that result in stability or compensation for age- or disease-related changes. Interventions associated with neuroplasticity that merit further preclinical and human study and that would have widespread applicability across neuropsychiatry conditions include epigenetic manipulations (histone deacelylase inhibitors), estrogen, and addressing neuro-inflammatory processes (Bewernick & Schlaepfer, 2013; Day & Sweatt, 2012), While there is a considerable focus on lifestyle and environmental factors associated with enhancing neuroplasticity, there are also modifiable factors that inhibit neuroplasticity and should be a focus of investigation and treatment development, particularly stress (Erickson & Gilders, 2013; Mora, 2013). Neuroplasticity associated with certain interventions (eg, TMS, MST and DBS) could restore the balance between functionally linked systems or induce a clinical response by having a greater effect on a neurotransmitter downstream from the primary effect (Chollet, 2013; Tison et al., 1991).

Cognitive Changes With Brain Aging

Associated with healthy aging is the loss of brain density and weight specifically in the frontal and temporal lobe volumes (including the hippocampus located in the medial temporal lobe region), about a 5-10 percent reduction, mostly due to water loss, between the ages of 50 and 90. Additionally, the aging brain also experiences select neuron death in the frontal lobes (the most recently evolved areas of the brain that is crucial for many intellectual functions) and parts of the brain related to movement (cerebellum and basal ganglia), widening of brain surface grooves (sulci) and shrinkage of the convolutions (gyri), 25 percent reduction in overall brain electrical activity, probably related to decreased blood flow as we age, increase in neuro-fibrillary tangles (i.e., abnormally hard clusters of damaged or dying neurons), formation of senile plaques (starch like deposits of amyloid protein), reduction in the amount of specific neurotransmitters (i.e., acetylcholine in the hippocampus, and other specific transmitter systems), and degradation of the myelin sheath (i.e., white matter) around neurons (Glisky, 2007; Whalley, 2001; Guttman, 2001). A recent study found some but not significant neuron death as a result of aging in healthy adults, contrary to a long-held view on the subject, suggesting the likelihood of subtler structural and molecular changes in the frontal lobes and hippocampal circuitry, the latter perhaps accounting for mild memory degradation that often appears late in life (Morrison & Hof, 1997). It is not yet known how or whether any of these observed physical changes listed above specifically affect cognition (Gazzalley, 2009), but it is clear that age-related structural brain alterations and declines in cognition are not uniform across the whole brain (known as selective abiotrophy) or across all mature adults (Glisky, 2007).

Characteristics of brain aging is loss of brain volume (white matter > gray matter) especially in the hippocampus and frontal lobes; loss of myelin; synapses and the dendritic arbor; cystoskeletal changes (accumulation of neurofibrillary tangles and deposition of amyloids in brain and blood vessels). Infarcts of various sizes and other evidence of cerebrovascular disease (Erten- Lyons et al., 2009). Aging is associated with progressive losses in function across multiple systems (sensation, cognition, memory, motor control and affect) and they occur with increasing age. Healthy ageing involves maintenance or improvement of cognitive performance, larger brain and hippocampal volumes were associated with preserved cognitive function, ability to make decisions and remain independent, avoidance of disease and disability by maintenance of physical, cognitive and sustained social engagement.

Gazzaley et al. (2008) identified the following Effects of Aging on Basic Adult Cognitive Functions:

- **Attention:** Some form of attention is involved in nearly all cognitive domains, and attentional declines have far-reaching impacts on functional human capacity. The attention categories listed here are constructs that correlate with active research streams on normal aging.
    - ***Selective Attention*:** Refers to the ability to attend to specific stimuli while disregarding others that are task irrelevant. Older adults tend to be slower than younger ones on such exercises reflecting, most likely, a general slowing of information processing ability.
    - ***Divided Attention/Attention Switching*:** Refers to the ability to process simultaneously two or more informational sources or tasks (e.g., driving a car). There are significant age-related declines in this capacity, particularly when information/task is complex. There is some evidence that age differences in attention switching can be reduced through practice, extended training, and aerobic exercise.
    - ***Sustained Attention*:** Refers to the ability to maintain task attention for an extended period of time. There appears to be no age-related decline in this domain.

In general, "The tasks on which older adults show impairments tend to be those that require flexible control of attention, a cognitive function associated with the frontal lobes. Importantly, these types of tasks appear to be amenable to training and show benefits of cardiovascular fitness" (p. 3).

- ***Working Memory:*** Refers to the active manipulation of a limited amount of information that is the current focus of attention. For example, in a task that involves learning a phone number and then providing the digits in reverse, which demands active reorganization of the information, adults show significant impairment with age. This deficit appears related to the divided attention deficit phenomenon, above, but there is currently little agreement among researchers on the mechanisms involved. However, Gazzaley et al. (2008) reported that older adults demonstrate a selective deficit in suppressing task irrelevant information when encoding which, in turn, reduces cognitive processing speed. What is clear is that active reorganization and manipulation of complex information by adults in problem solving, decision-making, and life planning is critical to the activities of daily living (ADL), underscoring the overall importance of intact working memory across the lifespan.

In contrast, short term memory involves the simple retention of information over a short period of time, like a telephone number that is rehearsed until it is used, and then forgotten. "Older adults show minimal or no deficits in short-term memory and can typically hold about 7 ± 2 digits in mind as long as the digits are being rehearsed" (p.4).

- ***Long Term Memory:*** Refers to the accurate retrieval of stored information that is no longer present in an active state of consciousness. Like attention, this is a multifaceted construct. Despite what many older adults may think, their remote memories of events in terms of specific detail are not as accurate as recent ones. Particularly problematic for older adults is remembering accurately the context or source of information, that is, where or when something was heard, seen, or read, or even whether something actually occurred or was just thought about, what has been termed by researchers as "reality monitoring" (Denburg et al., 2007).
- ***Semantic Memory*****:** Refers to the storage of general information, facts, and principles. The organization of this memory system, stored in the posterior neocortex, appears unaffected by age.
- ***Episodic Memory*****:** Refers to personal experiences connected to a particular place and time. It is considered the most advanced form of memory and may be uniquely human. It is affected by age and also appears to be the most susceptible to brain damage. At the input memory stage, older adults appear to encode some information less meaningfully and with less elaboration, such as, forgetting where they placed the car keys (locus: prefrontal lobes). Older adults also experience problems with memory storage or consolidation (locus: medial temporal lobe structures, including the hippocampus). Effortful memory retrieval is likewise impaired by aging (locus: prefrontal lobes and hippocampus).
- ***Autobiographical Memory:*** Refers to both semantic and episodic memories of one's personal past. More recent memories are easier to retrieve, and there is a general decrease in retention from the present to the most remote past. Autobiographical memories are largely preserved across the lifespan, however.
- ***Procedural Memory*****:** Refers to remembering how to do things, like riding a bike, driving a car, or reading. Generally, older adults show retention of acquired motor and cognitive domains until end-of-life (locus: several brain regions, including the basal ganglia and the cerebellum).
- ***Implicit Memory*****:** Refers to memory recall that occurs as a result of prior experience, even if one has no explicit recollection of that prior experience. This kind of "memory priming" remains relatively intact as adults age (loci: in the visual domain, priming involves extra-striate regions of the visual cortex; in the conceptual domain priming involves the left frontal and left temporal cortical regions).
- ***Prospective Memory*****:** Refers to remembering to do things in the future, such as, keeping appointments, paying bills, etc. Using a variety of external aids (e.g., lists, calendars) older adults retain functional prospective memory (locus: prefrontal cortex, but different from episodic memory).
- ***Perception:*** Refers to sensory processes that occur prior to cognition. Aging significantly impairs vision and hearing in most adults, much of which can be corrected and improved with re-training and practice. But to the extent that it is not, a broad range of cognitive functioning can be negatively impacted.
- ***Speech and Language:*** In normal aging, speech and language processing are largely intact in older adults, and can even improve with age, although processing time may be somewhat slower. Older adults have well structured, elaborate narratives and extensive vocabularies, and are usually judged as more interesting per se than younger people. But they can experience some text comprehension problems, which may be related to working memory deficits noted above (Buchman et al., 2014).
- ***Decision Making:*** Very little research has been done in this area, but there tends to be reliance by older adults on expert opinion.

- ***Executive Control:*** Refers to a range of different cognitive processes that are involved in the planning, organization, coordination, implementation, and evaluation of non-routine activities. Executive control plays a pivotal role in virtually all cognition, including allocating attentional resources, inhibiting task irrelevancies, formulating strategies for encoding and retrieving memories, and directing problem-solving, decision-making, and other higher order cognitive activities. This too is a multi-faceted research construct that has received considerable research attention in recent years. All executive control depends on the prefrontal cerebral cortex (aka, "frontal lobe hypothesis of aging"). Neuroimaging studies have revealed a preferential decline in older adults in both the volume and function of prefrontal brain regions (Gazzalley, 2009).
- ***Visual Perceptual Abilities*:** Principally the ability to understand spatial relationships, also show decline with age, especially after age 80. This weakness causes another driving-related problem, such as not knowing how far away a curb is or how much to turn to parallel-park a car. Visual scanning ability also can diminish so that, for example, it becomes more difficult to see a misplaced object among other items (Hartshorne et al., 2015).

MANAGEMENT AND FUTURE RESEARCH DIRECTIONS

Cognitive function in old age continues to be a focus of researchers interested in aging processes, not only with respect to health care issues, but also with respect to quality of life, human factors and issues of work and retirement in the elderly. Some of the aspects which effectively can help in either preventing pathological aging or enhancing positive ageing are discussed below:

Neuroplasticity, the capacity of brain cells to change in response to intrinsic and extrinsic factors, can have negative or positive influence at any age across the entire lifespan. Director of NIMH has encouraged "the 21st century discipline of clinical neuroscience" to include brain-plasticity based strategies in providing clinical care (White, 2011). In keeping with the increasing shift in focus from illness to what maximizes wellness, psychologists are uniquely trained to use evidence based behavioral techniques as effective methods for driving neuroplasticity in a positive direction. The researchers concluded that the performance of older adults is a reflection of predictable outcomes of increased learning on information processing and is not an indication of cognitive decline. Viewing cognitive differences across the lifespan as related to better awareness of details and accumulated learning is an example of a hopeful perspective which could effectively empower any individual to factor neuroplasticity into their efforts to promote improved business and health behaviors (Ramscar et al., 2014).

Music is a complex and multisensory form of enrichment that has a positive influence on neuroplasticity in several regions of the brain because it requires integration of audiovisual information as well as appreciation of abstract rules (Paraskevopoulos et al., 2012; Kuchenbuch et al., 2014). Magneto encephalography measures with individuals with an average age of 26.45 found that the anterior prefrontal cortex played a central role and that the neuro-plastic response was greater in musicians with long term training than was noted in those with short term training (Paraskevopoulos et al., 2014). After 4 months of piano lessons, people aged 60–84 years enjoyed improved mood as well as significant improvements in the cognitive skills of attention, control, motor function, visual scanning, and executive functioning (Seinfeld et al., 2013). A recent review (Benz et al., 2016) found music training associated with enhanced cognition in a variety of musical and non-musical skills "spanning from executive functions to creativity."

It is clear from various studies that physical exercise prescriptions need to be part of healthcare to enhance brain health (Hallal & Lee, 2013; Ryan & Nolan, 2016). Regular exercise can reinvigorate the immune system (Simpson et al., 2012). In elders without known cognitive impairment exercise can improve cognitive performance (Angevaren et al., 2008). Being aerobic up to 60 min can improve information processing, increase volume of the hippocampus (Niemann et al., 2014), energizes motor responses to improve the speed of reaction (Audiffren et al., 2008), increase gray brain matter in elders such that cognitive losses and behavioral problems associated with brain atrophy can be prevented (Erickson et al., 2014).

Total intake of food and fluid, frequency of intake and content consumed all factor into the molecular events of energy metabolism and neuroplasticity (Gomez-Pinilla & Tyagi, 2013). Several dietary choices that could be neuroprotective (Dauncey, 2014), could have positive effects on neuroplasticity (Murphy et al., 2014) including on adult neurogenesis (Chesnokova et al., 2016), and could influence the reduction of chronic inflammation (Barbaresko et al., 2013) which has deleterious effects on brain health and function.

Neuroplasticity and Cognitive Training

It is well-documented by scientists and well-recognized by the public that, as people age, they experience some diminishment of cognitive abilities. At some point, for many older adults, the decline becomes sufficiently serious that they are no longer able to live independently and manage their lives. Of course, when individuals decline cognitively to the point of inability to manage, they are experiencing significant neuropathology in the form of some type of dementia or other neurological disorder. In order to improve cognitive function, the aging brain must have plasticity that is, the ability to change structure or function in a sustained manner in response to some type of external stimulation. Most studies that have conducted interventions on older adults have focused on training some type of cognitive skill through practice, and, at the end of a training period, measuring improvement. The improvement is typically behavioral (eg, improved working memory capacity Buschkuehl et al. 2008; Li et al., 2008) but there are some studies that focus on actually changing neural activity or increasing neural tissue with training (Dahlin et al. 2008; Nyberg et al., 2003). Most studies also consider whether the observed improvement "transfers" to other tasks (Jaeggi et al., 2008).

The Alzheimer's Association estimates that if the onset of Alzheimer's disease could be delayed by 5 years due to successful interventions, this would result in a 50% decrease in Alzheimer's diagnoses (Alzheimer's Association, 2010). Moreover, many older adults are interested in staying in the work force past traditional retirement age. Participation in the work force for most adults would require that they maintain cognitive ability. Thus, slowing decline for this group could be very meaningful, as it would allow them to continue to work. There are few studies that have examined the effects of interventions over a period of years. Nevertheless, the ability to find effective techniques that will slow the process of aging is almost certainly more important than the demonstration of short-term improvements in cognitive function. Slowing decline of the aging mind is both an economic and quality of life issue that is central to controlling spiraling health costs as well as providing for the emotional well-being of both older adults and their families.

Cognitive Reserve in Aging

The idea of reserve against brain damage comes from the repeated observation of individuals who manage to function clinically in the face of brain pathology. There are two kinds of reserve that have been reported to make independent and interactive contributions to preserving functioning in the face of brain injury: brain reserve and cognitive reserve.

Brain reserve refers to quantitative measures such as brain size or neuronal count. Those with more brain reserve tend to have better clinical outcomes for any given level of pathology although for a negative report and dissenting view see (Helzner et al., 2007). According to the brain reserve model, there is some threshold at which clinical deficits will become apparent and those individuals with more brain reserve require more pathology to reach that threshold. That is, in the case of Alzheimer's for example, the disease will progress longer and more pathology will accumulate before deficits will be seen in those that start out with a bigger brain and/or more neurons. The brain reserve model is quantitative: a given brain injury will affect each individual the same way and brain injuries across the lifespan will sum together (Stern et al. 1999).

The brain reserve model is quantitative: a given brain injury will affect each individual the same way and brain injuries across the lifespan will sum together. There is some evidence that some injuries do accumulate across the lifespan such that Alzheimer's has been reported to be more likely with each psychiatric episode (Kessing & Andersen, 2004) and similarly that Alzheimer's is more likely in athletes that have sustained multiple concussions (Guskiewicz, et al., 2005). Yet, in this model individual differences are only observed in brain reserve, and damage either is or is not sufficient to reach the threshold needed to observe clinical symptoms. While the brain reserve model does explain some observations, the assumption that more is better is likely overly simple. In the context of aging, there are preliminary reports that the orbital prefrontal cortex may actually grow larger with aging and that this increase may be associated with decreased (i.e., worse) working memory performance (Salat et al., 2002). Thus, the assumption made by the brain reserve model that those with the biggest brain capacity are always at the biggest advantage may need to be tempered somewhat. A further limitation of this model is that it cannot explain why those with higher IQ and more education decline more quickly once Alzheimer's is diagnosed and progress to death sooner (Sternetet al., 1999; Scarmeas et al., 2006; Hall et al., 2007).

Cognitive reserve refers to how flexibly and efficiently one can make use of available brain reserve. Standard proxies for cognitive reserve include education and IQ although this has expanded to include literacy, occupational attainment, engagement in leisure activities, and the integrity of social networks (Barnett et al. 2006). Some recent evidence suggests that personality variables may be important as well. Indeed, Mortimer et al. (2003) reported that while those with a lower brain capacity, operationalized by a smaller head circumference, have a greater risk of Alzheimer's; yet, those with a lower brain capacity but higher cognitive reserve, as operationalized by more years of education, did not have a greater risk of Alzheimer's. Thus, cognitive reserve allowed people to compensate for pathology by making better use of that brain reserve which was still available.

Cognitive reserve is protective against brain injury in terms of cognitive and functional outcomes are established; yet it is unclear if cognitive reserve is similarly protective in terms of affective or psychiatric outcomes. One study suggested that higher cognitive reserve does not protect against the depressive symptoms that emerge early in the course of Alzheimer's (Geerlings et al., 2000); yet, other studies of healthy individuals have shown that higher cognitive reserve is protective against psychiatric diseases including depression (Koenen et al., 2009; Barnett et al., 2006). It may be assumed that restoration of neural activities, either by pharmacological or non-pharmacological stimuli, would lead to diminishment of cognitive impairment (Swaab, 1991; Swaab et al., 1998.) Following are the studies showing efficacy of pharmacological and non-pharmacological treatments in various disorders related to brain aging:

Pharmacological Stimuli

Tacrine Application

Cholinesterase inhibitors enhance acetylcholine content in the synaptic cleft, which results in restoration of cholinergic nicotinic receptor functioning and glucose metabolism. The application of moderately long-acting cholinesterase inhibitors such as tacrine (tetrahydroaminoacridine, THA), indeed has some positive effects on cognitive functioning in some AD patients and has even been claimed to slow down the course of the disease (Nordberg, 1995). Thus, even transmitter replacement may fit in the idea that enhanced functional brain activity can be obtained in Alzheimer's disease after application of the proper stimulus. The positive effects of tacrine were mainly obtained in mildly to moderately demented patients, suggesting that a too strong hippocampal atrophy or neuronal loss prevents the beneficial effects of such a treatment (Riekkinen et al., 1995).

Testosterone Supplementation

It was indeed shown to be able to restore the AVP innervation in old animals (Dobie et al., 1992). Furthermore, since testosterone is aromatized to estrogens in the brain, estrogens form a potentially important (re)stimulating factor as well. In view of the proposed decline in aromatase activity and decreased numbers and affinities of androgen receptors in senescent rat brain, estrogens or brain-specific estrogen receptor ligands may be even more effective than testosterone in stimulating sex-steroid dependent mechanisms in the senescent brain. Other animal studies also show stimulatory effects of estrogens, but not of testosterone, on e.g. choline acetyltransferase activity in several brain areas as well as on memory and learning tasks (McBee et al., 1997).

Estrogen Replacement Therapy

Estrogens are presently frequently prescribed to postmenopausal women, as they have beneficial effects on several features of female aging, such as bone loss (osteoporosis), hot flushes, nightly sweating, vaginal dryness and atrophy, heart disease and colon cancer as well as aging of the skin. Epidemiological evidence indicated that estrogen replacement therapy in postmenopausal women was effective in preventing and delaying the onset of AD (Costa et al., 1999). Several studies have shown beneficial effects of estrogens on memory in postmenopausal women (LeBlanc et al., 2001), to enhance mental functioning in women with mild to moderate Alzheimer's disease (Henderson, 1997), and to improve cognitive performance in patients with Alzheimer's disease by enhancing the response to the acetylcholinesterase inhibitor tacrine (Schneider et al., 1996).

NON-PHARMACOLOGICAL STIMULI

The conceptual framework introduced by Clare et al. (2003) suggested 3 main approaches in CI: cognitive training (computer-based or paper-and-pencil cognitive exercises); cognitive stimulation (cognitive and social group activities); and cognitive rehabilitation (individualized interventions addressing patients' key difficulties and goals).

Cognitive training delivered in individual or a group format focuses on specific cognitive functions. Health professionals deliver paper-and-pencil as well as computer-based exercises with different difficulty levels (additionally, if not stressful to the patient, caregivers might participate in the intervention sessions or assist with exercise delivery at home). Traditionally, in older adults this intervention mostly focuses on memory training, but it can also target or include other cognitive functions aiming primarily at improving the trained functions/skills and/or learning compensatory techniques and secondary generalized gains to other tasks as well as to daily life. While there is some evidence for cognitive improvements resulting from training cognitive functions in all populations (*i.e.*, healthy adults, pre-dementia, and mild-to-moderate dementia), generalization of effects is not yet evident (Buschert et al., 2010).

Cognitive stimulation, instead, adopts a more global and contextualized perspective on cognitive functioning, and assumes that cognitive functions work together and should be stimulated accordingly in a social setting. There is some evidence that this approach can benefit cognitive functioning in dementia patients (Clare et al., 2004). However, it is not yet clear whether the observed effects are due to cognitive or social components, since both are integral parts of cognitive stimulation. Cognitive rehabilitation aims to identify and work on personally relevant difficulties and goals. These difficulties may include memory or performance in daily tasks. For this method, a holistic approach is adopted with health professionals working with the patient as well as a family member or caregiver if needed. Although there are only few studies investigating intervention in age related cognitive impairment with the holistic approach, there is initial evidence that people in fact do benefit from cognitive rehabilitation (Buschert et al., 2010).

All three approaches can be useful for older adults with cognitive impairments while only cognitive training and stimulation are suitable for the healthy elderly.

1. *Reality Orientation*

Older studies already showed that reality orientation - a long-term program of formal didactic group therapy - improved cognitive functioning of demented elderly people. This shows that the nature of staff attention in a nursing home is crucial (Hanley et al., 1981). A more recent study confirmed the positive effects of reality orientation on Mini Mental States Examination and verbal fluency scores (Zanetti et al., 1995).

2. *Integrity-Promoting Care Program*

Exercise therapy improved cognition in institutionalized geriatric mental patients (Powell, 1974). In two studies, elderly demented patients, including AD patients, received an 'integrity-promoting care' program consisting of increased emotional and intellectual communication and physical activation (Widerlov et al., 1989). After applying this program for 2 months, short-term memory and visual perception had improved in the experimental group while they had deteriorated in the control group (Karlsson et al., 1985). Moreover, compared to the experimental group, concentration declined and absent-mindedness increased significantly in the control group.

3. *Transcutaneous Electrical Nerve Stimulation Therapy (TENS)*

A longitudinal study suggested that the engagement in leisure activities may reduce the risk of dementia (Scarmeas et al., 2001). In a series of experiments, E.J.A. Scherder examined the effects of increased somatosensory input by means of various types of peripheral nerve stimulation (i.e. transcutaneous electrical nerve stimulation (TENS), tactile nerve stimulation, and a combination of both types of stimuli) on memory, and on independent and affective functioning of patients in a relatively early stages of AD (Scherder et al., 1998). The results of these studies show that, compared to controls who received a placebo treatment, various aspects of non-verbal short-term memory, non-verbal and verbal long-term memory, and word fluency of stimulated AD patients improved. More specifically, these improvements imply that, after treatment, patients were better capable of: (1) learning new material;(2) retrieving familiar, categorized information from their memory store; and (3) storing, reversing and reproducing non-verbal information. With respect to independent and affective functioning, patients who were treated participated more independently in daily life, showed a better personal orientation and orientation in place, and enhanced their social interaction with fellow residents. In addition, stimulated patients felt less withdrawn, irritable, moody, dejected and gloomy and appeared to be more active and alert, possibly resulting in a decrease in forgetfulness. It is noteworthy though that TENS appeared to have a beneficial effect on the rest–activity rhythm, similar to the one observed in patients in an early stage of the disease (Scherder et al., 1999).

4. *Trans-Cranial Electro Stimulation (TCES or TES)*

A related type of stimulation is transcranial electro-stimulation (TCES or TES). In one study, TCES in elderly patients with multi-infarct dementia was also found to decrease wandering and nocturnal delirium and to enhance patients' interaction with others (Hozumi et al., 1996). The combined anatomical, physiological and behavioral findings suggest that a dysfunctional clock may underlie the sleep–wake pattern fragmentation (Swaab, 1999; Liu et al., 2000), strategies were designed to stimulate the circadian timing system in order to promote preservation of neuronal functioning of the circadian timing system, and thereby to enhance the functionality of the clock. Increased input to the circadian timing system can, among other things, be effectuated by means of bright environmental light, peripheral nerve stimulation and increased levels of physical activity.

The effect of additional physical activity in circadian rhythms was investigated in healthy elderly subjects, since fitness training was not a feasible option for most demented subjects. Fitness training improved the fragmentation of periods of rest and activity that occurs both during normal aging, and very pronounced after Supra-Chiasmatic Nucleus (SCN) (biological clock of the brain) lesions, as known from rat studies (Van Someren et al., 1997b). The anatomical and functional findings from the reported studies indicate that the SCN retains considerable plasticity in old rats, and, in functional terms, also in healthy and demented elderly subjects.

SUCCESSFUL BRAIN AGING

A growing body of scientific research is focused on determining what's different about people who age "successfully," that is, with the least declines in cognition and memory. It appears they share certain characteristics that may contribute to keeping them mentally sharp.

Physical Activity

Physical activity has a benefit for people of any age, regardless of their current fitness levels. Many experts contend that regular exercise is the single most important thing we can do to improve overall health and prevent disease. Exercise is strongly associated with successful brain aging. Exercise increases levels of brain chemicals that encourage the growth of neurons, which may be why aerobic activity (e.g., walking, biking, and swimming) seems to sharpen memory and enhance learning. A recent study found that strength training also improves cognition in older women. There is increasing evidence that regular exercise reduces the risk of dementia and Parkinson's disease. For optimal brain and body benefits, the National Institute on Aging suggests a well-rounded fitness program that incorporates four types of exercise:

- Endurance exercises, such as walking and other aerobic activities, increase stamina and appear to delay and help prevent diabetes, heart disease, colon cancer, and stroke. Research strongly suggests that this kind of exercise reduces the risk of dementia and Parkinson's disease. Studies showing improved mood and relief from depression due to exercise have generally involved endurance exercises, particularly walking.
- Strength exercises, done with free weights or resistance weights, help keep body weight down and regulate blood sugar by building lean tissue to increase metabolism. They may also help prevent osteoporosis. In recent years, experts have increasingly emphasized the importance of strength exercises in the prevention and treatment of diabetes—a major threat to brain health.
- Flexibility exercises, such as stretching or yoga, help forestall injuries and promote quicker recovery from injuries, so you can stay active, mentally and physically.
- Balance exercises, including yoga, tai chi, and such simple practices as standing on one foot, help prevent falls—a significant cause of head injury, particularly in older people.

Mental Exercise

Learning new things or pursuing activities that are intellectually stimulating, has been shown to strengthen brain cell networks and help preserve mental functions. Longer formal education, even if completed years earlier, is associated with mental sharpness among older people. Scientists theorize that learning creates a "cognitive reserve" of denser, stronger nerve-cell connections that increases the brain's ability to compensate for age-related changes in neural structure and function. It may also be that better-educated people tend to adopt more brain-healthy lifestyles, paying more attention to nutrition, for example.

Stepping Out of Old Habits

When we settle into daily routines that we repeat all but automatically, the brain is largely operating on auto-pilot, and its level of activity dwindles. By trying something fresh and different even approaching the day's tasks and chores in novel ways you can activate parts of the brain that have been falling into disuse. Some studies suggest that doing so may stimulate growth factors that support neurons and increase neurotransmitter production, among other beneficial effects on neural processes.

Social Connection

As we age, the more contact we have with others staying socially active and connecting regularly with family and friends the better we may become at preserving mental sharpness. Some evidence suggests that people who engage in more social activities are less likely to develop dementia. Conversely, social isolation is associated with faster decline and other health problems. In one study, people with the most limited social connections were twice as likely to die in a given period as those with the widest social networks. Many experts believe that social isolation can create a chronically stressful condition that accelerates aging. This may pose a particular risk for older people, who are more likely to lead solitary lives, especially if family and friends have moved away or died.

Self-Efficacy

Feeling good about ourselves and believing that what we do makes a difference, seems to prevent cognitive decline, according to several large studies that have chronicled lifestyle factors of people who stay mentally sharp into old age. The reasons are not entirely clear, but some experts believe it may be related to a greater resilience to stress (Scarmeas et al., 2006). Evidence suggests that a sense of purpose preserves mental edge and even reduces the risk of dementia. A recent study of nearly one thousand older people found those leading a more "purpose-driven" life retained their cognitive capacities significantly better over the next seven years and were far less likely than their peers to develop Alzheimer's disease.

Manage Stress

While acute, short-term stress can focus attention and improve memory, chronic stress takes a physical toll on the brain and body particularly for those ages 60 and over. Stress has been linked to anxiety and depression. Some research suggests it impairs memory and makes the hippocampus a key structure in memory formation vulnerable to injury.

To summarize, then following are considered as *Protective Factors* in promoting successful brain aging:

That diet may have a part to play in biological ageing and the development of cognitive decline is raised by studies showing that a diet higher in energy and lower in antioxidants is a risk factor alongside studies showing that energy restriction may prolong life, reduce oxidative damage, or ameliorate/ protect against cognitive decline. Increased consumption of fish and seafood, even only once a month, may be protective and reduce stroke (Budge et al. 2000) In addition to a healthy diet, low to moderate alcohol intake may reduce cardiovascular risk and may stimulate the hippocampus. Exercise is also beneficial, and studies have shown increasing executive functioning and even reduction in the ageing expected decline of white and grey tissue density with increased fitness (Piguet et al. 2002).

Yet there are other ways to maintain brain aging which are contributing factors to healthy ageing is:

- Stay away from smoking and limit alcohol consumption.
- Maintain a high level of physical activity through exercise.

- Exercise facilitates the maintenance of muscle flexibility, strength and mood (Friedland et al.,2001) patients with less cognitive and physically active at midlife had 250% increase risk for developing Alzheimer's Disease, highest activity group had 60% less incidence of AD.
- Routine medical care is also essential in maintaining good health.
- Extensive social support networks provide a good mechanism for sharing the aging process with other people who are experiencing the same challenges and joys of entering into the latter years of life.
- Gardening, playing bridge, walking, reading or other activities that are complicated enough to involve mind but don't add stress to life are examples of such activities.

CONCLUSION

The concept of "normal aging" may be an outdated and misleading concept, as we come to understand how differently our brains age and how many factors influence the process. Some of the body and mind changes normally associated with aging may not be normal at all, but are rather the result of treatable health conditions or a lifetime of poor health habits. What may seem like declining mental fitness in older people may actually be symptoms of an illness that should be medically evaluated and treated. Researchers suggest that only about 30 percent of physical aging can be traced to our genes the rest is up to us. There is a lot we can do to take charge of our brain health and maintain our cognitive fitness, no matter how old we are. Many of the scourges of aging might be prevented if we followed the old-fashioned advice of eating right, staying active, and getting plenty of rest.

REFERENCES

Alzheimer's Association. (2010). Retrieved November 25, 2012 from http://www.alz.org/alzheimers_disease_trajectory

Angevaren, M., Aufdemkampe, G., Verhaar, H. J. J., Aleman, A., & Vanhees, L. (2008). Physical activity and enhanced fitness to improve cognitive function in older people without known cognitive impairment. *Cochrane Database of Systematic Reviews*, *2*. doi:10.1002/14651858.CD005381

Audiffren, M., Tomporowski, P., & Zagrodnik, J. (2008). Acute aerobic exercise and information processing: Energizing motor processes during a choice reaction time task. *Acta Psychologica*, *129*(3), 410–419. doi:10.1016/j.actpsy.2008.09.006 PMID:18930445

Barbaresko, J., Koch, M., Schulze, M. B., & Nothlings, U. (2013). Dietary pattern analysis and biomarkers of low-grade inflammation: A systematic literature review. *Nutrition Reviews*, *71*(8), 511–527. doi:10.1111/nure.12035 PMID:23865797

Barnett, J. H., Salmond, C. H., Jones, P. B., & Sahakian, B. J. (2006). Cognitive reserve in neuropsychiatry. *Psychological Medicine*, *36*(08), 1053–1064. doi:10.1017/S0033291706007501 PMID:16854246

Benz, S., Sellaro, R., Hommel, B., & Colzato, L. S. (2016). Music makes the world go round: The impact of musical training on non-musical cognitive functions—a review. *Frontiers in Psychology*, *6*, 2023. doi:10.3389/fpsyg.2015.02023 PMID:26779111

Bewernick, B., & Schlaepfer, T. (2013). Chronic depression as a model disease for cerebral aging. *Dialogues in Clinical Neuroscience*, *15*(1), 77–85. PMID:23576891

Budge, M., Johnston, C., Hogervorst, E., De Jager, C., Milwain, E., Iversen, S. D., ... Smith, A. D. (2000). Plasma total homocysteine and cognitive performance in a volunteer elderly population. *Annals of the New York Academy of Sciences*, *903*(1), 407–410. doi:10.1111/j.1749-6632.2000.tb06392.x PMID:10818531

Buschert, V., Bokde, A. L. W., & Hampel, H. (2010). Cognitive intervention in Alzheimer disease. *Nature Reviews. Neurology*, *6*(9), 508–517. PMID:20717104

Buschkuehl, M., Jaeggi, S. M., Hutchison, S., Perrig-Chiello, P., Däpp, C., Müller, M., ... Perrig, W. J. (2008). Impact of working memory training on memory performance in old-old adults. *Psychology and Aging*, *23*(4), 743–753. doi:10.1037/a0014342 PMID:19140646

Chesnokova, V., Pechnick, R. N., & Wawrowsky, K. (2016). Chronic peripheral inflammation, hippocampal neurogenesis, and behavior. *Brain Behavior and Immunity, 22*. doi:1016/j.bbi.2016.01.017

Chollet, F. (2013). Pharmacologic approaches to cerebral aging and neuroplasticity: Insights from the stroke model. *Dialogues in Clinical Neuroscience*, *15*(1), 69–78. PMID:23576890

Clare, L., & Woods, R. T. (2004). Cognitive training and cognitive rehabilitation for people with early-stage Alzheimer's disease: A review. *Neuropsychological Rehabilitation*, *14*(4), 385–401. doi:10.1080/09602010443000074

Clare, L., Woods, R. T., Cook, E. D. M., Orrell, M., & Spector, A. (2003). Cognitive rehabilitation and cognitive training for early-stage Alzheimer's disease and vascular dementia. *Cochrane Database of Systematic Reviews*, *4*. PMID:14583963

Costa, M. M., Reus, V. I., Wolkowitz, O. M., Manfredi, F., & Lieberman, M. (1999). Estrogen replacement therapy and cognitive decline in memory-impaired post-menopausal women. *Biological Psychiatry*, *46*(2), 182–188. doi:10.1016/S0006-3223(98)00355-2 PMID:10418692

Dahlin, E., Neely, A. S., Larsson, A., Backman, L., & Nyberg, L. (2008). Transfer of learning after updating training mediated by the striatum. *Science*, *320*(5882), 1510–1512. doi:10.1126/science.1155466 PMID:18556560

Dauncey, M. J. (2014). Nutrition, the brain and cognitive decline: Insights from epigenetics. *European Journal of Clinical Nutrition*, *68*(11), 1179–1185. doi:10.1038/ejcn.2014.173 PMID:25182020

Day, J. J., & Sweatt, J. D. (2012). Epigenetic treatments for cognitive impairments. *Neuropsychopharmacology*, *37*(1), 247–260. doi:10.1038/npp.2011.85 PMID:21593731

Deary, I. J., & Johnson, W. (2010). Intelligence and education: Causal perceptions drive analytic processes and therefore conclusions. *International Journal of Epidemiology*, *39*(5), 1362–1369. doi:10.1093/ije/dyq072 PMID:20504860

Deary, I. J., Johnson, W., & Houlihan, L. M. (2009). Genetic foundations of human intelligence. *Human Genetics*, *126*(1), 215–232. doi:10.1007/s00439-009-0655-4 PMID:19294424

Deary, I. J., Penke, L., & Johnson, W. (2010). The neuroscience of human intelligence differences. *Nature Reviews. Neuroscience*, *11*, 201–211. PMID:20145623

Denburg, N. L., Cole, C. A., Hernandez, M., Yamada, T. H., Tranel, D., Bechara, A., & Wallace, R. B. (2007). The orbitofrontal cortex, real-world decision-making, and normal aging. *Annals of the New York Academy of Sciences*, *1121*(1), 480–498. doi:10.1196/annals.1401.031 PMID:17872394

Dobie, D. J., Miller, M. A., Raskind, M. A., & Dorsa, D. M. (1992). Testosterone reverses a senescent decline in extra hypothalamic vasopressin MRNA. *Brain Research*, *583*(1-2), 247–252. doi:10.1016/S0006-8993(10)80030-7 PMID:1504830

Erickson, K. I., Gildengers, A., & Butters, M. (2013). Physical activity and brain plasticity in late adulthood. *Dialogues in Clinical Neuroscience*, *15*(1), 99–108. PMID:23576893

Erickson, K. I., Leckie, R. L., & Weinstein, A. M. (2014). Physical activity, fitness, and gray matter volume. *Neurobiology of Aging*, *35*, 20–28. doi:10.1016/j.neurobiolaging.2014.03.034 PMID:24952993

Friedland, R. P., Fritsch, T., Smyth, K. A., Koss, E., Lerner, A. J., Chen, C. H., & Debanne, S. M. (2001). Patients with Alzheimer's disease have reduced activities in midlife compared with healthy control-group members. *Proceedings of the National Academy of Sciences of the United States of America*, *98*(6), 3440–3445. doi:10.1073/pnas.061002998 PMID:11248097

Gazzaley, A., Clapp, W., Kelley, J., McEvoy, K., Knight, R. T., & D'Esposito, M. (2008). Age related top-down suppression deficit in the early stages of cortical visual memory processing. *Proceedings of the National Academy of Sciences of the United States of America*, *105*(35), 13122–13126. doi:10.1073/pnas.0806074105 PMID:18765818

Gazzalley, A. (2009). Normal aging. UCSF Memory and Aging Center. Retrieved August 4, 2009 from http://memory.ucsf.edu/Education/Topics/normalaging.html

Geerlings, M. I., Bouter, L. M., Schoevers, R., Beekman, A. T. F., Jonker, C., & Deeg, D. J. H. (2000). Depression and risk of cognitive decline and Alzheimer's disease: Results of two prospective community-based studies in The Netherlands. *The British Journal of Psychiatry*, *176*(6), 56875. doi:10.1192/bjp.176.6.568 PMID:10974964

Glisky, E. L. (2007). Changes in cognitive function in human aging. In D.R. Riddle (Ed.), Brain aging: Models, methods, mechanisms. Boca Raton, FL: CRC Press. Retrieved July 30, 2009 from http://www.ncbi.nlm.nih.gov/bookshelf/br.fcgi?book=frbrainage&part=ch1

Gomez-Pinilla, F., & Tyagi, E. (2013). Diet and cognition: Interplay between cell metabolism and neuronal plasticity. *Current Opinion in Clinical Nutrition and Metabolic Care*, *16*(6), 726–733. doi:10.1097/MCO.0b013e328365aae3 PMID:24071781

Guskiewicz, K. M., Marshall, S. W., Bailes, J., McCrea, M., Cantu, R. C., Randolph, C., & Jordan, B. D. (2005). Association between recurrent concussion and late-life cognitive impairment in retired professional football players. *Neurosurgery*, *57*(4), 719–726. doi:10.1093/neurosurgery/57.4.719 PMID:16239884

Guttman, M. (2001). The aging brain. *USC Health Magazine*. Retrieved August 4, 2009 from http://www.usc.edu/hsc/info/pr/hmm/01spring/brain.html

Hall, C. B., Derby, C., LeValley, A., Katz, M. J., Verghese, J., & Lipton, R. B. (2007). Education delays accelerated decline on a memory test in persons who develop dementia. *Neurology*, *69*(17), 1657–1664. doi:10.1212/01.wnl.0000278163.82636.30 PMID:17954781

Hallal, P. C., & Lee, I. M. (2013). Prescription of physical activity: An undervalued intervention. *Lancet*, *381*(9864), 356–357. doi:10.1016/S0140-6736(12)61804-2 PMID:23199848

Hanley, I. G., McGuire, R. J., & Boyd, W. D. (1981). Reality orientation and dementia: A controlled trial of two approaches. *The British Journal of Psychiatry*, *138*(1), 10–14. doi:10.1192/bjp.138.1.10 PMID:7023589

Hanninen, T., Koivisto, K., Reinikainen, K. J., Helkala, E. L., Soininen, H., Mykkanen, L., & Riekkinen, P. J. (1996). Prevalence of ageing-associated cognitive decline in an elderly population. *Age and Ageing*, *25*(3), 201–205. doi:10.1093/ageing/25.3.201 PMID:8670552

Hartshorne, J. K., & Germine, L. T. (2015). When does cognitive functioning peak? The asynchronous rise and fall of different cognitive abilities across the life span. *Psychological Science*, *26*(4), 433–443. doi:10.1177/0956797614567339 PMID:25770099

Helzner, E. P., Scarmeas, N., Cosentino, S., Portet, F., & Stern, Y. (2007). Leisure activity and cognitive decline in incident Alzheimer disease. *Archives of Neurology*, *64*(12), 1749–1754. doi:10.1001/archneur.64.12.1749 PMID:18071038

Henderson, V. W. (1997). Estrogen replacement therapy for the prevention and treatment of Alzheimer's disease. *CNS Drugs*, *8*(5), 343–351. doi:10.2165/00023210-199708050-00001

Hozumi, S., Hori, H., Okawa, M., Hishikawa, Y., & Sato, K. (1996). Favorable effect of transcranialelectrostimulation on behavior disorders in elderly patients with dementia: A double-blind study. *The International Journal of Neuroscience*, *88*(1-2), 1–10. doi:10.3109/00207459608999809 PMID:9003961

Jaeggi, S. M., Buschkuehl, M., Jonides, J., & Perrig, W. J. (2008). Improving fluid intelligence with training on working memory. *Proceedings of the National Academy of Sciences of the United States of America*, *105*(19), 6829–6833. doi:10.1073/pnas.0801268105 PMID:18443283

Karlsson, I., Widerlöv, E., Melin, E. V., Nyth, A., Brane, G. A. M., Rybo, E., ... Nemeroff, C. B. (1985). Changes of CSF neuropeptides after environmental stimulation in dementia. *Nordisk Psykiatrisk Tidsskrift [Nordic Journal of Psychiatry]*, *39*, 75–81.

Kessing, L. V., & Andersen, P. K. (2004). Does the risk of developing dementia increase with the number of episodes in patients with depressive disorder and in patients with bipolar disorder? *Journal of Neurology, Neurosurgery, and Psychiatry*, *75*(12), 1662–1666. doi:10.1136/jnnp.2003.031773 PMID:15548477

Kirkwood, T. B. (2008). Gerontology: Healthy old age. *Nature*, *455*(7214), 739–740. doi:10.1038/455739a PMID:18843351

Koenen, K. C., Moffitt, T. E., Roberts, A. L., Martin, L. T., Kubzansky, L., Harrington, H., ... Caspi, A. (2009). Childhood IQ and adult mental disorders: A test of the cognitive reserve hypothesis. *The American Journal of Psychiatry*, *166*(1), 50–57. doi:10.1176/appi.ajp.2008.08030343 PMID:19047325

Kuchenbuch, A., Paraskevopoulos, E., Herholz, S. C., & Pantev, C. (2014). Audio-tactile integration and the influence of musical training. *PLoS One*, *9*(1), e85743. doi:10.1371/journal.pone.0085743 PMID:24465675

LeBlanc, E. S., Janowsky, J., Chan, B. K. S., & Nelson, H. D. (2001). Hormone replacement therapy and cognition. *Journal of the American Medical Association*, *285*(11), 1489–1499. doi:10.1001/jama.285.11.1489 PMID:11255426

Li, S. C., Schmiedek, F., Huxhold, O., Rocke, C., Smith, J., & Lindenberger, U. (2008). Working memory plasticity in old age: Transfer and maintenance. *Psychology and Aging*, *23*(4), 731–742. doi:10.1037/a0014343 PMID:19140644

Liu, R. Y., Zhou, J. N., Hoogendijk, W. J. G., Van Heerikhuize, J. J., Kamphorst, W., Unmehopa, U. A., ... Swaab, D. F. (2000). Decreased vasopressin gene expression in the biological clock of Alzheimer's disease patients with and without depression. *Journal of Neuropathology and Experimental Neurology*, *59*(4), 314–322. doi:10.1093/jnen/59.4.314 PMID:10759187

McBee, W. L., Dailey, M. E., Dugan, E., & Shumaker, S. A. (1997). Hormone replacement therapy and other potential treatments for dementias. *Menopause Hormone and Replacement Therapy*, *26*, 329–345. PMID:9193887

Mora, F. (2013). Successful brain aging: Plasticity, environmental enrichment, and lifestyle. *Dialogues in Clinical Neuroscience*, *15*(1), 45–52. PMID:23576888

Morrison, J. H., & Hof, P. R. (1997). Life and death of neurons in the aging brain. *Science*, *278*(5337), 412–419. doi:10.1126/science.278.5337.412 PMID:9334292

Mortimer, J. A., & Graves, A. B. (1993). Education and other socioeconomic determinants of dementia and Alzheimer's disease. *Neurology*, *43*, S39–S544. PMID:8389010

Murphy, T., Dias, G. P., & Thuret, S. (2014). Effects of diet on brain plasticity in animal and human studies: Mind the gap. *Neural Plasticity*, *14*, 563–160. PMID:24900924

Niemann, C., Godde, B., & Voelcker-Rehage, C. (2014). Not only cardiovascular, but also coordinative exercise increases hippocampal volume in older adults. *Frontiers in Aging Neuroscience*, *6*, 170. doi:10.3389/fnagi.2014.00170 PMID:25165446

Nordberg, A. (1995). Long-term treatment with tacrine: effects on progression of Alzheimer's disease as determined by functional brain studies. In K. Iqbal, J. A. Mortimer, B. Winblad, & H. M. Wisniewski (Eds.), *Research Advances in Alzheimer's Disease and Related Disorders* (pp. 293–298). New York: John Wiley and Sons.

Nyberg, L., Sandblom, J., Jones, S., Neely, A. S., Petersson, K. M., Ingvar, M., & Backman, L. (2003). Neural correlates of training related memory improvement in adulthood and aging. *Proceedings of the National Academy of Sciences of the United States of America*, *100*(23), 13728–13733. doi:10.1073/pnas.1735487100 PMID:14597711

Paraskevopoulos, E., Kuchenbuch, A., Herholz, S. C., & Pantev, C. (2012). Musical expertise induces audiovisual integration of abstract congruency rules. *The Journal of Neuroscience*, *32*(50), 18196–18203. doi:10.1523/JNEUROSCI.1947-12.2012 PMID:23238733

Paraskevopoulos, E., Kuchenbuch, A., Herholz, S. C., & Pantev, C. (2014). Multisensory integration during short-term music reading training enhances both Uni- and multisensory cortical processing. *Journal of Cognitive Neuroscience*, *26*(10), 2224–2238. doi:10.1162/jocn_a_00620 PMID:24669793

Penke, L., Valde ´s Hernande ´z, M. C., & Maniega, S. M. (2010). Brain iron deposits are associated with general cognitive ability and cognitive aging. *Neurobiology of Aging*. PMID:20542597

Piguet, O., Grayson, D., Broe, A., Tate, R. L., Bennett, H. P., Lye, T. C., ... Ridley, L. (2002). Normal ageing and executive functions in the 'old-old' community dwellers poor performance is not an inevitable outcome. *International Psychogeriatrics*, *14*(2), 139–159. doi:10.1017/S1041610202008359 PMID:12243206

Powell, R. R. (1974). Psychological effects of exercise therapy in institutionalized geriatric mental patients. *Journal of Gerontology*, *29*(2), 157–164. doi:10.1093/geronj/29.2.157 PMID:4811950

Rahimi, J., & Kovac, G. G. (2014). Prevalence of mixed pathologies in the aging brain. *Alzheimer's Research & Therapy*, *6*(9), 82. doi:10.1186/s13195-014-0082-1 PMID:25419243

Ramscar, M., Hendrix, P., Shaoul, C., Milin, P., & Baayen, H. (2014). The myth of cognitive decline: Non-linear dynamics of lifelong learning. *Cognitive Science*, *6*(1), 5–42. PMID:24421073

Riekkinen, P. Jr, Soininen, H., Helkala, E.-L., Partanen, K., Laakso, M. P., VanHanen, M., & Riekkinen, P. J. Sr. (1995). Hippocampal atrophy, acute THA treatment and memory in Alzheimer's disease. *Neuroreport*, *6*(9), 1297–1300. doi:10.1097/00001756-199506090-00017 PMID:7669991

Ryan, S. M., & Nolan, Y. M. (2016). Neuroinflammation negatively affects adult hippocampal neurogenesis and cognition: Can exercise compensate? *Neuroscience and Biobehavioral Reviews*, *61*, 121–131. doi:10.1016/j.neubiorev.2015.12.004 PMID:26695382

Salat, D. H., Kaye, J. A., & Janowsky, J. S. (2002). Greater orbital prefrontal volume selectively predicts worse working memory performance in older adults. *Cerebral Cortex*, *12*(5), 494–505. doi:10.1093/cercor/12.5.494 PMID:11950767

Scarmeas, N., Albert, S. M., Manly, J. J., & Stern, Y. (2006). Education and rates of cognitive decline in incident Alzheimer's disease. *Journal of Neurology, Neurosurgery, and Psychiatry*, *77*(3), 308–316. doi:10.1136/jnnp.2005.072306 PMID:16484637

Scarmeas, N., Levy, G., Tang, M.-X., Manly, J., & Stern, Y. (2001). Influence of leisure activity on the incidence of Alzheimer's disease. *Neurology*, *57*(12), 2236–2242. doi:10.1212/WNL.57.12.2236 PMID:11756603

Scarmeas, N., & Stern, Y. (2004). Cognitive reserve: Implications for diagnosis and prevention of Alzheimer's disease. *Current Neurology and Neuroscience Reports*, *4*(5), 374–380. doi:10.1007/s11910-004-0084-7 PMID:15324603

Scherder, E. J. A., Bouma, A., & Steen, A. M. (1998). Isolated transcutaneous electrical nerve stimulation in Alzheimer's disease. *Biological Psychiatry*, *43*, 417–424. doi:10.1016/S0006-3223(97)00208-4 PMID:9532346

Scherder, E. J. A., Van Someren, E. J. W., & Swaab, D. F. (1999). Transcutaneous electrical nerve stimulation (TENS) improves the rest–activity rhythm in midstage Alzheimer's disease. *Behavioural Brain Research*, *101*(1), 105–107. doi:10.1016/S0166-4328(98)00150-8 PMID:10342404

Seinfeld, S., Figueroa, H., Ortiz-Gil, J., & Sanchez-Vives, M. V. (2013). Effects of music learning and piano practice on cognitive function, mood and quality of life in older adults. *Frontiers in Psychology*, *4*, 810. doi:10.3389/fpsyg.2013.00810 PMID:24198804

Shenkin, S. D., Bastin, M. E., Macgillivray, T. J., Deary, I. J., Starr, J. M., & Wardlaw, J. M. (2009). Birth parameters are associated with late-life white matter integrity in community-dwelling older people. *Stroke*, *40*(4), 1225–1228. doi:10.1161/STROKEAHA.108.527259 PMID:19213950

Simpson, R. J., Lowder, T. W., Spielmann, G., Bigley, A. B., LaVoy, E., & Kunz, H. (2012). Exercise and the aging immune system. *Aging Research Review*, *11*(3), 404–420. doi:10.1016/j.arr.2012.03.003 PMID:22465452

Stern, Y., Albert, S., Tang, M.-X., & Tsai, W.-Y. (1999). Rate of memory decline in AD is related to education and occupation: Cognitive reserve? *Neurology*, *53*(9), 1942–1947. doi:10.1212/WNL.53.9.1942 PMID:10599762

Swaab, D. F. (1991). Brain aging and Alzheimer's disease: 'wear and tear' versus 'use it or lose it'. *Neurobiology of Aging*, *12*(4), 317–324. doi:10.1016/0197-4580(91)90008-8 PMID:1755879

Swaab, D. F. (1999). Biological rhythms in health and disease: the suprachiasmatic nucleus and the autonomous system. In P.J. Vinken and G.W. Bruyn, O. Appenzeller (Eds.), Handbook of Clinical Neurology (pp. 467–521). Amsterdam: Elsevier.

Swaab, D. F., Lucassen, P. J., Salehi, A., Scherder, E. J. A., Van Someren, E. J. W., & Verwer, R. W. H. (1998). Reduced neuronal activity and reactivation in Alzheimer's disease. In J. Verhaagen, F. W. Van Leeuwen, & A. Salehi et al. (Eds.), Progress in Brain Research (pp. 343–377). Amsterdam: *Elsevier*. doi:10.1016/S0924-977X(98)80078-3

Tang, M. X., Jacobs, D., Stern, Y., Marder, K., Schofield, P., Surland, B., ... Mayeux, R. (1996). Effect of estrogen during menopause on risk and age of onset of Alzheimer's disease. *Lance*, *348*(9025), 429–432. doi:10.1016/S0140-6736(96)03356-9 PMID:8709781

Tison, F., Mons, N., Geffard, M., & Henry, P. (1991). The metabolism of exogenous L-dopa in the brain: An immune histochemical study of its conversion to dopamine in non-catecholaminergic cells of the rat brain. *Journal of Neural Transmission. Parkinson's Disease and Dementia Section*, *3*(1), 27–39. doi:10.1007/BF02251134 PMID:2064729

Van Someren, E. J. W., Lijzenga, C., Mirmiran, M., & Swaab, D. F. (1997b). Long-term fitness training improves the circadian rest–activity rhythm in healthy elderly males. *Journal of Biological Rhythms*, *12*(2), 146–156. doi:10.1177/074873049701200206 PMID:9090568

Whalley, L. J. (2001). *The aging brain*. New York: Columbia University Press.

Whalley, L. J., Deary, I. J., Appleton, C. L., & Starr, J. M. (2004). Cognitive reserve and the neurobiology of cognitive aging. *Ageing Research Reviews*, *3*(4), 369–382. doi:10.1016/j.arr.2004.05.001 PMID:15541707

White, C. (2011). Brain circuitry model for mental illness will transform management, NIH mental health director says. *British Medical Journal*, *343*(2), d5581. doi:10.1136/bmj.d5581 PMID:21885534

Widerlöv, E., Bråne, G., Ekman, R., Kihlgren, M., Norberg, A., & Karlsson, I. (1989). Elevated CSF somatostatin concentrations in demented patients parallel improved psychomotor functions induced by integrity-promoting care. *Acta Psychiatrica Scandinavica*, *79*(1), 41–47. doi:10.1111/j.1600-0447.1989.tb09232.x PMID:2564721

Yaffé, K., Krueger, K., Sarkar, S., Grady, D., Barrett-Connor, E., Cox, D. A., & Nickelsen, T. (2001). Cognitive function in postmenopausal women treated with raloxifene. *The New England Journal of Medicine*, *344*(16), 1207–1213. doi:10.1056/NEJM200104193441604 PMID:11309635

Zanetti, O., Frisoni, G. B., De Leo, D., Della Buono, M., Bianchetti, A., & Trabucchi, M. (1995). Alzheimer Disorder. *Related Disorders*, *9*, 132–138.

KEY TERMS AND DEFINITIONS

Brain Aging: Brain aging is characterized by the formation of neurofibrillary tangles (NFTs) and senile plaques (SPs) as well as neuronal and synaptic loss in both cognitively intact individuals and patients with AD.

Brain Reserve: Brain reserve refers to a brain that has formed many cellular connections and is rich in brain cell density. The power of brain reserve is that we believe it has the ability to delay the clinical onset of neurodegenerative diseases such as Alzheimer's Disease (AD).

Cognitive Decline: Cognitive decline is among the normal processes of aging. It happens at different times and is noticed to affect different elements of people's lives, but it always has the same overall effect. It means that brain doesn't work as well as it used to. It is a response to the aging of neurons and the decreased speed at which the brain functions.

Cognitive Rehabilitation: Cognitive rehabilitation is a program to help brain-injured or otherwise cognitively impaired individuals to restore normal functioning, or to compensate for cognitive deficits. It entails an individualized program of specific skills training and practice plus metacognitive strategies.

Cognitive Reserve: The mind's resistance to damage of the brain. The mind's resilience is evaluated behaviorally, whereas the neuropathological damage is evaluated histologically, although damage may be estimated using blood-based markers and imaging methods.

Cognitive Stimulation: Cognitive stimulation is an intervention for people with dementia that offers a range of enjoyable activities providing general stimulation for thinking, concentration and memory, usually in a social setting such as a small group.

Cognitive Training: The term cognitive training (also called brain training or neurobics) reflects a hypothesis that cognitive abilities can be maintained or improved by exercising the brain, in an analogy to the way physical fitness is improved by exercising the body.

Neuroplasticity: The ability of the brain to form and reorganize synaptic connections, especially in response to learning or experience or following injury.

Protective Factors: Protective factors are conditions or attributes (skills, strengths, resources, supports or coping strategies) in individuals, families, communities or the larger society that help people deal more effectively with stressful events and mitigate or eliminate risk in families and communities.

Section 3
Medical Morbidity in Ageing

Chapter 10
Cardiovascular Disease in Elderly an Early Care:
Biopsychosocial Perspective

Barre Vijaya Prasad
Dharwad Institute of Mental Health and Neurosciences (DIMHANS), India

Shamsi Akbar
King George's Medical University, India

Ashwini R.
Dharwad Institute of Mental Health and Neurosciences (DIMHANS), India

ABSTRACT

This chapter describes how cardiovascular disease in industrialized nations the proportion is higher, reaching 90%. Ageing has a remarkable effect on the heart and arterial system, out of which leading to an increase in cardiovascular disease including atherosclerosis, hypertension, myocardial infarction, and stroke. Cardiovascular disease is one of the leading causes of Cardiovascular Disease morbidity and mortality today. Coronary heart disease accounts for 70 to 80 per cent of deaths in men and women in adults over 60 years of age. Congestive Heart Failure is the most common cause of hospitalization in the elderly. Since a significant proportion of the population is and will be elderly and the morbidity and mortality of cardiovascular disease in this population is so profound, it is important to understand the evaluation and treatment of cardiovascular disease in the elderly

INTRODUCTION

Aging-associated diseases are atherosclerosis and cardiovascular disease (CVD), cancer, arthritis, cataracts, osteoporosis, type 2 diabetes, hypertension and Alzheimer's disease. The incidence of all of these diseases increases rapidly with aging (increases exponentially with age, in the case of cancer) of the roughly 150,000 people who die each day across the globe, about two thirds 100,000 per day die of age-related causes. In industrialized nations, the proportion is higher, reaching 90%. Aging has a remarkable effect

DOI: 10.4018/978-1-5225-3480-8.ch010

on the heart and arterial system, out of which leading to an increase in CVD including atherosclerosis, hypertension, myocardial infarction, and stroke. Cardiovascular disease is one of the leading causes of Cardiovascular Disease morbidity and mortality today. Coronary heart disease accounts for 70 to 80 per cent of deaths in men and women in adults over 60 years of age. Congestive Heart Failure (CHF) is the most common cause of hospitalization in the elderly. Since a significant proportion of the population is and will be elderly and the morbidity and mortality of cardiovascular disease in this population is so profound, it is important to understand the evaluation and treatment of cardiovascular disease in the elderly. Deaths, at a given age, from CVD are more common and have been increasing in much of the developing world, while rates have declined in most of the developed world since the 1970s (Bridget, 2010; Moran, 2014). Coronary artery disease and stroke account for 80% of CVD deaths in males and 75% of CVD deaths in females (Mendis, Puska., & Norrving, 2011). Most cardiovascular disease affects older adults. In the United States 11% of people between 20 and 40 have CVD, while 37% between 40 and 60, 71% of people between 60 and 80, and 85% of people over 80 have CVD (Go et al., 2013). The average age of death from coronary artery disease in the developed world is around 80 while it is around 68 in the developing world (Bridget, 2010). Disease onset is typically seven to ten years earlier in men as compared to women (Mendis et al., 2011).

TYPES OF CVDS

Cardiovascular diseases (CVDs) are a group of disorders of the heart and blood vessels. There are many cardiovascular diseases involving the blood vessels. They are known as vascular diseases.

- Coronary artery disease (also known as coronary heart disease and ischemic heart disease).
- Peripheral arterial disease: disease of blood vessels that supply blood to the arms and legs.
- Cerebrovascular disease: disease of blood vessels that supply blood to the brain (includes stroke).
- Renal artery stenosis.
- Aortic aneurysm.
- There are also many cardiovascular diseases that involve the heart.
- Cardiomyopathy: diseases of cardiac muscle.
- Hypertensive heart disease: diseases of the heart secondary to high blood pressure or hypertension.
- Heart failure: a clinical syndrome caused by the inability of the heart to supply sufficient blood to the tissues to meet their metabolic requirements.
- Pulmonary heart disease: a failure at the right side of the heart with respiratory system involvement.
- Cardiac dysrhythmias: abnormalities of heart rhythm.
- Inflammatory heart disease.
    - Endocarditis: inflammation of the inner layer of the heart, the endocardium. The structures most commonly involved are the heart valves.
    - Inflammatory cardiomegaly.
    - Myocarditis: inflammation of the myocardium, the muscular part of the heart.
- Valvular heart disease.
- Congenital heart disease: heart structure malformations existing at birth.
- Rheumatic heart disease: heart muscles and valves damage due to rheumatic fever caused by streptococcus pyogenes a group a streptococcal infection.

RISK FACTORS FOR CVD IN AGEING

There are many risk factors for heart diseases: age, gender, tobacco use, physical inactivity, excessive alcohol consumption, unhealthy diet, obesity, genetic predisposition and family history of cardiovascular disease, raised blood pressure (hypertension), raised blood sugar (diabetes mellitus), raised blood cholesterol (hyperlipidemia), psychosocial factors, poverty and low educational status, and air pollution (Bridget, 2010). While the individual contribution of each risk factor varies between different communities or ethnic groups the overall contribution of these risk factors is very consistent (Yusuf, Hawken & Ounpuu, 2004). Some of these risk factors, such as age, gender or family history/genetic predisposition, are immutable; however, many important cardiovascular risk factors are modifiable by lifestyle change, social change, drug treatment for example prevention of hypertension, hyperlipidemia, and diabetes (Stephen, 2012). People with obesity are at increased risk of atherosclerosis of the coronary arteries (Eckel, 1997). In terms of age is by far the most important risk factor in developing cardiovascular or heart diseases, with approximately a tripling of risk with each decade of life (MacRae, Calum, & Vasan, 2016). Coronary fatty streaks can begin to form in adolescence (Finegold, Asaria, & Francis, 2012). It is estimated that 82 percent of people who die of coronary heart disease are 65 and older (D'Adamo et al., 2015). At the same time, the risk of stroke doubles every decade after age 55. Multiple explanations have been proposed to explain why age increases the risk of cardiovascular/heart diseases. One of them is related to serum cholesterol level (Mackay, Mensah & Mendis, 2004). In most populations, the serum total cholesterol level increases as age increases. In men, this increase levels off around age 45 to 50 years. In women, the increase continues sharply until age 60 to 65 years (Jousilahti & Tuomilehto, 1999). Aging is also associated with changes in the mechanical and structural properties of the vascular wall, which leads to the loss of arterial elasticity and reduced arterial compliance and may subsequently lead to coronary artery disease (Jani & Rajkumar, 2006).

PREVALENCE AND MORTALITY

World Scenario

Cardiovascular diseases are the leading cause of death globally. This is true in all areas of the world except Africa (Mendis et al., 2011). Together they resulted in 17.9 million deaths (32.1%) in 2015 up from 12.3 million (25.8%) in 1990 (GBD 2015 Mortality and Causes of Death, Collaborators (2016); GBD 2013 Mortality and Causes of Death, Collaborators. (2014). Deaths, at a given age, from CVD are more common and have been increasing in much of the developing world, while rates have declined in most of the developed world since the 1970s (Moran et al., 2014). Coronary artery disease and stroke account for 80% of CVD deaths in males and 75% of CVD deaths in females (Mendis et al., 2011). Most cardiovascular disease affects older adults. In the United States 11% of people between 20 and 40 have CVD, while 37% between 40 and 60, 71% of people between 60 and 80, and 85% of people over 80 have CVD. The average age of death from coronary artery disease in the developed world is around 80 while it is around 68 in the developing world. Disease onset is typically seven to ten years earlier in men as compared to women (Mendis et al., 2011). According to the National Institute of Aging (NIA), about 40% of all deaths in the elderly (age 65 and older) are related to cardiovascular disease (NIA, 2005). The risk for cardiovascular morbidity between the ages of 50 and 80 increases by about 10-fold.

ENDOTHELIAL DYSFUNCTION

In vascular diseases, endothelial dysfunction is a systemic pathological state of the endothelium (the inner lining of blood vessels) and can be broadly defined as an imbalance between vasodilating and vasoconstricting (see Figure 1) substances produced by (or acting on) the endothelium (Deanfield et al., 2005). Normal functions of endothelial cells include mediation of coagulation, platelet adhesion, immune function and control of volume and electrolyte content of the intravascular and extravascular spaces. Endothelial dysfunction can result from and/or contribute to several disease processes, as occurs in hypertension, hyper cholesterolaemia, diabetes, septic shock, and Behcet's disease and it can also result from environmental factors, such as from smoking tobacco products and exposure to air pollution (Munzel, 2008). Endothelial dysfunction is more prevalent in shift workers, a group known to have a higher risk for cardiovascular diseases (Suessenbacher, 2011).

Cellular senescence and vascular aging are perpetrated and/or accelerated by several factors that induce oxidative stress and DNA damage. Some of the common predisposing factors include aging, tobacco smoke, chemotherapeutic drugs and exposure to radiation. For example, ionizing radiation depopulates stem cell reserve and induces premature replicative senescence (i.e. arrests cell division) of somatic cells through increased generation of free radicals and subsequent DNA damage (Paris, Fuks,

Figure 1. Endothelial dysfunction

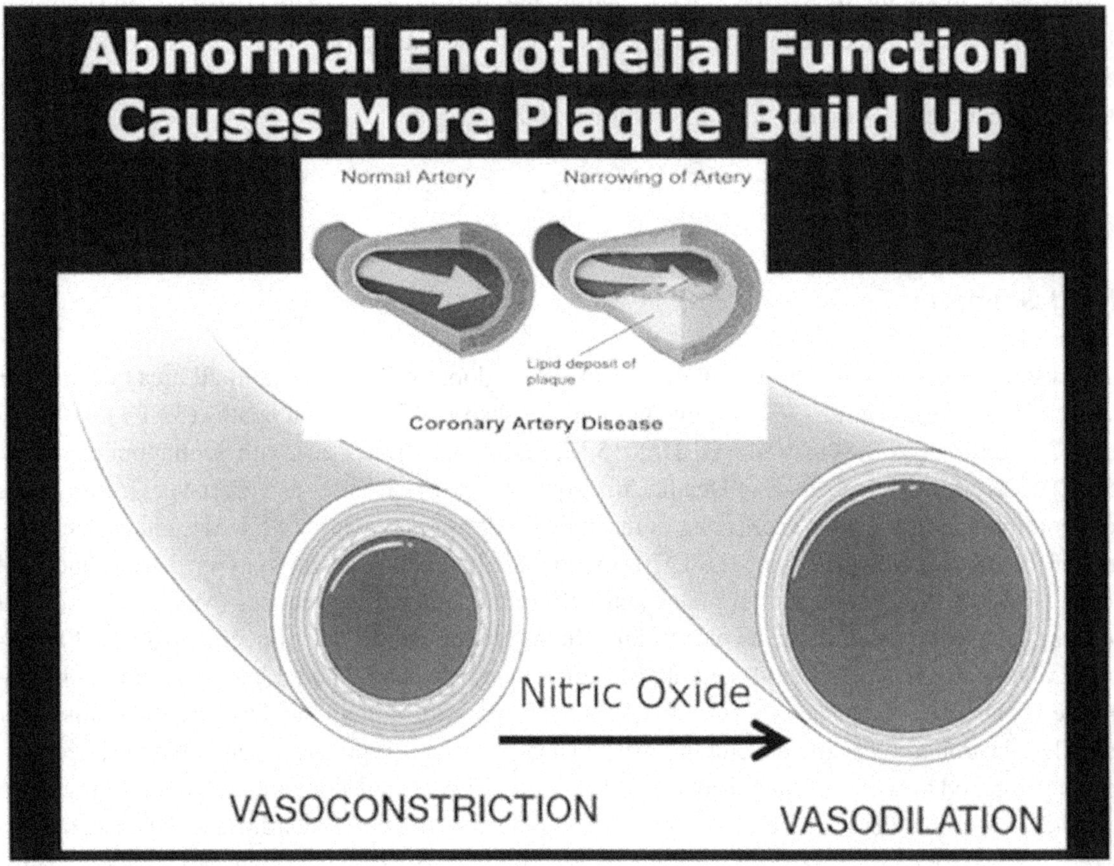

Kang, Capodieci., & Juan, 2001; Dong, Tong, Qian, Zhang., & Dong, 2015). In addition, some of the commonly used chemotherapeutic drugs such as doxorubicin and cisplatin induce cellular senescence by altering DNA structure and function (Yeh, Tong, Lenihan, Yusuf, &Swafford, 2004). In the cardiovascular system, some chemotherapeutic drugs and radiation therapy are associated with increased risk of cardiotoxicity and vascular damage (Yehet al., 2004; Patane, 2014)]. In particular, the administration of radiation therapy to the chest wall is a significant cause of vascular endothelial dysfunction including impaired perfusion, fibrous thickening of the pericardium and myocardial fibrosis (Brosius, Waller., & Robert, 1981; Veinot., &Edwards, 1996). These cardiac and vascular lesions culminate to senescence of resident cardiomyocytes and endothelial cells leading to hardening of the heart muscle and stiffening of vascular wall to trigger angina, dyspnea and heart failure that leads to sudden death (Orzan, Brusca, Conte, Presbitero., & Figliomeni, 1993). In the absence of history of exposure to chemotherapy or radiation therapy, traditional risk factors such as chronological aging play significant role in promoting processes involved in biological aging including oxidative stress, DNA methylation, telomere shortening, as well as structural and functional changes to the vasculature. As a result, the endothelium compromises its ability to secrete many of its vasoactive molecules such as growth factors, hormones, nitric oxide (NO) and microRNA (miRNA). In addition, the number and function of endothelial progenitor cells (EPCs) is reduced with advancing age. Taken together, the endothelium becomes senescent and prone to cardiovascular disease including hypertension, atherosclerosis and diabetes (Orzan et al., 1993; Pinto, 2007).

PSYCHOSOCIAL RISK FACTORS FOR CVD

Over the past three decades, a large and varied body of research has examined the role of chronic psychosocial stress in the development of CVD (Cohen, Janicki-Deverts, & Miller, 2007; Kaplan, Chen, & Manuck, 2009). Psychosocial stress may be defined as aversive or demanding conditions that tax or exceed the behavioral resources of the organism (Lazarus, 1966). The debilitating and often fatal complications of CVD are usually seen in middle-aged or elderly men and women. However, atherosclerosis the main pathological process leading to coronary artery disease, cerebral artery disease and peripheral artery disease begins early in life and progresses gradually through adolescence and early adulthood (Berenson, 1989; Mendis, 2005). It is usually asymptomatic for a long period. The rate of progression of atherosclerosis is influenced by cardiovascular risk factors: tobacco use, an unhealthy diet and physical inactivity (which together result in obesity), elevated blood pressure (hypertension), abnormal blood lipids (dyslipidaemia) and elevated blood glucose (diabetes). Continuing exposure to these risk factors leads to further progression of atherosclerosis, resulting in unstable atherosclerotic plaques, narrowing of blood vessels and obstruction of blood flow to vital organs, such as the heart and the brain. The clinical manifestations of these diseases include angina, myocardial infarction, transient cerebral ischaemic attacks and strokes. Given this continuum of risk exposure and disease, the division of prevention of cardiovascular disease into primary, secondary and tertiary prevention is arbitrary, but may be useful for development of services by different parts of the health care system. The concept of a specific c threshold for hyper-tension and hyperlipidaemia is also based on an arbitrary dichotomy. Recent reviews were indicated other behavioral and psychosocial risk factors for CVD are, behavioral factors, poor diet, overeating, physical inactivity, smoking, poor sleep, hygiene, depression, anxiety, pessimism, hostility/anger, chronic stress, job stress, marital strain, child abuse and trauma, chronic illness, poor social support and socioeconomic factors.

GENDER DIFFERENCES

Differences in CVD between men and women represent a very recent acknowledge in the field of cardiovascular medicine. Although extensive literature about atherosclerotic process and its consequences dates many decades by now, only recently researchers have proven that gender greatly impacts on pathophysiology and clinical manifestation of CVD. Paradoxically, the first step in the knowledge of gender differences has to be the awareness of similarities between men and women. In other words, it is time to recognize that CVD may occur in both sexes. Indeed, until a few years ago, coronary heart disease (CHD) has been extensively considered to typically affect male gender and most medical papers have passed the notion that female gender could suffer more from breast cancer than from CVD and CHD (Leonarda, & Gabriella, 2015). Nowadays, CHD constitutes the leading cause of mortality not only among men, but also among women, accounting for one third of all female deaths. Of note, such evidence still remains largely unknown by most physicians (Perk, De Backer, Gohlke, Graham, & Reiner, 2012). Most women are completely unaware about meaning of cardiovascular risk, often because the healthcare providers do not sufficiently advise them about it. Women appear less conscious than men of their own cardiovascular risk profile, but 1 in 2 women may eventually die of heart disease or stroke (compared with 1 in 25 who may potentially die of breast cancer (Mosca, Manson, Sutherland, Langer., & Manolio, 1997). In many Countries over the world, women are more likely than men to die every year of CVD. In the United States, since 1984, the number of CVD deaths for females has exceeded that for males (National Center for Health Statistics [NCHS], (2009). Similarly, the World Health Organization in 2004 reported an overall cardiovascular mortality in Europe of 55% of cases in women and 43% of cases in men. Ischemic heart disease, stroke and other CVD represented 23%, 18% and 15% of cases respectively in women and 21%, 11% and 11% of cases respectively in men (Stramba-Badiale, Fox, Priori, Collins, & Daly, 2006). The impact of female CVD on public health is definitively related also to morbidity, given that advances in science and medicine allow many women to survive heart disease and to be affected by chronic CVD. Nowadays, 1 in 3 female adults has some form of CVD (NCHS, 2009). As life expectancy in female gender is longer than in male gender, the loss of disability-adjusted life years in women is significantly growing up. In 2006 it has been estimated that 34% (> 38 million) of women in the United States lived with CVD. Nowadays it represents a global health issue: in most Countries, including China, the proportion of women 35 to 74 years of age affected by dyslipidemia and hypertension has reached 53% and 25%, respectively (Mosca, Banka, Benjamin, Berra, & Bushnell, 2007). Medical interventions tailored on individual patients can effectively prevent CVD. Such goal is in the first place in women, but needs an appropriate acknowledge of gender differences lying behind risk factors, pathophysiology and clinical manifestation of CVD.

Clinical manifestations of CVD also differ between sexes, thus making diagnosis challenging. Symptoms frequently experienced by men, such as oppressive or constrictive chest pain and dyspnoea have been traditionally recognized as typical of myocardial ischemia, in light of the strict correspondence with obstructive coronary artery disease. Conversely, women more often suffer from abdominal pain, dizziness, shortness of breath, frequent indigestion, unusual fatigue: in such cases, the absence of severe coronary artery disease has caused any important misperceptions, so that the term "atypical" symptoms has been commonly used as synonymous of "low probability of myocardial ischemia". Moreover, the evidence that both epicardial coronary artery disease and microvascular dysfunction in women may potentially manifest the same symptoms has greatly contributed to generate confusion. As consequence, the prognostic value of chest pain in women has been greatly underestimated. This derives partly by the evidence that women in the Framingham study developed chest pain more often than men, but it rarely progressed to myocardial infarction (Lerner., & Kannel, 1986). The predictive value of angina increased only among older subsets of women (Kannel., & Feinleib, 1972). According to the most recent literature data, we think that such important issue has to be focused by another point-of-view: irrespectively of the precise pathophysiological mechanisms, men and women may equally suffer from myocardial ischemia and are worthy to be properly treated. The acknowledge of gender differences by physicians is crucial for ensuring the most appropriate treatment strategy in both sexes. In keeping, symptoms should not be more categorized as "typical" and "atypical": a re-definition of clinical manifestations as "typical of men" and "typical of women" urges and might potentially improve prognosis. In Figure 2 presented schematic representations of symptoms, usually occurring in men and women, and pathophysiological mechanisms underlying myocardial ischemia in both sexes.

CVD RISK ASSESSMENT

Aims of Clinical Assessment

- To search for all cardiovascular risk factors and clinical conditions that may influence prognosis and treatment;
- To determine the presence of target organ damage (heart, kidneys and retina);
- To identify those at high risk and in need of urgent intervention;

Figure 2. Pathophysiological mechanisms myocardial ischemia in male and female
(Source: Leonarda & Gabriella, 2015)

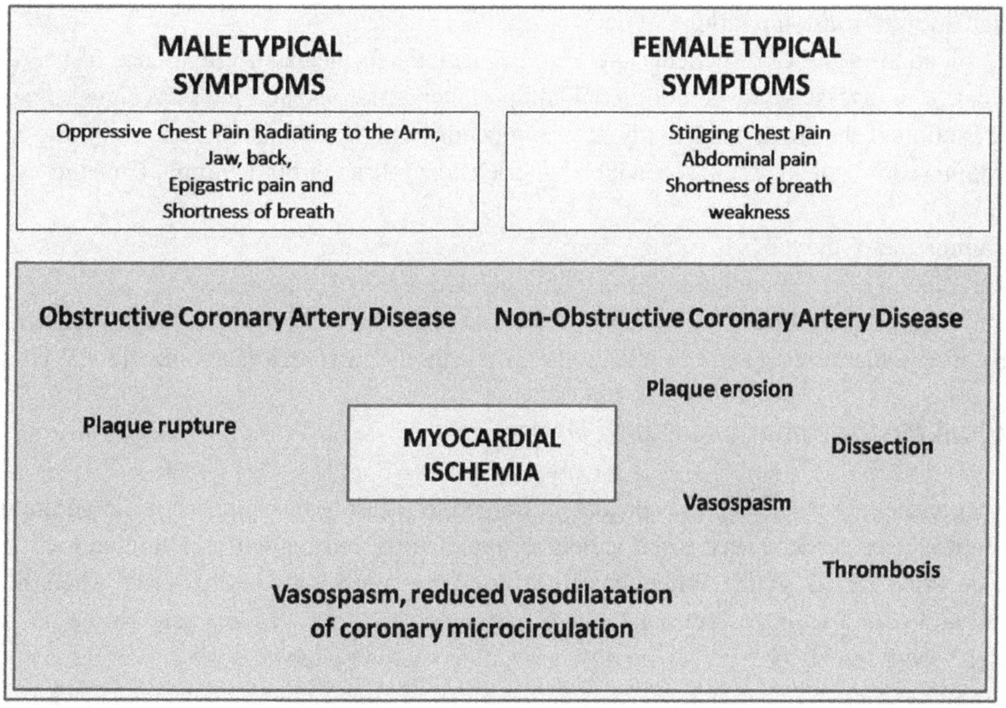

- To identify those who need special investigations or referral (e.g. those with secondary hypertension. A Comprehensive Clinical History:
- Current symptoms of coronary heart disease, heart failure, cerebrovascular disease, peripheral vascular disease, diabetes, and renal disease;
- Information on the use of drugs known to raise blood pressure (oral contraceptives, nonsteroidal anti-inflammatory drugs, liquorice, cocaine, amfetamine, erythropoietin, cyclosporins and steroids);
- The family history of high blood pressure, diabetes, dyslipidaemia, coronary heart disease, stroke and renal disease;
- The personal history of coronary heart disease, heart failure, cerebrovascular disease, peripheral vascular disease, diabetes, gout, bronchospasm, sexual dysfunction, and renal disease;
- Symptoms suggestive of secondary hypertension, i.e. hypertension caused by an underlying condition;
- Information on behaviour, including tobacco use, physical activity and dietary intake of fat, salt and alcohol;
- Personal, psychosocial, occupational and environmental factors that could influence the course and outcome of long-term care.

Physical Examination

A full physical examination is essential, and should include careful measurement of blood pressure, as described below. Other important elements of the physical examination include:

- Measurement of height and weight, and calculation of body mass index (BMI) (weight in kilograms divided by the square of height in meters); measurement of waist and hip circumference for calculation of waist–hip ratio;
- Examination of the cardiovascular system, particularly for heart size, evidence of heart failure, evidence of disease in the carotid, renal and peripheral arteries, and physical signs suggestive of coarctation of the aorta, particularly in young people with hypertension;
- Examination for features of secondary hypertension (phaeochromocytoma, Cushing syndrome, etc.)
- Examination of the lungs for congestion;
- Examination of the abdomen for bruits, enlarged kidneys and other masses;
- Examination of the optic fundi and of the central and peripheral nervous system for evidence of cerebrovascular disease and complications of diabetes (World Health Organization [WHO], 2005)

Periodical Measurement of Blood Pressure

Health care professionals need to be adequately trained to measure blood pressure. In addition, blood pressure measuring devices need to be validated, maintained and regularly calibrated to ensure that they are accurate (WHO, 2005). Where possible, blood pressure should be measured when the patient is relaxed and seated with the arm outstretched and supported. Two readings should be taken; if the average is 140/90 mmHg or more, an additional reading should be taken at the end of the consultation for confirmation. Blood pressure should be measured in both arms initially, and the arm with the higher reading used for future measurements. If the difference between the two arms is more than 20 mmHg for systolic pressure or 10 mmHg for diastolic pressure, the patient should be referred to the next level of care for examination for vascular stenosis. Patients with accelerated (malignant) hypertension (blood pressure ≥180/110 mmHg with papilloedema or retinal haemorrhages) or suspected secondary hypertension should be referred to the next level immediately.

PREVENTIVE STRATEGIES

Preventive strategies assist high-risk individuals to lower their cardiovascular risk by:

- Quitting tobacco use, or reducing the amount smoked, or not starting the habit.
- Making healthy food choices.
- Being physically active.
- Reducing body mass index (to less than 25 kg/m2) and waist–hip ratio (to less than 0.8 in women and 0.9 in men (these figures may be different for different ethnic groups).
- Lowering blood pressure (to less than 140/90 mmHg).
- Lowering blood cholesterol (to less than 5 mmol/l or 190 mg/dl).
- Lowering LDL-cholesterol (to less than 3.0 mmol/l or 115 mg/dl).
- Controlling glycaemia, especially in those with impaired fasting glycaemia and impaired glucose tolerance or diabetes.

The above goals represent the minimum that should be achieved. They are given for broad guidance in managing cardiovascular risk. In some subgroups of high-risk people, particularly those with established cardiovascular disease or diabetes, a case can be made for lower targets for blood pressure (< 130/80 mmHg), total cholesterol and LDL-cholesterol, which may require more intensive treatment. Similarly, in very high-risk patients, a total cholesterol of less than 4.0 mmol/l (152 mg/dl) and LDL-cholesterol of less than 2.0 mmol/l (77 mg/dl), or a reduction of 25% in total cholesterol and 30% in LDL-cholesterol, whichever achieves the lower absolute level, may be desirable goals (WHO, 2005)

MEDICAL MANAGEMENT

It is important to differentiate the cardiac manifestations of normal aging which do not require medical management from cardiac disease in the older patient. A rationale for greater utilization of diagnostic techniques can be made in the older patient who may present with atypical symptoms, multiple confounding medical problems, and age-related alterations in physical findings of some cardiac diseases. The management of most cardiac diseases in the older patient is similar to that of the younger patient, with the important recognition of the need to reduce medication dosages and be aware of the increased risk of adverse effects or drug interactions. Age should not be a contraindication to invasive procedures or surgical procedures or thrombolytic therapy, since when properly selected, they benefit older patients to the same or greater degree as younger patients.

MULTIDESCIPLAINARY TEAM APPROACH

The composition of a disease management team may vary both from centre to centre and from patient to patient, a suggested list of team members is given below:

- Nurse coordinator or case manager
- Dietitian
- Social services representative
- Clinical pharmacist
- Physical therapist/occupational therapist
- Exercise/rehabilitation specialist
- Clinical Psychologist
- Patient and family
- Primary care physician
- Cardiologist/other consultants.

Each team member provides their own unique expertise and/or perspective, and these are then woven into an integrated package tailored to meet each individual patient's needs, expectations, and circumstances. Importantly, not all patients will require the services of all team members, and it is therefore essential to identify a team leader. In most cases, this will be the nurse coordinator or case manager, who, in addition to being the patient's primary contact person and educator, is also responsible for coordinating the efforts of other team members, including the selective activation of appropriate consultations on an individualized basis. In addition to the team itself, several other components are essential for effective disease management. First, the patient and family should be provided with comprehensive information about heart disease, including common etiologies, symptoms and signs, standard diagnostic tests, medications, diet, activity, prognosis and the role of the patient and family in ensuring that heart disease remains under control. This information should be provided in a readily understandable patient-friendly format and several patient-oriented heart disease brochures are now commercially available. In addition to these materials, the patient should be given a scale (if not already owned) and a chart to record daily weights, an accurate and detailed list of medications supplemented by medication aids if needed (e.g. a pill box), and specific information about when to contact the nurse, physician, or other team member in the event that questions or new symptoms arise. In this regard, the importance of establishing an effective one-on-one nurse-to-patient relationship cannot be overemphasized, as this interaction will often be critical to the early diagnosis and effective outpatient treatment of heart disease exacerbations (Essays, 2013).

IMPORTANCE OF SOCIAL SUPPORT

Old age is accompanied by role change and often, role loss. Most people can expect transformation in occupational, family and community roles and for many the number of different roles declines in later life. Some of the major contributors to social and psychological challenges for seniors are as follows: loneliness from losing a spouse and friends, inability to independently manage regular activities of living difficulties coping and accepting physical changes of ageing, frustration with ongoing, medical problems and increasing number of medication social isolation as adult children are engaged in their own lives, feeling inadequate from inability to continue to work, boredom from retirement and lack of routine activities', financial stressors from the loss of regular income. In this context, social support is one the important component in ageing and their health behavior. Social support refers to the function and quality of social relationships, such as perceived availability of help or actually received support. It occurs through an interactive process and can be related to altruism, a sense of obligation, and the perception of reciprocity (Schwarzer, & Leppin, 1992). Holahan and colleagues (1995) define social support "…as the perception of emotional sustenance, informational guidance, and tangible assistance…" (p. 153). "Researchers have demonstrated a strong relationship between physical health, social support, and psychological problems in healthy populations as well as in a number of populations with chronic health conditions such as cardiovascular disease, cancer, diabetes and chronic pain…" (Hagedoorn et al., 2000). Social support may directly affect health or may work to buffer the effects of prolonged stress associated with managing a chronic illness (Cohen & Willis, 1985). Social support may increase one's coping resources, which in turn increase their beliefs about their control over the situation. It may also affect physiological arousal, immune functioning, as well as health maintains behaviors. Several types of social support have been investigated, such as instrumental support (e.g., assist with a problem), tangible support (e.g., donate goods), informational support (e.g., give advice), and emotional support (e.g., give reassurance), among others. Social support can assist coping and exert beneficial effects on various health outcomes. It has also been found to be advantageous for patients during recovery from heart surgery. Coronary artery bypass surgery patients who received many visits by their spouses were, on average, released earlier from hospital than those who received only few visits. Cardiac patients and their spouses were studied over a half-year period before and after heart surgery. It was found that resourceful spouses transferred their resiliency to the patients as part of a dyadic coping process (Schroder, Schwarzer., & Endler, 1997).

COMPREHENSIVE CARDIAC REHABILITATION (CCR)

Role of Psychologist

More people are living longer, and the biology of aging in this expanding senior population is intrinsically conducive to many types of CVD (e.g., CHD as well as heart failure [HF], valvular heart disease [VHD]) for which cardiac rehabilitation (CR) is now indicated (Thomas & King, 2010; Yancy, Jessup., & Bozkurt, 2013). Moreover, older adults are more likely to experience unique consequences from CVD and CVD management for which CR can be especially useful. Deconditioning, atypical symptoms, management conundrums, and poor adherence are all more likely in older age. Such vulnerabilities can arise when treatment goes smoothly (due to increased susceptibility to deconditioning and post-hospitalization syndrome with age) and they are especially likely if and when common difficulties arise (e.g., through the compounding effects of concurrent diseases, delirium, and prolonged lengths of stay), all of which are everyday scenarios among older CVD patients (Krumhol, 2013; Graf, 2006).

Comprehensive cardiac rehabilitation is a multi-component and coordinated intervention aimed at optimizing physical, psychological, and social functioning and reducing morbidity and mortality of patients with cardiovascular diseases [Majnemer, Limperopoulos, Shevell, Rosenblatt., & Rohlicek, 2006; Magomedova., & Damadaeva, 2014).Cardiac rehabilitation provides opportunities to contend with predictable geriatric intricacies in older patients with CVD, including 1) multimorbidity (multiple cardiac and non-cardiac diseases occurring in combination), 2) polypharmacy (multiple new medications in the context of age-related changes in pharmacokinetics and pharmacodynamics that predispose to side effects and iatrogenesis), 3) detrimental processes of care (harmful effects of hospitalizations and transitions, including delirium, deconditioning, disability, and to institutionalization thereafter), 4) sarcopenia (age-related atrophy and weakening of skeletal muscle), and 5) the challenge of education, decision making, and behavior changes in the context of declining cognition (especially given the common impairments in executive cognitive function that are associated with CVD and age). After shifting the focus from direct pathology to the identity of the patient, the psychologist is becoming an important member of the multidisciplinary team. He can help cardiologists in the following fields (Leon, Franklin, Costa, Balady, & Berra, 2005):

1. Maintaining a patient during the hospitalization, when it enters into a therapeutic alliance, aid in the modification of lifestyle, and the working out of traumatic events related to feeling a "victim" after a heart attack;
2. Personalization of therapy, which will improve the dialogue between a doctor and a patient;
3. If necessary, providing a differential diagnosis.

In Italian guidelines for psychological care in cardiorehabilitation (Sommaruga, Tramarin, Angelino, Bettinardi, & Cauteruccio, 2003) are reserved five phases of communication that characterize the interaction between cardiac patient and a psychologist:

1. **Selection:** Patients have the right to request and receive psychological counseling.
2. **Entry:** Reflects the first contact between the patient and the psychologist.
3. **Assessment:** The aim is to identify psychological problems, needs, resources, and a collection of all data necessary for appropriate intervention. In this phase it is important to focus on nonadaptive behaviors and habits of the patient in the pathopsychological aspects.
4. **Intervention:** Psychological support in the rehabilitation of the patient and a family. Activities include the following tasks:
    a. The recognition and expression of emotional experiences related to illness;
    b. Identification and implementation of mechanisms that help to control risk factors and modify lifestyle;
    c. Restore a satisfactory quality of life.

These psychological interventions contain group and individual counseling and psychotherapy (mainly cognitive-behavioral), learning strategies, stress management, and self-help activities.

SOLUTIONS AND RECOMMENDATIONS

Physical Activity

Physical activity (PA) frequently decreases with age due to a reduction in the pace of life. However, the importance of staying physically active cannot be underestimated. There is significant evidence, from a broad range of studies which suggest an inverse relationship between PA and CVD risk. This amelioration could be induced by an improvement in blood lipid profile. For example, in a classic meta-analysis Leon (2001) reviewed 51 human intervention studies examining the effects of at least 12 weeks of PA on blood lipid profile in men and women from 1987-2000 (Leon et al., 2001). The authors reported a lipid profile improvement in response to PA in nearly half of the studies reviewed. It has also been suggested that lipid profile is improved through the activation of lipoprotein lipase a key enzyme involved in fatty acid metabolism, which stimulates the clearance of triglyceride-rich lipoproteins to supply free fatty acids to exercising muscle.

Diet

Diet is a significant adaptable determinant of healthy ageing. The dietary habits of the population, changes have occurred in different areas. For example, the intake of salt and saturated fats has been reduced in most societies. The food industry has reduced the presence of trans fatty acids in different food items; this has been promoted by regulatory initiatives in some communities. However, the potential to prevent CVD through dietary adaptations is still poorly implemented. Adherence to a balanced diet is generally limited; the control of elevated blood pressure, dyslipidaemias and dysglycaemia can largely be improved through changes in lifestyle. Achieving better adherence with dietary recommendations requires the understanding of the determinants of poor compliance. At the population level, structural measures such as product information and consumer-friendly nutrition labeling may improve health-friendly choices. Energy-dense, nutrient-deficient foods are generally highly accessible and inexpensive; the marketing of such foods could be limited and taxed. On the other hand, fruits and vegetables tend to be more expensive; the subsidizing of their costs may be useful.

Quit Smoking

Smoking is a major cause of cardiovascular disease (CVD) and causes one of every three deaths from CVD, according to the 2014 Surgeon General's Report on smoking and health. CVD is the single largest cause of death in the United States, killing more than 800,000 people a year. More than 16 million Americans have heart disease. Almost 8 million have had a heart attack and 7 million have had a stroke (Smoking and heart health (2014). Even though we don't know exactly which smokers will develop CVD from smoking, the best thing all smokers can do for their hearts is to quit. Smokers who quit start to improve their heart health and reduce their risk for CVD immediately. Within a year, the risk of heart attack drops dramatically, and even people who have already had a heart attack can cut their risk of having another if they quit smoking. Within five years of quitting, smokers lower their risk of stroke to about that of a person who has never smoked.

Cut Down Alcohol

So far as alcohol concern people who drink heavily have a high mortality from all causes and cardiovascular disease, including sudden death and hemorrhagic stroke. In addition, they may suffer from psychological, social and other medical problems related to high alcohol consumption (Marmot, 2001; Donaldson, 2004).

Yoga and Yoganidra

The circulatory system plays a vital role in the nourishment of tissues. Elements necessary for nourishment of tissues are carried to them by blood. Practices of pranayama rejuvenate the tissues with a fresh supply of oxygen. Asanas improve cardiovascular efficiency. The yogic exercises give a good massage to the perpetually working heart. Asanas involve very little muscular activity. In such a condition, the heart has a tendency to slow down its speed and the heart beats in a controlled manner. When the muscular activity is less, there is minimum production of carbon dioxide. This reduces the levels of stress to the heart. Yoga enhances heart health, lowers blood pressure, reduces chronic stress, boosts immune system and enhances cognitive ability. Yoga has an important role in the prevention of cardiovascular diseases as well as recurrence of heart attacks, hypertension and coronary heart diseases. Yoga affects the hypothalamus directly the area of the brain, controlling the endocrine activity and it helps to prevent heart attacks. It is very obvious most of the aged people may not be habituated to practice yoga all of sudden, for them required yoga trainer or else they can practice more simple method like YogaNidra. YogaNidra is a state of conscious Deep Sleep. YogaNidra brings an incredible calmness, quietness and clarity. It has great Therapeutics values. Sankalpa can bring about even the impossible in life, therefore CVD even cancer and AIDS patients can benefit.

CONCLUSION

Currently there is an extensive set of interrelated psychosocial factors and CVD risk, and therefore there is a need for a thorough study. This will allow diverse preventive measures that will enhance the effect of cardiac treatment. Such events not only help to reduce the risk of recurrent episodes of acute forms of CVD, but also improve the quality of life of patients. Today there is a significant need in the development of differentiated methods of secondary prevention and rehabilitation of patients with cardiovascular diseases. While the psychological and social methods are very promising, there is also a need for the development of effective models to study the interaction between different psychosocial factors and the establishment of scientific basis for developing preventive medical, surgical as well as psychological interventions. Although an unavoidable cardiovascular risk factors in ageing, may overcome all the other risk factors collectively. Therefore, understanding fundamental mechanisms that dictate the pace of aging could lead to significant advancements into both preventative and therapeutic treatments of CVD that of enhancing quality of life of elderly.

REFERENCES

Berenson, G. S., Srinivasan, S. R., Hunter, S. M., Nicklas, T. A., Freedman, D. S., Shear, C. L., & Webber, L. S. (1989). Risk factors in early life as predictors of adult heart disease: The Bogalusa Heart Study. *The American Journal of the Medical Sciences*, *298*(3), 141–151. doi:10.1097/00000441-198909000-00001 PMID:2679086

Bridget, B. K. (2010). *Promoting Cardiovascular Health in the Developing World: A Critical Challenge to Achieve Global Health* (V. Fuster Ed.). Washington, D.C: National Academies Press.

Brosius, F. C. III, Waller, B. F., & Roberts, W. C. (1981). Radiation heart disease. Analysis of 16 young (aged 15 to 33 years) necropsy patients who received over 3,500 rads to the heart. *The American Journal of Medicine*, *70*(3), 519–530. doi:10.1016/0002-9343(81)90574-X PMID:6782873

Cohen, S., Janicki-Deverts, D., & Miller, G. (2007). Psychological stress and disease. *Journal of the American Medical Association*, *298*(14), 1685–1687. doi:10.1001/jama.298.14.1685 PMID:17925521

Cohen, S., & Willis, T. A. (1985). Stress, social support, and the buffering hypothesis. *Psychological Bulletin*, *98*(2), 310–375. doi:10.1037/0033-2909.98.2.310 PMID:3901065

D'Adamo, E., Guardamagna, O., Chiarelli, F., Bartuli, A., Liccardo, D., Ferrari, F., & Nobili, V. (2015). Atherogenic dyslipidemia and cardiovascular risk factors in obese children. *International Journal of Endocrinology*, *912047*. doi:10.1155/2015/912047 PMID:25663838

Deanfield, J., Donald, A., Ferri, C., Giannattasio, C., Halcox, J., Halligan, S., ... Lerman, A. (2005). Endothelial function and dysfunction. Part I: Methodological issues for assessment in the different vascular beds: a statement by the Working Group on Endothelin and Endothelial Factors of the European Society of Hypertension. *Journal of Hypertension*, *23*(1), 7–17. doi:10.1097/00004872-200501000-00004 PMID:15643116

Donaldson, I. M. (2004). Bon sante: Is wine good for your health? *International Medical Journal*, *34*(5), 221–223. doi:10.1111/j.1444-0903.2004.00583.x PMID:15151665

Dong, X., Tong, F., Qian, C., Zhang, R., Dong, J., Wu, G., & Hu, Y. (2015). NEMO modulatesradiation-induced endothelial senescence of human umbilical veinsthrough NF-kappaB signal pathway. *Radiation Research*, *183*(1), 82–93. doi:10.1667/RR13682.1 PMID:25536232

Eckel, R. H. (1997). *Obesity and Heart Disease: A Statement for Healthcare Professionals From the Nutrition Committee.* American Heart Association.

Essays, U. K. (2013). *Cardiovascular Disease.* Retrieved from https://www.ukessays.com/essays/health/cardiovascular-disease.php?cref=1

Finegold, J. A., Asaria, P., & Francis, D. P. (2012). Mortality from ischaemic heart disease by country, region, and age: Statistics from World Health Organisation and United Nations. *International Journal of Cardiology*, *168*(2), 934–945. doi:10.1016/j.ijcard.2012.10.046 PMID:23218570

GBD 2013 Mortality and Causes of Death, Collaborators. (2014). Global, regional, and national age-sex specific all-cause and cause-specific mortality for 240 causes of death, 1990-2013: a systematic analysis for the Global Burden of Disease Study 2013."*Lancet*, *385*(9963), 117–71. doi:10.1016/S0140-6736(14)61682-2

GBD 2015 Mortality and Causes of Death, Collaborators. (2016). "Global, regional, and national life expectancy, all-cause mortality, and cause-specific mortality for 249 causes of death, 1980-2015: a systematic analysis for the Global Burden of Disease Study 2015. *Lancet*, *388*(10053), 1459–1544. doi:10.1016/S0140-6736(16)31012-1

Go, A. S., Mozaffarian, D., Roger, V. L., Benjamin, E. J., Berry, J. D., Borden, W. B., ... Turner, M. B. (2013). Heart disease and stroke statistics--2013 update: A report from the American Heart Association. *Circulation*, *127*(1), e6–e245. doi:10.1161/CIR.0b013e31828124ad PMID:23239837

Graf, C. (2006). Functional decline in hospitalized older adults. *The American Journal of Nursing*, *106*(1), 58–67. doi:10.1097/00000446-200601000-00032 PMID:16481783

Hagedoorn, M., Kuijer, R. G., Buunk, B. P., DeJong, G. M., Wobbes, T., & Sanderman, R. (2000). Marital satisfaction in patients with cancer: Does support from intimate partners benefit those who need it most? *Health Psychology*, *19*(3), 274–282. doi:10.1037/0278-6133.19.3.274 PMID:10868772

Jani, B., & Rajkumar, C. (2006). Ageing and vascular ageing. *Postgraduate Medical Journal*, *82*(968), 357–362. doi:10.1136/pgmj.2005.036053 PMID:16754702

Jousilahti, V., & Tuomilehto, P. (1999). Sex, Age, Cardiovascular Risk Factors, and coronary heart disease. *Circulation*, *99*(9), 1165–1172. doi:10.1161/01.CIR.99.9.1165 PMID:10069784

Kannel, W.B., &Feinleib, M. (1972). Natural history of angina pectoris in the Framingham Institute (NHLBI), Women and Cardiovascular Diseases—Statistics.

Kaplan, J. R., Chen, H., & Manuck, S. B. (2009). The relationship between social status and atherosclerosis in male and female monkeys as revealed by meta-analysis. *American Journal of Primatology*, *71*(9), 732–741. doi:10.1002/ajp.20707 PMID:19452517

Krumholz, H. M. (2013). Post-hospital syndrome--an acquired, transient condition of generalized risk. *The New England Journal of Medicine*, *68*(2), 100–102. doi:10.1056/NEJMp1212324 PMID:23301730

Leon, A. S., Franklin, B. A., Costa, F., Balady, G. J., & Berra, K. A. (2005). Cardiac rehabilitation and secondary prevention of coronary heart disease. *Circulation*, *111*(3), 369–376. doi:10.1161/01.CIR.0000151788.08740.5C PMID:15668354

Leonarda, G., & Gabriella, L. (2015). Short communication, gender differences in cardiovascular disease. *Journal of Interventional Cardiology*, *1*(1), 20–22. doi:10.15761/JIC.1000107

Lerner, D. J., & Kannel, W. B. (1986). Patterns of coronary heart disease morbidity and mortality in the sexes: A 26-year follow-up of the Framingham population. *American Heart Journal*, *111*(2), 383–390. doi:10.1016/0002-8703(86)90155-9 PMID:3946178

Mackay, J., Mensah, G. A., Mendis, S., & Greenlund, K. (2004). The atlas of heart disease and stroke (tech. Rep.). World Health Organization, Geneva, Switzerland.

MacRae, C.A., & Vasan, R. S. (2016). The Future of Genetics and Genomics: Closing the Phenotype Gap in Precision Medicine. *Circulation, 133*(25), 2634–2639. doi:10.1161/CIRCULATIONAHA.116.022547

Magomedova, S., & Damadaeva, A. (2014). Application of physical education in the rehabilitation of patients with cardiovascular disease. *Biological Medicine*, 6.

Majnemer, A., Limperopoulos, C., Shevell, M., Rosenblatt, B., Rohlicek, C., & Tchervenkov, C. (2006). Long-term neuromotor outcome at school entry of infants with congenital heart defects requiring open-heart surgery. *The Journal of Pediatrics*, *148*(1), 72–77. doi:10.1016/j.jpeds.2005.08.036 PMID:16423601

Marmot, M. G. (2001). Alcohol and coronary heart disease. *International Journal of Epidemiology*, *30*(4), 724–729. doi:10.1093/ije/30.4.724 PMID:11511592

Mendis, S. (2005). For the Pathobiological Determinants of Atherosclerosis in Youth (PBDAY) Research group. Atherosclerosis in children and young adults. *Prevention and Control; the Official Journal of the World Heart Federation*, *1*, 3–15. doi:10.1016/j.precon.2005.02.010

Mendis, S., Puska, P., & Norrving, B. (2011). Global Atlas on Cardiovascular Disease Prevention and Control (PDF). World Health Organization.

Moran, A. E., Forouzanfar, M. H., Roth, G. A., Mensah, G. A., Ezzati, M., Murray, C. J., & Naghavi, M. (2014). Temporal trends in ischemic heart disease mortality in 21 world regions, 1980 to 2010: The Global Burden of Disease 2010 study. *Circulation*, *129*(14), 1483–1492. doi:10.1161/CIRCULATIONAHA.113.004042 PMID:24573352

Moran, A. E., Forouzanfar, M. H., Roth, G. A., Mensah, G. A., Ezzati, M., Murray, C. J., & Naghavi, M. (2014). Temporal trends in ischemic heart disease mortality in 21 world regions, 1980 to 2010: The Global Burden of Disease 2010 study. *Circulation*, *129*(14), 1483–1492. doi:10.1161/CIRCULATIONAHA.113.004042 PMID:24573352

Mosca, L., Banka, C. L., Benjamin, E. J., Berra, K., Bushnell, C., Dolor, R. J., ... Wenger, N. K. (2007). Evidence-Based Guidelines for Cardiovascular Disease Prevention in Women. *Circulation*, *115*(11), 1481–1501. doi:10.1161/CIRCULATIONAHA.107.181546 PMID:17309915

Mosca, L., Manson, J. A. E., Sutherland, S. E., Langer, R. D., & Manolio, T. (1997). Cardiovascular Disease in Women. *Circulation*, *96*, 2468–2482. doi:10.1161/01.CIR.96.7.2468 PMID:9337227

Munzel, T., Sinning, C., Post, F., Warnholtz, A., & Schulz, E. (2008). Pathophysiology, diagnosis and prognostic implications of endothelial dysfunction. *Annals of Medicine*, *40*, 180–196. doi:10.1080/07853890701854702 PMID:18382884

National Center for Health Statistics (NCHS). (2009). The National Heart, Lung, and Blood Study: Prognosis and survival. *The American Journal of Cardiology*, *29*, 154–163.

National Institutes of Aging. (2005). Blood Vessels and Aging: The Rest of the Journey in Health and Aging.

Orzan, F., Brusca, A., Conte, M. R., Presbitero, P., & Figliomeni, M. C. (1993). Severe coronary artery disease after radiation therapy of the chest and mediastinum: Clinical presentation and treatment. *British Heart Journal*, *69*(6), 496–500. doi:10.1136/hrt.69.6.496 PMID:8343315

Paris, F., Fuks, Z., Kang, A., Capodieci, P., & Juan, G. (2001). Endothelial apoptosis as the primary lesion initiating intestinal radiation damage in mice. *Science*, *293*(5528), 293–297. doi:10.1126/science.1060191 PMID:11452123

Patane, S. (2014). Cardiotoxicity: Cisplatin and long-term cancer survivors. *International Journal of Cardiology*, *175*(1), 201–202. doi:10.1016/j.ijcard.2014.04.238 PMID:24820740

Perk, J., De Backer, G., Gohlke, H., Graham, I., & Reiner, Z. (2012). European guidelines on cardiovascular disease prevention in clinical practice (version 2012). *International Journal of Behavioral Medicine*, *19*, 403–488. doi:10.1007/s12529-012-9242-5 PMID:23093473

Pinto, E. (2007). Blood pressure and ageing. *Postgraduate Medical Journal*, *83*(976), 109–114. doi:10.1136/pgmj.2006.048371 PMID:17308214

Schroder, K., Schwarzer, R., & Endler, N. S. (1997). Predicting cardiac patients' quality of life from the characteristics of their spouses. *Journal of Health Psychology*, *2*(2), 231–244. doi:10.1177/135910539700200219 PMID:22013006

Schwarzer, R., & Leppin, A. (1992). Possible impact of social ties and support on morbidity and mortality. In H.O.F. Veiel & U. Baumann (Eds.), The meaning and measurement of social support (pp. 65-83). Washington, DC: Hemisphere.

Smoking and Heart Health. (2014). Centre for disease control prevention office on smoking and health. Retrieved 05.10.2017 from https://www.cdc.gov/tobacco/data_statistics/sgr/50thanniversary/pdfs/fs_smoking_CVD_508.pdf

Sommaruga, M., Tramarin, R., Angelino, E., Bettinardi, O., & Cauteruccio, M. A. (2003). Guidelines on psychological intervention in cardiac rehabilitation- methodological process. *Monaldi Archives for Chest Disease*, *60*, 40–44. PMID:12827831

Stephen, J. M. (2012). *Current medical diagnosis & treatment 2012* (p. 430). New York: McGraw-Hill Medical.

Stramba-Badiale, M., Fox, K. M., Priori, S. G., Collins, P., & Daly, C. (2006). Cardiovasculardiseases in women: A statement from the policy conference of the European Society ofCardiology. *European Heart Journal*, *27*(8), 994–1005. doi:10.1093/eurheartj/ehi819 PMID:16522654

Suessenbacher, A., Potocnik, M., Dorler, J., Fluckinger, G., Wanitschek, M., Pachinger, O., ... Alber, H. F. (2011). Comparison of peripheral endothelial function in shift versus nonshift workers. *The American Journal of Cardiology*, *107*(6), 945–948. doi:10.1016/j.amjcard.2010.10.077 PMID:21247546

Thomas, R. J., & King, M. (2010). Writing Committee to Develop Clinical Performance Measures for Cardiac Rehabilitation. AACVPR/ACCF/AHA 2010 update. *Circulation*, *122*, 1342–1350. doi:10.1161/CIR.0b013e3181f5185b PMID:20805435

Veinot, J. P., & Edwards, W. D. (1996). Pathology of radiation-induced heart disease: A surgical and autopsy study of 27 cases. *Human Pathology*, *27*(8), 766–773. doi:10.1016/S0046-8177(96)90447-5 PMID:8760008

World Health Organization. (2005). *Affordable technology. Blood pressure measuring devices for low resource settings*. Geneva: WHO.

World Health Organization. (2014). Global Atlas on Cardiovascular Disease Prevention and Control 2011. Retrieved from www.who.int

Yancy, C. W., Jessup, M., & Bozkurt, B. (2013). ACCF/AHA guideline for the management of heart failure. *Journal of the American College of Cardiology*, *62*, e147–e239. doi:10.1016/j.jacc.2013.05.019 PMID:23747642

Yeh, E. T., Tong, A. T., Lenihan, D. J., Yusuf, S. W., & Swafford, J. (2004). Cardiovascular complications of cancer therapy. *Circulation*, *109*(25), 3122–3131. doi:10.1161/01.CIR.0000133187.74800.B9 PMID:15226229

KEY TERMS AND DEFINITIONS

Cardiovascular Disease: CVD is a class of diseases that involve the heart or blood vessels it includes coronary artery diseases (CAD) such as angina and myocardial infarction (commonly known as a heart attack

Cardiac Rehabilitation: (CR) is a commonly used treatment for men and women with cardiovascular disease.

Elderly: Ageing, an inevitable process, is commonly measured by chronological age and, as a convention, a person aged 65-years or more is often referred to as 'elderly.'

Social Support: Is the perception and actuality that one is cared for, has assistance available from other people, and that one is part of a supportive social network. These supportive resources can be emotional (e.g., nurturance), tangible (e.g., financial assistance), informational (e.g., advice), or companionship (e.g., sense of belonging) and intangible (e.g., personal advice).

Treatment: The treatment that is normally provided to people with a given condition. In many studies, a control group receives the standard treatment while a treatment group receives the experimental treatment. After the clinical trial, researchers compare the outcomes of the two groups to see if the experimental treatment is better than, as good as or not as beneficial as the standard treatment.

Chapter 11
Stroke in Geriatric Population

Pradeep Kallollimath
Dharwad Institute of Mental Health and Neurosciences (DIMHANS), India

ABSTRACT

This chapter describes how a stroke or 'brain attack' occurs when blood circulation to the brain fails. Although first recognized 2400 years ago by Hippocrates, the father of medicine, advances in treatment are made only in the last few decades. After a stroke, 8 out of 10 patients develop paralysis on the side of body opposite the side of brain damaged. There are other symptoms to look for such as drooping of face to one side, slurred or confused speech, sudden visual disturbance, sudden giddiness and imbalance or sudden severe headache. Incidence of stoke increases with age and elderly people are more likely to have more severe stroke. In addition, elderly people will have multiple comorbidities which make management more difficult. After a disabling stroke, easing back to life requires a positive attitude to overcome difficulties. A physiotherapist can help restore the strength and reduce stiffness of muscles. Regular follow up with a physician or neurologist, taking medicines as prescribed is important to improve the outcome and prevent the recurrence of stroke.

INTRODUCTION

Stroke is defined by WHO as "rapidly developing clinical signs of focal cerebral dysfunction, with symptoms lasting 24 hours or longer, of vascular origin" (WHO Project Investigators, 1988). It is a huge public health problem because of its high morbidity and disability. Stroke is the second commonest cause of mortality after coronary artery disease. Prevalence in India is about 200/lakh population. 17 million people experience stroke each year. 6 million of those strokes will be fatal. Every six seconds, someone dies from a stroke. Stroke is the second commonest cause of mortality after coronary artery disease and is responsible for more deaths annually than those attributed to AIDS, tuberculosis and malaria combined. The frequency of stroke increases significantly in elderly due to age, increased prevalence of risk factors like diabetes, hypertension, cardiac diseases and carotid disease. Furthermore strokes in elderly are more severe, especially in women. Larger proportions of strokes are cardioembolic which have worse prognosis. Recovery and rehabilitation after stroke in elderly requires prolonged time. (Emma, Phillip., & Christine 2017; Saposnik et al., 2008)

DOI: 10.4018/978-1-5225-3480-8.ch011

Types of Stroke

There are two broad categories of stroke. Ischemic stroke occurs when arteries are blocked by blood clots or fatty deposits. About 85% of all strokes are ischemic. Hemorrhagic stroke occurs when the blood vessel in the brain ruptures leaking blood into the brain. Hemorrhagic strokes account for 15% of all strokes. (Figure 1)

Classification of Acute Stroke

1. Ischemic stroke
    a. Atrial fibrillation (17%)
    b. Carotid disease (4%)
    c. Other (64%)
2. Hemorrhagic
    a. Aneurysmal (4%)
    b. Hypertensive (7%)
3. Others (4%)

Risk Factors for Stroke

Everyone has some stroke risk. Some risk factors are beyond our control like age, gender, race, family history etc. But other risk factors can be modified. These are: Hypertension, diabetes mellitus, dyslipedemia, carotid artery stenosis, cardiac disease, prior history of stroke, obesity, cigarette smoking, and alcohol consumption.

Figure 1. Stroke subtypes and incidence

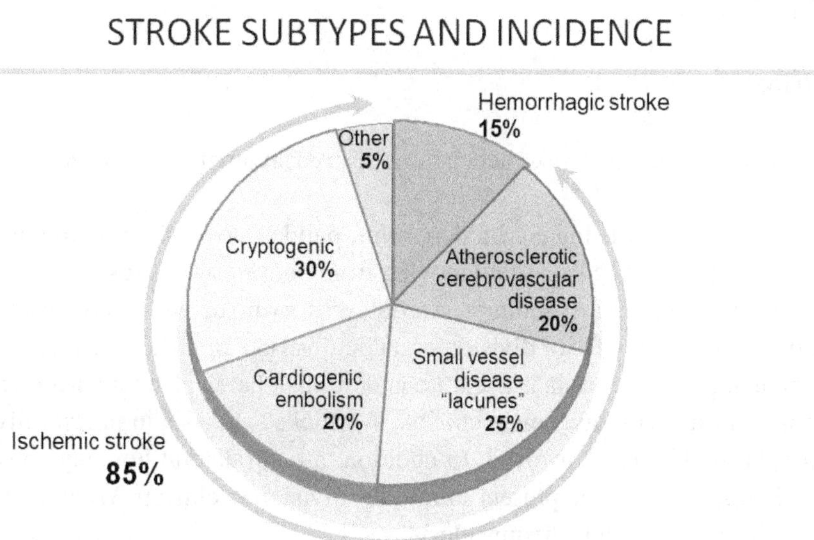

Environmental Factors

Environmental air pollution is associated with higher stroke admissions and mortality. Indoor air pollution from burning biomass fuels are a significant contributor in low and middle-income countries. The pathophysiologic mechanisms of air pollution's effects on cerebrovascular disease are unclear, but may be due to effects on vascular endothelium, blood pressure and increased risk of thrombosis. (Shah et al., 2015) Fossil fuel emissions from coal burning are regarded as the most harmful (Ostro et al., 2015) Exposure to toxic metals like lead, cadmium and mercury are also associated with increased risk of cerebrovascular disease (Menke et al., 2006; Tellez-Plaza, Jones, Dominguez-Lucas, Guallar, E., & Navas-Acien, 2013; Solenkova et al., 2014).

Behavioural Factors

- **Smoking:** Cigarette smoking is a causal risk factor for stroke that is dose and duration dependent (Woodward et al., 2005). Smoking cessation has been associated with decreased risk of stroke (Kawachi et al., 1993). Exposure to second-hand smoke is also associated with increased risk of stroke and mortality after stroke (Lin, Ovbiagele, Markovic., & Towfighi, 2016).
- **Alcohol:** The association between alcohol intake and stroke risk is J shaped. Moderate alcohol consumption is associated with reduced risk of strokes, while heavy alcohol consumption is associated with increased risk, probably by increasing the risk of hypertension, atrial fibrillation, cardiomyopathy and diabetes (Reynolds et al, 2003).
- **Obesity and Metabolic Syndrome:** Abdominal obesity and general obesity are associated with increased risk of cerebrovascular disease. Metabolic syndrome (abdominal obesity, hypertension, low HDL cholesterol, high triglycerides and insulin resistance) is a recognized risk factor for stroke (Hill & Towfighi, 2017).

ISCHEMIC STROKE

Clinical Features

Clinical features of acute ischemic stroke depend on the arterial territory involved.

- **Carotid Artery:** Amaurosis fugax: Sudden, brief, painless loss of vision in one eye, usually reported as fog, shade, blurring or curtain moving from above downwards.
- **Middle Cerebral Artery:** Most common arterial territory involved. Symptoms depend on whether stem, superior division, inferior division or lenticulostriate branches are involved. There will be contralateral hemiplegia. Aphasia is a feature in dominant hemisphere involvement. There will be Broca's aphasia in superior division occlusion, Wernicke's aphasia in inferior division occlusion and global aphasia if stem is involved. In addition, a contralateral homonymous hemianopia or inferior quadrantanopia may be present in inferior division occlusion. When nondominant hemisphere is involved, there will be hemineglect.
- **Anterior Cerebral Artery:** Uncommon. Contralateral weakness involving primarily lower extremity. There will be deviation of eyes towards the side of lesion, urinary incontinence. In bilat-

eral lesions, there will be abulia or akinetic mutism. Infarction in the territory of artery of Huebner (medial lenticulostriate artery) causes faces and arm weakness due to involvement of anterior limb of internal capsule. Anterior choroidal artery syndrome is characterized by hemiparesis, hemisensory loss and hemianopia.

- **Lacunar Syndromes:** Lacunar infarcts are small ischemic infarctions in deep regions of brain and brainstem that range from 0.5 to 15 mm in diameter. These result from occlusion of penetrating branches of major cerebral arteries. 5 best recognized lacunar syndromes are:
    - *Pure motor hemiparesis*
    - *Pure sensory stroke*
    - *Sensory-motor stroke*
    - *Ataxic hemiparesis*
    - *Clumsy hand dysarthria syndrome*
- **Vertebrobasilar Territory Syndromes:** Vertebrobasilar system supplies brainstem, cerebellum and portions of thalamus, temporal lobe and occipital lobes. Clinical features of vertebrobasilar insufficiency include vertigo, diplopia, vomiting, and ataxia. There are many named syndromes like Wallenberg syndrome (lateral medulla), Dejerine syndrome (medial medullary syndrome); Weber syndrome, Claude syndrome, Benedikt syndrome (midbrain), Miller syndrome, Foville syndrome (pons). Top of basilar syndrome is caused by occlusion of rostral basialar artery leading to infarctions of midbrain, thalamus, and portions of temporal and occipital lobes. Patients will have somnolence, peduncular hallucinosis, memory disturbance, agitated delirium, gaze abnormalities and visual field defects. To create awareness among public for early recognition of symptoms of stroke, mnemonic FAST has been used.
    - *F: Face drooping*
    - *A: Arm weakness*
    - *S: Speech disturbance*
    - *T: Time to call emergency*
- **Transient Ischemic Attack (TIA):** A TIA is a temporary and "non-marching" neurological deficit of sudden onset; attributed to focal ischemia of the brain, retina, or cochlea; and lasting less than 24 hours. Yet most TIAs last only a few minutes. TIA is also known as a "warning stroke" or "mini-stroke" that produces stroke-like symptoms. The difference between a TIA and a stroke is that the blockage is transient, or temporary. Symptoms are exactly the same as stroke, but usually last less than five minutes. A TIA is a prognostic indicator of stroke, with one-third of untreated TIA patients having a stroke within 5 years. About 1 in 10 patients with TIA experience a stroke in the next 3 months.

DIAGNOSIS

Ischemic strokes may result from (1) large-artery atherosclerotic disease resulting in stenosis or occlusion, (2) small-vessel or penetrating artery disease (lacunes), (3) cardiogenic or artery-to-artery embolism, (4) nonatherosclerotic vasculopathies, (5) hypercoagulable disorders, and (6) infarcts of undetermined causes.

Diagnosis of stroke is based on clinical features and brain imaging. Clinically stroke has to be differentiated from other conditions mimicking stroke. These stroke mimics include metabolic abnormalities like hypoglycaemia, hyponatremia; neuroinfections; brain tumors etc.

Figure 2. Magnetic resonance imaging (MRI) in acute ischemic stroke. FLAIR showing hyperintensity in left basal ganglia (a), DWI showing diffusion restriction (b) with corresponding reduced signal in ADC (c).

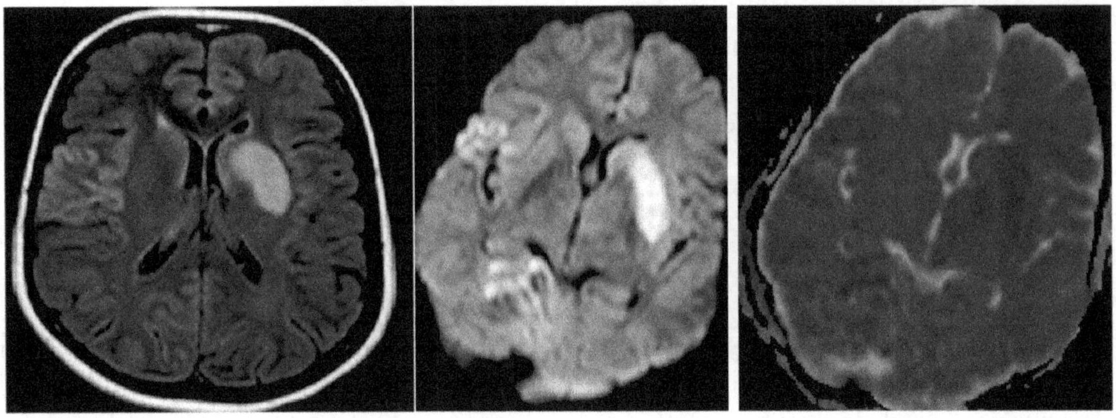

Fig 2 (a) (b) (c)

A CT (computed tomography) scan of brain or MRI(magnetic resonance imaging) will help in confirming the diagnosis of stroke, to differentiate ischemic from hemorrhagic strokes and to differentiate small vessel and large vessel ischemic strokes.

Blood investigations including blood glucose level, lipid profile, coagulation parameters will help in detecting the risk factors. Immediate diagnostic studies mandatory in evaluation of acute ischemic stroke are shown in Table 1.

Carotid and vertebral Doppler is done to look for carotid stenosis.

Atrial fibrillation is the most common cause of stroke in the very elderly age group (above 90 years of age). All elderly patients with stroke require cardiac evaluation including ECG and echocardiogram to look for atrial fibrillation. To detect paroxysmal atrial fibrillation, continuous 24-hour (Holter) ECG monitoring is recommended.

Cerebral angiography may be required to differentiate atherosclerotic from non-atherosclerotic vasculopathies like fibromuscular dysplasia, arterial dissections, moya moya disease, vasculitis, aneurysms and arteriovenous malformations.

Table 1. Immediate diagnostic studies in evaluation of a patient with Suspected Acute Ischemic Stroke

All Patients
Noncontrast brain CT or brain MRI
Blood glucose
Oxygen saturation
Serum electrolytes/renal function tests*
Complete blood count, including platelet count*
Markers of cardiac ischemia*
Prothrombin time/INR*
Activated partial thromboplastin time*
ECG*
**Although it is desirable to know the results of these tests before giving intravenous rtPA, fibrinolytic therapy should not be delayed while awaiting the results. Only blood glucose must precede intravenous tPA administration.*

PREVENTION

Prevention strategies include primordial, primary and secondary preventions. Primordial prevention is preventing onset of disease by strategies to counteract environmental and behavioural risk factors. Example: increasing urban green spaces, restricting smoking in public areas etc.

Primary prevention of stroke is directed at controlling established stroke risk factors like hypertension, diabetes mellitus, hyperlipidemia with use of proper medications, along with lifestyle modification by adopting a healthy lifestyle with regular exercise, healthy diet, stopping cigarette smoking.

Secondary prevention is aimed at controlling risk factors in individuals with established stroke or TIA and the use of medications like antiplatelet agents to prevent recurrence of stroke.

TREATMENT

Current treatment options for stroke are:

1. Conservative
2. IV thrombolysis
3. IA thrombolysis
4. Bridging therapy
5. Mechanical

All acute stroke patients should be given at least 150mg of aspirin immediately after brain imaging has excluded intracranial hemorrhage. In patients with t-PA, aspirin should be delayed until after 24 hours post thrombolysis. In patients with large hemispheric infarct (malignant MCA territory infarct), aspirin may be delayed until surgery or decision is made not to operate.

Thrombolysis in Acute Ischemic Stroke

The *ischemic penumbra*, or area of "misery perfusion," is the area of the ischemic brain in which there are some neurons that are functionally silent but structurally intact and potentially salvageable. Reperfusion by thrombolysis offers the potential to salvage ischemic penumbra and reduce the extent of ischemic injury. Thrombolysis with rtPA (recombinant tissue plasminogen activator) has revolutionized the treatment of acute ischemic stroke. Mechanism of action of rtPA: Thrombus is formed during ischemic stroke. Alteplase (rtPA) binds to fibrin in a thrombus and converts plasminogen to plasmin which directly attacks the fibrin mesh. This initiates local fibrinolysis with minimal systemic effects. All patients with disabling acute ischemic stroke presenting within 3 hours (up to 4.5 hours) after symptom onset should be evaluated for eligibility for thrombolysis.

Some of the prerequisites and inclusion criteria are:

1. Diagnosis of acute ischemic stroke
2. No evidence of hemorrhage on plane CT
3. Neurological deficit of NIHSS 4-25 severity
4. Onset of symptoms within 4.5 hours of beginning treatment

Absolute and relative exclusion criteria for thrombolysis are given in tables 2 and 3. These exclusion criteria are mainly to reduce the risk of hemorrhage. rt-PA 0.9 mg/kg (maximum dose of 90mg) is given over 60 min with 10% of the dose given as IV bolus over 1 minute. Patient should be admitted in an intensive care/dedicated stroke unit and monitored over 24 hours.

Therapeutic Window in Treatment of Acute Ischemic Stroke

About 1.9 million neurons are destroyed each minute treatment is delayed. Hence there is a narrow therapeutic window time in treatment of ischemic stroke. For IV thrombolysis, therapeutic window is 3 hours, which can be extended up to 4.5 hours with additional exclusion criteria (Table 4). Endovascular treatments like clot removal using MERCI or solitaire device can be done up to 8 hours or even up to 12 hours if ischemic penumbra can be demonstrated using advanced imaging techniques (Figure 3).

Table 2. Exclusion criteria

■ Significant head trauma/prior stroke in previous 3 months.
■ Symptoms suggesting SAH
■ H/O previous intracranial haemorrhage.
■ Arterial puncture at noncompressible site in previous 7 days
■ Intracranial neoplasm, AVM or aneurysm.
■ Recent intracranial or intraspinal surgery.
■ Elevated BP>185mmHg systolic or >110mmHg diastolic
■ Active internal bleeding
■ Acute bleeding diathesis, including Platelet count <100000/mm3,
■ Heparin received within 48hours, resulting in elevated aPTT
■ Current use of anticoagulant with INR>1.7 or PT>15 seconds
■ Current use of direct thrombin inhibitors with abnormal aPTT, INR, platelet count.
■ Blood glucose concentration <50mg/dL
■ CT demonstrating multilobar infarction (hypodensity > 1/3 cerebral hemisphere)

Table 3. Relative exclusion criteria

■ Only minor or rapidly improving stroke symptoms (clearing spontaneously)
■ Pregnancy
■ Seizure at onset with postictal residual neurological impairments
■ Major surgery or serious trauma within previous 14 days
■ Recent gastrointestinal or urinary tract hemorrhage (within previous 21 days)
■ Recent acute myocardial infarction (within previous 3 months)

Table 4. Eligibility for intravenous tPA may be extended from 3 to 4.5 hours, with additional exclusion criteria for

■ (a) patients > 80 years of age
■ (b) patients taking oral anticoagulants
■ (c) patients with baseline National Institutes of Health Stroke Scale (NIHSS) score > 25
■ (d) those with ischemic injury to more than one third of the middle cerebral artery territory
■ (e) those with history of both stroke and diabetes.

Figure 3. Therapeutic window periods for different interventions in stroke

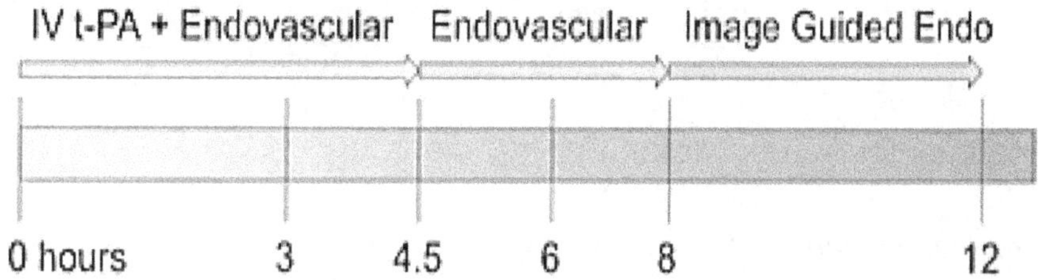

Given the narrow therapeutic window for treatment of acute ischemic stroke, timely ED evaluation and diagnosis of ischemic stroke are paramount. The time targets recommended by NINDS for emergency management of acute ischemic stroke patients are shown in table 5.

Benefits and Risks of Thrombolysis

For every 8 patients treated with rtPA, 1 patient has excellent recovery, and for every 15 patients treated, 1 patient has symptomatic intracranial haemorrhage There is overall favourable outcome with sustained benefit at 6 and 12 months compared to placebo.

The risk and benefit ratio for thrombolysis is less well defined in elderly, as elderly patients with significant comorbidities are often not included in clinical trials. Decision to thrombolyse should be made on individual basis in the very elderly.

Acute Stroke-Ready Hospitals (Stroke-Capable Hospitals)

Acute stroke ready hospitals are the hospitals that have made an institutional commitment to effectively and efficiently evaluate, diagnose, and treat most ED stroke patients but that do not have fully organized inpatient stroke systems of care.

These have:

- Written emergency stroke care protocols
- Ability to administer intravenous rtPA
- Ability to perform emergency brain imaging (e.g., CT scan) at all times

Table 5. NINDS recommended time targets for potential candidates for thrombolysis

Time Interval	Time Target
Door to doctor	10 minutes
Access to neurologic expertise	15
Door to CT initiation	25
Door to CT interpretation	45
Door to drug	60
Admission to monitored bed	3 hours

- Ability to conduct emergency laboratory testing at all times
- Suggested protocol for acute stroke management:

Suggested Protocol for Acute Stroke Management

Step 1. *History and examination and stabilization of the patient*

- ABC's of emergency
- Establish onset time
- Differentiate stroke from stroke mimics like seizure, hypoglycemia, and migraine.
- Identify red flags for IC hemorrhage
- Check for vascular risk factors
- Check historical findings for rt-PA contraindications

Inform unit consultant on call, neuroradiology resident on duty

Step 2. *Get Urgent Non-Contrast CT, do GRBS and Send Stat Investigations*

- CBC, Biochemistry
- PT, aPTT, INR
- Blood group and cross match
- Take ECG after CT

Step 3

- Rule out IC hemorrhage
- Check indications and contraindications for IV thrombolysis
- Perform Baseline NIHSS (National institute of health stroke scale)
- Check reports

Step 4

- If eligible for thrombolysis, start thrombolysis as 0.9 mg/kg with 10% as bolus over 1-2 min followed by remaining 90% over 60 min
- If there is contraindication, check
- If contraindication is modifiable e.g. hypertension, blood sugars
- If not look for alternative reperfusion therapies e.g. endovascular approaches especially after 3 hrs.
- Arrange for MRI

Step 5. *Monitor Vitals and NIHSS as per Standard NINDS Trial Protocol*

- Be watchful for intracranial hemorrhage- headache, vomiting rising BP, deteriorating patient/ NIHSS
- Stop infusion, get immediate CT, arrange for FFP and platelets
- Get neurosurgery consultation if hemorrhage present
- On completion of rt-PA, shift the patient to stroke ward/ICU for close monitoring

General care of acute stoke patient is equally important. Admission of patients in specialized stroke units has been shown to reduce mortality and reduce the length of hospital stay. Attention should be given to airway protection to avoid obstruction, hypoventilation and aspiration pneumonia. Pneumonia contributes to up to 25% of mortality in bedridden stroke patients. Enteral feeding through Ryle's tube is advised to prevent aspiration in patients with oropharyngeal dysfunction. To reduce intracranial pressure, head end of the bed should be elevated to 15 degrees and mannitol infusion is given. Endotracheal intubation is required if Glasgow coma scale is less than 8. Deep vein thrombosis of lower extremities is prevented by low molecular weight heparin or intermittent pneumatic compression. Care should be taken to avoid bedsores. Fluid and nutritional status of the patient should be assessed and treated accordingly.

HEMORRHAGIC STROKE

Intracerebral hemorrhage accounts for about 15% of strokes. It has high mortality rate.

The most common cause of intracerebral hemorrhage is hypertension. Non-hypertensive causes include aneurysms, arteriovenous malformations, tumors, bleeding disorders, antithrombotic treatment, cerebral amyloid angiopathy etc.

Clinical features of intracerebral hemorrhage are those secondary to raised intracranial pressure like headache altered sensorium and those specific to location of bleed. Hypertensive intracerebral hemorrhage commonly occurs in basal ganglia and lead to contralateral hemiparesis.

A CT scan of brain will help in detecting the bleed, location and size of the bleed.

Treatment includes measures to reduce intracranial pressure like mannitol, hyperventilation. Surgical intervention is required if there is significant mass effect and brainstem compression.

Hypertension is treated with intravenous and oral drugs.

RESEARCH

Regarding stroke prevention, areas of future research include: determining specific target outcomes for secondary stroke prevention, health system changes that are needed to implement complex interventions for patients poststroke (Hill & Towfighi, 2017).

Despite our aging demography, very little is known about the fastest growing age group. As the number of elderly with stroke is increasing, stroke specialists and teams will need to develop specific skills in managing such patients. This approaching phenomenon is being recognized as "stroke silver Tsunami". Including more elderly subjects in clinical trials and other research will help in improving survival and quality of life in the elderly (Saposnik et al., 2008).

CONCLUSION

The incidence of stroke increases with age, and elderly people tend to have more severe strokes with increased morbidity and mortality. Management of elderly patients with stroke poses unique challenges due to associated comorbidities and factors specific for geriatric population. Clinical trials on stroke should include more and more elderly subjects to gain insight into the factors unique for geriatric population, which in turn will help in providing better treatment and care of such patients.

REFERENCES

Emma, P., Phillip, F., & Christine, R. (2017). Management of Acute Stroke in the Older Person. *Geriatrics*, *2*(3), 27. doi:10.3390/geriatrics2030027

Hill, V., & Towfighi, A. (2017). Factors for Stroke and Strategies for Stroke Prevention. *Seminars in Neurology*, *37*(3), 237–258. doi:10.1055/s-0037-1603685 PMID:28759906

Kawachi, I., Colditz, G. A., Stampfer, M. J., Willett, W. C., Manson, J. E., Rosner, B., & Hennekens, C. H. (1993). Smoking cessation and decreased risk of stroke in women. *Journal of the American Medical Association*, *269*(2), 232–236. doi:10.1001/jama.1993.03500020066033 PMID:8417241

Lin, M. P., Ovbiagele, B., Markovic, D., & Towfighi, A. (2016). Association of Second hand Smoke with Stroke Outcomes. *Stroke*, *47*(11), 2828–2835. doi:10.1161/STROKEAHA.116.014099 PMID:27729574

Menke, A., Muntner, P., Batuman, V., Silbergeld, E.K., & Guallar, E. (2006). Blood lead below 0.48 micromol/L (10 microg/dL) and mortality among US adults. *Circulation, 114*(13), 1388-1394.

Ostro, B., Hu, J., Goldberg, D., Reynolds, P., Hertz, A., Bernstein, L., & Kleeman, M. J. (2015). Associations of mortality with long-term exposures to fine and ultrafine particles, species and sources: Results from the California Teachers Study Cohort. *Environmental Health Perspectives*, *123*(6), 549–556.

Reynolds, K., Lewis, B., Nolen, J.D., Kinney, G.L., & Sathya, B., & He, J. (2003). Alcohol consumption and risk of stroke: a meta-analysis. *Journal of the American Medical Association, 5*;289(5):579-88.

Saposnik, G., Cote, R., Phillips, S., Gubitz, G., Bayer, N., Minuk, J., & Black, S. (2008). Stroke outcome in those over 80: A multicenter cohort study across Canada. *Stroke*, *39*(8), 2310–2317. doi:10.1161/STROKEAHA.107.511402 PMID:18556583

Shah, A. S., Lee, K. K., McAllister, D. A., Hunter, A., Nair, H., Whiteley, W., & Mills, N. L. (2015). Short term exposure to air pollution and stroke: systematic review and meta-analysis. *BMJ,* 24 350. PMID:25633926

Solenkova, N. V., Newman, J. D., Berger, J. S., Thurston, G., Hochman, J. S., & Lamas, G. A. (2014). Metal pollutants and cardiovascular disease: Mechanisms and consequences of exposure. *American Heart Journal*, *168*(6), 812–822. doi:10.1016/j.ahj.2014.07.007 PMID:25458643

Tellez-Plaza, M., Jones, M. R., Dominguez-Lucas, A., Guallar, E., & Navas-Acien, A. (2013). Cadmium exposure and clinical cardiovascular disease: A systematic review. *Current Atherosclerosis Reports*, *15*(10), 356. doi:10.1007/s11883-013-0356-2 PMID:23955722

WHO MONICA Project Investigators. (1988). The World Health Organization MONICA Project (Monitoring trends and determinants in cardiovascular disease. *Journal of Clinical Epidemiology*, *41*(2), 105–114. doi:10.1016/0895-4356(88)90084-4 PMID:3335877

Woodward, M., Lam, T. H., Barzi, F., Patel, A., Gu, D., Rodgers, A., & Suh, I. (2005). Asia Pacific Cohort Studies Collaboration. Smoking, quitting, and the risk of cardiovascular disease among women and men in the Asia-Pacific region. *International Journal of Epidemiology*, *34*(5), 1036–1045. doi:10.1093/ije/dyi104 PMID:15914503

KEY TERMS AND DEFINITIONS

Elderly: People above 80 years of age.

Stroke: Rapidly developing clinical signs of focal cerebral dysfunction, with symptoms lasting 24 hours or longer, of vascular origin.

Thrombolysis: Treating patients with acute stroke within window period with rtPA.

Transient Ischemic Attacks: A temporary and "non-marching" neurological deficit of sudden onset; attributed to focal ischemia of the brain, retina, or cochlea; and lasting less than 24 hours.

Chapter 12
Ageing and Cancer:
The Epigenetic Basis, Alternative Treatment, and Care

Srijan Goswami
Indian School of Complimentary Therapy and Allied Sciences, India

Kongkoan Mahanta
Institute of Genetic Engineering, India

Swagata Goswami
Institute of Genetic Engineering, India

Trecy Jigdung
Indian School of Complimentary Therapy and Allied Sciences, India

Trishna Priya Devi
Indian School of Complimentary Therapy and Allied Sciences, India

ABSTRACT

This chapter describes how cancer is the disorder of immune system and is epigenetically controlled. As a person grows older the cells in their body become weaker. The defense system of the body and genetic repair mechanisms becomes more delicate. Loss of control in these protective mechanism leads to cancer. Thus, cancer and ageing are entwined in an intricate and abstruse relationship. This chapter explores the demographic changes, biological theories and clinical considerations that link cancer and ageing. It highlights the implications of these associations in the context of population and health system, with a focus on preventative strategies, research imperatives and delivery of cancer services. Furthermore, the chapter discusses how to best prepare the most junior of the medical profession to manage a growing number of senior cancer patients. Overall, it underscores how all elements in the relationship of cancer and ageing need to be considered and incorporated into a framework that facilitates a holistic approach to cancer control.

DOI: 10.4018/978-1-5225-3480-8.ch012

INTRODUCTION

Any understanding of human illness or wellness has to be in totality and not in bits and pieces, because human body does not work in bits and pieces but functions as a whole. (Hedge, 2014)

Physiological ageing implies a gradual loss of cellular and body vitality associated with atrophy of tissues or organs. This process is aggravated or mimicked by the degenerative diseases of the old age so that the physiological and pathological states tend to merge. Healthcare personnel should attempt to identify the distinctions between ageing and disease. In old age multiple disease often coexist and interact with one another and drug induced disorders are also common in this age groups (Cotran & Robbins,1997).Cancer is considered as genetic disorder expressed at cellular level, totally controlled by environment. Genetic Control System is the most intricate one. It operates in each and every cell in the body for controlling intracellular and extracellular functions. As a person grows older the cells in their body becomes weaker. The defence system of the body and genetic repair mechanisms becomes more delicate. Loss of control in these protective mechanism leads to cancer. Thus, cancer and ageing are entwined in an intricate and abstruse relationship. Epidemiological data demonstrate that both cancer incidence and mortality increase exponentially with age and thus age is regarded as a prime risk factor for cancer (Cassel, Leipzig, Cohen, & Larson, 2003). It is the connection between death and disease that makes cancer much more frightening. However, the biological mechanisms that underpin this correlation are still being uncovered. Additionally, the unique aspects of cancer management in an elderly cohort, relating to decision making, co-morbidities, prevention, diagnosis, treatment and clinical trial representation, continue to be recognised at the interface of geriatrics and oncology. For understanding how ageing is related with cancer it is crucial that one must understand how human system actually works. The reductionist science of the human body that are taught through mainstream medical education system is totally wrong. Human body and its functions are holistic phenomena.

Human body is a complex combination of various extremely specialized systems. All these specialized system functions in two major ways. First each and every system performs their functions at individual level and second, they work together with other systems of the body thus making the life possible. The ultimate goal of these specialized systems is to maintain the Homeostasis of the body. As it is known that Homeostasis is the maintenance of nearly constant condition in the internal environment of the body. Disturbance of any form caused to the homeostasis of the body leads to disease. Thus, a disease can be interpreted as the dynamic destruction of the homeostasis of the body. There are several complex biochemical reactions working together as a chain system in the body for maintaining the constant condition of the internal environment. One component from a biochemical pathway is related to some other biochemical pathway and so on. So, fault in a single component of a biochemical pathway may lead to the collapse of the entire system. There are various control systems in our body that are the contributing factor(s) in the maintenance of homeostasis (Goswami, 2017).

This chapter explores the demographic changes, biological theories and clinical considerations that link cancer and ageing. It highlights the implications of these associations in the context of population and health system, with a focus on preventative strategies, research imperatives and delivery of cancer services. Furthermore, the chapter discusses how to best prepare the most junior of the medical profession to manage a growing number of senior cancer patients. Overall, it underscores how all elements in the relationship of cancer and ageing need to be considered and incorporated into a framework that facilitates a holistic as well as personalized approach to cancer control. This chapter points out those issues and facts of cancer research that are not taught through mainstream medical education system, the truth that are kept hidden from people for financial gain at the expense of patient's life.

LITERATURE ON CANCER RESEARCH

The healthcare sector that was once considered as a service has become healthcare industry. This section does not contain false promises about chemotherapy, radiation therapy and surgery research and conventional cancer treatment and associated diagnostic procedures promoted by business minded pharmaceutical industries and their supported institutions. There are lots of texts and medias that are available that describes how safe and important chemotherapy, radiation therapy or surgery is, and essential for the survival of the cancer patients. Truth is always the truth even if no one believes it, and a lie is always lie even if everyone believes it. This section points out some of the truths about cancer research and management industry, brought forth by several scientists, doctors, professors and even patients about the reality of cancer research industries, that the people are not allowed to know. These facts and research findings are never taught through mainstream medical education systems. Most of the papers that address the lies of cancer research industry, those research papers never get published. The below table presents the comments and reviews about the reality of a disease called Cancer and its associated research.

MOLECULAR BIOLOGY OF CANCER AND AGEING

The Epigenetic Phenomena

Everyone should know that The War on Cancer is largely a fraud and that the National Cancer Institute &The American Cancer Society are derelict in their duties to the people who support them (The Pauling Blog, 2008)

For understanding what cancer actually is, how it progresses and how it can be prevented, it is crucial that the readers must keep an open mind towards the facts that the authors presented in this chapter. The facts presented here are exactly opposite of what everyone is taught to believe without question. Aging is associated with a number of events at the molecular, cellular, and physiologic levels that influence carcinogenesis and subsequent cancer growth. But that does not mean that studying each of these aspects in an isolated manner in the laboratory settings, under the microscope is going to solve the issue, for cancer is not the disease it is the result of the disease. There are two aspects of cancer and its associated concepts:

Table 1. Cancer and its associated research

Comments	Name of the Scientists
Cancer patients who refuse chemotherapy and radiation actually live up to four times longer as compared to treated cases. (Jones, n.d.)	Dr. Hardin Jones. Cancer Researcher
Everyone should know that most cancer research is largely a fraud and that the major cancer research organizations are derelict in their duties to the people who support them. (Pauling, 1986; The Pauling Blog, 2008)	Linus Pauling Ph.D. (1901-1994), two times Nobel Prize winner
The ably exploited fear of this dread disease, caused mainly by the products issuing from chemical and industrial laboratories, has become an inexhaustible source of income for the researchers, for the pharmaceutical industry, and the medical establishment. In the course of our century, so-called cancer research and cancer therapy have become a source of solid gold without precedent. (Ruesch, 1986)	Hans Ruesch in Naked Empress or The Great Medical Fraud, 1986
Cancer is by no means a mystery disease, the secrets of which can only be discovered by scientists, armed with microscopes, test tubes, etc. Unfortunately, the researchers have obscured the causation of this commonplace malady by the investigation of countless relatively unimportant scientific details which they have discussed in papers and books, in language quite incomprehensible to the general public and to the great majority of medical men themselves... Cancer is a disease of civilization. It is practically unknown to the primitive races leading primitive lives (Healing Cancer Naturally, 2004).	Sir Arbuthnot Lane, Bart., C.B., M.B., M.S., F.R.C.S., speaking in the House of Commons
The use of animals in cancer research has been attacked as unnecessary cruelty to animals, and defended as absolutely essential for research progress. From a scientific standpoint, what is pertinent is that what are called 'animal model systems' in cancer research have been a total failure....The moral is that animal model systems not only kill animals, they also kill humans. There is no good factual evidence to show that the use of animals in cancer research has led to the prevention or cure of a single human cancer. The money granted for animal research was spent for two reasons: • First it was a highly profitable undertaking for certain medical school and certain research institution which were incapable of doing any genuine cancer research. • Second it was sustained by a superstitious belief in a grossly unscientific notion: mice are miniature men. (Doctors against Vivisection, n.d.).	Dr. Irwin D. Bross Ph.D. The Lancet Medical Journal
For over two hundred years the inmates of the vivisection laboratories have tormented to death hundreds of millions of animals. Over 800 ways of inducing tumours in animals have been found, not one of which is remotely related to a cancer which has developed spontaneously in a human. Tumours are implanted under the skin, and then observed as the growth takes over the body, animals are radiated, limbs become gangrenous and fall off, force feeding large amounts of toxic substances causes vomiting and fits - until death intervenes... Animal-based "cancer research" fund-raisers include: Cancer Research UK (formerly The Imperial Cancer Research Fund and The Cancer Research Campaign), The Leukaemia Research Fund, Tenovus Cancer Research, The Yorkshire Cancer Research Campaign, Cancer and Leukaemia in Childhood Trust, Institute of Cancer Research, World Cancer Research Fund. If you support animal-based "cancer research" you are supporting the biggest fraud, medical or otherwise, in history, and the cruel and senseless torture and killing of your fellow beings; both human and animal. (Healing Cancer Naturally, n.d.)	British Anti-Vivisection Association
To the cancer establishment, a cancer patient is a profit center. The actual clinical and scientific evidence does not support the claims of the cancer industry. Conventional cancer treatments are in place as the law of the land because they pay, not heal, the best. Decades of the politics-of-cancer-as-usual have kept you from knowing this, and will continue to do so unless you wake up to their reality. (Defy your Doctor & be Healed, 2013, p. 352)	John Diamond, M.D.
The cancer establishment is the not-too-shadowy association of the American Cancer Society, the leading cancer hospitals, the National Cancer Institute, and the FDA. The shadowy part is the fact that these respected institutions are very much dominated by members and friends of members of the pharmaceutical industry, which profits so incredibly much from our profession-wide obsession with chemotherapy (Henderson, n.d.).	Robert C. Atkins, M.D., Author, *Dr. Atkins New Diet Revolution* and founder, The Atkins Center in New York.
Chemotherapy is an incredibly lucrative business for doctors, hospitals, and pharmaceutical companies. The medical establishment wants everyone to follow the same exact protocol. They don't want to see the chemotherapy industry go under, and that's the number one obstacle to any progress in oncology. (Defy your Doctor & be Healed, 2013, p. 352)	Glen Warner, M.D.
You wouldn't believe how many FDA officials or relatives or acquaintances of FDA officials come to see me as patients in Hanover. You wouldn't believe this, or directors of the AMA, or ACA, or the presidents of orthodox cancer institutes. (Defy your Doctor & be Healed, 2013, p.352)	Hans Nieper, M.D. Alternative medicine practitioner
When Dr. Hamer was arrested in 1997 for having given three people medical advice without a medical license, the police confiscated his patients' files and had them analyzed. Subsequently, one public prosecutor was forced to admit during the trial that, after five years, 6,000 out of 6,500 patients with mostly 'terminal cancer' were still alive. But with conventional treatment, the figures are generally just the reverse. (Total Health Institute, n.d.)	Dr. Caroline Markolin, Ph.D.
As a chemist trained to interpret data, it is incomprehensible to me that physicians can ignore the clear evidence that chemotherapy does much, much more harm than good. (WeeksMD, 2011)	Alan Nixon, Ph.D., Past President of the American Chemical Society
We have a multi-billion dollar industry that is killing people, right and left, just for financial gain. Their idea of research is to see whether two doses of this poison is better than three doses of that poison. (Havasi, 2012, p. 59)	Glen Warner, M.D., Oncologist

continued on following page

Table 1. Continued

Comments	Name of the Scientists
The FDA protects the big drug companies, and is subsequently rewarded, and using the government's police powers, they attack those who threaten the big drug companies. The thing that bugs me is that the people think the FDA is protecting them. It isn't. What the FDA is doing, and what the public thinks it is doing are as different as night and day (Defy your Doctor & be Healed, 2013, p. 7).	Dr. Herbert Ley, former Commissioner of the F.D.A.
Most cancer patients in this country die of chemotherapy. Chemotherapy does not eliminate breast, colon or lung cancers. This fact has been documented for over a decade. Yet doctors still use chemotherapy for these tumors. Women with breast cancer are likely to die faster with chemo than without it. (Cancer Tutor, 2017)	Alan Levin, M.D.
When a patient is found to have a tumor, the only thing the doctor discusses with that patient is what he intends to do about the tumor. If a patient with a tumor is receiving radiation or chemotherapy, the only question that is asked is, 'How is the tumor doing'? No one ever asks how the patient is doing. In my medical training, I remember well seeing patients who were getting radiation and/or chemotherapy. The tumor would get smaller and smaller, but the patient would be getting sicker and sicker. At autopsy, we would hear, 'Isn't that marvelous! The tumor is gone!' Yes, it was, but so was the patient. How many millions of times are we going to have to repeat these scenarios before we realize that we are treating the wrong thing? (Volker, 2016, p. 131)	Dr. Philip Bin, Cancer Researcher
According to medical associations, the notorious and dangerous side effects of drugs have become the fourth main cause of death after infarction, cancer, and apoplexy. (Cure Naturali Cancro, n.d.)	Journal of the American Medical Association, April 15, 1998
97 percent of the time chemotherapy does not work. So why is it still used? There's one reason and one reason only… money. (Glidden, 2010)	Peter Glidden, n.d.
Many oncologists recommend chemotherapy for almost any type of cancer, with a faith that is unshaken by the almost constant failures. (Braverman, 1991, p. 901)	Albert Braverman, MD, *Medical Oncology in the 90s*, Lancet, 1991, Vol. 337, p. 901
Since the 1950s, evidence has steadily accumulated that surgery, radiation, and chemotherapy are far less effective than the public is being led to believe. Investigative journalist Daniel Greenberg, writing in the Columbia Journalism Review in 1975, produced the first widely reported expose showing that cancer survival rates since the 1950s had not progressed, and that improvements from 1930 to 1950 were mainly a consequence of improved hospital nursing care and support systems. Greenberg found that even the valid improvements were very, very small, and that there had been no significant advancements in treating any of the major forms of cancer. (Ausubel, 2000)	When Healing Becomes a Crime –Kenny Ausubel, 2000
The majority of the cancer patients in this country die because of chemotherapy, which does not cure breast, colon or lung cancer. This has been documented for over a decade and nevertheless doctors still utilize chemotherapy to fight these tumors. (Lynes, 1990)	*The Healing of Cancer*, Marcus Books, 1990
If I were to contract cancer, I would never turn to a certain standard for the therapy of this disease. Cancer patients who stay away from these centres have some chance to make it. (Cure Naturali Cancro, n.d.)	Prof. Gorge Mathe, *Scientific Medicine Stymied,* Medicines Nouvelles, Paris, 1989
After all, and for the overwhelming majority of the cases, there is no proof whatsoever that chemotherapy prolongs survival expectations. And this is the great lie about this therapy, that there is a correlation between the reduction of cancer and the extension of the life of the patient. (Day, 2000)	Philip Day, *Cancer: Why we're still dying to know the truth,* Credence Publications, 2000
The majority of publications equate the effect of chemotherapy with (tumour) response, irrespective of survival. Many oncologists take it for granted that response to therapy prolongs survival, an opinion which is based on a fallacy and which is not supported by clinical studies. To date there is no clear evidence that the treated patients, as a whole, benefit from chemotherapy as to their quality of life. (Null, 2010)	Dr. Ulrich Abel.1990
The five year cancer survival statistics of the American Cancer Society are very misleading. They now count things that are not cancer, and because we are able to diagnose at an earlier stage of the disease, patients falsely appear to live longer. Our whole cancer research in the past 20 years has been a failure. More people over 30 are dying from cancer than ever before... More women with mild or benign diseases are being included in statistics and reported as being 'cured'. When government officials point to survival figures and say they are winning the war against cancer they are using those survival rates improperly. (Ryan, 1997)	Dr John Bailer, who spent 20 years on the staff of the U.S. National Cancer Institute and was editor of its journal, speaking at the Annual Meeting of the American Association for the Advancement of Science in May 1985
Approximately 1500 people (in Germany alone) die each day from cancer, treated to death in an atrocious manner with chemo and morphine ... According to the official statistics published by the German research centre on cancer in Heidelberg (Professor Abel), 98% of patients treated with chemo die within 7 years; 95% ... within 5 years. With the Germanische Neue Medizin however, 98% of those patients who did not previously receive treatments with chemo and morphine, survive. To deprive our patients of a 98% chance of survival is not worthy of medicine and criminal! (Total Health Institute, n.d.)	Dr. Ryke Geerd Hamer, founder of German New Medicine
Doctors are too busy to dig into the statistics of cancer treatments, they assume that what they are taught at school or what is demonstrated in the pages of briefing journals is the best treatment. They cannot afford to suspect that these treatments are only the best for the pharmaceutical companies that influence their 'institutions of higher learning'. (Healing Cancer Naturally, n.d.)	Paul Winter, The Cancell Home Page Webmaster.

continued on following page

Table 1. Continued

Comments	Name of the Scientists
After one recent survey two pathologists reported that after carrying out 400 post-mortem examinations they had found that in more than half the patients the wrong diagnosis had been made. This presumably also means that in more than half the patients the wrong treatment had been given. And since so many modern treatments are undeniably powerful it also presumably means that a large proportion of those patients died because of their treatment. The two pathologists reported that potentially treatable disease was missed in one in seven patients. They found that 65 out of 134 cases of pneumonia had gone unrecognised while out of 51 patients who had suffered heart attacks doctors had failed to diagnose the problem in 18 cases (Healing Cancer Naturally, n.d.).	Dr. Vernon Coleman, M.D., D. Sc., author of 114 books with translations into 23 languages selling in over 50 countries, excerpted from Dr. Vernon Coleman's article Modern Medicine is not a science
Oncologist Dr. Simoncini who developed a "gentle" and frequently very effective cancer treatment based on sodium bicarbonate was asked how he came to abandon the conventional cancer treatments of chemotherapy and radiation he had been trained to administer. He said that the reason was that he saw all his patients dying under this standard oncological care, so he prayed for God to show him a better way to treat those cancer victims he couldn't help with the best treatments he had known before. (Healing Cancer Naturally, n.d.)	Healing Cancer Naturally
Drugs affect the aura a great deal. I have seen dark energy forms in the liver left from drugs taken for various previous diseases. Hepatitis leaves an orange-yellow color in the liver years after the disease is supposedly cured. I have seen the radiopaque dye used to observe the spine that was injected into the spinal column to diagnose injury ten years after injection although it is supposed to be cleared by the body in a month or two. Chemotherapy clogs the whole auric field but especially the liver, with greenish-brown mucus-like energy. Radiation therapy frays the structured layers of the auric field like a burned nylon stocking. Surgery causes scars in the first layer of the field and sometimes all the way to the seventh layer. These scars, disfigurations and clogs can be healed by helping the physical body heal itself; if they are left distorted, the physical body will have a much more difficult time healing itself. When an organ is removed, the etheric organ can still be reconstructed and serve to keep harmony in the auric bodies above the physical body. I would imagine that someday, with more knowledge of the auric field and biochemistry, we may be able to cause organs that have been removed to grow again. (Barbara, 1988)	Ex-NASA physicist Barbara Ann Brennan in her book "Hands of Light" More in On the effects of drugs, chemotherapy and radiation on the human energy field or aura
Each time a patient comes in and needs cancer therapy, you could say it was a failure of prevention. (Raymond, 2011, p.14)	Dr. Samuel Broder, former Director of the National Cancer Institute.
The most promising approach to the control of cancer is a national commitment to prevention, with a concomitant rebalancing of the focus and funding of research. (Bailer, 1997)	John C. Bailar, MD, PhD, Former Deputy Associate Director for Cancer Control of the National Cancer Institute & Professor at the University of Chicago
No medical man during his student days is taught to think. He is expected to assimilate the thoughts of others and to bow to authority. Throughout the whole of his medical career he must accept the current medical fashions of the day or suffer the loss of prestige and place. No public appointments, no coveted preferment are open to the medical man who declines to parrot the popular shibboleths of his profession. (Healing Cancer Naturally, n.d.)	Dr. Hadwen in his book 'The Difficulties of Dr. Deguerre' on why most doctors will accept and perpetuate the status quo in medical treatment, no matter how unsatisfying or unsuccessful.
It's not the results of the "bone scans" or "CTs" which are of crucial importance ... but whether the cancer can be gotten under control or not. While many of the test methods used by us physicians are certainly scientific, they say nothing about the patient's state of health. (Healing Cancer Naturally, n.d.)	Dr Armin Grunewald, MD
Cutting away each and every cells thought to be cancerous, in order to "prevent metastases", as done today, is both unnecessary and maiming. Either way, the canceration will continue in the area, since the conflict is still unresolved, so it's important to focus entirely on conflict solution afterwards - something conventional medicine doesn't care about. (Stahel, n.d.)	A. Stahel in My Interpretation of New Medicine: A Revolutionary Biological Paradigm

- The first one being the manipulated story containing half-truth about cancer and its associated treatment procedures that conventional healthcare system controlled by pharmaceutical industries wants people to know and blindly believe in without question, so that their annual profits keeps on increasing.
- On the other hand, suppressing by every means possible, the reality about cancer and its associated curative treatment procedures that conventional healthcare system controlled by pharmaceutical industries does not wants people to know, because they are aware that a patient cured means a customer lost.

INTERACTION OF AGING AND CARCINOGENESIS: WHAT THE DRUG COMPANY WANTS RESEARCHERS AND DOCTORS TO BE BUSY WITH

Molecular Level

One of the more developed theories of aging is the free radical theory proposed in 1954 by Harman. This theory postulates that various oxidative reactions occurring in the organism generate free radicals as a by-product. This causes multiple lesions in macromolecules (nucleic acids, proteins, and lipids), leading to their damage and aging. The key mechanisms of both aging and cancer are linked via endogenous stress-induced DNA damage caused by reactive oxygen species. The links include oxidative nuclear and mitochondrial DNA damage and repair, telomere shortening, and telomere- driven cellular senescence. These have been discussed in a number of comprehensive reviews.

The intensity of natural damages to DNA is high. In a human cell, spontaneous depurinization takes place at a rate of up to 10,000 events per day and spontaneous deamination of adenine and cytosine at a rate of hundreds of events per day. As a result, permanently active mechanisms of DNA repair have evolved. However, both of the most intensive natural mutation processes (depurinization and deamination) rarely involve thymidine, and therefore the reparation schemes for thymidine may have evolved less intensely. Hence, if one wants to induce uniformly distributed point mutations in laboratory animals, it is suitable to use analogs of thymidine as a mutagen (Casson et al., 2003).

Cellular Level

The term "cellular senescence," originally defined as a series of cellular changes associated with aging, now refers more commonly to a signal transduction program leading to irreversible arrest of cell growth, accompanied by a distinct set of changes in the cellular phenotype. Senescence is a potent anti-carcinogenic program, and the process of neoplastic transformation involves a series of events that allow cells to bypass senescence. Senescent cells were demonstrated capable of stimulating the malignant progression of premalignant keratinocytes and mammary gland epithelial cells. Senescent cells have also been detected at sites of age-related pathology, including benign hyperplastic prostate and atherosclerotic lesions.

Cellular senescence is controlled by the tumor suppressor proteins p53 and pRb. Inactivation of these proteins results in bypass of senescence. Due to its essentially irreversible growth arrest and the requirement for p53 and pRb function, cellular senescence is considered a potent tumor suppressor mechanism. The natural history of spontaneous tumors in humans and the survival of cancer patients newly diagnosed at different ages provide information on the effects of age on tumor growth in humans (Casson, 2003).

Physiologic Level

The potential link between aging and insulin/IGF-1 signaling has attracted substantial attention during recent years based on evidence such as the age-related increase in the incidence of insulin resistance and type 2 diabetes in accelerated aging syndromes or lifespan extension by caloric restriction in rodents. Concomitant reduction in plasma insulin and plasma glucose levels, which implies increased sensitivity to insulin, emerges as a hallmark of increased longevity. Hyperglycemia is an important aging factor involved in the generation of advanced glycosylation end products (AGEs). There is evidence that hyperinsulinemia favors the accumulation of oxidized proteins by reducing their degradation as well as facilitating protein oxidation by increasing the steady-state level of oxidative stress.

It is proposed that ageing can influence carcinogenesis through several molecular mechanisms. Telomeres, the non-coding DNA caps that protect the end of chromosomes, are thought to play a crucial role. With each cell division there is continued shortening of telomere length until a critical limit is reached and the cell enters senescence, a state of growth arrest. This process is considered to be a driver of ageing as well as an important tumor suppressive mechanism. Several studies indicate that shorter telomeres are a risk for cancer and telomere dysfunction is believed to promote malignancy. Additionally, it is speculated that the accumulation of senescent cells with age creates a tissue environment permissive to cancer. The age-related deterioration of mitochondria is thought to promote the production of reactive oxygen species that interfere with DNA and protein function, facilitating cancer development. Changes in the activity of enzymes involved in the activation of carcinogens are postulated to make older tissues more receptive to the effects of carcinogens. Other age-associated genetic modifications including DNA hyper methylation, point mutations and chromosomal translocation are thought to groom ageing tissues for neoplastic development (Casson et al., 2003).

INTERACTION OF AGING AND CARCINOGENESIS: WHAT THE DRUG COMPANY DOES NOT WANT RESEARCHERS AND DOCTORS TO REALIZE

The researchers are being misled by the powerful drug companies controlling the cancer research. The central dogma of molecular biology that are being taught to everyone is in fact not true. The word dogma itself means a set of religious principle laid down by an authority as incontrovertibly true or unquestioning belief. Conventional central dogma portrays Genetic Determinism, in short organisms are victims of their genes. But the reality is it's not the genes that controls us, but the environment. Environment controls gene expression, and by extension environment itself controls human life. So, human are not victims of the bad genes. Wrong or mutated genes are the result, faulty proteins are the result and strictly not the cause (Lipton, 2016).

Dr. Bruce Lipton in his book titled The Biology of Belief writes about the stem cell research under the guidance of the great scientist, Dr. Irv Konigsberg, the first cell biologist to master the art of cloning stem cells. During their research, when they provided healthy environment for the stem cells, they thrived. When the environments were less than optimal, the cells faltered. When they adjusted the environment, these sick cells revitalized. Dr. Konigsberg suggested that if one is studying an ailing cell, then the researcher must first look to the cell's environment and not inside the cell for the cause. Even Charles Darwin himself conceded near the end of his life, that his evolutionary theory had short-changed the role of environment. In the year 1876 Darwin wrote a letter to Moritz Wagner and the author quotes...

In my opinion, the greatest error which I have committed has been not allowing sufficient weight to the direct action of the environment that is food, climate, lifestyle etc. independently of the natural selection. When I wrote the Origin of Species, and for some years afterwards, I could find little good evidence of the direct action of the environment, now there is a large body of evidence. (Darwin, 1876)

Even Darwin acknowledged and admitted that genes do not control one's life, environment does but still this fact is never mentioned in mainstream textbooks. Neither have they taught the students these

Figure 1. Central Dogma of Molecular Biology as per Conventional Science. Science of Genetics

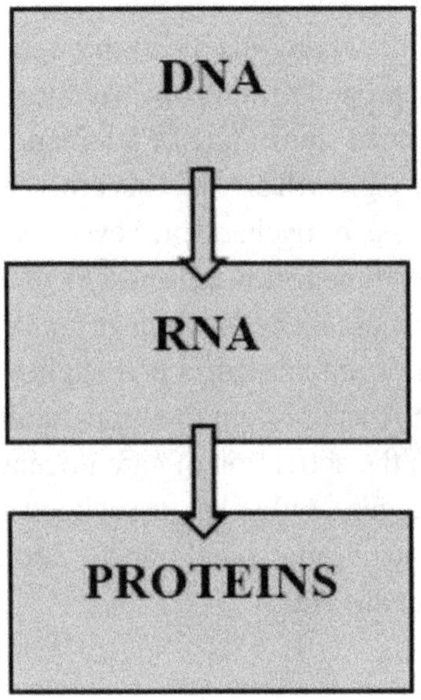

facts. The young researchers and doctors are being misled to believe that if something goes wrong, if any disease occurs look inside the cells, stay busy with studying the behavior of already expressed proteins and their interactions. In short, they are made to run blindly after the symptoms while purposefully distracting them form the direction that will lead to the actual cause and lead to discovery of cure.

Young researchers and doctors are made to believe that genes controls life because it brings profit to the pharmaceutical industry controlling cancer research. Nijhout (1990) provided evidence that the notion that genes control biology has been so frequently repeated for such a long period of time that the scientists have forgotten that it is actually a hypothesis and not a proven truth. In reality, the ideology that genes controls life of an organism has never been proven. Nijhout (1990) summarizes the truth as and the author quotes…

When a gene product is needed, a signal from its environment, not an emergent property of the gene itself, activates expression of that gene.

According to a paper published by Hegde (2014) the scientific communities hide the truth about diseases like cancer just for profit and that cancer is not a disease. It is just a process of ageing. Some people age faster than others. He mentioned that the ageing was not morphological ageing but at a cellular level. Depending on the rate of growth of cancer, it could either outlive the person or precede him (Massague & Norton, 2006; Hegde, 2014). When the cancer starts growing inside human body, the body's natural defence system and healing mechanisms continuously attempts to suppress it or to overcome it. If during the process the body's immune system takes over, the cancer cells dies prematurely. The unusually high rate of cancers in AIDS patients are perfect example. Biologically a cancer cell is nothing but the normal cell that have outlived its appointed time of death. These appointed times of death of cells are known as Apoptosis or Programmed Cell Death. The entire process of apoptosis is controlled by suicide genes, which transmits signal to every cell, when it's time for the cell to die. If for any reason the suicide

Figure 2. The way in which genes are actually controlled. Science of Epigenetics

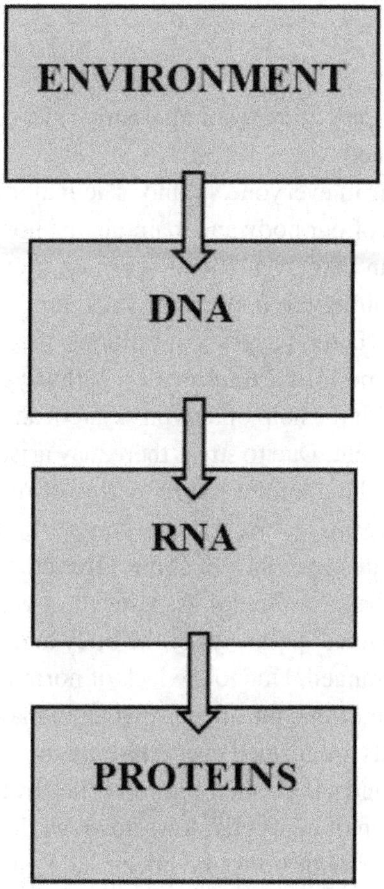

gene either fails to send the signals, or the associated messenger proteins and enzymes fails to perform their activities, the target cell might not receive the message at all. In this kind of situation that cell could outlive its lifespan, but cannot divide any further, since there is an upper limit for cellular replication in every situation, which in today's date known as Hayflick's Law or Hayflick's Limit (Hegde, 2014).

The Hayflick's Limit is a concept that helps to explain the mechanism behind cellular aging. The law states that a normal human cell can only replicate and divide about 60 times before it cannot divide anymore and will be taken down by programmed cell death or apoptosis (Bartlett, 2014). The cell that escapes this mechanism of apoptosis at right time mutates to change its DNA. This is the beginning of the potential future cancer if and only if it chooses to do so (Coffey et al., 2006).Every human being harbours some sort of potential cancer or the other at all times. It is only epigenetic factor(s) that one such biological cancer could transform into clinical cancer. In an consecutive post-mortem study of two hundred and fifty deaths due to suicide, where the researchers found the presence of biological cancer in every one of them. Depression was the cause of suicide and not those biological cancers (Michael, McFarlane, Feinstein., & Wells., 1987; Eddy, 1989).

CANCER AND ITS RELATIONSHIP WITH AGEING

The Holistic Level

The ideology of epigenetic is what practitioners of alternative systems of medicine follow strictly. The concept is known as holistic approach.

Cancer is a term that brings fear in everyone's mind. The major function of our brain is to regulate the normal physiological functions of our body and maintain the homoeostasis. As long as the homoeostasis is maintained no diseases can take over. But as a person grows old his brain has to take care of lots of other issues than just controlling the bodily activities. It is our brain that is actually controlling and regulating the functional and structural aspects of millions of cells that makes up our body and also the numerous chemical reactions and signal transduction pathways occurring in our body. The entire process is regulated by our brain with the help of nervous system and its associated components directly controlled by surrounding environment. Due to stress there may arise a situation in any one of the cell in our body that lost the control from the brain for a brief period of time. This causes disruption of integrity of the numerous biochemical reactions occurring at a time in our body that are interdependent on each other. In that particular moment due to lack of control from the brain, one of the numerous healing mechanisms working in our body becomes faulty. As a result, it will create chemical components that are not recognized by the other chemical pathways of the body and thus the entire biochemical process inside the cell dynamically gets deranged. Due to the lack of normal functioning of the cellular healing processes the cell may enter a stage of uncontrolled growth and may lead to cancers.

In our body millions of new cells are formed every day and they replace the old worn out cells. This process is carried out by the spleen and it is cleaned and controlled by the Lymph glands. When we neglect our body, the process of regeneration of new cells slows down while the process of decaying-destroying of cells-increases, more toxins gather in the body, the spleen and Lymph glands are overburdened. Slowly but steadily, there is a malignant growth in the body, but it is not easily noticed. Meanwhile, these toxins/wastes gather in the body in the part which is most damaged e. g. for a smoker, these toxins gather in the lungs or in the mouth. When these toxins are gathered in a large quantity, it forms a duct and starts developing fast. In the meantime, the weak Lymph gland is greatly damaged and through it other glands are damaged. And a stage is reached when these glands become tired and stop secreting the most vital hormones in the body. At that time, this malignant growth becomes fast and the final signal is given by Nature. There is a change in metabolism, severe headache, loss of weight, change of voice, color of the spots on the body changes, and constant fever. At this time, this disease is diagnosed as cancer.

With age, comes an increased risk of cancer because the cells of the brain become weaker and its control over various portions of the body gets less prompt. Older adults account for 60% of incidences of cancer and 70% of cancer related deaths. The process of ageing favors two essential processes in cancer development: the acquisition of mutations and the formation of a molecular and cellular environment which favors carcinogenesis. As one ages, processes like DNA repair become less active and efficient, allowing DNA adduct formation, hypo methylation of DNA and more frequent mutations, chromosomal breaks and translocations. Mutations can inactivate anti proliferative and apoptotic tumor suppressor genes, cause proto oncogenes to become oncogenes or hinder the function of DNA repair genes. The accumulation of such non-lethal genetic damage is the basis of cancer.

SCREENING AND PREVENTION OF CANCER IN AGEING POPULATION

The fundamental goals of modern medicine (allopathic) are the prevention or early detection of disease through screening. Screening can lead to interventions that may decrease morbidity and mortality. In short screening is done for safety. This is what people are taught to believe from the very first day of medical education and each and every conventional textbooks or mainstream media addresses the same. But the fact is cancer is not a reductionist phenomenon, it is holistic phenomena. The lump or tumor that are being screened are not the disease, they are the result of the disease. So screening and removing the result of the disease does not cure the cancer. No screening process can detect the underlying cause that lead to cancer, they can only detect the lump or the bump.The author points out some of the incidences pointed out my eminent scientists around the world about the cancer screening and the risks associated with it. Prof. B.M. Hegde mentioned in an interview that when a cancer cell is detected in human body, what modern or conventional medicine does is they take a bit of the cells, kills the cells, stains them with toxic chemicals and then observe them under microscope for diagnosis and interpretation. This generates false positive results. Because what they are observing is a tombstone of the dead cells. So, there is no way one can determine what the cells are doing by this procedure. It is impossible to know anything from the slide about the cancer cells. Any understanding of human illness or wellness has to be in totality and not in bits and pieces, because human body does not work in bits and pieces but functions as a whole (Hegde, 2014).

Albert Szent Gyorgyi, (1960) a Hungarian Biochemist, who won Noble Prize in Physiology or Medicine in 1937 published the reality of cancer biochemistry in his book called Introduction to Sub Molecular Biology. In his book the great scientist writes and the author quotes…

I do not know what cancer is, because the cancer cells acts exactly like a normal cells. It may look morphologically different but works exactly like a normal cell. And I do not know how anybody could kill a cancer cell without killing the normal cells of the body.

One of the most common methods of cancer screening is PET scan. In this method radiated sugar is injected inside the patient's body because, it is known to conventional medical system that cancerous cells takes on sugars efficiently as compared to normal healthy cells. As the cancer cells takes up the radio labelled sugar, the doctors can view the cancer cells on the screen. They use the sugar to pinpoint where the lump is. Dr. Roby Mitchell, MD, well known orthomolecular medicine specialist reported in an interview (TTAC, 2017).

Dr. David C Jockers, DC, reported in an interview that sugar is a fuel for cancer cells. They have an altered metabolism, altered physiology and they are not able to produce energy from aerobic metabolism, so mitochondria itself is damaged. So cancer cells depends on anaerobic metabolism which is basically is breaking down of sugar. They utilize sugar and generate huge amounts of toxic wastes that make the body system more and more acidic. So by injecting sugars in patients with suspected cancers are like adding gasoline to the fire. It makes the condition worse for the patient but profitable for healthcare industries (TTAC, 2017).

Most of the Cancer patients die of nutrition deficiency….. Dr. Rashid Buttar.

Conventional medical fraternity talks about prevention and screening of cancer patients. This is why they claim to perform the screening tests that itself possesses the capability to worsen the cancer but the question is how many oncologists are addressing malnutrition? One will never hear an oncologist addressing proper nutrition to cancer patients. Instead they recommend the patients nutritional supplement powders advertised by the drug companies, that contains extremely high levels of sugars, to the cancer patients even after knowing that cancer cells are Obligate Glucose Metabolizer, which means sugar gives extra life and power to cancer cells. Evidently, they are creating more and more cancer patients for drug companies in the name of screening and prevention (TTAC, 2017). Sugar is like gasoline and cancer is like fire.

Bob Wright, founder of American Anticancer Institute (AACI) reported in an interview that for preventing cancer in real one need to strictly check the nutrition of the patient. He reported that average amount of sugar in a diet cold drinks is about ten tablespoons. That is enough to efficiently shut down a minimum of 50% of the total immune system for about four hours. Diet cold drinks have pH of around 2.5 to 2.7, which is highly acidic. When a cancer patient consumes such amount of sugar, it will require 11 liters of water having pH around 9.5, to neutralize the toxic effect (TTAC, 2017).

Burton Goldberg, The Voice of Alternative Medicine, reported in an interview that the oncologists use sugar to carry the radiologic molecules into the cancer cells, to show up in the PET scan. The oncologist knows that sugar feeds cancer, because that is why they use it as Trojan horse. And when one finishes chemotherapy or radiation therapy or surgery under conventional settings, the patients are given cookies, ice creams, candies. It is like putting out the fire and when the fire goes out they start adding the gasoline again. That means these oncologists are guilty of crimes against humanity, they are killing their patients slowly (TTAC, 2017)

According to a famous immunologist A. J. Lanigan, to overcome cancer, it is best to stop it before it begins or to reverse it. Immune system and body's natural healing mechanisms are the only thing that stands between an organism and all those things that are trying to destroy the organism's health, including cancer (TTAC, 2017).

Dr. Tony Jiminez, explained in an interview that for prevention, treatment and curing cancers the best thing one can do is enhance the patient's immune system, because it is the immune system that takes care of cold to cancer and everything in between. Chemotherapy, Radiation therapy and surgery are worst thing one can do to a cancer patient. Because of all these conventional or allopathic treatment destroys immune system. And patient dies of the after effects of chemotherapy, radiation therapy and surgery while the entire blame is given on the cancer. The patient receiving chemo or radiation dies because of the chemo and radiation and not because of the cancer the patient was suffering from because

- In one cubic centimeter of a tumor there are one billion cancer cells.
- 65% of those cells at any one time or the other were dormant, 35% of those were active.
- So, they are in the synthesis phase of the cell cycle and not in the resting phase.
- Of all those active cells 99% of the cells are non-cancerous stem cells.
- About 1% is cancer stem cells.

So, when someone undergoes chemo or radiation therapy, they are not only suppressing the immune system but they are making the cancer stem cells more and more aggressive.

- Chemotherapy and radiation therapy effects and kills only the non-cancerous stem cells.
- Chemotherapy and radiation therapy does not kill cancerous stem cells but instead activates them by destroying the immune system.

In short good cells get killed and bad cells get strengthened and above all the body's natural defense and healing capacity is damaged for lifetime. The lump of cancer that contained no harmful, non-cancerous stem cells gets killed and the lump gets smaller and smaller in size as detected by the conventional diagnostic methods. The doctor gets the impression that chemo or radiation cured the cancer. But they do not acknowledge the very fact that it did not kill the harmful cancer stem cells and instead it converted them into more powerful and aggressive form (TTAC, 2017).

CANCER THERAPIES SUITABLE FOR AGEING POPULATION

The FDA protects the big drug companies, and is subsequently rewarded, and using the government's police powers, they attack those who threaten the big drug companies. The thing that bugs me is that the people think that FDA is protecting them. It isn't. What the FDA is doing, and what the public thinks it is doing are as different as night and day..... .... Dr. Herbert Ley. Former Commissioner of FDA.

The methods of detection of cancer and its subsequent treatment by the procedures of chemotherapy, radiation therapy or surgery is in a way time consuming, expensive, lethal and by no means suitable for the old aged persons as their body system is already weak and the person's body may not be able to take the stress and side effects imposed by the treatment. People at the extremes of life are delicate so as a medical practitioner one must practice great caution. Early diagnosis is essential for planning of the proper treatment procedures. Following are brief idea of several Alternative therapies and techniques that can lead to detection of cancer at early stage and if the pathology is in the reversible state then the condition may be cured. With Alternative therapies there is a slight chance of curing the cancer which is never possible by conventional treatments. Administering chemotherapy and destroying the cancer cells, along with destroying the homoeostasis permanently without fixing the root cause that lead to the cancer stage will never help. Instead of that the medical practitioners should try to identify and fix the deranged chemical pathway, imbalance of which lead to cancers.

Cancer is not the disease, it is the result of the disease, but the Medical Doctors are taught to see it as disease, and this is the wrong approach. Approximately 10 years ago The American Cancer Society (ACS) stopped using the word "Cure" with respect to cancer and converted it to "Five years survivality". So as far as ACS is concerned, if one is diagnosed with cancer and receives conventional treatment like Chemotherapy, radiation therapy and surgery and the patient lives for five years and one day and then die of cancer, it is considered as a successful treatment and it goes into the statistical record book as a positive result. In a research performed by a group of scientists by performing the meta-analysis of the outcomes of 11 years of conventional cancer treatment performed on adult person and published them in American Journal of Clinical Oncology in the year 2004 stating that 97% of the time chemotherapy, radiation and surgery does not work (Glidden, 2010).

Then why the mainstream healthcare sector prescribes chemotherapy, radiation and surgery for cancer when it is proven that 97% of the time it does not work, and instead it makes the case much worse?

The one and only reason is money. The healthcare which was once a service sector now converted to healthcare industry and involves huge amount of money, finances and profits associated with cancer management. Dr. Peter Glidden, Naturopathic Physician in his book titled "The MD Emperor Has No Clothes" and in several of his interviews advised the cancer patient and their family to ask the doctor the list of questions before selecting cancer therapies like chemotherapy, radiation or surgery prescribed by conventional medical practitioner. The list of fundamental questions pointed out by Glidden (2010) that every cancer patient should ask their doctors before selecting treatment methods are as follows:

- Doctor, as the patient is diagnosed with a particular type of cancer, does the therapy you are recommending cures the patient's cancer?
- What actually caused the cancer in the patient under consideration?
- If the treatment you are recommending does not cure the cancer, what can the patient expect from the treatment?
- What are the side effects from the treatment that the doctors are prescribing to the patient?
- Can the cancer treatment give the patient cancer?
- How are the doctors going to manage the side effects of the treatment after the patient goes through the prescribed treatment methods?
- What is going to be the quality of the patient's life while he or she is going through the treatment and after the treatment is complete or better to say the rest of the life?
- How much are the doctors and institutions going to profit from this treatment?
- Finally, last question which the author quotes, "I would like to talk to five of your past patients who have had the same type of cancer that I have, who have had undergone the exact same treatment that I will be receiving, to see how that goes?" (Glidden, 2010).

ACUPRESSURE THERAPY FOR CANCERS

As published by various researchers and practitioners of acupressure around the world in several journals and books of repute that cancer is a man-made disease. The major cause for cancer is the continuous negligence to the organs of the body by the patient. For example, the lungs of a chain-smoker are continuously irritated. The cancer of the mouth or vocal cords is due to the habit of chewing tobacco, drinking hot tea, etc. In the case of cancer of the uterus, negligence about internal hygiene is the root cause. It has been observed that women, who take great care of their internal organs, do not get cancer of the uterus.

Cancer of the breast is due to non-feeding of the baby by mother, and suppression of the sexual desire by unmarried women. Cancer of the stomach and intestines is due to overuse of refined flour and rice, coffee, sugar and tea and the habit of overdrinking of alcohol. It has been observed that laborers in the sugar factory in the West Indies use brown sugar molasses-jaggery and so they are immune to cancer. And cancer of colon is due to continuous constipation caused by wrongful habits of food and sedentary life. It has been observed and documented by several researchers that the people, who are vegetarian and use more of milk and milk products like curd, buttermilk, etc., do not generally get this type of cancer (Nancy, 1999).

One should understand that the diseases are nothing but the signals given by the body that there is something wrong in that organ. It is just body's reaction to certain stress one should identify what component is causing that stress and must try to replenish the same. Instead of removing the root cause of the disease, either the signal, tonsils or appendix is removed by operation or the disease is suppressed like common cold with powerful antibiotics. The body is to be treated as a temple-a seat of God and each and every corner of this temple, body, should be kept neat and clean. Instead, the body is treated like a dustbin wherein useless things are dumped and instead of cleaning out the waste or toxins, they are suppressed; with the result it becomes a duct and which after a time results into a malignant growth (Nancy, 1999).

The long-term cause of cancer is the imbalance and disturbance caused to the metabolism of the body through:

- Foods grown with the help of inorganic manure and pesticides, etc.
- Increased use of canned foods, bottled pickles, etc.
- Unchecked use of fluoride.
- Working under unhygienic conditions e. g. working in asbestos factory without protection.
- Pollution of the environment by excessive use of diesel, cutting down of trees, etc.
- Polluting the water sources through chemical wastes, etc.
- Going against the laws from Nature.

It was documented in several literatures of acupressure that these root causes of cancer can be removed and thus cancer can be prevented. It was observed and documented by several researchers independently that in the animal world this dreaded disease is rarely found. The obvious reason is that they follow laws of Nature.

According to the science of acupressure, any minor disturbance of any organ is reflected on the palms or soles. When there is a continued complaint the first gland to be disturbed is the Thyroid/Parathyroid gland. The second gland to be disturbed in case of problems of degeneration leading towards cancer is the Lymph gland. As mentioned above, this important gland works to remove the toxins and dead cells from the body. When the process of regeneration of the cells of the body slows down, there is increase in the activity of clearing the dead cells and preventing pus formation. This gland, thus, gives ALARM. If Point No. 16 is touched, on hands and feet, and if these points are found to be tender and when one presses them, and the person will feel pain. Another pointer for detection is that the organ where, cancer is developing is disturbed and there is pain in the corresponding point on palms and soles. For example, in case of cancer of the breast, there is pain in the middle point on the back of palm as or in case of cancer of colon, there is pain in Point No. 20. For details about the location of pressure points on hand and feet, refer to any standard acupressure hand and feet maps.

The same way, for cancer in table 2 (Nancy, 1999):

If these signals are ignored, the declining process starts disturbing other glands also and reaches a dangerous point where these endocrine glands become tired and stop secreting hormones. During that time, more and more wastes or toxins get accumulated forming a duct and start multiplying and thus a fast malignant growth starts in that part of the body damaging the very metabolism of the body. Thus, it was observed and documented that cancer can be detected at a very early stage, and it can be controlled very easily. Moreover, it can be observed that if regular acupressure treatment is taken daily or at least 3 times a week the lethargic spleen or lymph gland can be reactivated, and factors leading to cancer can be checked. Thus, acupressure can prevent cancer.

Table 2. Types of Cancer and corresponding acupressure points.

Type of Cancer	Acupressure Points
Throat Cancer	Pain at Point No. 6
Windpipe Gullet Cancer	Pain between Point No. 6 and 27
Stomach Cancer	Pain at Point No. 7
Small Intestine Cancer	Pain at Point No. 9
Large Intestine & Colon Cancer	Pain at Point No. 10 and 20
Liver Cancers	Pain at Point No. 22 and 23
Lung Cancers	Pain at Point No. 30
Brain Cancers	Pain at Point No. 1 to 5
Blood Cancers	Pain at Point No. 37
Bone Cancers	Pain at Point No. 9 and 37
Uterus Cancer	Pain at Point No. 11 and 15

(Nancy, 1999)

HOMOEOPATHY FOR CANCERS

Homeopathy is a holistic system of medicine which has been used by many practitioners to treat cancer patients. There are historical accounts about homeopathy treatment of cancer and modern literature also gives several case studies of homeopathy for cancer treatment. Homeopathy treats the person as a whole. It means that homeopathic treatment focuses on the patient as a person, as well as his pathological condition. The homeopathic remedies for cancer are selected after a full individualizing examination and case-analysis, which includes the medical history of the patient, physical and mental constitution etc. A tendency of predisposition and susceptibility, also termed as miasms is also often taken into account for the treatment of chronic conditions. The homeopathic remedies for cancer given below indicate the therapeutic affinity but this is not a complete and definite guide to the treatment of this condition. The symptoms listed against each remedy may not be directly related to this disease because in homeopathy general symptoms and constitutional indications are also taken into account for selecting a remedy. Following is the list of some common used homeopathic remedies for cancer.

- **Calcarea Fluorica or Fluoride of Lime:** According to Dr. J.B. Bell and Dr. W.H. Suchessler, homeopathic remedy for cancer is most useful for knots, kernels or hardened lumps in the female breast, accompanied with indurated glands of stony hardness; the enlargements may occur in the fasciae. It will prevent the development of cancer, and should be considered always in the cases where the breasts present suspicious lumps (Boericke, 1927).
- **Lapis Albus:** According to Dr. V. Grauvogl several cases of incipient scirrhus (cancer) of the breasts, presenting retraction of the nipple, and the other characteristic symptoms have been cured with this remedy. Dr. E. G. Jones recommends Lapis in malignant diseases of the uterus where the discharges are black and offensive and intense burning pains all through the diseased part (Boericke, 1927).

- **Silicea or Silica:** According to Dr. W.H. Suchessler and Dr. Samuel Hahnemann silecea will often abate the pains of cancer. Lupus and sarcoma with a thick yellow and offensive discharge (Boericke, 1927).
- **Hecla Lava:** According to Dr. C. Hering this may be a remedy for Osteomata (Bone Cancer), not so-called ivory tumours, but those of spongy nature (Boericke, 1927).
- **Conium:** Proven by Dr. Samuel Hahnemann. Great hardness of the infiltrated glands, with flying stitches in them worse at night. Cancer, mammary tumors of beginning of scirrhus; chief remedy, especially useful after contusions and bruises, it corresponds particularly to glandular bruises. Here it is an absolute specific, and the writer advises the 30th potency. Dr. O. S. Haines has verified this statement. The irritability seems the characteristic. Epithelioma, enlarged testicles or uterus (Boericke, 1927).
- **Condrango:** Proved by Dr. J.C. Burnett and Dr. J.P. Dinsmore. This homeopathic remedy for cancer has achieved considerable reputation is cancer of the stomach and various forms of carcinoma. Many cases have improved under the Ix; open cancer and cancerous ulcers; it modifies the pain. Bernstein believes the field of this remedy to be in Epithelioma, especially in open and ulcerated types. He recommends the 6x potency, and has had remarkable results from its use (Boericke, 1927).
- **BarytaCarbonica:** Proved by Dr. Samuel Hahnemann. Applied for Fatty tumours appearing here and there over the body (Boericke, 1927).
- **Phytolacca:** As proven by Allentown College, it has a tendency to fat formation, and may prove useful in fatty tumors as well as in hard, painful nodosities in the breast. Cancers of the breast when the tumors is hard, painful and purple. It acts as an absorbent in fibroid tumors of the uterus (Boericke, 1927).
- **Plumbumiodatum:** As per Hartlub, it is indicated in inflamed indurated masses in the female breast slowly developing. The hard, unchangeable character, the slow development and the supervening of painful inflammations therein are the elements of decision (Boericke, 1927).
- **Arsenicum:** According to Dr. Hahnemann this homeopathic remedy corresponds to the general phenomena of the cancerous diathesis, though Bayes notes that we have other remedies which may possess more power over cancer indicated. It is said to be almost a specific for lupus, and its special indications in any form of tumour, be it cancer or not, the sharp burning and lancinating pain, the weakness and debility and the general Arsenicum symptoms known so well. In other words, the patient is to be treated, not the disease (Boericke, 1901).
- **Thuja:** According to Dr. Hahnemann it is a remedy for polypoid growths in the nose and ears. The epithelial variety of cancer, and cauliflower excrescences would seem to correspond to this remedy. Dr. Helmuth also considered Thuja as a valuable remedy in sarcoma. Palpillomata also comes within its field.
- **Hydrastis:** Proven by Burt. This remedy corresponds to what Jousset terms the epithelial diathesis and is of undoubted and special value in epithelioma and uterine cancer. Our English confreres praise this remedy in simple glandular tumors of the breast; here it allays the pain retards the growth and improves the patient generally. The dyspeptic symptoms of the remedy lead to its choice. The hydrastis treatment is one of the best known in cancer.
- **Radium:** Introduced by Dr. J.H.C. Clarks. The use of this substance has been heralded as a homeopathic remedy for cancer. Though it produces actually and pathologically that disease, it has never

cured in any dosage or in any stage of that affection. It uses all doses save those of Homoeopathy is dangerous and should be avoided. However, Dieffenbach has proven its use and it may indicate therefore, not in Cancer, but in what Vannier so happily the terms that "Cancerinique" dyscrasia, which means the abnormal blood conditions which tend toward that disease, and always precede it. Thus, it use is confined to the pre-growth manifestations when we have such symptoms as aching pains, itching over the body, pains resembling a chronic arthritis, apprehension, mentally tired and irritable patients, pimples on the skin and spots which itch and burn. Restlessness, heat in stomach, flatulence and constipation. The 30th potency is as low as it should be used. We can never be certain whether a patient has not been subjected in some unknown way to radium emanations and by giving the remedy in the lower strengths we may add to the trouble. A recent finding of the New York Health Department (1932) says: "In regions where radio-active minerals were mined an increased incidence of cancer, especially of cancer of the lungs, had been noted." It also condemned the use of so-called radium waters as elements of danger. A study of the "cancerinique' or pre-growth symptoms will give positive information as to the approach of this disease, and positive indications for the remedies that should be used to prevent the same.

These are some of the numerous cancer remedies used in homoeopathy. And since these treatment is personalized the healing will be prompt and with no side effects. Because all the complementary therapy acts by boosting up the body's natural healing mechanisms. Here the medicine substances boost up the body's natural healing mechanism and then the body's mechanisms cure itself. These systems are more personalized (Boericke, 1901).

BIOCHEMIC OR CELL SALTS REMEDIES FOR CANCER

The Biochemic System of Medicine was proved and introduced by Dr. Wilhelm Heinrich Schuessler in the year 1973. According to Schuessler (2013), when a cell gets all the nutrients and salts that are necessary for performing their regular biochemical activities, the cell stays healthy and no disease can take over the cell, but if somehow there occurs deficiency of the required amount of nutrients or inorganic salts, the cells fails to perform their normal biochemical processes and functions, thus becomes weak and the disease takes over. So somehow if one can maintain or restore the nutrient and salt requirements of the cell, no diseases can take over. Schuessler (2013) explained in his research and the authors quote…

The relationship between the blood and the body is same as that of soil and plant. It is common phenomena that poor exhausted soil will produce only weak, sickly plants. In the same way poor blood lacking its essential constituents will produce disease prone and weak sickly bodies. By enriching the soil, the sick plants can be made to recover and flourish. The recovery of ailing human body can be achieved by a similar process that is by restoring to the blood the constituent in which it is lacking.

The following section contains a brief idea about the importance of the twelve tissue salts, and for detailed knowledge about the cell salts it is advised to consult Biochemic Materia Medica and Biochemic Practice of Medicine:

- **CalcareaFluorica or Calcium Fluoride (Calc Flour):** It gives tissues the quality of elasticity. It combines with the organic substances such as albumin to form elastic tissue and is found in the walls of blood vessels, in muscular tissues in connective tissues, in the surface of bones and in enamel of teeth. Its deficiency results in a loss of elasticity and consequent relaxed condition. Its main function is preservation of contractile power of elastic tissues. Whenever the symptoms are traceable to relaxed condition, for example, relaxed condition of veins and arteries, sluggish circulation, piles, tendency to cracks on skin, this tissue salt is needed. It is also useful in the treatment of diseases affecting the surface of the bones and joint and when teeth become loose in their socket and decay rapidly. The elasticity of muscular tissue and supporting membranes becomes impaired when this tissue salt is deficient, resulting in muscular weakness, bearing down pains etc. The symptoms are generally worse in humid condition and are relieved by massage and warmth (Boericke, 1901).
- **Calcarea Phosphorica or Calcium Phosphate (CalcPhos):** It is a tissue salt concerned with nutrition. It combines with albumin and is indicated when there are albuminous discharges. Without Calcarea Phosphorica there could be no blood coagulation. It will assist the action of a more directly indicated tissue salts and thus produce more rapid results. It promotes healthy cellular activity and restores tone to weakened organs and tissues. This tissue salt is concerned with the formation of bone and teeth and thus becomes an important remedy for children. It aids in normal growth and development and should be given in cases of backwardness more particularly where there is bone weakness or recurring tooth troubles. It is the Biochemic remedy for rickets. Calcarea Phosphorica is a constituent of saliva and gastric juices. It assists in digestion and assimilation and favors the building up of a sturdy, robust constitution. The restorative power of these inorganic salts will speed up recovery and replenish the body's reserves of strength. It is the tissue salt for weak blood and condition associated with weak and imperfect circulation. It is a great restorative remedy (Boericke, 1901).
- **Calcarea Sulphurica or Calcium Sulphate (CalcSulph):** It is the blood purifier and restorer. It is found in the liver where it helps in the removal of waste products from the blood stream and it has a cleansing and purifying influence throughout the system. It cleans out the accumulation of non-functional organic matter in the tissues and causes infiltrated parts to discharge their contents readily, throwing off decaying organic matter, so that it may not lie dormant or slowly decay and thus injure the surrounding tissues. This inorganic salt is indicated in conditions arising from impurities in the blood stream. It supplements the action of Kalium Muraticum in the treatment of catarrh, acne etc. and it should always be given when pimples occur in adolescence. It checks the weakening drain of suppuration too long continued for example, abscess and wounds which will not heal readily and tend to become septic. If taken in early stage, it prevents a sore throat from developing and in the same way it will often cut short a threatening cold. The symptoms are generally worse after getting wet and are better in a warm, dry atmosphere (Boericke, 1901).
- **Ferrum Phosphorica or Iron Phosphate (FerrumPhos):** It is classified as Biochemic first aid. It is the oxygen carrier. It enters into the composition of hemoglobin, the red coloring matter of the blood. It takes up oxygen from the air inhaled by the lungs and carries it in the blood stream to all parts of the body thus furnishing the vital force that sustains life. It gives strength and toughness to the circular walls of the blood vessels, especially the arteries. Freely circulating, oxygen rich blood is essential to health and life and for this reason Ferrum Phosphate is always considered

as a supplementary remedy, no matter what other treatment may be indicated by the symptoms. Congestion, inflammatory pain, high temperature, and quickened pulse all calls for more oxygen and it is iron phosphate that is the major component through which oxygen is taken up by the blood stream and carried into the affected area. This tissue salts can be given with advantage in the early stage of most acute disorders and it should be administered at frequent intervals until the inflammatory symptom subsides. It is also indicated where there is a lack of RBC as in anemia and as a first aid remedy for hemorrhages. Bleeding from wounds cuts and abrasions can be controlled with a little powdered Ferrum Phosphate applied directly to the injured parts. It should also be thought of as a first aid in cases of muscular strains and sprains, etc. (Boericke, 1901).

- **Kalium Muraticum or Potassium Chloride (Kali Mur):** It is the remedy for sluggish conditions. It combines with the organic substance fibrin. Thus, a deficiency of this tissue salt causes fibrin to become nonfunctional, and to be thrown off in the form of thick white discharges giving rise to catarrhs and similar symptoms affecting the skin and mucous membranes. Its action is complementary of Calcarea Sulphurica as both are concerned with cleansing and purifying the blood. In conditions calling for Kalium Muraticum, the blood the blood thickens and forms clot. It is the remedy for white, thick fibrinous discharges. Other prominent symptoms are white coated tongue and light-colored stools along with torpidity of liver. It is frequently needed in the treatment of inflammatory diseases, particularly those affecting respiration – coughs, cold, sore throat, tonsillitis, bronchitis etc. and also for measles, mumps, chicken pox etc. The inorganic salt is concerned with the production of saliva and is therefore important in the early stages of digestion. The symptom may be worse after eating fatty or rich foods and there may be lack of appetite. With Natrum Muraticum it is utilized in the production of hydrochloric acid and is thus an essential link in the process of digestion. This tissue salt is useful as a first aid for treatment of burns (Boericke, 1901).
- **Kalium Phosphorica or Potassium Phosphate (Kali Phos):** It is a nutrient for nerves. It is the remedy for ailments of a truly nervous character. School children often needs this tissue salt, it helps to maintain a happy, contented disposition and sharpens the mental faculties. There may be fretfulness, ill humor, bashfulness, laziness and similar indications. It is the remedy for nervous headaches, nervous dyspepsia, sleeplessness, depression, weariness, low vitality, and several other conditions. It covers all those ailments caused by nervous issues. It is also indicated in the treatment of irritating skin ailments, for restoring underlying nerve conditions. It is helpful for breathing in nervous asthma. The symptoms are usually worse from mental and physical exertion and from cold (Boericke, 1901).
- **Kalium Sulphurica or Potassium Sulphate (Kali Sulph):** It works with Ferrum Phosphate as oxygen carrier. It assists in exchange of oxygen from the blood stream to the tissue cells thereby completing the respiratory processes initiated by Ferrum Phosphate. Internal breathing of tissues depends upon Kalium Sulphurica, external breathing is the function of Ferrum Phosphate, if the exchange of gases in the lungs is designated in this manner. It is beneficial on respiration and is indicated in those cases where there is a feeling of stuffiness or desire for cool air. It is also considered as an anti-friction salt, ensuring the smooth working of all organs thus acting as a lubricant. This inorganic salt is indicated where there is a sticky yellowish discharge from skin and mucous membrane. Eruptions on the skin and scalp, with scaling, calls for this remedy. Chilliness, shifting or moving pain are some other striking indications. It is very useful in cases of stomach derangements and in inflammatory condition for promoting perspiration (Boericke, 1901).

- **Magnesia Phosphorica or Magnesium Phosphate (Mag Phos):** It is known as anti-spasmodic remedy. Its main function is in nervous system where it supplements the action of Kalium Phosphorica. When a deficiency of Magnesium Phosphate occurs the white nerve fibers contract causing spasms and cramps. This tissue salt is vital to muscular tissues. It quickly relieves pain especially of cramping, shooting, and spasmodic nature. It is indicated for nerve pains such as neuralgia, neuritis, sciatica headaches etc. this inorganic salt is indicated in cases of muscular twitching, cramps, hiccups, convulsive fits, menstrual pains etc. It acts on every kind of pain. The doses are to be taken in frequent intervals with warm water (Boericke, 1901).
- **Natrum Muraticum or Sodium Chloride (Natrum Mur):** It is the tissue salt that regulates water balance. It enters into the composition of every fluid and solid of the body. Because of its strong affinity for water it controls and regulates the electrolyte balance and flow of the body fluids. Its prime function is to maintain the moisture equilibrium in the body. In absence of this tissue salt cell division and normal growth could not proceed. It is closely associated with nutrition, glandular functioning and bodily secretions which play such an important part of the physiological processes. Excessive moisture or excessive dryness in any part of the system is a clear indication of the deficiency of the mineral salt. An important function of this cell salt is production of hydrochloric acid, so imbalance in the cell salt concentration will result in faulty secretion of the acid and thus causing illness (Boericke, 1901).
- **Natrum Phosphorica or Sodium Phosphate (Natrum Phos):** It is an acid neutralizer. It is the basic remedy for wide group of diseases arising from an acid condition of the blood. This tissue salt is also of importance for its action on digestive organs. The assimilation of fats and other nutrient is dependent on the action of this remedy. A deficiency of this mineral in blood allows uric acid to form salts which becomes deposited around the joints and tissues and giving rise to stiffness and swelling and other painful symptoms like that of rheumatism. This salt is indicated whenever symptoms of acidity are present, highly colored urine, golden yellow or creamy coating at the root of the tongue, intestinal worms etc. (Boericke, 1901).
- **Natrum Sulphurica or Sodium Sulphate (Natrum Sulph):** It regulates the density of the intercellular fluids by eliminating excess water. This tissue salt largely controls the healthy functioning of the liver, it ensures an adequate supply of free flowing, healthy bile essential for several stages of digestion. The removal of toxic metabolic products which are the normal result of the chemical exchange constantly taking place in the tissue cells, is brought about by the action of this particular inorganic salts. If conditions arise which allow these toxic fluids to accumulate in the blood stream and tissues, may lead to self-poisoning. This inorganic salt ensures the disposal of these toxic fluids and its importance in the healing of rheumatic complaints is self-evident. This salt is indicated in the healing of diseases affecting the liver, presence of sandy substance in urine, greenish brown coating on tongue and marked bitter taste of mouth are few of the guiding symptoms. It is the principal remedy in the treatment of influenza. It treats complaints aggravated by humidity (Boericke, 1901).
- **Silecea or Silica Oxide (Sil):** This salt is categorized as cleanser and eliminator. It is a deep acting remedy and is also known as Surgeon's Knife. It helps the body to eliminate nonfunctional organic matter from the body system. It initiates the healing process by promoting suppurations and breaking up pathological accumulations. This inorganic salt is a constituent of hair, skins, nails and surfaces of the bones. It also acts as in the manner of insulator for the nerves. In conditions of checked perspiration, this inorganic salt restores the activity of the skin, thereby aiding this

important cleansing process. It is the Biochemic remedy for offensive perspiration of the feet and armpits. Silecea is indicated in cases of pus formation or threatened suppuration. It is promising in the cases of tonsillitis associated with pus formation, brittle nails etc. This particular mineral salt should be used with caution. This salt should not be given to people having medical implants in their body. For example, people with implanted pacemaker or steel plates on bones etc. Since this salt is an eliminator it may try to eliminate the foreign object present in the body (Boericke, 1901).

All of the body's cells are made up of combinations of the 12 basic mineral cell salts and are activated in fusion by the mineral salt Iron Phosphate, also known as Ferrum Phos. In the presence of an Acidic PH level, stress, toxins, lack of proper oxygen supply and other conditions the fluids of the body and blood become depleted in Iron (Iron Phosphate, Ferrum Phos) and three forms of Potassium known as Kali Sulph (Sulphate of Potassium), Kali Phos (Potassium Phosphate) and Kali Mur (Chloride of Potassium). In cases of stomach cancer, Natrum Phosphate (sodium Phosphate) will also be lacking.

When this happens, the corpuscles of the body slowly suffocate and "putrefy". THIS IS THE TRUE CAUSE OF CANCER on a biochemical level. Without Iron, cellular combustion cannot go on in the body. A mix of the correct mineral cell salts and Iron are the legitimate cure for this complex disease. Normally these mineral cell salts and Iron are abundant in raw, uncooked fruits, vegetables, legumes, herbs and certain spices. Most modern diets are lacking in these things or the modern body is too Acidic in PH and lacking proper nutrients and oxygen to perform cellular combustion, hence putrefaction of the cells. Table salt (sodium) is not a healthy salt and should be avoided. These are mineral cell salts which make up the parts of the body's cellular tissues, table salt is not one of the recommended cancer fighting salts and the grains are too course to be assimilated into the cells unless specially prepared and crushed in micro homeopathic quantities. It cannot be overstated that it is essential when fighting cancer to supplement your diet with the following mineral cell salts to replenish the putrefied cells and get corpuscle combustion started. These mineral cell salts can be found in your local health store in tablets that can be chewed or easily dissolved in water or herbal tea and drank. They should all be taken together, three times daily with the prescribed amount of tablets listed on the bottles.

- The form of Potassium mixed with Ferrum is the biochemical cancer healing agent. **KaliumPhosphorica**(Potassium Phosphate)
- **KaliumMuraticum** (Chloride of Potassium)
- **KaliumSulphurica** (Sulphate of Potassium) The most crucial of the three Potassium mineral cell salts
- **FerrumPhosphorica** (Iron Phosphate) absolutely necessary for the corpuscles and cellular combustion needed with the preceding Potassium cell salts.
- **Natrum Phosphorica-** for cases of stomach cancer, along with the three Potassium mineral salts and the Iron Phosphate (Carey, 1894).

CONCLUSION

Everyone has doctor in him or her. We just have to help it in its work. The natural healing force within each one of us is the greatest force in getting well..." (Hippocrates, n.d.)

Even great Hippocrates, taught people that body heals itself, all we have to do is strengthen it, and the body's own healing mechanism will cure the fault. But in reality, what we actually do is follow what pharmaceutical industries want us to do and that is doing exactly opposite of what great Hippocrates taught us. In one hand we take oath to protect mankind on the other hand we are poisoning people, just because of money. It is the author's request to all those readers who are associated with cancer research, education and treatment, that if you are genuinely looking for evidences. If all the facts presented here in this chapter about the failures of conventional treatment methods are true or not then instead of looking into the conventional textbooks or medical journals, make time and talk to the family of the patients suffering from cancer. Those people who are undergoing chemo therapy, and also with the family members of those patients who died because of chemotherapy or radiation therapy and also going through the list of books and documentaries listed in the references section of this chapter. The reality will be in front of you. One cannot learn anything about how human system actually works just by spending all the time studying bits and pieces inside a laboratory as we are trained and taught to do. Great physician Hahnemann himself gave the definition of an ideal cure inspired by the vision of Hippocrates and the author quotes,

The ideal cure or ideal curative procedures are those that restores health rapidly, gently, permanently, possess ability to remove and destroy whole disease in shortest, surest, least harmful way, without causing any drug dependency and are clearly based on natural laws of healing (Hahnemann, Para 2, Organon).

So if one really wishes to find cure for cancer and also design the appropriate prevention strategies, the following points need to be considered;

- Cancer is not a disease, they are the symptoms of the disease.
- Cancer and immune system are interlinked. If one has a healthy immune system the person cannot have cancer. If the person has cancer then the person surely have weak immune system.
- They best way to fight cancer is to prevent it from happening.
- Cancer cells are epigenetically controlled, and with proper approach the damage can be reversed to some extent.
- Studying molecular interactions inside the cells are essential for academic and research purposes, but it has very little or no significance when it comes to curative treatments.
- Spending all the research grants, efforts and valuable time on studying a faulty protein that are already produced by a faulty gene does not going to solve the issue. It is essential to look inside outwards. It is crucial that one must search for the factors that forced the genes to mutate in the first place. If that causative agent is found and addressed, the faulty gene expression will be turned off and will start producing normal proteins.
- Fix the environment, cell knows how to fix itself, much better than we do. Because environment controls gene expression. Intelligence of each cell is much higher as compared to all the wisdom of human mind combined.
- Cancer cells needs anaerobic condition to survive. So supplying the body with fresh oxygen will kill cancer cells faster. Because oxygen means aerobic, and cancer cells cannot survive aerobic conditions.
- Pranayama, the scientific way of breathing and bathing each and every cell with natural oxygen on a regular basis is a great way of preventing cancer. It promotes aerobic respiration of the cells.

- Sugar suppresses the immune system. Any food or drugs that suppress the immune system should be avoided. Because only the immune system possesses the power to protect us from cancer.
- The relationship between sugar and cancer cells are sugar is the gasoline and cancer cells are fire. By avoiding sugar one is cutting out the power supply of cancer cells.
- Cancer cells thrive well in acidic environment. So maintaining the body pH to a basic level is a good preventive measure.
- Each and every person has cancer cells in their body. That does not mean those cells will cause cancer.
- Unnecessary diagnosis and cancer screening activates cancer and makes it more progressive.
- 98% of the time chemotherapy and radiation therapy does not work.
- The patient receiving chemo or radiation dies because of the chemo and radiation and not because of the cancer the patient was suffering from.
- Chemotherapy and radiation therapy effects and kills only the non-cancerous stem cells.
- Chemotherapy and radiation therapy does not kill cancerous stem cells but instead activates them by destroying the immune system.
- In short good cells get killed and a bad cell gets strengthened and above all the body's natural defense and healing capacity is damaged for lifetime. The lump of cancer that contained nonharmful, non-cancerous stem cells gets killed and the lump gets smaller and smaller in size as detected by the conventional diagnostic methods. The doctor gets the impression that chemo or radiation cured the cancer. But they do not acknowledge the very fact that it did not kill the harmful cancer stem cells and instead it converted them into more powerful and aggressive form.

So, it is high time that the research communities must acknowledge the fact that the war against cancer cannot be won using allopathic medicine system. Chemotherapy, Radiation therapy or surgery has already failed to do so, and repeating the same mistake again and again knowingly just because they bring profit at the end of the day is a crime against mankind. Money is essential, but not in expense of someone's life. Researchers, doctors, professors, medical personnel, all are in a profession together that calls for service to mankind. We are the ones who take the oath of doing no harm to our patients, these oaths are not just words, and it's a great responsibility. A responsibility that we are failing to perform each and every day. Every time a patient becomes a victim of health-care system and medical clap trap and dies of the faulty treatment procedures like chemotherapy, radiation or surgery, it is because we failed to perform our responsibility, we did not had courage to do what is right, because all the cancer research is funded directly or indirectly by the industries, and it is not acceptable to generate results that exposes the lies of the funding organization. Let us take a look at the original Hippocratic Oath (Ludwig, 1943), not the version tampered by drug companies that are taught in present days, with the hope of reminding ourselves of our responsibilities towards service of humanity.

I swear by Apollo Physician and Asclepius and Hygieia and Panaceia and all the gods and goddesses, making them my witnesses, that I will fulfill according to my ability and judgment this oath and this covenant:

To hold him who has taught me this art as equal to my parents and to live my life in partnership with him, and if he is in need of money to give him a share of mine, and to regard his offspring as equal to my brothers in male lineage and to teach them this art—if they desire to learn it—without fee and cov-

enant; to give a share of precepts and oral instruction and all the other learning to my sons and to the sons of him who has instructed me and to pupils who have signed the covenant and have taken an oath according to the medical law, but no one else.

I will apply dietetic measures for the benefit of the sick according to my ability and judgment; I will keep them from harm and injustice.

I will neither give a deadly drug to anybody who asked for it, nor will I make a suggestion to this effect. Similarly I will not give to a woman an abortive remedy. In purity and holiness I will guard my life and my art.

I will not use the knife, not even on sufferers from stone, but will withdraw in favor of such men as are engaged in this work.

Whatever houses I may visit, I will come for the benefit of the sick, remaining free of all intentional injustice, of all mischief and in particular of sexual relations with both female and male persons, be they free or slaves.

What I may see or hear in the course of the treatment or even outside of the treatment in regard to the life of men, which on no account one must spread abroad, I will keep to myself, holding such things shameful to be spoken about.

If I fulfill this oath and do not violate it, may it be granted to me to enjoy life and art, being honored with fame among all men for all time to come; if I transgress it and swear falsely, may the opposite of all this be my lot. (Ludwig, 1943)

Let us remember the oath and progress together forgetting all the differences towards creating an integrated system of treatment for better future. And it is only possible when all the medical fields unite as one. Be it conventional or alternative or complementary, the war against cancer can only be won if and only if the best of all these three systems are combined to form an Integrated System of Medicine that will be personalized, more scientific and free from adverse effects. Because it's not the bits and pieces, it is the whole that matters.

REFERENCES

Albert, S. G. (1960). *Introduction to a Submolecular Biology*. New York: AP.

Ausubel, K. (2000). *When Healing Becomes a Crime: The amazing Story of Hoxsey Cancer Clinics and the Return of Alternative Therapies*. Healing Arts Press.

Bailer, J. C., & Gornik, H. L. (1997). Cancer Undefeated. *The New England Journal of Medicine, 336*(22), 1569–1574. doi:10.1056/NEJM199705293362206 PMID:9164814

Barbara, A. (1988). Hands of Light: A Guide to Healing Through the Human Energy Field. Bantam publishers.

Bartlett, Z. (2014). The Hayflick Limit. In *The Embryo Project Encyclopaedia*. Arizona State University.

Boericke, W. (1901). *Pocket Manual of Homeopathic Materia Medica* (1st Ed.), San Francisco: Retrieved from www.materiamedica.info/en/materia-medica/william-boericke/index

Boericke, W. (1927). Pocket manual of homoeopathic materia medica: comprising the characteristic and guiding symptoms of all remedies (clinical and pathogenetic).

Braverman, A. (1991). Medical Oncology in the 90s. *Lancet*, *337*(8746), 901–902. doi:10.1016/0140-6736(91)90218-E PMID:1672980

Cancer Tutor. (2017). Death by doctoring, Fraught with risks and side effects. Retrieved from https://www.cancertutor.com/deathbydoctoring4/

Carey, G. W. (1894). *Biochemic System of Medicine*. The Theory, Pathological Action, Therapeutical Application, MateriaMedica, and Repertory of Schuessler's Twelve Tissue Remedies.

Cassel, C. K., Leipzig, R. M., Cohen, H. J., & Larson, E. B. (2003). Geriatric Medicine: An Evidence-Based Approach (4th ed.). Springer-Verlag.

Cassels, A., & Moyninan, R. (2005). *Selling Sickness: How Drug Companies Are Turning Us All into Patients*. Greystone Books.

Casson, A. G., Evans, S. C., Gillis, A., Porter, G. A., Veugelers, P., Darnton, S. J., ... Hainaut, P. (2003). Clinical implications of p53 tumor suppressor gene mutation and protein expression in esophageal adenocarcinomas: Results of a ten-year prospective study. *The Journal of Thoracic and Cardiovascular Surgery*, *125*(5), 1121–1131. doi:10.1067/mtc.2003.176 PMID:12771886

Coffey, D. S. (2006). Hyperthermic biology and Cancer therapies. *Journal of the American Medical Association*, 296. PMID:16868303

Corriher, C. T., & Corriher, S. G. (2013). *Defy Your Doctor and Be Healed*. Health Wyze Media.

Corriher, C. T., & Corriher, S. G. (2013). *Defy Your Doctor and Be Healed*. Health Wyze Media.

Cotran, R. S., & Robbins, S. L. (1997). Basic Pathology (6th ed.). W.B. Saunders Company.

Cure Naturali Cancro. (n.d.). 75% of the physicians refuses chemotherapy themselves. Retrieved from http://www.curenaturalicancro.com/en/75-percent-of-the-physicians-refuses-chemotherapy-themselves/

Darwin, C. (1888). *The life and letters of Charles Darwin*. New York: D. Appleton and Company.

Day, P. (2000). *Cancer: Why we're still Dying to Know the Truth*. Credence Publications.

Doctors Against Vivisection. (n.d.). Doctors Against animal Research Experiments. Retrieved from https://doctorsagainstvivisection.wordpress.com/

Eddy, D. M. (1989). Screening for lung cancer. *Annals of Internal Medicine*, 111. PMID:2665590

Glidden, P. (2010). *The MD Emperor has No Clothes*.

Goswami, S. (2017). Proteomics in Personalized Medicine: An Evolution Not a Revolution. In Applying big Data Analytics in Bioinformatics & Medicine. Hershey, PA: IGI Global.

Gyorgyi, A. S. (1960). Introduction to a Submolecular Biology (1st ed.). Academic Press.

Havasi, P. (2012). The Education of Cancer Healing (Vol. 2: Specialists).

Healing Cancer Naturally. (2004). Cancer causes statistics drugs. Retrieved from http://www.healingcancernaturally.com/cancer-causes-statistics-drugs.html

Healing Cancer Naturally. (n.d.). Quotes animal models of human disease. Retrieved from http://www.healingcancernaturally.com/quotes-animal-models-of-human-disease.html

Healing Cancer Naturally. (n.d.). Quotes on cancer diagnosing. Retrieved from http://www.healingcancernaturally.com/quotes-on-cancer-diagnosing.html

Hegde, B. M. (2014). What Doctors Don't Get to Study. In *Medical School* (4th ed.). Paras Medical Publisher.

Henderson, B. (n.d.). Cancer-Free. Retrieved from http://www.beating-cancer-gently.com/doctors-comments.html

Hering, C. (1836). Preface to the first American edition. In the Organon of Homeopathic Medicine. New-York: William Radde.

Hering, C. (1879). *The Guiding Symptoms of our MateriaMedica*. Philadelphia: The American Publishing Society.

Jones, H. (n.d.). Cancer cures more deadly than disease. Rethinking Cancer, Foundation for Advancement in Cancer Therapy. Retrieved from http://www.rethinkingcancer.org/resources/magazine-articles/2_1-2/cancer-cures-more-deadly-than-disease.php

Kent, J. T. (1929). *Lectures on Homeopathic Philosophy* (2nd ed.). Chicago: Ehrhardt & Karl.

Lipton, B. (2015). *The Biology of Belief*. Hay House Publishers Pvt. Ltd.

Lipton, B. H. (2017). *The Biology of belief: Unleashing the power of consciousness, Matter & Miracles*. New York: Hay House, Inc.

Ludwig, E. (1943). *The Hippocratic Oath: Test, Translation and Interpretation*. Baltimore: John Hopkins Press.

Lynes, B. (1990). *The Healing of Cancer: the Cures the cover ups and the solution now*. Marcus Books.

Markolin, C. (n.d.). Total Health Institute. Dr. Hammer's Medical Paradigm. Retrieved from http://www.totalhealthinstitute.com/german-new-medicine/

Massague, L., & Norton, L. (2006). Is cancer a disease of self seeding? *Nature Medicine*, *12*(8), 875–878. doi:10.1038/nm0806-875 PMID:16892025

Michael, J., McFarlane, A.R., & Feinstein, C. K., & Wells. (1987). "The epidemiologic necroscopy": Unexpcted detections, demographic selections and changing rate of lung cancer. *Journal of the American Medical Association*, 258.

Nancy, A. (1999). *"The Illustrated Encyclopedia of Body Mind Disciplines", the Rosen Publishing Group Inc. New York. New York Health Department. (1932). Practical Homeopathic Therapeutics.* New York: Oxford University Press.

Nijhout, H. F. (1990). Metaphors and the role of genes in development. *BioEssays*, *12*(9), 441–446. doi:10.1002/bies.950120908 PMID:1979486

Null, G. (2010). Death by Medicine (DVD ed.). Axios Press.

Pauling, L. (2008). The Pauling Blog. Clarifying Three Widespread Quotes. Retrieved from https://paulingblog.wordpress.com/2008/10/28/clarifying-three-widespread-quotes/

Raymond, A. (2011). *Never Fear Cancer Again: How to Prevent & Reverse Cancer* (p. 14). Health Communications Inc.

Ryan, R. (1997). Cancer Research-A super fraud? Retrieved from http://www.pnc.com.au/~cafmr/online/research/cancer.html

Schuessler, W. H. (2013). The *Biochemic Handbook*. CMG Archives. Retrieved from http://www.campbellmgold.com

Stahel, A. (n.d.). Healing Cancer Naturally. German New Medicine: A Revolutionary Biological Paradigm. Retrieved from http://www.healingcancernaturally.com/hamer-new-medicine-interpretation-part2.html

LiveT. T. A. C. (2017). Retrieved from https://www.cancertutor.com/ttac-live-2017-hope-cancer-free-future/

Volker, H. (2016). *Lies in the Medical Profession* (Vol. 2).

WeeksMD. (2011). Sober Reflection up on Chemotherapy……? The Economist! Retrieved from http://weeksmd.com/2011/12/sober-reflection-upon-chemotherapy-source-the-economist/

ADDITIONAL READING

Abramson, J. (2008). *Overdosed America: The Broken Promise of American Medicine (P.S).* Harper Perennial.

Angell, M. (2005). *The Truth about The Drug Companies: How they Deceive Us and What To Do About It*. Random House Publisher.

Bollinger. (2016). *The Truth About Cancer: What you need to know about cancer's History, Treatment and Prevention*. Hey House Inc.

Geriatric Medicine. (2017). *An Evidence-Based Approach* (4th ed.). Retrieved Oct 08 2017 from https://www.researchgate.net/publication/245662227_Geriatric_Medicine_An_Evidence-Based_Approach_4th_Ed

Guyton, A., & Hall, J. (2009). *Biochemistry. Human Metabolism in Health and Disease* (11th ed.). Wiley.

Hahnemann, S. (1982). *Organon of Medicine*. Germany: The Hahnemann Foundation.

Molony, E. (2014). Ageing and Cancer: A Complex Relationship.

Owen, D. (2007). *Principles and Practice of Homoeopathy. The therapeutic and Healing Process*. London: Elsevier.

Roberts, H. A. (1942). The Principles and Art of Cure by Homeopathy (2nd rev. ed.). Rustington: Health Science Press.

Ruesch, H. (1986). *Naked Empress or The Great Medical Fraud*. Civis Publications.

KEY TERMS AND DEFINITIONS

Acupressure: A form of alternative therapy in which manual pressure is used to stimulate specific points on the body along what are considered to be lines of energy.

Biochemic Medicine: A system of alternative medicine created by W. H. Schuessler, also known as Mineral Salt Therapy.

Complementary / Alternative Therapy: Umbrella term used to denote those treatment procedures that aims in treating patients, rather than treating diseases. They may or may not use drugs to cure the person. One form of personalized form of treatments.

Geriatrics: Branch of medicine dealing with the health and care of old people.

Homoeopathy: is a system of alternative medicine created in 1796 by Samuel Hahnemann, based on his doctrine of like cures like (similiasimilibuscurentur which means like cures like).

Oncology: Study and treatment of tumors.

Chapter 13
Aging and Cancer:
Intervention Strategies

Shailendra Prasad Verma
King George's Medical University, India

Pooja Mahour
King George's Medical University, India

ABSTRACT

This chapter describes aging and the resultant effects of aging. According to WHO report 8.8 million people died from cancer worldwide in 2015. The incidence of cancers increases with age. This increase incidence may be due to biological factors, prolonged exposure to carcinogens and incidence of mutations etc. Cancers in elderly may have poor biological vulnerability, presence of various co-morbidities and poor tolerance of therapy hence treatment got compromised. Elderly cancer patients also are neglected in various trials and strong data lacks for optimal management. Other important aspect is psychosocial state of these patients. Discipline of Psycho-oncology deals with patients with cancer, their lifestyle related difficulties, negligence by self, family members and society, Lack of emotional support, poor financial assistance and treatment monitoring etc. leading to various psychological problems. This chapter will address issues of cancers in elderly including disease biology, disease characteristics, management, their quality of life etc. with reference to elderly patients suffering from cancer.

INTRODUCTION

Aging and cancers are closely interrelated. Incidence of most cancers increases with age. Most of the cancer patients are in there 60's or 70's. As the average life span of a population increases with availability of better healthcare, more and more elderly population and more cancers are expected in this group. Recent SEER data estimates that 60% of all cancers and 69% of all cancer related deaths occur above 65 years of age in US (Ries et al., 1996). Both solid and haematological malignancies increase with aging. To understand it deeply we should be able to understand biology of aging and cancer at cellular and molecular level and see their interrelation.

DOI: 10.4018/978-1-5225-3480-8.ch013

AGING AT CELLULAR AND MOLECULAR LEVEL

Aging is a complex process many theories have evolved over a time period in quest of explanation to the aging process. None of the theories proposed till date could explain it in a holistic way. It is increasingly becoming apparent that the molecular and subcellular processes of aging are also relevant in cancer and tumorogenesis.

Genetics and Aging

Experiments have shown that there are defined genes in low evolutionary animals like yeast, nematodes and drosophila which affect the life span of these organisms (Orr et al., 1994; Sun et al., 1994). Probably certain critical genes also relate to aging and life span in humans. Genetic regulation of aging comes from analysis of clinical syndromes with accelerated aging like progeria. Accelerated aging is seen in early onset progeria, late onset progeria and Down syndrome (Yu et al., 1996). Identification of genes in these patients is at least a beginning towards understanding of molecular mechanisms involved in aging process. Werner syndrome is a disease of adolescent onset characterised by short stature and probability of development of cancers of mesenchymal origin. Yu et al. (1996) published a data on etiology of Werner syndrome caused by mutation in a single gene located on human chromosome 8 that encodes a helicase –like protein (Yu et al.,1997). Functional characterisations of these genes may be of great significance in understanding physiology of aging.

Telomere Biology and Aging

Cells have their genetic code in form of DNA which is a part of the chromosome. Telomeres are part of our chromosomes which cap their terminal ends and protect chromosomes from damage. With each cell division the telomere gets shortened. Ultimately it comes to a critical level where cell senescence occurs and cell dies. This process gives a defined life span to an individual. Telomerase is an enzyme which tries to protect the telomeres from shortening (Harley & Villeponteau, 1995). During this process cancers can arise due to chromosomal instability. If telomere shortening can be prevented life can be extended which is area of current research too. Many cells of our body like stem cells, sperm cells and T lymphocytes have high replicative power and express telomerase.

There is evidence that many key genes may be involved in maintenance of telomeres. TERC (Telomere RNA complex gene) and TERT (Telomere reverse transcriptase gene) mutations have been implicated in rapid shortening of telomeres in inherited and acquired aplastic anaemia, a process where bone marrow fails producing hematopoietic stem cells. Dyskeratosiscongenita (DKC) is an inherited bone marrow failure syndrome characterized by extremely short telomeres. It has X- linked, autosomal recessive and autosomal dominant patterns of inheritance. Mutation in a gene called DKC1 which codes dyskerin protein is responsible for X-linked type of DKC. Autosomal dominant type of DKC is associated with mutation in TERC gene. This syndrome presents with bone marrow failure (cytopenias), dystrophic nails and skin changes. Patients with DKC are at increased risk myelodysplastic syndrome, leukemia, primarily acute myeloid leukemia and squamous cell carcinomas. This is a classic example of a group of relatively recententity i.e. telomeropathy (Dokal, 2000).

Free Radical Damage and Aging

Aging is not a disease itself, but it is a change in physiology and physiological processes which makes aging persons exposed to cancer development. Major sites of generation of ROS are mitochondria, peroxisomes and the cytochrome P450 enzyme system. Mitochondria serve as a source as well as target of reactive oxygen species (ROS)(Harman,1956). Oxidative stress, free radical mediated damage and accumulation of oxygen free radicals is considered one of the prevailing factors in physiology of aging. Free radicles derived from oxygen and nitrogen act as an important chemical effector that links inflammation to carcinogenesis by inducing oxidative stress (Harman, 1971).

Oxygen free radicals can cause protein and DNA damage, abrogation of cell cycle checkpoints and lead to carcinogenesis. Reactive nitrogen products are known to activate signal transduction of cell survival pathways including MAPK signaling leading to activation of proto-oncogenes including c-fos, c-Jun and AP-1. Current data reinforces that free radicals play important roles in genetic alterations as well as damaging cellular structure and chemical components leading to cancer initiation, promotion and promotions.

Experiments in transgenic Drosophila, genetically engineered to express higher amount of free radical scavenging enzymes superoxide dismutase or catalase live on average one third longer than control fruit flies (Orr & Sohal.,1994). This proves the genetic influence on life span. This effect has been well studied in less evolutionary complex species like yeast and nematodes but same holds true in higher organisms is still to be proven.

Autophagy

Recently it has been recognised that autophagy plays an important role in the processes of aging. Originally described in yeast, macroautophagy is the process where cells accumulate macromolecules, organelles and oxidatively damaged proteins with passage of time. These proteins and organelles are sequestered in a double membrane organelle known as autophagosome. These results in declining cellular function and altered pathways. Autophagy is the process by which these cells are removed. Loss of autophagy may be considered as a major reason for accumulation of such damaged cellular machinery in aging cells. Experiments in *C. elegans* and Drosophila have shown that loss of function in autophagy genes leads to accumulation of these damaged proteins and accelerated aging. Conversely increased autophagy leads to increased life span. Mitochondrial function and ATP production also declines in aging cells. Various molecular pathways are involved in regulation of autophagy and have been reviewed in detail (Ohsumi, 2001; Liang et al.1999).

DNA Repair Defect

DNA repair is an integral part of cell survival. Various DNA damaging agents exist including radiation, environmental factors and drugs. Cell has many sensors to respond to DNA damage and repair it. Defect in factors responsible for sensing and responding to DNA damage can lead to DNA instability, tumorogenesis and cell death. Multiple mechanisms exist in body for underlying DNA repair and genomic instability. Somatic mutations get accumulated in the mother cell with repeated divisions and can lead to genetic instability (Gilchrest & Bohr, 1997).

Cell Cycle and Check Points

Every cell has to go through defined phases of growth to finally divide and give rise to daughter cells. These phases are G0, G1, S, G2 and M. There are various checkpoints at these stages which control the rate of cell cycle. If cell cycle is uncontrolled it will give rise to uncontrolled growth of cells and malignant potential (Sherr & Roberts, 1995). For example, Retinoblastoma gene (RB) is a tumor suppressor gene and prevents cancer genesis but if it gets mutated it can give rise to malignancy. RB gene encodes a protein (pRb) that actively inhibits the E2F growth stimulating transcription factor. pRb gets phosphorylated by a cyclin dependent kinase (Cdk) when appropriate growth stimulatory signal is present. Phosphorylation inhibits function of pRb and E2F is able to bind with DNA and cell cycle progresses (Hara et al., 1996).

Stem Cells, Cellular Senescence, Aging and Cancer

Many checks and balances are important in the maintenance of homeostasis in multicellular organisms. Sustained damage can trigger cell death so that damaged cell can be removed. If damaged cell is not removed it may be in part responsible for development of cancer. Stem cells are capable of replacing the lost cells by maintaining homeostasis. Stem cells play a very important role in tissue maintenance, homeostasis and development of the organism. The role of stem cells in the process of aging is area of ongoing research. Emerging evidence suggest that diverse tissue specific stem cell reserve decline with advancing age. This gives rise to pathophysiological changes compatible with aging (Rossi et al., 2008). A meta-analysis of National Marrow Donor Program (NMDP) registry clearly shows that advanced donor age was associated with reduced overall survival (Kollman et al., 2001). Some of these stem cells transform to cancer stem cell or leukaemia stem cells (Clarke & Fuller, 2006). These cells become excellent target for cancer therapy if normal stem cells can be spared. Experiments have shown that replicative potential of cells from old animals is less than that of young animals. Derangement of pathways leading to replicative senescence can lead to uncontrolled proliferation of cells and cancer. Senescent cells usually get arrested in G1 phase and mutations involving this phase are very common in human cancers.

Angiogenesis

Angiogenesis is an integral part of tumor expansion and metastasis. Tumors secrete many angiogenic factors like fibroblast growth factor (FGF) and vascular endothelial growth factor (VEGF). These factors promote neoangiogenesis and tumor progression (Folkman & Shing, 1992). There is age dependent less angiogenesis in elderly patients with tumours. This explains reduced rate of tumor growth and spread in aged population.

Aging and Inflammation

Aging process can be visualised as time driven worn out process of efficient working machinery. Aging leads to marked abnormalities in multiple cellular and molecular events that translate to various chronic ailments and diseases. This ultimately leads to impairment of quality of life (morbidity) and demise of living beings (mortality). Inflammation is a defence mechanism against invasive organisms or non- biological xenobiotic agents or response to trauma. Inflammation is characterized by redness, pain, swelling and temperature. This subsides when the act of wound healing, tissue repair or defence is completed. Many inflammatory cells like neutrophils, macrophages, monocytes and dendritic cells invade the site of infection or wound and establish an inflammatory microenvironment. This leads to death and degeneration of the organism. Chronic inflammation is mediated by few important key molecular players like prostaglandins, cytokines, nuclear factor-B (NF-kB), angiogenic factors and chemokine (Li et al., 2005).

Chronic inflammatory state or inflammatory etiology can result in cancer genesis in approximately 20% of all cancer cases (Lu et al., 2006). H.pylori infection is a classic example of genesis of cancer by chronic inflammation. This is known to cause gastric mucosa associated lymphoid tissue (MALT) lymphomas and even gastric carcinoma (Peek & Crabtree, 2006). Crohn's disease and ulcerative colitis are inflammatory bowel diseases of colon which have potential to give rise to colon cancer (Vagefi & Longo, 2005). Failure of complex regulation of inflammatory process to resolve cellular damage could lead to sustained antigenic stimulation in aging patient leading to chronic diseases like cancer.

Although, initiation events like acquired or inherited mutations initiate carcinogenesis by altering cell cycle, programmed cell death and differentiation, secondary event like inflammation is also important in promotion to full malignant potential. In tumour niche inflammatory cells produce various substances that contribute to tumour growth and survival. TNF-α, colony stimulating factor-1 (CSF-1), PGE-2, COX-2 are some of these substances. Moreover, macrophages within the tumour may also release reactive oxygen species which can provide carcinogenic potential. NF-kB is a transcription factor which is critical for the regulation of innate immune response, inflammation, cell proliferation and apoptosis. NF-kBexists in a latent state in cytoplasm bound to specific inhibitory proteins, IkBs. Activated NF-kB migrates into the nucleus to regulate the transcription of multiple target genes. TNFα is a strong regulator of NF-kB activation. Inhibition of apoptosis and several angiogenic factors are regulated by NF-kB (Karin & Greten, 2005).

AGING AND CANCER

Clinical Aspects

Aging is a normal physiological phenomenon. Organ functions like renal function and bone marrow reserve and immunity declines normally with age (Miller, 1991, 1996). This does not indicate any disease but they can predispose older individuals to diseases like reactivation of tuberculosis, herpes zoster or poor antibody formation to vaccination (Dubrow,1976). Physiological alterations or decline in reserve with time does not lead to carcinogenesis. It is accumulation of carcinogens over time which gives rise to malignancies. Concept of multiple hits is also very important. A cell needs multiple hits to turn into malignant cell. Initial mutations make the cell unstable but driver mutation acquired later provides it a malignant potential.

Tumour Aggressiveness

Tumor aggressiveness is a debatable issue in elderly patients. Common concept is that aged people have less aggressive tumours, but the outcome is poor in elderly (Kaesberg & Ershler, 1989; Ershler et al., 1984). This is contradictory to the common belief. Many underlying reasons may be there like underlying comorbidities, availability of services, selection of treatment options and psychological and family support. Immunogenic tumours are highly aggressive because of lower immunity and immune mediated anticancer effect.

Performance Status

Performance status decreases with age, co-morbidities and disease progression. This is a measure of physical functionality. Elderly have a poor performance status and this becomes important issue in all cancer chemotherapies. Patients with very poor performance status cannot receive very toxic chemotherapy. This reduces their chances of cure and long-term survival. Eastern Co-operative Oncology Group (ECOG) performance scale or WHO performance status scale is most commonly used scales in cancer patients.

Tumor Resistance and Adverse Cytogenetics

Some hematological malignancies are common in elderly. Acute myeloid leukemia (AML), myelodysplastic syndromes (MDS), myeloproliferative neoplasms (MPN) and Chroniclymphocytic leukemia (CLL) are few to name. Resistance to chemotherapy is high in elderly because of underlying nature of disease. Aging population has complex karyotype, high risk karyotype and multiple mutations leading to poor outcome (Taylor et al., 1995). A classic example is Philadelphia chromosome positivity in cases of acute lymphoblastic leukemia. In children its positivity is 5% but reaches above 25% in adults and elderly (Burnett & Eden, 1997). This cytogenetic abnormality is considered as ultrahigh risk disease. Multi drug resistance (MDR-1) expression is common in elderly with leukemias (Leith et al., 1997). It is an independent negative prognostic factor in management of leukemia in elderly.

Immune Senescence in the Development of Cancer

Aging is associated with functional compromise of various organs and systems including immune system. Immune surveillance is one of the major protective barriers in development of cancer. Our body is exposed to numerous aggregations and challenges like infection, inflammation, free radicals and various carcinogens present in environment, food and water. This continuous exposure leads to progressive waning of our immune defences. Innate immune system includes dendritic cells, macrophages and natural killer cells. These cells have the capability to eliminate cancer cells by themselves, but innate immunity goes down with aging predisposing elderly persons to cancer development (Fulop et al., 2011).

With aging there is impairment of macrophage function, cytokine dysregulation and reduced NK cell cytotoxicity. Although, the number of macrophages are preserved but their function is grossly impaired (Shaw et al., 2013). Decreased immune functions are common with aging. T cell function is compromised in elderly while B cell function (antibody formation and secretion) is largely preserved. Increased PGE2 production by macrophages is one of the factors for impaired T cell function.

T cell mediated immunity belongs to adaptive immunity. This is second line of immune defence against development of cancers. Chronic antigenic stress and thymic involution is one of the important phenomenon. This leads to decrease in naive CD4+ CD45RA+ and CD28+ T cells and increase in memory CD45RO+CD95+, CD152+ cell population (Larbi & Fulop,2014). Infection with persistent viruses like CMV, HSV, EBV and VZV can lead to chronic antigenic stimulation. CD4/CD8 ratio is altered due to increased CD8 positive T cells. Impaired T cell function gives rise to various viral activations and reactivation of tuberculosis. Some key cytokines are also altered. IL-2 is decreased while IL-6 levels increase with aging. Increased IL-6 is implicated in many diseases associated with aging while low IL-2 indicated decreased T cell function. During chemotherapy also this cellular immunity is further compromised. As we know the bone marrow reserve is also compromised, chemotherapy induced marrow suppression is prolonged and severe leading to fatal infections and even death. B lymphocyte function is also altered in the elderly with a reduced production of specific antibodies. Most of the produced antibodies are low affinity.

Aging and Malignant Haematological Disorders

Haematological malignancies are a heterogenous group of tumors arising from lymphatic system and bone marrow. They are divided into three main groups: Leukemias, lymphomas and plasma cell disorders. Almost 45% of all haematological malignancies occur in people aged 70 or more (Ferlay et al., 2010). As most cancers also some tumours of this group of malignancies is closely linked to age and incidence increases with age.

Leukemias are further subdivided into acute and chronic leukemias. Acute leukemias mainly comprise of acute myeloid leukemia (AML), acute lymphoblastic leukemias (ALL) and chronic leukemias comprise of chronic myeloid leukemia (CML) and chronic lymphocytic leukemia (CLL). Incidence of AML increases with age with a median age of 64 years. Similarly, CML and CLL are also diseases of elderly and seldom seen in children and adolescents. Median age for CLL is 70 years. Lymphomas can be broadly divided into aggressive and low-grade lymphomas. Most of the low-grade lymphomas like follicular lymphomas, marginal zone lymphomas, lymphoplasmacytic lymphomas have median age >50 years at presentation. Even in aggressive lymphomas mantle cell lymphomas and many cases of diffuse large B cell lymphomas present in elderly age group. Multiple Myeloma is malignancy of plasma cells and most consistently associated with older age group with median age of diagnosis between 65-70 years.

Other important malignant haematological disorders of elderly comprise of myelodysplastic syndromes (MDS) and myeloproliferative neoplasms (MPN). MDS is a group of disorders having ineffective erythropoiesis, dysplasia in different cell lines and increase in immature cells in marrow or peripheral blood with tendency to convert in overt leukemia over time. MDS is rare in children and its incidence increase with age and markedly above 70 years of age. MPNs are a group of disorders where there is marked proliferation of myeloid cells. This includes 4 classical MPNs namely polycythemiavera (PV), essential thrombocytosis (ET), primary myelofibrosis (PMF) and chronic myeloid leukemia (CML). All MPNs are disorders of elderly and rarely seen below 50 years of age.

Aetiology of Haematological Malignancies

Development of haematological tumours is favoured by aging process but strictly etiology is largely unknown. Epidemiological studies have revealed several risk factors and some associations have been found and assessed. Environmental risk factors and genetic susceptibilities combined lead to development of haematological cancers. Lack of equilibrium between renewal and death of blood cells is the most general mechanism proposed. Hematopoietic cells begin to age and lose their physiological functions with aging. This also leads to loss of check for homeostasis and to repair DNA damages. Immunosuppressant, autoimmunity and chronic inflammation also plays important role in development of lymphoproliferative disorders. Many viruses have been implicated in pathogenesis of lymphomas. Human immunodeficiency virus [HIV] (Seaberg et al., 2010), Hepatitis C Virus (Marcucci, 2011), Epstein Barr Virus [EBV] (Kuppers, 2003) and HTLV-1 are some of them (Franchini et al., 2003). Chemical compounds like benzene, formaldehyde, organic solvents, and agricultural pesticides have been associated with increased risk. Ionising radiation, socioeconomic status, obesity and overweight have been associated with increased risk of haematological cancers.

Treatment and Outcome

Effect of age and age-related tumour biology, underlying molecular and cytogenetic risk, and performance status decide outcomes in elderly patients. Acute myeloid leukemia is a prototypic example of haematological malignancy in elderly. Optimal treatment strategy is still debatable between supportive care and standard aggressive therapies. The main reason behind this confusion is low survival rates and substantial risk of treatment toxicity. Therefore only 40% of older adults receive chemotherapy after AML diagnosis in United States. This proportion is even more in developing countries. Complete remission (CR) rates are also lower in elderly population. CR rates of 64%, 46%, 39%, and 33% were found in age group <56, 56-65, 66-75 and >75 years respectively. Among patients who achieved remissions median disease-free survivals were 21.6, 7.4, 8.3 and 8.9 months respectively (Appelbaum et al., 2006). Treatment related deaths (deaths within 30 days of initiation of chemotherapy) are high (15-30%) in elderly and increases progressively with age. Other haematological malignancies like lymphomas, chronic leukaemia's and myeloma have better survivals in era of current chemotherapy still the outcomes worsen with advancement of age compared to young individuals.

Clinical Trials: Involved Issues

Today we have treatment data for all cancers based on randomized clinical trials (RCT). These trials are considered best for making recommendation of treatment in a specific situation. But RCTs have their limitations and most important limitation is that trials put elderly age as exclusion criteria and drop these patients. We lack RCTs and strong recommendations regarding management of most cancers in elderly.

Precisely older people need special attention regarding the disease and treatment options, evaluation of organ functions and goals of treatment. Aggressiveness of therapy depends on performance status, comorbidities personal and family preferences. In this regard a caution should be made that the disease physiology, treatment options, and outcomes including possibility of cure should be well explained to the patient and family members and they should be provided adequate time to decide.

PSYCHOLOGICAL ASPECTS

Issues Related to Quality of Life of Cancer Patient's

Cancer is the second leading cause of death globally and accounts for 8.8 million deaths in 2015. The most common type of cancers among men are Lung, prostate, colorectal, stomach and liver cancer, and among women, breast, colorectal, lung, cervix and stomach cancer are the most common as reported by WHO (2016). Cancer is a life-threatening disease, and being diagnosed with cancer is an extremely stressful experience (White & Macleod, 2002). The morbidity as well as mortality of cancer depends upon the severity of cancer which is measured by the 'Cancer stages'. In advanced stage of cancer many difficulties could be faced by the patients such as inability to stand treatment due to poor physical status, high co-morbidities, limitation of the treatment options etc. (Henoch et al., 2007).

Health related quality of life (QOL) is one of the biopsychosocial concepts which include health related physical, psychological and social care of the individual under pathology as well as in normal course of life. Especially with an illness like cancer where a patient needs more and more physical and mental strength, QOL, sense of wellbeing, support system, long term care etc. might work as boosters to fight with the illness. Some studies suggested that QOL may improve patient–physician communication, and that emotional functioning in particular may be discussed more frequently during consultation (Dirven et al., 2013; Taphoorn et al., 2015).

National Comprehensive Cancer Network (NCCN, 2014) has given list of significant difficulties at various levels to the diseased and his/ her caregivers.

- **Physical Problems:** Common physical problems occur in the form of appearance, bathing/dressing, changes of urination, constipation, diarrhea, eating, fatigue, swelling, fevers, getting around, indigestion, impairment in memory and concentration, mouth sores, nausea, dry/congestion in nose, pain, skin dry/itchy, sleep disturbance, substance abuse, tingling in hands/feet.
- **Emotional Problems:** Emotional difficulties can be seen more in the form of mental health problems like depression, anxiety, fears, nervousness, sadness, spiritual/religious, worry, loss of interest in usual activities.
- **Family Problems:** Family of patient with cancer also got certain difficulties like dealing with children, dealing with partner, ability to have children, family health issues etc.
- **Practical Problems:** like how to do a child care along with cancer patient or self as a cancer patient, insurance/financial, transportation, work/school and treatment decisions.

Since cancer causes multiple kinds of impairment in the individual, it is imperative to be mentally healthy to handle these many difficulties. Studies have suggested mental disturbances as co-morbidity in cancer. A meta-analysis on co- morbidity with cancer patients has suggested that approximately one-third of persons with cancer in acute care hospitals are affected by common mental disorders (Singer et al., 2010, Arden et al., 2008). Psychiatric co-morbidity was present in 47% of the studied patients. There was predominance of major depressive disorder and the adjustment disorder, both of which constituted approximately 80% of the total diagnoses (Hans & Dar, 2015). The most common diagnosis is depression among cancer patients (Mitchell et al., 2011; Honda & Goodwin, 2004).

Psychological assessment is important in such an illness, as brain and behaviour work in a unit and influences each other. Psychological assessment helps to form that connection of brain and behaviour and eventually helps in identification of specific problems and to develop a treatment plan. Any kind of mental health problem may aggravate the primary illness, hence its early identification and prevention becomes significant for treatment plan. Cancer being a terminal illness, patients of which may have several health-related issues; so, it is important to know their quality of life (QoL). QoL is a subjective, multidimensional construct surrounding several aspects of physical and psychosocial well-being there are several measures which can assess quality of life of cancer patients.

In table 1, there are different measures of QOL. Some of them are specific to the cancer related quality of life and some of them measures general quality of life. After knowing the areas and level of difficulties at psychological as well as functional level, treating team can make a realistic treatment plan. If the

Table 1. Various quality of life measurement tools

Tools	
HRQOL	Health Related Quality Of Life
QLQ-15 PAL	Quality of Life of Palliative Cancer
VAS-C	Visual Analog Scale - Cancer
POMS	Profile of Mood States- Cancer specific
EORTC QLQ-C30	European Organisation for Research and Treatment of Cancer QoL Questionnaire -C30.
FACT-G	Functional Assessment of Cancer Therapy – General
QLIC-ON Profile	QoL in Childhood Oncology-Profile
PediQUEST	Pediatric QoL and Evaluation of Symptom Technology
ESRA-C	Electronic Self-report Assessment-Cancer
PROMIS	Patient-Reported Outcomes Measurement Information System
RSCL	Rotterdam Symptom Checklist for cancer patients
SF- 36	Short Form- 36 for Health Survey
Prostate QOL	International Prostate Symptom Score (I-PSS), with QOL due to urinary symptoms.

Source: (Chaturvedi, 1991; Ware & Sherbourne, 1992; Sprangerset al.,1993)

diseased person would be well worse with his/her illness conditions and treatment pattern and needs, then this can make the process of healing comparatively easy.

Psychological Intervention of Patients and Their Family

To reduce the impairment, agony and mortality due to cancer globally, an effective and meaningful intervention and palliative care is required. The treatment may include surgery, medicines and/or radiotherapy etc. The intervention should include not only the patient but their families too. Palliative care, which focuses on improving the quality of life of patients and their families, is an essential component of cancer care, which includes a multidimensional approach such as symptom relief, pain management, physical and mental stress management, all in all improving quality of life of the patient and their care givers. Palliative care interventions are helpful for improving perceptions of care of patient and their caregiver (Dy et al., 2013). A powerful action plan is needed to improve cancer care; global targets to reduce cancer deaths and to provide health care for all consistent with universal health coverage (WHO, 2016). A mentally strong person can handle the situations more efficiently comparative to a weaker one, thus some psychotherapeutic interventions are also required to cater their psychological difficulties, following are the intervention techniques which have been discussed by Spiegel (2002, p. 360).

Social Support

The basic concept of enhancing social support refers to be in contact of survivors, self-help groups or organizations which are aiming to intervene for this particular disorder. Social support may help the individual for hope for survival, self-confidence, motivation enhancement, awareness of many treatment modalities. Regarding supportive group intervention for patients with metastatic cancer psychological benefit in the form of lower mood disturbance, fewer maladaptive coping and fewer phobic reactions were reported by Spiegel et al. (1981).

Emotional Expression

This mode of intervention aims to enhance the emotional ventilation in patients. The metaphor of cancer is assumed as death, thus patients affected by it may present with grief reaction, depression, hopelessness, fear and anxiety soon after knowing this news for the first time. Lack of expression and emotional ventilation might maintain or aggravate the problem or cause hindrance in treatment process. Hence with the help of treating doctor or intervention team these issues should be handled first. Patients advised to be in self-help groups where many others has similar distress which might normalizes their own extreme emotional reactions, and making them less strange and overwhelming. They get examples, learning how to change their perception from emotion to practical difficulties, improve their coping for managing symptoms.

Reorganizing Life Priorities and Living in the Present

"A realistic evaluation of the future can help those with life-threatening illness make the best use of remaining time" (Spiegel, 2002, p. 360). When the cost is time, then it can be best to plan his/her time more judiciously, prioritizing the time and task, focus of thinking can be future oriented rather past, life goals can be reframed with realistic approach, clear communication with the supportive environment can facilitate the treatment process, family support can become a real asset in healing process.

Detoxifying Dying: Processing Existential Concerns

Knowledge about the fact that self-strength is deteriorating day by day rather faster than any other healthy individual; is very distressing and anxiety provoking. By far all this emotional trauma causes a vicious cycle of negative perception, lack of fighting spirit, induction of death anxiety, fear of losing loved ones, feelings of helplessness/ loneliness and things like that. Negative emotions do weaken the resilience of the individual and contaminate the overall health. Few coping strategies can be helpful for the individual with cancer such as positive reappraisal, distraction, self-positive reinforcement, problem solving, reframing the life goal, involvement in to self-help groups, coping strategies can be more cognitive and action focus rather emotion focus.

Enhancing Family Support

This is the time when one needs support at max; not only perceived but also tangible support also, which means a person with cancer may require help from various resources like financial, medical, legal, social, emotional etc. Family is one of the vital health care support which can facilitate with all other kind of support, like in adapting the new requirement of treatment, in sharing the work responsibility, help in developing realistic goal, can provide more mobility for treatment needs, they also can provide clarity in communication and expressing the problems of the patients regarding which the patient is guarded/ restrained with the treating team, emotional support as well. Hence from the diagnosis to all treatment process, family remains a crucial part of treatment. It does not imply that those who don't have much family support, they would not get treatment, but yes one who has good family support comparatively, they may handle the illness related difficulties more effectively than the patients without such support.

Improving Communication With Physicians

Correct and timely communication is a key factor for the treatment and adherence. The nature of illness requires constant efforts from all the people involved directly or indirectly. The primary unit is the patient itself, thus it is crucial that the patient would be able to communicate his/her apprehension, fear, problems in adherence of the treatment etc. without any hesitation to the physician. Support group can be helpful in channelizing the interaction, providing information as rightly stated by Spiegel (2002, p. 361) "Groups provide mutual encouragement to get questions answered, to participate actively in treatment decisions, and to consider alternatives carefully".

Symptom Control

During the course of illness patients may develop many co-morbidities such as mental and physical health related problems, like anxiety, depression, panic, pain, nausea, bathing/dressing, bowel and bladder disturbances, etc. due to their lack of awareness, acceptance or grief reaction one finds it difficult in dealing with this fatal illness. Psychotherapeutic intervention might be a helpful tool in dealing with such difficulties. Relaxation techniques, physical exercise, Individual psychotherapy, group and supportive psychotherapy, family counselling, emotional ventilation, behavioural intervention, problem solving approaches can make the individual and their family members more functional.

CONCLUSION

Aging is a complex biological process. Aging and cancer are intimately related. Incidence of cancers steeply increases as age increases. DNA damage, abnormal DNA repair mechanisms, deregulated telomere biology, oxidative stress and reactive oxygen species cause protein and DNA damage and strongly implicated in aging and cancer biology. Role of stem cells is important in renewal of damaged cells, tissue maintenance and homeostasis. When a molecular defect or damage occurs to these stem cells they can be converted to cancer stem cells leading to development of cancers. Although inflammation is a protective mechanism it can be deleterious if persists for long. Organ functions, Immunity and performance status progressively declines with aging and instituting intensive chemotherapy becomes impossible. Complex abnormal karyotype and multidrug resistance mechanisms further complicates the issues. Elderly population is often excluded from these trials due to multiple co-morbidity and poor performance status. Haematological malignancies and myelodysplasias are quite common in elderly population and their incidence increases with age.

Older people need special attention regarding disease and treatment option, tailoring treatment according to comorbidities and performance status. Family members have great responsibilities of physical, mental and monitory support to this elderly population. Considering the severe nature of the illness a multimodality treatment is requiring with skilled professionals. Not only the patient but their family members also needs to be take into treating team to make the process realistically functional, although with advancement of treatment, treatment rule and regulation facilities physical, biological, economical, professional, legal needs had been taken care of. As many researches has suggested that improvement of mental health co-morbidities, improvement in quality of life of the patient, active participation in treatment process, social support, motivation and hope for the life gives rise to the improvement in cancer patients.

FUTURE RESEARCH DIRECTIONS

Current research in tumor biology has led to more and more precise and targeted chemotherapy. Use of tyrosine kinase inhibitor imatinib in chronic myeloid leukemia is the best example of targeted therapy. This avoids unnecessary toxicity of chemotherapy and at the same time maintaining comparative or ever better responses. Reduced intensity conditioning has led to stem cell transplant in fair number of elderly patients who need it. Newer biologicals (antibodies and antibody conjugates) are coming up and many of them are already very well established in haematological as well as solid cancers. Anti CD20 (Rituximab) is a very good example of it being used in almost all CD20 positive lymphomas and chronic lymphocytic leukaemia. Future seems to be very promising in elderly with cancers and we can expect good survival in these patients with multimodality and comprehensive management in current research context.

REFERENCES

Appelbaum, F. R., Gundacker, H., Head, D. R., Slovak, M. L., Willman, C. L., & Godwin, J. E. (2006). Age and acute myeloid leukemia. *Blood*, *107*(9), 3481–3485. doi:10.1182/blood-2005-09-3724 PMID:16455952

Arden Close, E., Gidron, Y., & Moss Morris, R. (2008). Psychological distress and its correlates in ovarian cancer: A systematic review. *Psycho-Oncology*, *17*(11), 1061–1072. doi:10.1002/pon.1363 PMID:18561287

Burnett, A. K., & Eden, O. B. (1997). The treatment of leukemia. *Lancet*, *349*(9047), 270–275. doi:10.1016/S0140-6736(96)08086-5 PMID:9014927

Chaturvedi, S. K. (1991). What's important for quality of life to Indians—in relation to cancer. *Social Science & Medicine*, *33*(1), 91–94. doi:10.1016/0277-9536(91)90460-T PMID:1882246

Clarke, M. F., & Fuller, M. (2006). Stem cells and cancer: Two faces of eve. *Cell*, *124*(6), 1111–1115. doi:10.1016/j.cell.2006.03.011 PMID:16564000

Dirven, L., Reijneveld, J. C., Aaronson, N. K., Bottomley, A., Uitdehaag, B. M., & Taphoorn, M. J. (2013). Health-related quality of life in patients with brain tumors: Limitations and additional outcome measures. *Current Neurology and Neuroscience Reports*, *13*(7), 359. doi:10.1007/s11910-013-0359-y PMID:23666388

Dokal, I. (2000). Dyskeratosis congenital in all its forms. *British Journal of Haematology*, *110*(4), 768–779. doi:10.1046/j.1365-2141.2000.02109.x PMID:11054058

Dubrow, E. L. (1976). Reactivation of tuberculosis: A problem of aging. *Journal of the American Geriatrics Society*, *24*(11), 481–487. doi:10.1111/j.1532-5415.1976.tb03269.x PMID:972234

Dy, S. M., Apostol, C., Martinez, K. A., & Aslakson, R. A. (2013). Continuity, coordination, and transitions of care for patients with serious and advanced illness: A systematic review of interventions. *Journal of Palliative Medicine*, *16*(4), 436–445. doi:10.1089/jpm.2012.0317 PMID:23488450

Ershler, W. B., Stewart, J. A., Hacker, M. P., Moore, A. L., & Tindle, B. A. (1984). B16 melanoma and aging: Slower growth and longer survival in old mice. *Journal of the National Cancer Institute*, *72*(1), 161–164. doi:10.1093/jnci/72.1.161 PMID:6582296

Ferlay, J., Shin, H. R., & Bray, F. (2010). GLOBOCAN 2008 v2.0, Cancer incidence and mortality worldwide. Lyon: *International agency for Research on Cancer*. Retrieved from http://globocan.iarc.fr

Folkman, J., & Shing, Y. (1992). Angiogenesis. *The Journal of Biological Chemistry*, *267*, 10931–10934. PMID:1375931

Franchini, G., Fukumoto, R., & Fullen, J. R. (2003). T-Cell control by human T cell leukemia/lymphoma virus type 1. *International Journal of Hematology*, *78*(4), 280–296. doi:10.1007/BF02983552 PMID:14686485

Fulop, T., Larbi, A., Kotb, R., de Angelis, F., & Pawelec, G. (2011). Aging, immunity, and cancer. *Discovery Medicine*, *11*(61), 537–550. PMID:21712020

Gilchrest, B. A., & Bohr, V. A. (1997). Aging processes, DNA damage, and repair. *The FASEB Journal*, *11*, 322–330. PMID:9141498

Hans, G., & Dar, M. M. (2015). Psychiatric co-morbidity in patients suffering from cancer and its relationship to disease awareness. *Delhi Journal of Psychiatry*, *18*(1), 40–47.

Hara, E., Smith, R., Parry, D., Tahara, H., Stone, S., & Peters, G. (1996). Regulation of p16CDKN2 expression and its implications for cell immortalization and senescence. *Molecule Cell Biology*, *16*(3), 859–867. doi:10.1128/MCB.16.3.859 PMID:8622687

Harley, C. B., & Villeponteau, B. (1995). Telomeres and telomerase in aging and cancer. *Current Opinion in Genetics & Development*, *5*(2), 249–255. doi:10.1016/0959-437X(95)80016-6 PMID:7613096

Harman, D. (1956). Aging: A theory based on free radical and radiation chemistry. *Journal of Gerontology*, *11*(3), 298–300. doi:10.1093/geronj/11.3.298 PMID:13332224

Harman, D. (1981). The aging process. *Proceedings of the National Academy of Sciences of the United States of America*, *78*(11), 7124–7128. doi:10.1073/pnas.78.11.7124 PMID:6947277

Henoch, I., Bergman, B., Gustafsson, M., Gaston-Johansson, F., & Danielson, E. (2007). The impact of symptoms, coping capacity, and social support on quality of life experience over time in patients with lung cancer. *Journal of Pain and Symptom Management*, *34*(4), 370–379. doi:10.1016/j.jpainsymman.2006.12.005 PMID:17616335

Honda, K., & Goodwin, R. D. (2004). Cancer and mental disorders in a national community sample: Findings from the National Comorbidity Survey. *Psychotherapy and Psychosomatics*, *73*(4), 235–242. doi:10.1159/000077742 PMID:15184718

Kaesberg, P. R., & Ershler, W. B. (1989). The importance of immune senescence in the incidence and malignant properties of cancer in hosts of advanced age. *Journal of Gerontology*, *44*(6), 63–66. doi:10.1093/geronj/44.6.63 PMID:2681365

Karin, M., & Greten, F. R. (2005). NF-kappaB: Linking inflammation and immunity to cancer development and progression. *Nature Reviews. Immunology*, *5*(10), 749–759. doi:10.1038/nri1703 PMID:16175180

Kollman, C., Howe, C. W., Anasetti, C., Antin, J. H., Davies, S. M., & Filipovich, A. H. (2001). Donor characteristics as risk factors in recipients after transplantation of bone marrow from unrelated donors: The effect of donor age. *Blood*, *98*(7), 2043–2051. doi:10.1182/blood.V98.7.2043 PMID:11567988

Kuppers, R. B. (2003). Cells under influence: Transformation of B cells by Epstein –Barr virus. *Nature Reviews. Immunology*, *3*(10), 801–812. doi:10.1038/nri1201 PMID:14523386

Larbi, A., & Fulop, T. (2014). From "truly naïve" to "exhausted senescent" T cells: When markers predict functionality. *Cytometry. Part A*, *85*(1), 25–35. doi:10.1002/cyto.a.22351 PMID:24124072

Leith, C. P., Kopecky, K. J., Godwin, J., McConnell, T., Slovak, M. L., & Chen, I. M. (1997). Acute myeloid leukemia in the elderly: Assessment of multidrug resistance (MDR1) and cytogenetics distinguishes biologic subgroups with remarkably distinct responses to standard chemotherapy. A Southwest Oncology Group study. *Blood*, *89*, 3323–3329. PMID:9129038

Liang, X. H., Jackson, S., Seaman, M., Brown, K., Kempkes, B., Hibshoosh, H., & Levine, B. (1999). Induction of autophagy and inhibition of tumorigenesis by beclin1. *Nature*, *402*(6762), 672–676. doi:10.1038/45257 PMID:10604474

Lu, H., Ouyang, W., & Huang, C. (2006). Inflammation, a key event in cancer development. *Molecular Cancer Research*, *4*(4), 221–233. doi:10.1158/1541-7786.MCR-05-0261 PMID:16603636

Marcucci, F., & Mele, A. (2011). Hepatitis viruses and non-Hodgkin lymphoma: Epidemiology, mechanism of tumorigenesis and therapeutic opportunities. *Blood*, *117*(6), 1192–1198. doi:10.1182/blood-2010-06-275818

Miller, R. A. (1991). Aging and immune function. *International Review of Cytology*, *124*, 187–215. doi:10.1016/S0074-7696(08)61527-2 PMID:2001916

Miller, R. A. (1996). The aging immune system: Primer and prospectus. *Science*, *273*(5271), 70–74. doi:10.1126/science.273.5271.70 PMID:8658199

Mitchell, A. J., Chan, M., Bhatti, H., Halton, M., Grassi, L., Johansen, C., & Meader, N. (2011). Prevalence of depression, anxiety, and adjustment disorder in oncological, haematological, and palliative-care settings: A meta-analysis of 94 interview-based studies. *Lancet*, *12*(2), 160–174. doi:10.1016/S1470-2045(11)70002-X PMID:21251875

NCCN. (2014). NCCN Distress thermometer and problem list of patients. Retrieved on 25 February 2015 from https://www.nccn.org/patients/resources/life_with_cancer/pdf/nccn_distress_thermometer.pdf

Ohsumi, Y. (2001). Molecular dissection of autophagy: Two ubiquitin-like systems. *Nature Reviews. Molecular Cell Biology*, *2*(3), 211–216. doi:10.1038/35056522 PMID:11265251

Orr, W. C., & Sohal, R. S. (1994). Extension of life-span by overexpression of superoxidedismutase and catalase in *Drosophila melanogaster. Science*, *263*(5150), 1128–1130. doi:10.1126/science.8108730 PMID:8108730

Peek, R. M. Jr, & Crabtree, J. E. (2006). Helicobacter infection and gastric neoplasia. *The Journal of Pathology*, *208*(2), 233–248. doi:10.1002/path.1868 PMID:16362989

Ries, L. A., Kosary, C. L., Hankey, B. F., Harras, A., Miller, B. A., & Edwards, B. K. (1996). *SEER cancer statistics review, 1973–1993: tables and graphs*. Bethesda, MD: National Institutes of Health.

Rossi, D. J., Jamieson, C. H., & Weissman, I. L. (2008). Stems cells and the pathways to aging and cancer. *Cell*, *132*(4), 681–696. doi:10.1016/j.cell.2008.01.036 PMID:18295583

Seaberg, E. C., Wiley, D., Martinez-Maza, O., Chmiel, J. S., Kingsley, L., Tang, Y., ... Jacobson, L. P. (2010). Cancer incidence in the multicentre AIDS cohort study before and during HAART era: 1984 to 2007. *Cancer*, *116*(23), 5507–5516. doi:10.1002/cncr.25530 PMID:20672354

Shaw, A. C., Goldstein, D. R., & Montgomery, R. R. (2013). Age-dependent dysregulation of innate immunity. *Nature Reviews. Immunology*, *13*(12), 875–887. doi:10.1038/nri3547 PMID:24157572

Sherr, C. J., & Roberts, J. M. (1995). Inhibitors of mammalian G1 cyclin-dependent kinases. *Genes & Development*, *9*(10), 1149–1163. doi:10.1101/gad.9.10.1149 PMID:7758941

Singer, S., Das-Munshi, J., & Brahler, E. (2010). Prevalence of mental health conditions in cancer patients in acute care—a meta-analysis. *Annals of Oncology: Official Journal of the European Society for Medical Oncology*, *21*(5), 925–930. doi:10.1093/annonc/mdp515 PMID:19887467

Spiegel, D. (2002). Cancer Patients: Psychotherapy. In M. Hersen & W. Sledge (Eds.), Encyclopedia of Psychotherapy (1st ed., pp. 359-364). USA: Elsevier Science, Academic Press.

Spiegel, D., Bloom, J. R., & Yalom, I. (1981). Group Support for Patients With Metastatic Cancer A Randomized Prospective Outcome Study. *Archives of General Psychiatry*, *38*(5), 527–533. doi:10.1001/archpsyc.1980.01780300039004 PMID:7235853

Sprangers, M. A., Cull, A., Bjordal, K., Groenvold, M., & Aaronson, N. K. (1993). The European Organization for Research and Treatment of Cancer. Approach to quality of life assessment: Guidelines for developing questionnaire modules. EORTC Study Group on Quality of Life. *Quality of Life Research: An International Journal of Quality of Life Aspects of Treatment, Care and Rehabilitation*, *2*(4), 287–295. doi:10.1007/BF00434800 PMID:8220363

Sun, J., Kale, S. P., Childress, A. M., Pinswasdi, C., & Jazwinski, S. M. (1994). Divergent roles of RAS1 and RAS2 in yeast longevity. *The Journal of Biological Chemistry*, *269*, 18638–18645. PMID:8034612

Taphoorn, M. J., Sizoo, E. M., & Bottomley, A. (2015). Review on quality of life issues in patients with primary brain tumors. *The Oncologist*, *15*(6), 618–626. doi:10.1634/theoncologist.2009-0291 PMID:20507891

Taylor, P. R., Reid, M. M., & Stark, A. N. (1995). *De novo* acute myeloid leukaemia in patients over 55-years-old: A population-based study of incidence, treatment and outcome. *Leukemia*, *9*, 231–237. PMID:7532766

Vagefi, P. A., & Longo, W. E. (2005). Colorectal cancer in patients with inflammatory bowel disease. *Clinical Colorectal Cancer*, *4*(5), 313–319. doi:10.3816/CCC.2005.n.003 PMID:15663834

Ware, J. E., & Sherbourne, E. C. (1992). The MOS 36-Item Short Form Health Survey 1: Conceptual framework and item selection. *Medical Care*, *30*, 473–483. doi:10.1097/00005650-199206000-00002 PMID:1593914

White, C. A., & Macleod, U. (2002). Cancer. *BMJ (Clinical Research Ed.)*, *325*(7360), 377–380. doi:10.1136/bmj.325.7360.377 PMID:12183312

WHO. (2016). Cancer. Retrieved from http://www.who.int/cancer/en/

Yu, C. E., Oshima, J., Fu, Y. H., Wijsman, E. M., Hisama, F., Alisch, R., ... Schellenberg, G. D. (1996). Positional cloning of the Werner's syndrome gene. *Science*, *272*(5259), 258–262. doi:10.1126/science.272.5259.258 PMID:8602509

Yu, C. E., Oshima, J., Wijsman, E. M., Nakura, J., Miki, T., & Piussan, C. (1997). Mutations in the consensus helicase domains of the Werner syndrome gene. Werner's Syndrome Collaboration Group. *American Journal of Human Genetics*, *60*, 330–341. PMID:9012406

KEY TERMS AND DEFINITIONS

Angiogenesis: Angiogenesis is formation of new blood vessels usually mediated by some chemicals in body.

Cell Cycle: Cell Cycle is a highly regulated process of events occurring inside the cell leading to cell division (mitosis) and formation of new cells.

Cellular Senescence: Generally defined as an irreversible state of G1 cell cycle arrest in which cells are refractory to growth factor stimulation.

DNA Repair Defect: A limited number of rare hereditary diseases characterized by genetic defect of DNA repair mechanisms is known as DNA repair defect for example: comprising ataxia telangiectasia, Nijmegen breakage syndrome, Werner syndrome, Bloom Syndrome, Fanconianemia, xerodermapigmentosum.

Malignant Hematological Disorders: Refers to cancers of hematological origin like lymphomas and leukemias.

Psychological Management in Cancer: Taking care of psychological aspects of treatment of cancer. Emotional and social support can help patients learn to cope with psychological stress. Such support can reduce levels of depression, anxiety, and disease- and treatment-related symptoms among patients.

Quality of Life: The standard of health, comfort, and happiness experienced by an individual or group.

Resistance Cytogenetic: Adverse cytogenetic abnormalities leading to poor response to chemotherapy.

Stem Cells: An undifferentiated cell of a multicellular organism which is capable of giving rise to indefinitely more cells of the same type, and from which certain other kinds of cell arise by differentiation.

Tumour Aggressiveness: Describes a tumor or disease that forms, grows, or spreads quickly usually associated with adverse biological and clinical features without intense chemotherapy.

Chapter 14
Sensory Impairments and Challenges in Ageing

Ashwini R.
Dharwad Institute of Mental Health and Neurosciences (DIMHANS), India

Barre Vijaya Prasad
Dharwad Institute of Mental Health and Neurosciences (DIMHANS), India

ABSTRACT

This chapter describes how sensory impairment is often regarded from a medical/disability point of view and its effects on mental health can be poorly recognized. Communication is a key issue for deaf and deaf-blind people and difficulties here underlie developmental, psychological and emotional problems and delay or prevent appropriate assessment and treatment. Sensory related issues are seen as medical problems and as disabilities. 95% of the information about the world around us comes from our sight and hearing. However, the main concerns of visual and hearing affected by the total or partial absence of sight and/or hearing are usually how to live, how to learn and how to communicate. Their difficulties are often as much to do with society's attitudes towards them as with the direct effect of sensory impairment.

INTRODUCTION

The best way to keep something bad from happening is to see it ahead of time... and you can't see it if you refuse to face the possibility." William S. Burroughs

Ageing is the process of becoming older. Ageing can refer to single cells within an organism which have ceased dividing (cellular senescence) or to the population of a species (population ageing). In humans, ageing represents the accumulation of changes in a human being over time (Bowen, & Atwood 2004), encompassing physical, psychological, and social changes. Ageing is among the greatest known risk factors for most human diseases (Dillin, Gottschling, & Nyström 2014), of the roughly 150,000 people who die each day across the globe, about two thirds die from age-related causes. The causes of ageing are uncertain; current theories are assigned to the damage concept, whereby the accumulation of damage (such as DNA oxidation) may cause biological systems to fail, or to the programmed ageing concept,

DOI: 10.4018/978-1-5225-3480-8.ch014

whereby internal processes (such as DNA methylation) may cause ageing. Programmed ageing should not be confused with programmed cell death (apoptosis). Human behaviour is highly dependent on the reception and integration of information derived from sensory organs, such as the eye and ear, as well as from nerve endings in skin, muscle, joints, and internal organs. There is, however, no direct relation between the sensitivity of receptors and the adequacy of behaviour, because the usual level of stimulation is considerably greater than the minimum required for stimulation of the sense organs. In addition, an individual adapts to gradual impairments in one sensory organ by using information available from other sense organs. Modern technology has also provided glasses and hearing aids to compensate for reduced acuity in the sense organs.

Age can result in visual impairment, whereby non-verbal communication is reduced (Worrall, & Hickson, 2003) which can lead to isolation and possible depression. Macular degeneration causes vision loss and increases with age, affecting nearly 12% of those above the age of 80 (Mehta, 2015). This degeneration is caused by systemic changes in the circulation of waste products and by growth of abnormal vessels around the retina (Nussbaum, Thompson., & Robinson, 1989).

Ageing is a complex multifactorial process leading to loss of function and a very broad spectrum of diseases. Sensory impairment is often regarded from a medical/disability point of view and its effects on mental health can be poorly recognised. Communication is a key issue for deaf and deaf–blind people and difficulties here underlie developmental, psychological, and emotional problems and delay or prevent appropriate assessment and treatment. Sensory functions are the critical means by which individuals gain access to information and connect to their physical environment and the people around them. Unfortunately, many older people and their families, as well as the professionals who serve them, accept sensory loss as a "normal" part of the Ageing process. Furthermore, few are fully aware of the range of rehabilitation interventions available for older adults with sensory impairments. 95% of the information about the world around us comes from our sight and hearing. Sensory impairment is when one of the senses; sight, hearing, smell, touch, taste and spatial awareness, is no longer normal. Communication is the greatest challenge. A sighted and hearing person will explore their surroundings, a person with sensory impairments will need encouragement to explore and interact. Normal progress to language is hard and intensive education and support is needed throughout the person's lifetime. Ageing has long been associated with decline in sensory function, a critical component of the health and quality of life of older people.

Sensory functions are the critical means by which individuals gain access to information and connect to their physical environment and the people around them. Unfortunately, many older people and their families, as well as the professionals who serve them, accept sensory loss as a "normal" part of the Ageing process. Furthermore, few are fully aware of the range of rehabilitation interventions available for older adults with sensory impairments. Sensory impairment is often regarded from a medical/disability point of view and its effects on mental health can be poorly recognised. Dual sensory impairment is the combination of both hearing and sight impairment. It is not necessarily a total loss of both senses – indeed the majority of dual sensory impaired people do have some degree of sight and/or hearing. Those with a less severe degree of both sight and hearing impairment may also be referred to as having a dual sensory impairment or loss. Sensory impairment is often regarded from a medical/disability point of view and its effects on mental health can be poorly recognised. Sensory impairment is the most common health problem that the elderly experience and could occur or increase as a result of disease or Ageing (Kim, Kim., & Kim, 2011; Saunders, & Echt, 2007).

Any temporary or permanent loss or abnormality of body structure or function, whether physiological or psychological. An impairment is a disturbance affecting functions that are essentially mental (memory, consciousness) or sensory, internal organs (heart, kidney), the head, the trunk or the limbs. The term sensory impairment is therefore often used when referring to damage that occurs to the structure of the eyes or ears affecting the normal functioning of our vision and hearing senses.

TYPES OF SENSORY IMPAIRMENTS

The latest prevalence estimates on vision, hearing, and dual impairment come from the National Health and Examination Surveys 1999 to 2006 (Schiller, Lucas, & Peregoy, 2012; Swenor, Ramulu, Willis, Friedman, & Lin, 2013). Vision impairment was considered best corrected visual acuity of 20/40 or worse in the better eye, and hearing impairment was considered pure-tone average >25 decibels in the better ear. Dual impairment in their study was a combination of vision impairment and hearing impairment. It is true that sensory impairment particularly vision and hearing impairment is common in Ageing. These normal age-related sensory impairments are common, as are vision and hearing impairments due to multifactorial etiologies such as chronic diseases (e.g., diabetes, hypertension) as well as exposure to excessive noise, ultraviolet sun light, and excessive tobacco use (Agrawal, Platz, & Niparko, 2008; Dillion, Gu, Hoffman, & Ko, 2010). There are three major types of sensory impairments were discussed in following order namely; visual impairment, hearing impairment and Deaf-blindness (dual sensory impairment).

VISUAL IMPAIRMENT

Among the various issues that affect the elderly, common health problems including age related visual Impairment will be one of the major concerns. Demographic studies have consistently shown that age is the best predictor of blindness and visual impairment (Padula, 1982). It was also reported that legal blindness (best corrected visual acuity of less than 20/200 in the better eye) occurs in up to 3% of the world population by the age of 60 (Padula, 1982; Patterson, 1994). Visual impairment among the elderly is a major health problem. With advancing age, the normal function of eye tissues decreases and there is an increased incidence of ocular pathology. Demographic studies have shown that age is the best predictor of blindness and visual impairment. The most common causes of age related visual impairment in the elderly are presbyopia, cataracts, age related macular degeneration, primary open angle glaucoma and diabetic retinopathy. Untreated visual impairment leads to physical handicap, increased incidence of fall, depression, social isolation and dependency. Active screening for visual loss in the elderly should be part of the health examination. The elderly should be encouraged to come for formal 1-2 yearly eye assessment for early detection of visual impairment and to treat all associated problems in order to prevent permanent visual loss. People who are blind or have low vision can use technology aids, equipment and strategies to lead fairly independent and safe lives at home and in the community. Blindness and low vision can occur as a result of disease or infection, conditions or accidents. Symptoms of vision impairment are central vision loss, peripheral vision loss, contrast impairment, glare, reduced depth perception and blur. Vision loss among the elderly is a major health care problem. Approximately one person in three has some form of vision-reducing eye disease by the age of 65. The most common causes of vision loss among the elderly are age-related macular degeneration, glaucoma, cataract and diabetic retinopathy. Age-related macular degeneration is characterized by the loss of central vision. Primary open-angle glaucoma results in optic nerve damage and visual field loss. Because this condition may initially be asymptomatic, regular screening examinations are recommended for elderly patients. Cataract is a common cause of vision impairment among the elderly, but surgery is often effective in restoring vision. Diabetic retinopathy may be observed in the elderly at the time of diagnosis or during the first few years of diabetes. Patients should undergo eye examinations with dilation when diabetes is diagnosed.

HEARING IMPAIRMENTS

Age-related hearing loss (presbycusis) is the loss of hearing that gradually occurs in most of us as we grow older. It is one of the most common conditions affecting older and elderly adults. Approximately one in three people in the United States between the ages of 65 and 74 has hearing loss, and nearly half of those older than 75 have difficulty hearing. Having trouble hearing can make it hard to understand and follow a doctor's advice, respond to warnings, and hear phones, doorbells, and smoke alarms. Hearing loss can also make it hard to enjoy talking with family and friends, leading to feelings of isolation. Age-related hearing loss most often occurs in both ears, affecting them equally. Because the loss is gradual, if you have age-related hearing loss you may not realize that you've lost some of your ability to hear. There are many causes of age-related hearing loss. Most commonly, it arises from changes in the inner ear as we age, but it can also result from changes in the middle ear, or from complex changes along the nerve pathways from the ear to the brain. Certain medical conditions and medications may also play a role.

Many factors can contribute to hearing loss as you get older. It can be difficult to distinguish age-related hearing loss from hearing loss that can occur for other reasons, such as long-term exposure to noise. Noise-induced hearing loss is caused by long-term exposure to sounds that are either too loud or last too long. This kind of noise exposure can damage the sensory hair cells in your ear that allow you to hear. Once these hair cells are damaged, they do not grow back and your ability to hear is diminished. Conditions those are more common in older people, such as high blood pressure or diabetes, can contribute to hearing loss. Medications that are toxic to the sensory cells in your ears (for example, some chemotherapy drugs) can also cause hearing loss. Rarely, age-related hearing loss can be caused by abnormalities of the outer ear or middle ear. Such abnormalities may include reduced function of the tympanic membrane (the eardrum) or reduced function of the three tiny bones in the middle ear that carry sound waves from the tympanic membrane to the inner ear. Older people who experience hearing loss have a combination of both age-related hearing loss and noise-induced hearing loss. Age-related hearing loss is also known as presbycusis. Although age-related hearing loss is not a life-threatening condition, it can have a significant impact on your quality of life if left untreated.

Age-related hearing loss occurs gradually over time. Various changes in the inner ear can cause the condition, these include:

- Changes in the structures of the inner ear.
- Changes in blood flow to the ear.
- Impairment in the nerves responsible for hearing.
- Changes in the way that the brain processes speech and sound.

- Damage to the tiny hairs in the ear that are responsible for transmitting sound to the brain.

Age-related hearing loss can also be caused by other issues, including:

- Diabetes
- Poor circulation
- Exposure to loud noises
- Use of certain medications
- Family history of hearing loss
- Smoking

Symptoms of age-related hearing loss typically begin with an inability to hear high-pitched sounds. Typical we may notice that they have difficulty hearing the voices of females or children. They also have difficulty hearing background noises or difficulty hearing others speak clearly.

Other symptoms that may occur include:

- Certain sounds seeming overly loud.
- Difficulty hearing in areas that are noisy.
- Difficulty hearing the difference between "s" and "th" sounds.
- Ringing in the ears.
- Turning up the volume on the television or radio louder than normal.
- Asking people to repeat themselves being unable to understand conversations over the telephone.

These are the early symptoms for hearing impairment. They could be signs of other medical conditions and should be checked out by a doctor. Hearing loss or hearing impairment is a partial or total inability to hear. It can be caused by genetics, Ageing, exposure to noise, illness, chemicals and physical trauma. It is usually described as mild, mild-moderate, moderate, moderately severe, severe, or profound. Hearing loss exists when there is diminished sensitivity to the sounds normally heard. Deafness is defined as a degree of impairment that a person is unable to understand speech even in the presence of amplification. Many in the deaf community view it as a condition, rather than an illness.

DUAL SENSORY IMPAIRMENT

Dual sensory impairment (DSI), or deaf-blindness, is a combination of vision and hearing impairment that interferes with the person's ability to acquire information and communicate with others (Watters, Owen., & Munroe, 2005) DSI encompasses a spectrum of sensory loss and individuals may be completely deaf and completely blind or they may have some residual hearing and/or vision. The widely used Nordic definition states that "deaf-blindness is a combined vision and hearing disability. It limits activities of a person and restricts full participation in society to such a degree that society is required to facilitate specific services, environmental alterations and/or technology." (Puts, Deeg, Hoeymans, Nusselder., & Schellevis, 2008). The loss of functioning in one sense cannot be compensated for with the other sense, resulting in a distinct disability. Those with DSI can be broadly classified into two main groups based on when the sensory losses occurred: a) congenital (individuals who experience the onset of hearing and visual impairment before the age of two years, including onset at birth) (Munroe, 2001) acquired (onset later in life). Common causes of congenital DSI include intra-uterine infections (e.g., congenital rubella syndrome), (Dammeyer, 2010) congenital brain damage and chromosomal abnormalities such as CHARGE syndrome (Lew, Weihing, Myers, Pogoda., & Goodrich, 2010; Kramer, Kapteyn., & Kuik, 2002). Acquired DSI can be related to Ageing, post-natal infections/early childhood infections and acquired brain injury, (Lew, Weihing, Myers, Pogoda., & Goodrich, 2010; Saunders, & Echt, 2007; Spandau & Rohrschneider, 2002). Among older persons with DSI, vision loss is often a result of presbyopia, decreased pupil size, cataracts and glaucoma, (Saunders, & Echt, 2007; Watson, 2001) and causes of hearing loss include age-related changes in the inner ear and a reduction in blood flow and loss of neurons that result in a diminished capacity within the central auditory system (Saunders, & Echt, 2007).

The occurrence of DSI is particularly prevalent among the Ageing population, with studies showing between 9% and 21% of adults older than 70 years having some degree of DSI. (Campbell, Crews, Moriarty, Zack., & Blackman, 1999; Jee, Wang, Rose, Lindley, Landau., & Mitchell, 2005), Despite this, there is little direction regarding recommended clinical practice and rehabilitation of individuals with DSI. It is assumed that the problems encountered by individuals with DSI are considerably greater than the effects of vision impairment or hearing impairment alone, because when these two sensory impairments are combined, the individual is seriously deprived of compensatory strategies that make use of the nonimpaired sense. In this article, the literature available regarding DSI is summarized, and research needs regarding rehabilitation strategies are outlined and discussed. Simple suggestions for addressing DSI are provided that use available tools and technology.

Impaired vision and hearing are common among older adults, (Watters, Owen., & Munroe, 2005; Puts, Deeg, Hoeymans, Nusselder., & Schellevis, 2008), and can occur separately or in combination (Munroe, 2001). Visual loss impacts negatively on functional independence, mental health and cognition, and reduces quality of life, as well as increasing the need for support services (Dammeyer, 2010; Saunders, & Echt, 2007). Age-related hearing loss is more frequent and is associated with an increased risk of depression, and impairs quality of life and the ability to conduct activities of daily living, as well as leading to an increased reliance on community and informal supports (Puts, Deeg, Hoeymans, Nusselder., & Schellevis, 2001; Spandau, & Rohrschneider, 2002; Fisher et al., 2014). Hence, strategies include the provision of corrective lenses, hearing aids, assistive devices (e.g., magnifiers, listening devices) and rehabilitative services such as visual, auditory and communication training should be encouraged and/ or implemented by clinicians in order to promote both longevity and an improved quality of life in their older sensory impaired patient.

PHYSIOLOGY OF SENSORY IMPAIRMENT IN AGEING

Physiological Ageing refers to the changes in structure and functioning of the body that occur over a lifespan. Many of these changes are involuntary and occur very gradually while others occur over a short period. After the age of 70 other sense organs may show a reduction in sensitivity. Reduced taste sensitivity is associated with atrophy and loss of taste buds from the tongue in the elderly. Human Ageing, physiological changes that take place in the human body leading to senescence, the decline of biological functions and of the ability to adapt to metabolic stress. In humans the physiological developments are normally accompanied by psychological and behavioural changes, and other changes, involving social and economic factors, also occur. Ageing begins as soon as adulthood is reached and is as much a part of human life as are infancy, childhood, and adolescence. Gerontology (the study of Ageing) is concerned primarily with the changes that occur between the attainment of maturity and the death of the individual. The goal of research in gerontology is to identify the factors that influence these changes. Application of this knowledge is expected to reduce the disabilities now associated with Ageing. The biological-physiological aspects of Ageing include both the basic biological factors that underlie Ageing and the general health status. Since the probability of death increases rapidly with advancing age, it is clear that changes must occur in the individual which make him more and more vulnerable to disease. For example, a young adult may rapidly recover from pneumonia, whereas an elderly person may die. Physiologists have found that the performance of many organs such as the heart, kidneys, brain, or lungs shows a gradual decline over the life span. Part of this decline is due to a loss of cells from these organs, with resultant reduction in the reserve capacities of the individual. Furthermore, the cells remaining in the elderly individual may not perform as well as those in the young. Certain cellular enzymes may be less active, and thus more time may be required to carry out chemical reactions. ultimately the cell may die.

Ageing also brings about a reduction in the ability to change the focus of the eye for viewing near and far objects (presbyopia), so that distant objects can ordinarily be seen more clearly than those close at hand. This change in vision is related to a gradual increase in rigidity of the lens of the eye that takes place primarily between the ages of 10 and 55 years. After age 55 there is little further change. Many people in their 50s adopt bifocal glasses to compensate for this physiological change. The primary age change in the skin is a gradual loss of elasticity. Although this basic change plays a role, other factors, such as exposure to the weather and familial traits, also contribute to the development of wrinkles and the pigmentation associated with senescence. The ability of the skin to take up slack and remain closely adherent to the underlying structures is due to the presence of fibres of the proteins elastin and collagen. Because of the importance of hormones in the regulation of many physiological systems, impairments in endocrine (ductless) glands have traditionally been cited as important determinants in Ageing. With Ageing, the bones gradually lose calcium. As a result, they become more fragile and are more likely to break, even with minor falls. Healing of fractures is also slower in the old than in the young.

PREVALENCE OF SENSORY IMPAIRMENT IN AGEING

Prevalence estimates indicate the burden of a condition (e.g., visual impairment) at a defined location at a point or period in time. Accurate prevalence estimates are needed to plan for availability of health care services, associated monetary costs, and quality of life connected with having the condition. Such data are also of importance in planning future studies, such as controlled clinical trials of prevention and treatment of the disease. Periodic estimates of prevalence enable the tracking of temporal trends; this is important especially in situations where new, costly interventions are being introduced.

Vision impairment has been identified as the second most prevalent physical impairment observed within the elderly population (U.S. Department of Health and Human Services, 1995). Prevalence rates of blindness and visual impairment for elderly persons have been consistently demonstrated to increase sharply and monotonically with increasing age. Like vision impairment, hearing impairment has been identified as a major chronic condition in old age (U.S. Department of Health and Human Services, 1995). Recent studies have shown that hearing impairment among elderly people has doubled in prevalence over the past 30 years in the United States, based on self-reported data on trouble hearing (Strawbridge, Wallhagen, Shema, and Kaplan, 2000). Millions of Americans are affected by sensory impairments, with vision and hearing loss being two with the highest prevalence. Vision and hearing loss are particularly prominent in the older adult population. While vision loss has a negative impact on a person's perception of the world, hearing loss diminishes a person's mode of communication and can lead to social isolation. The World Health Organization (WHO) estimates approximately 360 million or 5% of the world's population has at least a moderate hearing loss (WHO). An estimated half of these hearing loss cases result from a lack of preventative measures, including but not limited to immunizations or noise exposure reduction. In the United States, an analysis of data from 2001 to 2010 estimated 60.7 million individuals aged 12 years or older have hearing loss in at least one ear. The prevalence of hearing loss in the US is even higher in the older adult population; 75% of individuals aged 70 years or older have hearing loss, defined by pure-tone thresholds as mild (>25 through 40 dB HL), moderate (>40 through 55 dB HL), moderately severe (>55 through 70 dB HL), severe (>70 through 90 dB HL), or profound (>90 dB HL) (Goman, & Lin, 2016; American Speech-Language-Hearing Association, 2016) . Despite this high prevalence of hearing loss in the elderly population, less than 30% of those who could benefit from hearing aids (HA).

Vision loss is another sensory impairment with a high prevalence in the elderly population. The WHO estimated in 2014 that 285 million people are estimated to have a visual impairment, with 39 million classified as blind and 246 million as low vision (World Health Organization, 2014). Low vision is defined as the grouping of moderate and severe visual impairments. Approximately 65% of these individuals are aged 50 years and older. Reportedly, the treatment of visual impairment over the past 20 years has improved significantly worldwide. Unlike the prevalence of hearing loss, the prevalence of visual impairment has decreased despite an increasingly larger population of older adults globally. This is primarily due to a decline in vision loss caused by infectious diseases worldwide. The high prevalence of dual sensory impairment in the older adult population, there continues to be a lack of awareness and resources not only among those affected but also among professionals in these fields. Increased collaboration among the interdisciplinary fields is crucial to lessen the impact of undiagnosed or untreated dual sensory impairment.

CHALLENGES IN AGEING

For many of us, it can be unpleasant to grow older. Our society and culture value youth, and being old is sometimes treated like a disease that has no cure. Of course, it's a reality that all of us have to face at some point, so Ageing is a huge topic of study for sociologists. Among other things, they observe patterns of social activity and identify the challenges we all face as we age. Three of the larger challenges that have been identified are retirement, ageism and social isolation. Challenge of Ageing that may seem more obvious is ageism. Although it can target any age group, ageism generally refers to prejudice and/or discrimination against older people. Ageism can be blatant or subtle. For example, it involves anything from refusing to hire an elderly worker to assuming an older woman needs help crossing the road. The elderly are often given a negative stereotype: slow, confused, helpless, resistant to change, and/or generally unhappy. Like racism and sexism, discrimination can happen when unfair generalizations like this are made. Although the stereotype is not true of every older individual, age-related bias, unfortunately, exists in practically every setting. Another challenge of Ageing is that of social isolation. Being alone can be extremely unpleasant at any age. It's something that many people fear about growing old because, unfortunately, social isolation is common amongst the elderly.

Our journey through the second half of life requires each one of us to adapt to a variety of age-related challenges. The physical challenges of Ageing result in various forms of functional decline in the body. The psychological challenges of Ageing impact our sense of identity, independence, and purpose in life. The spiritual challenges of Ageing demand reflection on difficult issues such as loss, grief, death, and impermanence. The cultural challenges of Ageing include retirement, financial planning, ageism, inclusion, and contribution. And finally, the environmental challenges of Ageing include dealing with change, transition, transience, thresholds, and liminality. The challenge of Ageing is a means to cultivate clarity, understanding, and self-compassion. The challenges and choices of Ageing impact our quality of life. It is important to understand the essential characteristics and influences that Ageing has on our body, mind, spirit, culture, and environment so that we give ourselves an opportunity to meet the challenges ahead with the spirit of creativity.

The major challenges of Ageing conjure doubt, despair, difficulty, discomfort, uncertainty, and anxiety. Our tendency is to approach Ageing with a sense of enmity. Our tendency is to avoid, deny, or hide ourselves from the raw realities of Ageing. Perhaps this is the most significant challenge of all that is, overcoming our fear of Ageing.

CONSEQUENCES IN AGEING

Impairment is the effect of any problem associated to any body part. These are reflected as the cause of disabilities; this means that they act as symptom prior to the disability, which could be treated or would be attempted to stop by consulting a doctor or prescribing a treatment. The Ageing of our societies is one of the greatest success stories of the twentieth century. More than three decades have been added to the lives of hundreds of millions of people over the last hundred years. This is an accomplishment well worth celebrating; but we must also bear in mind that with increased longevity come significant long-term economic consequences – and that many societies are ageing at a record speed.

One of the most recognized consequences of ageing is a decline in immune function. While elderly individuals are by no means immunodeficient, they often do not respond efficiently to novel or previously encountered antigens. This is illustrated by increased vulnerability of individuals 70 years of age and older to influenza, a situation that is exacerbated by their poor response to vaccination.

Hearing loss affects more than 8 million people in the UK. About 5 million people could benefit from hearing aids, but over half of these are reluctant to use an aid because of the associated stigma.

Multiple psychosocial factors have been associated with poor vision in elderly people. Visual impairment among elderly people has been correlated with psychological distress, low morale, and depression.

Empirical evidence that documents the full sequence of events involving the indirect effects of sensory impairment on quality of life and well-being is lacking. Only one previous study (Lee et al. 1999) has examined the impact of both vision and hearing impairment on psychological well-being. Ageing of the population affects all aspects of the society including health, social security, education, socio-cultural activities and family life.

SENSORY IMPAIRMENT AND DISABILITIES

A disability is a condition in which there is a lack of an individual's mental, mobile or moving functions of its respective organ or part. In this condition, the individual is not able to function or complete any task which is associated to its absent part or organ. It can also entail to any sensory, physical, cognitive or intellectual impairment and various types of chronic disease and mental illnesses. It's not compulsory in disability that the condition should occur from birth; it can rather occur at any time in an individual's life span. The term broadly classifies the illness or irregular capacity of any functioning of a body part, then it may relate to any associative physical, cognitive, mental, sensory, emotional, developmental, or some combination of problems.

Sensory disabilities dramatically increase with age and may seriously compromise an older person's ability to carry out routine daily activities. In 1991, visual and hearing impairments were reported by over 10% and 17% of persons aged 65 years and over, respectively (Raina, Wong, Dukeshire, Chambers., & Lindsay, 2000). Given the projected growth of the older adult population, it is particularly important to continue understanding the relationship between visual and hearing impairment and functional independence.

Impairment is a cause of Disability. According to the federal government, the term impairment is defined as: an "inability to engage in any substantial gainful activity by reason of any medically determinable physical or mental impairment which can be expected to last or has lasted for a continuous period of not less than 12 months." Medically, it is a condition which leads to disability in an individual. It can be stated as the basic root cause of any disability. It's an abnormality associated with the physiological, psychological, or anatomical structure or function of a body part or organ. Impairment can relate to the permanent or temporary loss of functioning of an organ. It acts as an alerting symbol to identify an affected problem in an individual. The problem when diagnosed at the specific time can be cured by consulting or taking a prior treatment.

SCREENING AND IDENTIFICATION

Timely screening of hearing and vision will: (1) facilitate identifying those in need of referral to a hearing or vision professional; (2) enable individually tailored care for residents, thus promoting the health and well-being of older adults with sensory impairments; (3) identify sensory impairments and, by addressing them to whatever extent possible, care plans can be adapted to accommodate for these impairments.

Simple approach that can be used by general internists to routinely screen the functional status of elderly patients in office practice. The approach relies on checking a limited number of targets that are commonly dysfunctional but often unappreciated when conventional histories and physical examinations are done for elderly patients. The new focus is on carefully selected tests of vision, hearing, arm and leg function, urinary incontinence, mental status, instrumental and basic activities of daily living, environmental hazards, and social support systems. Brief questions and easily observed tasks are used to obtain the information needed for a suitable, effective screening while minimizing the time for administration.

Visual impairment is common among older people and is associated with falls and reduced quality of life. Visual problems in older people are often not reported to medical services. Screening has been recommended because vision could be improved by encounter ageing treatment in the majority of older people with impaired vision. There are several ways to screen for hearing impairment. For example, there are a number of physical measures and scales that seem to correlate reasonably well with pure tone audiometry, the current "gold standard." (Dupuis et al., 2015; Moher, Shamseer., & Clarke, 2015). Pure tone audiometry can be made more or less sensitive and specific depending on the frequencies tested and the decibel threshold used to define hearing loss. Third, there are hearing handicap scales (Carpenter & Hirdes, 2013; Schow, & Nerbonne, 1980; The American Speech-Language-Hearing Association, 2016).

REHABILITATION SERVICES

Rehabilitation services for older adults with age-related sensory loss need to accommodate these difficulties. Improved staff education and rehabilitation programmes providing clients and carers with strategies to overcome communication breakdown is required. A multidisciplinary perspective to the assessment and remediation of older adults is recommended.

Vision rehabilitation services can vastly improve quality of life and help them live more independently. Vision rehabilitation services include:

- Communication skills: reading, writing, Braille and assistive computer technology.
- Counselling: to help you, your spouse, family members and friends adjust to your vision loss.
- Independent living and personal management skills: home management, home modifications, personal self-care, financial management.
- Occupational therapy.
- Independent movement and travel skills: orientation and mobility training.
- Low vision evaluation and training with low vision devices.
- Vocational evaluation and training.

Hearing loss services include:

- Comprehensive hearing evaluations.
- Cochlear implants.
- Speech and language therapy.
- Assistive devices (e.g. audio loops).
- Training on hearing aids, assistive devices.
- Supportive workshops.
- Recreational/social activities.

In current practice, rehabilitation of sensory impairments in the ageing population is divided into separate rehabilitation services for impairments in vision (low vision rehabilitation centres) and in hearing (audiology centres and hearing aid providers). Concurrent hearing impairment could affect the success of low vision rehabilitation (Leonard, & Horowitz, 2004) and vice versa. Moreover, healthcare providers do not automatically deal with impairment of the 'other sense', which may lead to less effective rehabilitation.

Educating our peers and using these guidelines in our practice will enhance the quality of life of the geriatric patient. One of the greatest challenges in the geriatric population is their ability to communicate their problems, needs, and desires in a medical setting. Hearing and visual impairments can hamper a patient's ability to express himself or herself clearly or to understand questions or commands. This is an enormous burden on the patient, the caregiver, and the physiatrist as they work to achieve rehabilitation goals. Addressing these issues on the patient's initial visit can ameliorate problems and prevent frustration and further difficulties.

Rehabilitation comprises the provision of a custom-fitted hearing aid and instruction on its use and maintenance. Progress during rehabilitation depends on patient and family education to help the patient adjust to the hearing loss and the use of hearing aids. Family training with a speech therapist is also crucial to teach them about auditory enhancement techniques and communication skills. Improving the geriatric patient's ability to hear can lead to significant gains in terms of rehabilitation and the patient's overall quality of life. Physicians should evaluate their patient's hearing on a regular basis and consider the management of hearing deficits as they care for their patients. Utilization of healthcare resources and assistance increases in the geriatric population with visual impairment because of their decreased level of function overall.

RESEARCHES ON SENSORY IMPAIRMENT IN AGEING

Researchers have discovered that sensory impairment is more dangerous than previously thought, particularly in regard to mortality. Vision loss has been associated with a 5% to 29% increased mortality rate in older adults (Cugati et al., 2007; Karpa et al., 2010). Hearing impairment alone has been linked to all-cause mortality through three mediating variables: disability in walking, cognitive impairment, and self-rated health (Karpa et al., 2010). A recent cohort study from Australia documented that dual sensory impairment increases risk of mortality over 10 years by 62% compared to older adults without sensory impairment (Gopinath et al., 2013). In addition, older adults with best corrected vision impairment and moderate to severe hearing loss had a two-fold increase in 10-year mortality (Gopinath et al., 2013). A strength of this population study was the objective measurement of sensory impairment through pure tone audiometry and distance visual acuity. Asking older adults about their vision and hearing impairment is often not sufficient. The researchers also controlled for smoking, body mass index, systolic blood pressure, diabetes, cancer history, angina, stroke, acute myocardial infarction, and cognitive impairment (Gopinath et al., 2013). Additional steps to improve the care of older adults with sensory impairment include: (a) reconsideration of the "lack of evidence" supporting population screening for vision and hearing impairment; (b) development and testing of primary care models of interventions for hearing and vision screening and referrals; (c) development of safe environmental designs; (d) technology designed and tested for this population; and (e) neuro-imging studies to investigate brain changes due to sensory impairment.

FUTURE RESEARCH DIRECTIONS

Future research will need to examine the influence of other concurrent health conditions on sensory impairment. Asking the elderly about their overall hearing and visual function is not sufficient in detecting sensory impairment. To detect hearing and vision impairments among elderly home care patients, standardized measurements of their hearing and vision are necessary. Today's practitioners should focus on the use of screening tools in the clinic, risk assessments, programs for fall prevention, and rehabilitation after a fall.

CONCLUSION

Impairments of vision and hearing are common in this frail older outpatient population. Combined vision and hearing impairments have a greater effect on function than single sensory impairments and influence functional status independent of mental status and comorbid illness. Elderly home-care patients cannot be expected to take the necessary actions to meet their sensory impairments themselves; they need close assistance and help. With the increasing need for and use of health care services due to an ageing population, the major goal in public health and medicine is to keep elderly individuals living independently and to prevent institutionalisation. Small improvements in vision and hearing impairment may enhance physical and psychological functioning in older adults.

REFERENCES

Agrawal, Y., Platz, E. A., & Niparko, J. K. (2008). Prevalence of hearing loss and differences by demographic characteristics among US adults: Data from the National Health and Nutrition Examination Survey, 1999-2004. *Archives of Internal Medicine*, *168*(14), 1522–1530. doi:10.1001/archinte.168.14.1522 PMID:18663164

Bowen, R. L., & Atwood, C. S. (2004). Living and Dying for Sex. *Gerontology*, *50*(5), 265–290. doi:10.1159/000079125 PMID:15331856

Campbell, V.A., Crews, J.E., Moriarty, D.G., Zack, M.M., & Blackman, D.K. (1999). Surveillance for sensory impairment, activity limitation, and health-related quality of life among older adults – United States.

Carpenter, I., & Hirdes, J. P. (2013). Using interRAI assessment systems to measure and maintain quality of long-term care. In A Good Life in Old Age. Monitoring and Improving Quality in Long-term Care (pp. 93–139). OECD Health Policy Studies. doi:10.1787/9789264194564-7-en

Cugati, S., Cumming, R. G., Smith, W., Burlutsky, G., Mitchell, P., & Wang, J. J. (2007). Visual impairment, age-related macular degeneration, cataract, and long-term mortality: The Blue Mountains Eye Study. *Archives of Ophthalmology*, *125*(7), 917–924. doi:10.1001/archopht.125.7.917 PMID:17620571

Dammeyer, J. (2010). Prevalence and aetiology of congenitally deafblind people in Denmark. *International Journal of Audiology*, *49*(2), 76–82. doi:10.3109/14992020903311388 PMID:20151880

Dillin, A., Gottschling, D. E., & Nyström, T. (2014). The good and the bad of being connected: The integrons of aging. *Current Opinion in Cell Biology*, *26C*, 107–112. doi:10.1016/j.ceb.2013.12.003 PMID:24529252

Dillion, C. F., Gu, Q., Hoffman, H. J., & Ko, C. (2010). Vision, hearing, balance, and sensory impairment in Americans aged 70 years and over. *United States, 1999–2006* (Data Brief No. 31). Retrieved from http://www.cdc.gov/nchs/data/databriefs/db31.pdf

Dupuis, K., Pichora-Fuller, M. K., Chasteen, A. L., Marchuk, V., Singh, G., & Smith, S. L. (2015). Effects of hearing and vision impairments on the Montreal Cognitive Assessment. *Neuropsychological Development Cognition Brain Aging Neuropsychol Cognition*, *22*(4), 413–437. doi:10.1080/13825585.2014.968084 PMID:25325767

Fisher, D., Li, C.-M., Chiu, M. A., Themann, C. L., Petersen, H., & Jonasson, F. (2014). Impairments in hearing and vision impact on mortality in older people. *International Journal of Audiology*, *54*(9), 634–641. doi:10.3109/14992027.2015.1024889 PMID:25816699

Gopinath, B., Schneider, J., McMahon, C. M., Burlutsky, G., Leeder, S. R., & Mitchell, P. (2013). Dual sensory impairment in older adults increases the risk of mortality: A population-based study. *PLoS One*, *8*(3), e55054. doi:10.1371/journal.pone.0055054 PMID:23469161

Jee, J. J., Wang, J. J., Rose, K. A., Lindley, R., Landau, P., & Mitchell, P. (2005, January). Wang, K. A. Rose, R. Lindley, P. Landau, & P. Mitchell, "Vision and hearing impairment in aged care clients. *Ophthalmic Epidemiology*, *12*(3), 199–205. doi:10.1080/09286580590969707 PMID:16036479

Karpa, M. J., Gopinath, B., Beath, K., Rochtchina, E., Cumming, R. G., Wang, J. J., & Mitchell, P. (2010). Associations between hearing impairment and mortality risk in older persons: The Blue Mountains Hearing Study. *Annals of Epidemiology*, *20*(6), 452–459. doi:10.1016/j.annepidem.2010.03.011 PMID:20470972

Kim, H. J., Kim, B. H., & Kim, O. S. (2011). The Effect of Visual and Hearing Impairment on Depression and Cognitive Function in Community-dwelling Elderly. *Journal of Aging and Health*, *19*(7), 658–665.

Kramer, S. E., Kapteyn, T. S., Kuik, D. J. H., & Deeg, D. J. H. (2002). The association of hearing impairment and chronic diseases with psychosocial health status in older age. *Journal of Aging and Health*, *14*(1), 122–137. doi:10.1177/089826430201400107 PMID:11892756

Lee, D. C., Artero, E. G., Sui, X., & Blair, S. N. (2010). Mortality trends in the general population: The importance of cardiorespiratory fitness. *Journal of Psychopharmacology (Oxford, England)*, *24*(4 Suppl.), 27–35. doi:10.1177/1359786810382057 PMID:20923918

Leonard, R., & Horowitz, A. (2004). Hearing problems of and the need for hearing services by consumers of vision rehabilitation services. *Journal of Visual Impairment & Blindness*, *98*, 168–172.

Lew, H. L., Weihing, J., Myers, P. J., Pogoda, T. K., & Goodrich, G. L. (2010). Dual sensory impairment (DSI) in traumatic brain injury (TBI)- an emerging interdisciplinary challenge. *NeuroRehabilitation*, *26*, 213–222. doi:10.3233/nre-2010-0557 PMID:20448311

Mehta, S. (2015). "Age-Related Macular Degeneration.". Primary care. Clinics in office. *Practice*, *42*(3), 377–391.

Moher, D., Shamseer, L., Clarke, M., Ghersi, D., Liberati, A., Petticrew, M., ... Stewart, L. A. (2015). Preferred reporting items for systematic review and meta-analysis protocols (PRISMA-P) 2015 statement. *Systematic Reviews*, *4*(1), 1. doi:10.1186/2046-4053-4-1 PMID:25554246

Munroe, S. (2001). *Developing a National Volunteer Registry of Persons with Deafblindness in Canada. Results from the study, 1999-2001*. Port Morien, Nova Scotia: Canadian Deafblind and Rubella Association.

Nussbaum, J. F., Thompson, T. L., & Robinson, J. D. (1989). Barriers to conversation. In J. F. Nussbaum, T. Thompson, & J. D. Robinson (Eds.), *Communication and aging*. New York: Harper & Row.

Padula, W. V. (1982). Low vision related to function and service delivery for the elderly. In *Ageing and Human Visual Function* (pp. 315–322). Alan R Lis Color Inc.

Patterson, C. (1994). Screening for visual impairment in the elderly. In Canadian Guide to Clinical Preventive Health Care (pp. 932-942). Ottawa: Health Canada.

Puts, M. T., Deeg, D. J., Hoeymans, N., Nusselder, W. J., & Schellevis, F. G. (2008). Changes in the prevalence of chronic disease and the association with disability in the older Dutch population between 1987 and 2001. *Age and Ageing*, *37*(2), 187–193. doi:10.1093/ageing/afm185 PMID:18250095

Raina, P., Wong, M., Dukeshire, S., Chambers, L. W., & Lindsay, J. (2000). Prevalence, risk factors and self-reported medical causes of seeing and hearing-related disabilities among older adults. *Canadian Journal on Aging*, *19*(02), 260–278. doi:10.1017/S0714980800014045

Saunders, G. H., & Echt, K. V. (2007). An overview of dual sensory impairment in older adults: Perspectives for rehabilitation. *Trends in Amplification*, *11*(4), 243–258. doi:10.1177/1084713807308365 PMID:18003868

Schiller, J. S., Lucas, J. W., & Peregoy, J. A. (2012). Summary health statistics for U.S. adults: National health interview survey. *Vital and Health Statistics*, *10*(252), 1–207. PMID:22834228

Schow, R. L., & Nerbonne, M. A. (1980). Hearing levels among elderly nursing home residents. *The Journal of Speech and Hearing Disorders*, *45*(1), 124–132. doi:10.1044/jshd.4501.124 PMID:7354624

Spandau, U. H. M., & Rohrschneider, K. (2002). Prevalence and geographical distribution of Usher syndrome in Germany. Graefe's archive for clinical and experimental ophthalmology. *Graefes Archive for Clinical and Experimental Ophthalmology*, *240*(6), 495–498. doi:10.1007/s00417-002-0485-8

Strawbridge, W. J., Wallhagen, M. I., Shema, S. J., & Kaplan, G. A. (2000). Negative consequences of hearing impairment in old age: A longitudinal analysis. *The Gerontologist*, *40*(3), 320–326. doi:10.1093/geront/40.3.320 PMID:10853526

Swenor, B. K., Ramulu, P. Y., Willis, J. R., Friedman, D., & Lin, F. R. (2013). The prevalence of concurrent hearing and vision impairment in the United States. Investigative Ophthalmology and Visual Science, 54(12), 7683-7690.

The American Speech-Language-Hearing Association. (ASHA) (2016). Hearing Screening. Retrieved from http://www.eventsinamerica.com/events/2016-asha-convention-american-speech-language-hearing-association/ev51362a573a0ed/

U.S. Department of Health and Human Services. (1995). Vital and health statistics, Current estimates from the National Health Interview Survey.

Watson, G. R. (2001). Low vision in the geriatric population: Rehabilitation and management. *Journal of the American Geriatrics Society*, *49*(3), 317–330. doi:10.1046/j.1532-5415.2001.4930317.x PMID:11300245

Watters, C., Owen, M., & Munroe, S. (2005). *A Study of Deaf-Blind Demographics and Services in Canada*. North York, ON: Canadian National Society of the Deaf Blindness.

World Health Organization (WHO). (2014). Visual Impairment and Blindness. Retrieved from http://www.who.int/mediacentre/factsheets/fs282/en/

Worrall, L., & Hickson, L. M. (2003). Theoretical foundations of communication disability in aging. In L.E. Worrall & L.M. Hickson (Eds.), Communication disability in aging: from prevention to intervention.

KEY TERMS AND DEFINITIONS

Ageing: Ageing is the process of becoming older.

Consequences: It is a result of a particular action or situation often one that is bad or not convenient.

Physiology: It is the scientific study of normal mechanisms and their interactions which works with in a living system.

Rehabilitation: It is a treatment or treatments designed for psychosocial aspects to facilitate the process of recovery from injury, illness or disease to as normal condition as possible.

Sensory Impairment: It refers to a defect in sensing and passing on the imulse. This leads to absense of sensation and neuronal coordination.

Chapter 15
Diabetes Mellitus and Aging

Jyoti Mishra Pandey
Government Medical College Chandigarh, India

Preeti Mishra
SMI Medical College and Hospital, India

ABSTRACT

Aging mirrors all the changes that occur over the period of life. It comes with various changes both positive and negative. Among all medical illnesses, Diabetes Mellitus is one of the most common and serious medical condition that has affected not only the aging population but also the young children and adults as well. Diabetes and its complications can contribute to aging process in a number of ways and the complications can speed up the aging process as well. For people with type 2 diabetes managing their emotional health can be as important as keeping their blood sugar under control. Patients with diabetes mellitus need psychological support throughout their life span from the time of diagnosis. However, provision of psychosocial support is generally inadequate due to its challenging nature of needs and demands on the healthcare systems. The present chapter will cover different aspects of diabetes mellitus and its impact on human life and also how with healthy coping mechanism one can prevent the distressing effect of diabetes on aging and vice versa.

INTRODUCTION

Health is a crown that the healthy wears, but only the sick can see it (Imam Shafiee)

Diabetes is a major health concern in both developing and developed countries. A person with diabetes under goes significant emotional and psychological turmoil like distress, anxiety and depression. This illness which is chronic in nature requires a constant effort for healthy life management. Among all medical illnesses, Diabetes Mellitus is one of the most common and serious medical condition that has affected not only the aging population but also the young children and adults as well. For people with diabetes managing their emotional health can be as important as keeping their blood sugar under control. Patients with diabetes mellitus need psychological support throughout their life span beginning from the time of diagnosis. The psychological make-up of the patients with diabetes mellitus plays a

DOI: 10.4018/978-1-5225-3480-8.ch015

central role in self-management behaviors. Without patient's adherence to the effective therapies, there would be persistent sub-optimal control of the disease, increased diabetes-related complications, causing deterioration in quality of life, resulting in increased healthcare utilization and burden on healthcare systems. So, preventing the disastrous effect of diabetes especially in elderly becomes important as they are more prone to various bio-psychosocial changes and its consequences.

India had more than 91.6 million elderly in 2010 with an annual addition of 2.5 million elderly between 2005 and 2010. The number of elderly in India is projected to reach 158.7 million in 2025 (United Nations Department of Economic and Social Affairs, 2008), and is expected, by 2050, to surpass the population of children below 14 years (Raju, 2006). Genetic loading, unhealthy life styles and obesity remain significant contributors towards developing diabetes. The disease burden is huge as exemplified by the World Health Organization report of 2016 which states that diabetes caused 1.5 million deaths in 1 year. Higher-than-optimal blood glucose caused an additional 2.2 million deaths, by increasing the risks of cardiovascular and other diseases. Forty-three percent of these 3.7 million deaths occur before the age of 70 years. The percentage of deaths attributable to high blood glucose or diabetes that occurs prior to age 70 is higher in low- and middle-income countries than in high-income countries (WHO, 2016). The global prevalence of type 2 diabetes mellitus is rapidly growing as a consequence of life-style changes, urbanization and population aging (Chen et al., 2011). The American Diabetes Association (ADA, 2014) has classified diabetes into four categories: Type 1 diabetes mellitus, caused by autoimmune destruction of the pancreatic beta cells; type 2 diabetes mellitus, itself a highly diverse group of disorders involving insulin resistance combined with relative insulin deficiency; gestational diabetes mellitus; and other specific types, another heterogeneous group which includes, among others, forms of diabetes resulting from the inheritance of a mutation in a single gene (monogenic diabetes). The majority of people with diabetes are affected by type 2 diabetes. It is a chronic illness that occurs either when the pancreas does not produce enough insulin or when the body cannot efficiently use the insulin it produces. Children normally suffer from type 1 diabetes whereas adult and elderly often suffers from type 2 diabetes. The ground of type 1 diabetes is unknown and is currently not preventable. The symptomatology of type 1 DM includes excessive urination, thirst, constant hunger, weight loss, fatigability and vision changes. The sign and symptoms of type 2 diabetes may be similar to those of type 1 diabetes, but are often less manifested or even absent. Therefore, the disease may go undiagnosed for several years, until complications have already takes place.

Diabetes mellitus is among those hazardous factors that affects the aging person. Since aging itself brings various physical and psychological changes in the person, diabetes mellitus becomes an additional factor to their overall physical and psychological changes. Aging as a whole causes changes throughout the entire body; basal metabolic rate, the amount of energy required declines with age. As they age and more the time passes, their body slowly becomes less adaptive at using glucose from the bloodstream, their visual acuity declines and so as the hearing ability. Other cognitive abilities and higher executive functioning, such as spatial ability, complex problem solving, and working memory, reasoning, planning all tend to decline to some extent with age.

Diabetes and aging are often associated with various psychological and emotional states. This is a condition where people know that there is no looking- back followed by various emotional symptoms like;

- Difficulty in accepting the diagnosis
- Don't want to discuss
- Decrease self-care

- Sleep disturbances
- Weight loss
- Difficulty in concentration
- Fatigability
- Thought of diabetes is overpowering
- Losing interest in pleasurable activities
- Withdrawal from near and dear ones
- Suicidal ideation and self-destructive behavior

AGING AND DIABETES

There are multiple factors that contribute to aging. Aging in-turn itself contributes to various illnesses and to its complications. Diabetes' input to the aging process occurs in a number of ways; cardiovascular disease can age nearly any tissue in the body by diminishing its blood supply, eye disease related to diabetes, including retinopathy, macular edema, and cataracts, can worsen already fading eyesight, diabetes related nerve disease can complicate the arthritis that comes with age, sometimes allowing greater joint erosion in the foot, and kidney disease can speed the decline in kidney function often seen with age. Hypoglycemia (low blood glucose) is one of the important concerns in elderly with diabetes. This population is prone to low blood glucose level because of the multiple drugs intake which may cause hypoglycemia, impaired glucose counter regulation, greater risk for an age-related decline in liver and kidney function, poor appetites and infrequent meals, all these factors may predispose to the elderly diabetics in developing hypoglycemia. It is one of those conditions that also speed up the aging process. On the other side, aging can make diabetes more difficult to control. One factor for this could be that insulin resistance increases and glucose tolerance decreases with age. With age, a person finds it difficult to focus attention and also faces difficulty in sustaining attention. As a result, they face difficulty in paying attention to the management required in diabetes, for example; meal planning, blood glucose monitoring, carbohydrate counting and intake of insulin and its correct doses. However, in today's scenario because of the better health approaches and services people with diabetes now have more opportunity to live longer than ever before.

CONSEQUENCES OF DIABETES ON AGING

Negligence in diabetes can have lethal consequences. Acute complications are a significant contributor to death, costs and poor quality of life. Significantly low blood glucose can occur in all types of diabetes and may result in seizures or loss of consciousness. There are various consequences of diabetes that affects aging;

Medical/Physical Consequences

Diabetes, a medical condition, affects various part of the body. It can damage the heart, blood vessels, eyes, kidneys and nerves. It can also increase the risk of heart attack, stroke, kidney failure, limb amputation, vision loss and nerve damage. Diabetes is one of the leading causes of kidney failure. Overweight, obesity and physical inactivity are estimated to cause a large percentage of the global diabetes burden (Global Burden of Disease (GBD), 2013). Studies have found an association between diabetes and cognitive decline on repeated neuropsychological tests in elderly (Gregg et al., 2000; Fontbonne et al., 2001). Additionally, diabetes doubles the overall risk of dementia. The specific association with Alzheimer's disease may be weaker and the association with stroke mediated dementia considerably stronger (Gregg et al., 2000; Fontbonne et al., 2001; Ott et al., 1996 & Luchsinger et al., 2001). It is also seen that diabetic women became physically disabled at approximately twice the rate of non-diabetic women and have an increased risk of falls and hip fractures (Schwartz et al., 2001; Gregg et al., 2002). The medical consequences in elderly with diabetes doubles because of the influence of behavioral factors like physical inactivity, inadequate sleep and poor life style. Uncontrolled diabetes can lead to poor health status and has been associated with disability, various other conditions like micro and macrovascular complications, and can also result in premature death as well (Krag et al., 2016). The management of this elderly population will be difficult because of the several other diseases and necessitation of numerous medications, however, prevention of secondary cardiovascular disease, weight loss and screening for depressive disorder and its treatment may help prevent disability that occurs in elderly with diabetes.

Psychological Consequences

Physical and medical condition of diabetes affects the mental health of the individual. Co-occurring psychiatric disorders in patients with diabetes are associated with impaired quality of life (Goldney et al., 2004), increased cost of care (Hutter et al., 2010), poor treatment adherence (Gonzalez et al., 2007), poor glycemia control (evidenced by elevated HbA1c levels) (Lustman, 2000), increased emergency room visits due to diabetic ketoacidosis, (Bryden, 2003), higher frequency of hospitalization, and higher rate of absenteeism (Das-Munshi et al., 2007).Co-morbidity of diabetes and depression correspond to a major clinical challenge as the outcomes of each condition are worsened by the presence of the other (Holt &Katon, 2012).Prevalence rates for elevated depressive symptoms range from 12–27% across studies of people with type 1 and type 2 diabetes, while rates of depressive disorders, as assessed by psychiatric interview protocols, range from 8–15% in adults with type 1 and type 2 diabetes (Anderson & Freedland, 2001; Pouweret al., 2013). Rates of diabetes-related distress have been shown to be higher (54%) than rates of psychiatrically diagnosed depression (Weissberg-Benchell & Antisdel-Lomaglio, 2011). As the elderly with diabetes and other co-morbid chronic conditions increases, outcomes such as cognitive and physical disability will become a greater distress because of their effect on their quality of life, loss of independence and demands on families or caregivers.

Psychological wellbeing and health are closely related and become more essential with older people because the chance for the occurrence of chronic illness increases with advancing age. Similarly, psychological state is affected by many factors other than health such as environmental conditions, social and family relationships, social roles and activities, these factors also change with age. Psychological wellbeing may even be a protective factor in health, reducing the risk of chronic physical illness and promoting longevity. It has also been argued that psychological wellbeing should be addressed in measures of health appraisal, and be considered in health care resource allocation (Dolan & White, 2007).

Social Consequences

There is a complex relationship between Type 2 diabetes and social determinants of health. Social factors are often related with the unequal development of chronic conditions and challenges encountered when managing medical conditions, particularly in Type 2 diabetes (Bryant et al. 2010).The major social factors affecting diabetes mellitus include; socioeconomic status (Krishnam et al., 2009), health education (Cooper et al., 2003; Brown et al., 1996), religion (Naeem, 2003), ethnicity (Bastid& Pagan, 2002), family (Grunnet, 2008), age (Kumar et al., 2008), education, locality or location (Azuamah et al., 2013). Earlier the main focus of diabetes management remained the behavioral and biologic such as diet and physical activity but now it is equally important to tackle the influence of physical and social environments, such as; poor income, unemployment or employment insecurity, low educational attainment and poor living conditions, on health outcomes. The main factor that contributes to Type II diabetes in lower status is nutrition, education and physical inactivity. The socially and economically disadvantaged are also at elevated risk for diabetes (Jacobs & Johnson 2001). It is seen that unemployment affects the physical health of the individual. It is reported that among adults aged 45 to 64 years, for example, 49% of diabetics are unemployed, compared with only 28% of non-diabetics (Krishnam et al., 2009). Religion, itself, has also a significant role to play in various physical health conditions. It has seen that more religious people had lower pressure, less hypertension, more compliance to treatment and follow-up and minimal utilization of healthcare (Naeem, 2003).

Social stigma is also associated with diabetes like losing jobs, not being employed or promoted, or experiences difficulty with insurances. The qualitative studies showed that they experience unjustified unequal treatment and exclusion due to their diabetes also in other contexts of their lives (Gredig & Bartelsen-Raemy, 2016), Other experiences include travel restrictions, broken friendships and restrictions against becoming an adoptive parent (Browne et al. 2013). High quality care is crucial but faces many institutional and financial barriers, particularly for individuals in long-term care (Huskamp et al., 2011). Growing number of recognition to the social determinants of health and their contribution to health disparities accepted the need to consider the social determinants of diabetes and health along with other individual factors.

Economic Consequences

Diabetes has a significant contribution in economic burden. Medical costs in diabetes comprise expenses for preventing and treating diabetes and its related complications. In a recent systematic review, it has been estimated that the direct annual cost of diabetes to the world is more than US$ 827 billion (NCD Risk Factor Collaboration, 2009; Seuring & Archangelidi, 2015). Federation (IDF) estimates that total global health-care spending on diabetes more than tripled over the period 2003 to 2013 – the result of increases in the number of people with diabetes and increases in per capita diabetes spending (International Diabetes Federation, 2013).Cost of care for non-mental health conditions among patients with co-occurring psychiatric disorders and endocrinal disorders is twofold or even higher (depending on the treatment setting) than the population without co-occurring psychiatric disorders (Centorrino et al., 2009). The average medical expenses for patients with diabetes are nearly twice as high as those for patients who do not have diabetes (National diabetes statistics, 2011). These increased financial pressures put burden not only to the care takers but also have a significant impact upon the elderly. The finances involved in managing elderly with aging are not only related to medications but also to the additional support or care they require.

FACTORS AFFECTING DIABETES AND AGING

There are various factors that contribute to diabetes. These are:

Personality

Personality of the individual remains an essential factor to study while dealing with any medical and psychiatric illnesses. Personality factors emerge as potential vulnerability factor for adverse health outcomes. Individuals with type-2 diabetes had higher levels of depressive and anxiety symptoms. Individuals with type-2 diabetes experience more psychological distress and have different personality traits compared to individuals without type-2 diabetes (Van Dooren, 2016). A study has shown that Type D personality refers to the combination of negative affectivity, a tendency to experience negative emotions and social inhibition, a tendency to inhibit self-expression (Denoll et al., 2005). Few studies have explored the potential behavioral and biological mechanisms that may link Type D with adverse health outcomes in individuals with type 2 diabetes (Nefs et al., 2012; Conti, et al., 2016). Study showed that type D personality was more prevalent in type 2 diabetes, while personality traits like extraversion, agreeableness, consciousness and emotional stability were slightly less prevalent (Van Dooren et al., 2016). The relationship between personality traits and diabetes were mediated by body mass index (BMI), alcohol intake, physical inactivity and dietary habits or life style.

Medication and other treatments improve symptoms of most common chronic diseases to some extent, but a considerable percentage of individuals with chronic diseases do not follow their prescribed treatments (Osterberg & Blaschke, 2005), which weakens the effectiveness of available medical care. Some people even after available treatment care are sloppy in its use but some are able to adjust to the illness over a period of time, which means diabetes is not always associated with psychiatric and psychological problems. Many studies have shown that people tend to regain their earlier levels of well-being after negative life events (Clark et al. 2008; Powdthavee, 2009; Davydov et al., 2010), although this is not always the case (Headey, 2010). Previous studies have reported declining levels of extraversion, conscientiousness and openness to experience with age (Lucas & Donnellan, 2011; Wortman et al. 2012). On the other hand, emotional stability and related traits have been shown to increase (Wortman et al., 2012) or remain stable (Lucas & Donnellan, 2011) in adulthood at least up to the age of 70 years, after which levels of negative affectivity may increase again (Baird et al., 2010; Jokela et al., 2013). This could be because of difficulty in coping with the emotional, behavioral and cognitive challenges. Therefore, understanding personality and its relation to disease onset and management is of supreme importance in planning successful intervention strategies in person with diabetes. Personality traits also help a clinician to understand whether the person will be successful in managing diabetes and its aging related consequences or not because as we age our personality forms a rigid habit and changing these habits in old age is another complicated task as they are already facing additional problems because of aging. However, knowing about personality and its consequences can help a person to prevent perilous complication because of diabetes.

Comorbid Conditions

Diabetes is often accompanied with a range of other illnesses and conditions, which further have a significant impact on its management. Dementia, Cognitive decline (Velayudhan et al., 2010), reduced muscle strength and quality (Volpato et al., 2012), disability (Volpato et al., 2003; Gregg et al., 2000), falls and fall-related morbidity (Schwartz et al. 2002; Strotmeyer et al., 2005), urinary incontinence (Brown et al., 2006), these conditions are very frequent in older diabetic people, especially in the weak ones. When present they exert a negative effect on the mental health, quality of life and mortality. It is a known risk factor for tuberculosis (Jeon & Murray, 2008) and is associated with poorer tuberculosis outcomes, while tuberculosis is associated with worsening glycemic control (Riza et al., 2014).Diabetes Mellitus is one of the leading causes of kidney failure, non-traumatic lower-limb amputations, and new cases of blindness among adults and is the seventh leading cause of death in the United States, killing more than 1.4 million people worldwide in 2011 (WHO, 2013).Ageing-related conditions such as decline in cognitive abilities and physical disability or decline in physical strength have emerged as frequent co-morbid conditions with diabetes.

Depression is two to three times more common in people with diabetes than in those without depression (Roy & Lloyd, 2012). Nefs et al. (2012) showed that 66% of individuals with type 2 diabetes who had a high depression score, still had a high score two to three years later. Furthermore, multiple studies have linked depression to a variety of adverse health outcomes among individuals with type 2 diabetes, like a reduced quality of life (Schram et al., 2009), less optimal self-care behaviors and higher HbA_{1c} levels (Pouwe et al., 2013), a higher risk of micro- and macrovascular complications (De Groot et al., 2001), higher mortality rates (Van Dooren et al., 2013) and increased health care costs (Hutter et al., 2010). Similar to depression, anxiety disorders typically have a chronic and recurrent life course, elevated anxiety symptoms and disorders in type 2 diabetes have been associated with reduced quality of life (Chyun et al., 2006), poor glycemic control (Lloyd et al., 2000; Balhara&Sagar, 2011) and diabetes complications (Collins et al., 2009).

The increasing longevity of HIV/AIDS patients is accompanied by a rising incidence and prevalence of insulin resistance and type 2 diabetes, some of which may be related to antiretroviral treatment (Oni et al. 2015; Reid et al., 2012). Co-morbidity of psychiatric disorder with diabetes shares a bidirectional association. Both the disorder can be present independently or can be co-morbid. Various biological and psychological conditions contribute to the emergence of psychiatric disorders.

Life Style

Poor life style such as; poor nutrition, overweight, increased rates of poor health behaviors such as smoking and alcohol consumption, stress, and limited access to health care, particularly in middle age when many individuals are at highest risk for developing diabetes (Buddy, 2006; Klein, 2011). Most lifestyle factors are related to depression as well and have adverse health outcomes in diabetes. Adults with Diabetes are generally seen as a high-risk group partially because they experience many stressful changes in their lives, such as searching for a job, adjustment and establishing relationships (Peters &

Laffel, 2011; Arnett, 2000). Such demands could interfere and even distract from focused diabetes management and a particular life style. Preventing complications and minimizing the risk of early mortality require modifications of lifestyle behaviors (Mondesir et al., 2015; Lipscombe et al., 2016). This treatment involves adherence to medication, improved diet, active lifestyle, self-monitoring blood glucose level, and good communication with health-care professionals.

DIABETICS AND MENTAL HEALTH

Diabetes is a life-long chronic medical condition that requires regular self-management. This situation affects the emotional and psychological well-being of the individual. Whole life pattern changes when a person comes to know about his illness; alteration in the pattern of eating habits, self-care, how much insulin is required, when and what kind of exercise to be done, how to interpret a glucose reading and so on. The "psychological burden hypothesis" states that the burden of knowing that one has diabetes, the management of having a chronic illness, or having complications to cope with, contribute to higher levels of depression (Talbot &Nouwen, 2000). A meta-analysis showed that the occurrence of depression was particularly increased in known type 2 diabetes, but not in persons with screen-detected type 2 diabetes (who were unaware about the diabetes) (Nouwen et al., 2011). Self-management in diabetes is known to be burden to the elderly person, as it requires constant effort to adapt every day activities like diet, exercise and rest, to medication use and glucose levels (Sullivan et al., 2005). Insulin therapy may be associated with increased psychological distress (Delahanty et al., 2007) because it becomes difficult to accept that they have to shift from oral medication to insulin. This can also cause functional limitations like reduced mobility, visual impairments, fatigue, pain and also poor quality of life (Rubin et al., 1999).

Managing diabetes in everyday of life is not an easy task, it makes a person more frustrated and depressed. When we talk about mental health, families and relationships have a significant role to play. However, having Type II diabetes changes life and affects the relationships as well. Diabetes management requires a lot of focus and attention which further becomes a responsibility for a spouse or a partner. A recent study of people whose partner had type II diabetes found that those who tried to exert control over their partner's dietary habit felt particularly stressed and burdened (Cornelis et al., 2013). The emotional strain of dealing will diabetes can cause stress and anxiety as well as communication difficulties that can lead to sexual dysfunction in relationship (Azuamah et al., 2012). People with diabetes seek mental health professional's help because of the difficulty to deal with the diabetes changes and the way it hampers the mental health. Staying with the treatment plan and taking care of themselves becomes important for some people but for other people it becomes an obstacle in living a life, the way they want to, which results in depression, anxiety, frustration and helplessness.

GENDER PERSPECTIVE

Type 2 diabetes mellitus is a chronic disease affecting 9.7 million women and 10.9 million men among middle age and older adults in United States (Correa-de-Araujo et al., 2006; Mondesir et al., 2015). Middle aged diabetics are more than half and incidence rises with increasing ages in both genders, reaching highest rates in the very old women. However, globally more males are diagnosed with diabetes.

Social factors, like low educational level, occupation and income largely contribute to unhealthy lifestyle behavior and thus are related to higher risk of diabetic mellitus particularly in women (Lee et al., 2013; Kautzky-Willer et al., 2012). The psychological component like unpaid housework and responsibilities in the family may contribute to feelings of conflicting demands and sustained stress levels in females, even in highly educated groups of employees (Lundberg, 2005; Berntsson et al., 2006). Discrimination, biasness, roles and responsibilities may further increase the environmental psychosocial stress and stress responses especially in women.

There is a significant difference in the way both genders experiences and manages diabetes, particularly in their beliefs, attitudes, fears and concerns about the disease. Women more often than men, view diabetes as negatively affecting their lives. At diagnosis, more women reported fearing loss of health, diabetes-related morbidity, and early mortality compared to men. Women report significantly more depressive symptoms, which can lower their participation in diabetes education and medication compliance (Park et al., 2004). Men are more concerned that diabetes will limit their lifestyles but also believes that it is controllable. Men report being more concerned about how diabetes affects their role, whereas women worry more about how self-care will hinder their familial responsibilities, and they also tend to sacrifice their dietary regimen for their family's food preferences (Mathew et al., 2012). So, the biggest hurdle to the diabetes management among women might include lack of self-confidence, aging related other complications and inadequate family and social support.

MANAGEMENT OF DIABETES IN AGING

A person diagnosed with diabetic mellitus can live a healthy and well-balanced life if proper and healthy life style has been followed. In comparison to type 1 diabetes, type 2 diabetes is largely preventable. There are some pharmacological and non-pharmacological approaches for the management of diabetes in aging:

Pharmacological Approach

Type 1 diabetes cannot be prevented with current knowledge. Effective therapeutic techniques are available to prevent or to cope with type 2 diabetes. Evidence suggests that both aging and environmental factors contribute to the high prevalence of diabetes in the elderly. Clinical management of diabetes in elderly presents challenges because of the multifaceted geriatric scenario. It significantly lowers the chances of "successful" aging. So, optimizing medicine approach is essential in the care of an older person with diabetes. In line with the Quality Use of Medicines Framework, three key steps should be considered in drug prescription: 1) to identify the best treatment (considering non-pharmacological measures whenever possible); 2) to select medicines cleverly (considering the possibility of serious adverse effects or drug-to-drug interactions); and 3) to use medicines based on the strongest clinical evidences (Hilmer et al., 2007). Likewise, three subgroups of older patients should be considered: 1) those who are relatively healthy; 2) those with complex medical histories in whom self-care may be difficult, and 3) those with a significant comorbidities and functional impairment (Blaum et al., 2010; Laiteerapong et al., 2012). Thus, clinicians caring for older diabetic patients have to solve a therapeutic dilemma: balancing the patient's needs while taking into consideration health profile and glycemic goals and avoiding adverse effects.

Non-Pharmacological Approach

Aging mirrors all the changes that occur over the course of life. We grow and reach to maturity. To the young, aging is exciting but middle age also is the time when people begin to notice a fair amount of physical decline. Even the physically fit cannot escape from these changes. These process of aging goes through various physical and mental changes and also accompany various medical and mental health complications. Diabetes is so prevalent that aging and developing diabetes is almost synonymous in current scenario. So, when we talk about the non-pharmacological management of diabetes the primary input to this is healthy life style for everyone similar to primary prevention, regardless of any age or any medical condition like diabetes, such as, exercising regularly, healthy eating habit, avoiding smoking, and controlling blood pressure and lipids can prevent various complications in patients with diabetes. Another form of managing diabetes in elderly is psychotherapy in which various therapeutic approaches like CBT, relaxation exercises, mindfulness meditations, stress and tension reduction techniques can improve the mental health of the person aging with diabetes. Family therapy can play a vital role in reducing the care giver burden, helping them to understand the diabetic condition associated with aging. Solutions focused and behavioral management can be helpful in handling the present condition or problem where the issues of financial burden can be managed. Healthy coping and positive attribution can be incorporated in the management plan. Personality is dynamic in nature and not a static component. So, working on unhealthy personality traits and habits can improve the diabetic condition in elderly. Studies have shown that group-based diabetes self-management education (DSME) in people with type 2 diabetes results in improvements in clinical, lifestyle and psychosocial outcomes (Steinsbekk et al., 2012). So, psychotherapeutic management for diabetes and associated conditions can prevent various catastrophic consequences of diabetes mellitus in elderly.

SOLUTIONS AND RECOMMENDATIONS

There are number of ways to offset some of the venomous effects of diabetes and aging, further can add healthy days in the older years. Before following the below mentioned recommendations it is important to understand that elderly with diabetes is not the only condition that affects the physical and mental health because there are many associated old age changes and diabetes is only one additional factor to the fixed changes that occurs in aging. These recommendations are;

- It is Important to have a regular monitoring of blood glucose levels of elderly, especially for those who are prone to additional complications of diabetes.
- Maintain a standard body weight because obesity contributes significantly to not only diabetes, but also to various other medical conditions like heart disease, stroke, and osteoarthritis.
- Be physically and mentally active because that can counter many effects of aging. Physical activities like regular exercises such as running, walking, bicycling, and swimming, is known to help maintaining blood glucose levels in people with diabetes. Similarly, staying mentally active is important too. It incorporates staying connected with your surroundings, maintaining good interpersonal relationships, and an effort to learn new things. The physical exercises of the elderly should be under consulting physician's supervision.

- It is recommended by WHO (2010) that adults aged 18–64 years should do at least 150 minutes of moderate-intensity aerobic physical activity (for example brisk walking, jogging, gardening) spread throughout the week, or at least 75 minutes of vigorous-intensity aerobic physical activity throughout the week, or an equivalent combination of moderate- and vigorous-intensity activity.
- For older adults the same amount of physical activity is recommended, but should also include balance and muscle strengthening activity tailored to their ability and circumstances (WHO, 2010).
- Maintain or practice healthy eating style because what you eat will determine how you age. Elderly with diabetes should maintain a proper meal plan in order to maintain appropriate weight, improve the blood glucose level and control the blood lipid levels.
- Practicing meditation and yoga helps improve the mental and physical health of all ages. Adding this habit to aging population can prevent various additional hurdles to healthy aging.
- Have a sound sleep because inadequate sleep can directly affect the physical health because sleep deprivation can lead to insulin resistance, which can make diabetes more difficult to control and may even raise the risk of heart disease.
- Keep a check on medicines and the prescribed doses and related side effects. This will require a regular check up to the consulting doctor because this can prevent any major catastrophe. This includes regular medical checkups, eye examinations, kidney tests, foot exams, dentist office visits, and vaccinations etc.
- Stick to a particular doctor because he will be aware of your disease progress report. Changing the doctors affects the routine management that an elderly diabetic requires.
- Stop unhealthy practices like smoking and drinking because smoking ages the tissues of the body and drinking may cause various cardiovascular disease, bone loss and psychiatric conditions such as depression, sleep problems and anxiety.
- Cognitive Behavior Therapy (CBT) can be an effective mode of management for treating co-morbid depression and other psychiatric and psychological conditions in diabetic patients.
- Mindfulness-based stress reduction techniques can also be an effective mode of management in elderly.
- Provide a supportive environment (family and social) to the aging population with diabetes which can play an essential role to have a healthy aging with diabetes. All that they required is affection, care and respect.

CONCLUSION

Aging is unavoidable and so are some diseases or medical conditions. However, a person can have some control over how well he/she can age. Access to adequate health care plays an even stronger role in controlling diabetes, preventing the development of complications to aging. By doing few things a person can stop or decrease the devastating effects associated with age and diabetes and can live an energetic life. There is no single policy or intervention that can ensure or prevent the effect of diabetic mellitus. It requires a holistic approach. Social, psychological and economical determinants of health and diabetes need to be considered when focusing on improving diabetes outcomes.

You're going to carry this illness for the rest of your life. So you can either wallow in the weight of that, or you can fight for your only life and make it a good story. ...LyssTrayers

REFERENCES

American Diabetes Association. (2014). Diagnosis and classification of diabetes mellitus. *Diabetes Care, 37*(1), 81-90.

Anderson, R. J., Freedland, K. E., Clouse, R. E., & Lustman, P. J. (2001). The prevalence of comorbid depression in adults with diabetes: A meta-analysis. *Diabetes Care*, *24*(6), 1069–1078. doi:10.2337/diacare.24.6.1069 PMID:11375373

Arnett, J. J. (2000). Emerging adulthood: A theory of development from the late teens through the twenties. *The American Psychologist*, *55*(5), 469–480. doi:10.1037/0003-066X.55.5.469 PMID:10842426

Azuamah, Y. C., Imaseun, A. F., Onoseta, O. H., & Onuoha, P. C. (2013). A review of sociological factors associated with diabetes mellitus. *The International Journal of Social Sciences (Islamabad)*, *11*(1), 131–137.

Baird, B. M., Lucas, R. E., & Donnellan, M. B. (2010). Life satisfaction across the lifespan: Findings from two nationally representative panel studies. *Social Indicators Research*, *99*(2), 183–203. doi:10.1007/s11205-010-9584-9 PMID:21113322

Balhara, Y. P., & Sagar, R. (2011). Correlates of anxiety and depression among patients with type 2 diabetes mellitus. *Indian Journal of Endocrinology and Metabolism*, *15*(5 Suppl. 1), S50–S54. doi:10.4103/2230-8210.83057 PMID:21847456

Bastid, E., & Pagan, J. A. (2002). Impact of Diabetes on adult employment and earning of Mexican American finding from a community based study. *Health Economics*, *11*(5), 403–413. doi:10.1002/hec.676 PMID:12112490

Berntsson, L., Lundberg, U., & Krantz, G. (2006). Gender differences in work-home interplay and symptom perception among Swedish white-collar employees. *Journal of Epidemiology and Community Health*, *60*(12), 1070–1076. doi:10.1136/jech.2005.042192 PMID:17108304

Blaum, C., Cigolle, C. T., Boyd, C., Wolff, J. L., Tian, Z., Langa, K. M., & Weir, D. R. (2010). Clinical complexity in middle-aged and older adults with diabetes: The Health and Retirement Study. *Medical Care*, *48*(4), 327–334. doi:10.1097/MLR.0b013e3181ca4035 PMID:20355264

Brown, J. S., Vittinghoff, E., Lin, F., Nyberg, L. M., Kusek, J. W., & Kanaya, A. M. (2006). Prevalence and risk factors for urinary incontinence in women with type 2 diabetes and impaired fasting glucose: Findings from the National Health and Nutrition Examination Survey (NHANES) 2001-2002. *Diabetes Care*, *29*(6), 1307–1312. doi:10.2337/dc05-2463 PMID:16732013

Brown, S. A., Upchurch, S., Anding, R., Winter, M., & Ramirez, G. (1996). Promoting weight loss in Type II diabetes. *Diabetes Care*, *19*(3), 613–624. doi:10.2337/diacare.19.6.613 PMID:8725861

Browne, J. L., Ventura, A., Mosely, K., & Speight, J. (2013). I call it the blame and the shame disease: A qualitative study about perceptions of social stigma surrounding type 2 diabetes. *BMJ Open*, *3*(11), 1–10. doi:10.1136/bmjopen-2013-003384 PMID:24247325

Bryant, T., Daiski, I., & Lines, E. (2010). Type 2 diabetes: poverty, priorities and policy: the social determinants of the incidence and management of Type 2 diabetes [monograph on the Internet] Toronto, Ontario, Canada: York University School of Health Policy and Management; Retrieved March 16, 2017 from www.hpclearinghouse.ca/pdf/Diabetes%20Fact%20Sheet%202010%20-%20March%2016%20-%20 final%20.pdf

Bryden, K. S., Dunger, D. B., Mayou, R. A., Peveler, R. C., & Neil, H. A. (2003). Poor prognosis of young adults with type 1 diabetes: A longitudinal study. *Diabetes Care*, *26*(4), 1052–1057. doi:10.2337/diacare.26.4.1052 PMID:12663572

Buddy, T. (2006). Drinking alcohol and diabetes. Retrieved from http://alcoholism.about.com

Centorrino, F., Mark, T. L., Talamo, A., Oh, K., & Chang, J. (2009). Health and economic burden of metabolic comorbidity among individuals with bipolar disorder. *Journal of Clinical Psychopharmacology*, *29*(6), 595–600. doi:10.1097/JCP.0b013e3181bef8a6 PMID:19910727

Chen, L., Magliano, D. J., & Zimmet, P. Z. (2011). The worldwide epidemiology of type 2 diabetes mellitus--present and future perspectives. *Nature Reviews. Endocrinology*, *8*(4), 228–236. doi:10.1038/nrendo.2011.183 PMID:22064493

Chyun, D. A., Melkus, G. D., Katten, D. M., Price, W. J., Davey, J. A., & Grey, N. (2006). The association of psychological factors, physical activity, neuropathy, and quality of life in type 2 diabetes. *Biological Research for Nursing*, *7*(4), 279–288. doi:10.1177/1099800405285748 PMID:16581898

Clark, A. E., Diener, E., Georgellis, Y., & Lucas, R. E. (2008). Lags and leads in life satisfaction: A test of the baseline hypothesis. *Economic Journal (London)*, *118*(529), F222–F243. doi:10.1111/j.1468-0297.2008.02150.x

Collins, M. M., Corcoran, P., & Perry, I. J. (2009). Anxiety and depression symptoms in patients with diabetes. *Diabetic Medicine*, *26*(2), 153–161. doi:10.1111/j.1464-5491.2008.02648.x PMID:19236618

Conti, C., Carrozzino, D., Patierno, C., Vitacolonna, E., & Fulcheri, M. (2016). The Clinical Link between Type D Personality and Diabetes. *Frontiers in Psychiatry*, *7*, 113. doi:10.3389/fpsyt.2016.00113 PMID:27445869

Cooper, H. C., Booth, K., & Gill, G. (2003). Patients' perspectives on diabetes health care education. *Health Education Research*, *18*(2), 191–206. doi:10.1093/her/18.2.191 PMID:12729178

Cornelis, M. C., Glymour, M., Kawachi, I., & Chivue, S. (2013). Marital status and risk of type 2 diabetes in the health professionals. *American Heart Foundation*. Retrieved from http://www.ahajournals.org

Correa-de-Araujo, R., McDermott, K., & Moy, E. (2006). Gender differences across racial and ethnic groups in the quality of care for diabetes. *Women's Health Issues*, *16*(2), 56–65. doi:10.1016/j.whi.2005.08.003 PMID:16638522

Das-Munshi, J., Stewart, R., Ismail, K., Bebbington, P. E., Jenkins, R., & Prince, M. J. (2007). Diabetes, common mental disorders, and disability: Findings from the UK National Psychiatric Morbidity Survey. *Psychosomatic Medicine*, *69*(6), 543–550. doi:10.1097/PSY.0b013e3180cc3062 PMID:17636148

Davydov, D. M., Stewart, R., Ritchie, K., & Chaudieu, I. (2010). Resilience and mental health. *Clinical Psychology Review*, *30*(5), 479–495. doi:10.1016/j.cpr.2010.03.003 PMID:20395025

Delahanty, L. M., Grant, R. W., Wittenberg, E., Bosch, J. L., Wexler, D. J., Cagliero, E., & Meigs, J. B. (2007). Association of diabetes-related emotional distress with diabetes treatment in primary care patients with Type 2 diabetes. *Diabetic Medicine*, *24*(1), 48–54. doi:10.1111/j.1464-5491.2007.02028.x PMID:17227324

Denollet, J. (2005). DS14: Standard assessment of negative affectivity, social inhibition, and Type D personality. *Psychosomatic Medicine*, *67*(1), 89–97. doi:10.1097/01.psy.0000149256.81953.49 PMID:15673629

Dolan, P., & White, M. P. (2007). How can measures of subjective well-being be used to inform public policy? *Perspectives on Psychological Science*, *2*(1), 71–84. doi:10.1111/j.1745-6916.2007.00030.x PMID:26151920

Fontbonne, A., Berr, C., Ducimetiere, P., & Alperovitch, A. (2001). Changes in cognitive abilities over a 4-year period are unfavorably affected in elderly diabetic subjects: Results of the epidemiology of vascular aging study. *Diabetes Care*, *24*(2), 366–370. doi:10.2337/diacare.24.2.366 PMID:11213894

Global Burden of Disease (GBD). (2013). Risk Factors Collaborators. Global, regional, and national comparative risk assessment of 79 behavioral, environmental and occupational, and metabolic risks or clusters of risks in 188 countries, 1990–2013: a systematic analysis for the Global Burden of Disease Study 2013. *Lancet, 386*, 2287–323.

Goldney, R. D., Phillips, P. J., Fisher, L. J., & Wilson, D. H. (2004). Diabetes, depression, and quality of life: A population study. *Diabetes Care*, *27*(5), 1066–1070. doi:10.2337/diacare.27.5.1066 PMID:15111522

Gonzalez, J. S., Safren, S. A., Cagliero, E., Wexler, D. J., Delahanty, L., Wittenberg, E., ... Grant, R. W. (2007). Depression, self-care, and medication adherence in type 2 diabetes: Relationships across the full range of symptom severity. *Diabetes Care*, *30*(9), 2222–2227. doi:10.2337/dc07-0158 PMID:17536067

Gredig, D., & Bartelsen-Raemy, A. (2016). Diabetes-related stigma affects the quality of life of people living with diabetes mellitus in Switzerland: implications for healthcare providers. *Journal of Health & Social Care in the Community*. doi.10.1111/hsc.12376

Gregg, E. W., Beckles, G. L., Williamson, D. F., Leveille, S. G., Langlois, J. A., Engelgau, M. M., & Narayan, K. M. (2000). Diabetes and physical disability among older U.S. adults. *Diabetes Care*, *23*(9), 1272–1277. doi:10.2337/diacare.23.9.1272 PMID:10977018

Gregg, E. W., Mangione, C. M., Cauley, J. A., Thompson, T. J., Schwartz, A. V., Ensrud, K. E., & Nevitt, M. C. (2002). Diabetes and incidence of functional disability in older women. *Diabetes Care*, *25*(1), 61–67. doi:10.2337/diacare.25.1.61 PMID:11772902

Gregg, E. W., & Narayan, K. M. V. (2000). Type 2 diabetes and cognitive function: Are cognitive impairment and dementia complications of type 2 diabetes? *Clinics in Geriatric Medicine*, *8*, 57–72.

Grunnet, J. (2008). Heredity and Diabetes. *Annals of Internal Medicine*, *6*(10), 1272–1274.

Headey, B. (2010). The set point theory of well-being has serious flaws: On the eve of a scientific revolution? *Social Indicators Research*, *97*(1), 7–21. doi:10.1007/s11205-009-9559-x

Hilmer, S. N., McLachlan, A. J., & Le Couteur, D. G. (2007). Clinical pharmacology in the geriatric patient. *Fundamental & Clinical Pharmacology*, *21*(3), 217–230. doi:10.1111/j.1472-8206.2007.00473.x PMID:17521291

Holt, R. I., & Katon, W. J. (2012). Dialogue on Diabetes and Depression: Dealing with the double burden of co-morbidity. *Journal of Affective Disorders*, *142*, S1–S3. doi:10.1016/S0165-0327(12)00632-5 PMID:23062852

In Holt, R. I. G., de Groot, M., & Huang, E. S. (2007). Appropriate application of evidence to the care of elderly patients with diabetes. *Current Diabetes Reviews*, *3*(4), 260–263. doi:10.2174/157339981070304026 0 PMID:18220684

Huskamp, H. A., Kaufmann, C., & Stevenson, D. G. (2011). The intersection of long-term care and end-of-life care. *Medical Care Research and Review*, *69*(1), 3–44. doi:10.1177/1077558711418518 PMID:21903662

Hutter, N., Schnurr, A., & Baumeister, H. (2010). Healthcare costs in patients with diabetes mellitus and comorbid mental disorders--a systematic review. *Diabetologia*, *53*(12), 2470–2479. doi:10.1007/s00125-010-1873-y PMID:20700575

International Diabetes Federation (IDF). (2013). *Diabetes* (6th ed.). Brussels: Atlas.

Jacobs, P., & Johnson, J. A. (2001). Productivity Losses Associated with Diabetes in the US. *Diabetes Care*, *24*(3), 257–261. PMID:11213875

Jeon, C. Y., & Murray, M. B. (2008). Diabetes mellitus increases the risk of active tuberculosis: A systematic review of 13 observational studies. *PLoS Medicine*, *5*(7), e152. doi:10.1371/journal.pmed.0050152 PMID:18630984

Jokela, M., Batty, G. D., & Kivimäki, M. (2013). Ageing and the prevalence and treatment of mental health problems. *Psychological Medicine*, *43*(10), 2037–2045. doi:10.1017/S0033291712003042 PMID:23324208

Kautzky-Willer, A., Dorner, T., Jensby, A., & Rieder, A. (2012). Women show a closer association between educational level and hypertension or diabetes mellitus than males: A secondary analysis from the Austrian HIS. *BMC Public Health*, *12*(1), 392. doi:10.1186/1471-2458-12-392 PMID:22646095

Klein, J. (2011). How lifestyle habits affect diabetes. Retrieved from http://www.Life.guiam.com

Krag, M. O., Hasselbalch, L., Siersma, V., Nielsen, A. B., Reventlow, S., Malterud, K., & de Fine Olivarius, N. (2016). The impact of gender on the long-term morbidity and mortality of patients with type 2 diabetes receiving structured personal care: A 13 year follow-up study. *Diabetologia*, *59*(2), 275–285. doi:10.1007/s00125-015-3804-4 PMID:26607637

Krishnam, S., Cozier, Y., Rosenberg, L., & Palmer, J. (2009). Socioeconomic status and incidence of type 2 diabetes: Results from the black women's health study. *American Journal of Epidemiology*, *171*(5), 564–570. doi:10.1093/aje/kwp443 PMID:20133518

Kumar, V., Fausto, N., & Abbas, A. (2008). *Pathologic Basis of Disease* (7th ed., pp. 1189–1206). Saunders Company.

Laiteerapong, N., Iveniuk, J., John, P. M., Laumann, E. O., & Huang, E. S. (2012). Classification of older adults who have diabetes by comorbid conditions, United States, 2005-2006. *Preventing Chronic Disease*, *9*, 3–8. PMID:22595321

Lee, D. S., Kim, Y. J., & Han, H. R. (2013). Sex differences in the association between socio-economic status and type 2 diabetes: Data from the 2005 Korean National Health and Nutritional Examination Survey (KNHANES). *Public Health*, *127*(6), 554–560. doi:10.1016/j.puhe.2013.02.001 PMID:23706862

Lipscombe, C., Smith, K. J., Gariepy, G., & Schmitz, N. (2016). Gender differences in the association between lifestyle behaviors and diabetes distress in a community sample of adults with type 2 diabetes. *Journal of Diabetes*, *8*(2), 269–278. doi:10.1111/1753-0407.12298 PMID:25850582

Lloyd, C. E., Dyer, P. H., & Barnett, A. H. (2000). Prevalence of symptoms of depression and anxiety in a diabetes clinic population. *Diabetic Medicine*, *17*(3), 198–202. doi:10.1046/j.1464-5491.2000.00260.x PMID:10784223

Lucas, R. E., & Donnellan, M. B. (2011). Personality development across the life span: Longitudinal analyses with a national sample from Germany. *Journal of Personality and Social Psychology*, *101*(4), 847–861. doi:10.1037/a0024298 PMID:21707197

Luchsinger, J. A., Tang, M., Stern, Y., Shea, S., & Mayeux, R. (2001). Diabetes mellitus and risk of Alzheimer's disease and dementia with stroke in a multiethnic cohort. *American Journal of Epidemiology*, *154*(7), 635–641. doi:10.1093/aje/154.7.635 PMID:11581097

Lundberg, U. (2005). Stress hormones in health and illness: The roles of work and gender. *Psychoneuroendocrinology*, *30*(10), 1017–1021. doi:10.1016/j.psyneuen.2005.03.014 PMID:15963652

Lustman, P. J., Anderson, R. J., Freedland, K. E., de Groot, M., Carney, R. M., & Clouse, R. E. (2000). Depression and poor glycemic control: A meta-analytic review of the literature. *Diabetes Care*, *23*(7), 934–942. doi:10.2337/diacare.23.7.934 PMID:10895843

Mathew, R., Gucciardi, E., De Melo, M., & Barata, P. (2012). Self-management experiences among men and women with type 2 diabetes mellitus: A qualitative analysis. *BMC Family Practice*, *13*(1), 122. doi:10.1186/1471-2296-13-122 PMID:23249410

Mondesir, F. L., White, K., Liese, A. D., & McLain, A. C. (2015). Gender, illness-related diabetes social support, and glycemic control among middle-aged and older adults. *The Journals of Gerontology. Series B, Psychological Sciences and Social Sciences*, *71*(6), 1081–1088. doi:10.1093/geronb/gbv061 PMID:26307487

Naeem, A. G. (2003). The role of culture and religion in the management of diabetes: A study of Kashiri men in Leeds. *The Journal of the Royal Society for the Promotion of Health*, *123*(2), 110–116. doi:10.1177/146642400312300216 PMID:12852196

National Diabetes Statistics. (2011). *Department of Health and Human Services*. National Institutes of Health.

Hill, J., Nielsen, M., & Fox, M. H. (2013). Understanding the Social Factors That Contribute to Diabetes: A Means to Informing Health Care and Social Policies for the Chronically Ill. *The Permanente Journal*, *17*(2), 67–72. doi:10.7812/TPP/12-099

NCD Risk Factor Collaboration (NCD-RisC). (2016). Worldwide trends in diabetes since 1980: a pooled analysis of 751 population-based studies with 4*4 million participants. *Lancet*. doi:.10.1016/S0140-6736(16)00618-8

Nefs, G., Pouwer, F., Denollet, J., & Pop, V. (2012). The course of depressive symptoms in primary care patients with type 2 diabetes: Results from the Diabetes, Depression, Type D Personality Zuidoost-Brabant (DiaDDZoB) Study. *Diabetologia*, *55*(3), 608–616. doi:10.1007/s00125-011-2411-2 PMID:22198261

Nefs, G., Pouwer, F., Pop, V., & Denollet, J. (2012). Type D (distressed) personality in primary care patients with type 2 diabetes: Validation and clinical correlates of the DS14 assessment. *Journal of Psychosomatic Research*, *72*(4), 251–257. doi:10.1016/j.jpsychores.2012.01.006 PMID:22405217

Nouwen, A., Nefs, G., Caramlau, I., Connock, M., Winkley, K., Lloyd, C. E., ... Pouwer, F. (2011). Prevalence of depression in individuals with impaired glucose metabolism or undiagnosed diabetes: A systematic review and meta-analysis of the European Depression in Diabetes (EDID) Research Consortium. *Diabetes Care*, *34*(3), 752–762. doi:10.2337/dc10-1414 PMID:21357362

Oni, T., Youngblood, E., Boulle, A., McGrath, N., Wilkinson, R. J., & Levit, N. S. (2015). Patterns of HIV, TB, and noncommunicable disease multi-morbidity in peri-urban South Africa – a cross sectional study. *BMC Infectious Diseases*, *15*(1), 20. doi:10.1186/s12879-015-0750-1 PMID:25595711

Osterberg, L., & Blaschke, T. (2005). Adherence to medication. *The New England Journal of Medicine*, *353*(5), 487–497. doi:10.1056/NEJMra050100 PMID:16079372

Ott, A., Stolk, R. P., Hofman, A., van Harskamp, F., Grobbee, D. E., & Breteler, M. M. (1996). Association of diabetes mellitus and dementia: The Rotterdam Study. *Diabetologia*, *39*(11), 1392–1397. doi:10.1007/s001250050588 PMID:8933010

Park, H., Hong, Y., Lee, H., Ha, E., & Sung, Y. (2004). Individuals with type 2 diabetes and depressive symptoms exhibited lower adherence with self-care. *Journal of Clinical Epidemiology*, *57*(9), 978–984. doi:10.1016/j.jclinepi.2004.01.015 PMID:15504641

Peters, A., & Laffel, L. (2011). Diabetes care for emerging adults: Recommendations for transition from pediatric to adult diabetes care systems. *Diabetes Care*, *34*(11), 2477–2485. doi:10.2337/dc11-1723 PMID:22025785

Pouwer, F., Nefs, G., & Nouwen, A. (2013). Adverse effects of depression on glycemic control and health outcomes in people with diabetes: A review. *Endocrinology and Metabolism Clinics of North America*, *42*(3), 529–544. doi:10.1016/j.ecl.2013.05.002 PMID:24011885

Powdthavee, N. (2009). What happens to people before and after disability? Focusing effects, lead effects, and adaptation in different areas of life. *Social Science & Medicine*, *69*(12), 1834–1844. doi:10.1016/j.socscimed.2009.09.023 PMID:19833424

Raju, S. (2006). *Ageing in India in the 21st Century: A Research Agenda*. Mumbai: The Harmony Initiative.

Reid, M. J. A., Tsima, B. M., & Kirk, B. (2012). HIV and diabetes in Africa. *African Journal of Diabetes Medicine*, *20*(2), 28–32.

Riza, A. L., Pearson, F., Ugarte-Gil, C., Alisjahbana, B., van de Vijver, S., Panduru, N. M., ... van Crevel, R. (2014). Clinical management of concurrent diabetes and tuberculosis and the implications for patient services. *The Lancet. Diabetes & Endocrinology*, *2*(9), 740–753. doi:10.1016/S2213-8587(14)70110-X PMID:25194887

Roy, T., & Lloyd, C. E. (2012). Epidemiology of depression and diabetes: a systematic review. *Journal of Affective Disorders, 142*(Suppl.), S8-21.

Rubin, R. R., & Peyrot, M. (1999). Quality of life and diabetes. *Diabetes/Metabolism Research and Reviews*, *15*(3), 205–218. doi:10.1002/(SICI)1520-7560(199905/06)15:3<205::AID-DMRR29>3.0.CO;2-O PMID:10441043

Schram, M. T., Baan, C. A., & Pouwer, F. (2009). Depression and quality of life in patients with diabetes: A systematic review from the European depression in diabetes (EDID) research consortium. *Current Diabetes Reviews*, *5*(2), 112–119. doi:10.2174/157339909788166828 PMID:19442096

Schwartz, A. V., Hillier, T. A., Sellmeyer, D. E., Resnick, H. E., Gregg, E., Ensrud, K. E., ... Cummings, S. R. (2002). Older women with diabetes have a higher risk of falls: A prospective study. *Diabetes Care*, *25*(10), 1749–1754. doi:10.2337/diacare.25.10.1749 PMID:12351472

Schwartz, A. V., Sellmeyer, D. E., Ensrud, K. E., Cauley, J. A., Tabor, H. K., Schreiner, P. J., ... Cummings, S. R. (2001). Older women with diabetes have an increased risk of fracture: A prospective study. *The Journal of Clinical Endocrinology and Metabolism*, *86*(1), 32–38. doi:10.1210/jcem.86.1.7139 PMID:11231974

Seuring, T., Archangelidi, O., & Suhrcke, M. (2015). The economic costs of type 2 diabetes: A global systematic review. *PharmacoEconomics*, *33*(8), 811–831. doi:10.1007/s40273-015-0268-9 PMID:25787932

Steinsbekk, A., Rygg, L., Lisulo, M., Rise, M. B., & Fretheim, A. (2012). Group based diabetes self-management education compared to routine treatment for people with type 2 diabetes mellitus. A systematic review with meta-analysis. *BMC Health Services Research*, *12*(1), 213. doi:10.1186/1472-6963-12-213 PMID:22824531

Strotmeye, E. S., Cauley, J. A., Schwartz, A. V., Nevitt, M. C., Resnick, H. E., Bauer, D. C., ... Newman, A. B. (2005). Nontraumatic fracture risk with diabetes mellitus and impaired fasting glucose in older white and black adults: The health, aging, and body composition study. *Achieves International Medicine*, *165*(14), 1612–1617. doi:10.1001/archinte.165.14.1612 PMID:16043679

Sullivan, P. W., Morrato, E. H., Ghushchyan, V., Wyatt, H. R., & Hill, J. O. (2005). Obesity, inactivity, and the prevalence of diabetes and diabetes-related cardiovascular comorbidities in the U.S., 2000–2002. *Diabetes Care*, *28*(7), 1599–1603. doi:10.2337/diacare.28.7.1599 PMID:15983307

Talbot, F., & Nouwen, A. (2000). A review of the relationship between depression and diabetes in adults: Is there a link? *Diabetes Care*, *23*(10), 1556–1562. doi:10.2337/diacare.23.10.1556 PMID:11023152

United Nations Department of Economic and Social Affairs, Population Division. (2008). World Population Prospects (2008 Revision). Retrieved from http://esa.un.org/unpp/index.asp?panel=2

Van Dooren, F. E., Nefs, G., Schram, M. T., Verhey, F. R., Denollet, J., & Pouwer, F. (2013). Depression and risk of mortality in people with diabetes mellitus: A systematic review and meta-analysis. *PLoS One*, *8*(3), e57058. doi:10.1371/journal.pone.0057058 PMID:23472075

Van Dooren, F. E. P., Denollet, J., Verhey, F. R. J., Stehouwer, C. D. A., Sep, S. J. S., Henry, R. M., ... Schram, M. T. (2016). Psychological and personality factors in type 2 diabetes mellitus, presenting the rationale and exploratory results from The Maastricht Study, a population-based cohort study. *BMC Psychiatry*, *16*(1), 17. doi:10.1186/s12888-016-0722-z PMID:26817600

Velayudhan, L., Poppe, M., Archer, N., Proitsi, P., Brown, R. G., & Lovestone, S. (2010). Risk of developing dementia in people with diabetes and mild cognitive impairment. *The British Journal of Psychiatry*, *196*(1), 36–40. doi:10.1192/bjp.bp.109.067942 PMID:20044657

Volpato, S., Bianchi, L., Lauretani, F., Lauretani, F., Bandinelli, S., Guralnik, J. M., ... Ferrucci, L. (2012). Role of muscle mass and muscle quality in the association between diabetes and gait speed. *Diabetes Care*, *35*(8), 1672–1679. doi:10.2337/dc11-2202 PMID:22596176

Volpato, S., Ferrucci, L., Blaum, C., Ostir, G., Cappola, A., Fried, L. P., ... Guralnik, J. M. (2003). Progression of lower-extremity disability in older women with diabetes: The Women's Health and Aging Study. *Diabetes Care*, *26*(1), 70–75. doi:10.2337/diacare.26.1.70 PMID:12502660

Weissberg-Benchell, J., & Antisdel-Lomaglio, J. (2011). Diabetes-specific emotional distress among adolescents: Feasibility, reliability, and validity of the problem areas in diabetes-teen version. *Pediatric Diabetes*, *12*(4 Pt 1), 341–344. doi:10.1111/j.1399-5448.2010.00720.x PMID:21443583

World Health Organization (WHO). (2010). *Global recommendations on physical activity for health.* Geneva.

World Health Organization (WHO). (2016). *Global report on diabetes.* Geneva.

Wortman, J., Lucas, R. E., & Donnellan, M. B. (2012). Stability and change in the Big Five personality domains: Evidence from a longitudinal study of Australians. *Psychology and Aging*, *27*(4), 867–874. doi:10.1037/a0029322 PMID:22775362

KEY TERMS AND DEFINITIONS

Aging: A process of becoming older.
Coping: The process of contending with life difficulties.
Diabetes: A group of metabolic diseases.
Life Style: The way in which a person lives.
Medical Illness: Unhealthy condition of the body.
Physical: Relating to things perceived through the senses and concrete in nature.
Positive Psychology: An applied approach to optimal functioning.

Chapter 16
Obesity Physical and Mental Health Consequences in Ageing

Gagan Chooramani
King George's Medical University, India

Barre Vijaya Prasad
Dharwad Institute of Mental Health and Neurosciences (DIMHANS), India

Shamsi Akbar
King George's Medical University, India

ABSTRACT

This chapter describes the prevalence of obesity which is rising in all age groups. The World Health Organization declared obesity as a Global epidemic. There has been the abundance of research in all over the world that provides evidence for physical and mental health consequences of obesity. Obesity is considered as one of the leading cause of various non-communicable diseases. Higher body mass index and abdominal obesity are considered to be an independent risk factor that significantly contribute to the increased prevalence of Type 2 diabetes, cardiovascular diseases and hypertension, metabolic disorders along with various mental health problems among elderly. Geriatric obesity further affects the treatment process, outcome, quality and quantity of life older adults. It also increases the risk of disability among older adults.

INTRODUCTION

Obesity is defined as abnormal or extensive fat accumulation that negatively affects health (Han & Bchir, 2013). According to the World Health Organization (WHO), obesity is defined as Body Mass Index (BMI) ≥ 30 kg/m2 and central obesity as a waist circumference greater than 102 cm in men and 88 cm in women (WHO, 2000). But in older adults, body composition changes that accompany aging make BMI less appropriate for use. This is because BMI relies on muscle mass to influence the ratio of height-to-weight, and aging is accompanied by a decline in muscle mass. BMI also relies on height, and there is often height reduction in older adults due to osteoporosis-related vertebral compression fractures and

DOI: 10.4018/978-1-5225-3480-8.ch016

kyphosis. Better measures in older adults are waist circumference and waist-to-hip ratio. Both correlate well with measures of visceral fat as determined by computed tomography (CT) and with the rates of obesity-related diseases. Waist circumference, which is easy to measure, is a stronger predictor than BMI of mortality in older women (Keller, Shaw-Snyder, & Ainsworth, 2015).

It is a complex multifactorial disease arises from the interactions between genetic, environmental and behavioral factors together with other factors results in energy imbalance and promotes excessive fat deposition (Farooqi et al., 2010). Obesity is now recognized as the most prevalent metabolic disease worldwide, reaching epidemic proportions in both developed and developing countries and affecting all age group (Michalakis, Mintziori, Kaprara, Tarlatzis, & Goulis, 2013). Over the past several decades, the proportion of obese elderly increased. Improvements in health care have contributed to a significant increase in life expectancy and have influenced the growth of the elderly population. Projection indicates that by the year 2020 there will be 470 million people aged 65 and above in developing countries which will be more than double the number of the developed world (WHO, 1992). This increase is accompanied by a similar rise in the occurrence of age- and nutrition-associated diseases including obesity, cardiovascular disease, and diabetes mellitus (Westendorp, 2006). Elderly people who belong to middle and higher income groups are prone to develop obesity and its related complications due to a sedentary lifestyle and decreased physical activity. Obesity is a significant risk factor for coronary artery disease, hypertension, cholelithiasis, diabetes, osteoarthritis (Swami, Bhatia, Gupta, & Bhatia, 2005). The rate of dementia is also higher among obese older adults. Moreover, older persons who are obese (BMI $\geq$ 30) have a greater rate of nursing home admissions than non-obese seniors (BMI: 18.5 - 24.9) (Salihu, Bonnema, & Alio, 2009). The body mass index associated with the lowest mortality falls within the range of 18.5 to 24.9 in men & women between the ages of 30 and 74 (Stevens, 2000). It was found that BMI of 26 or more is a significant risk factor for diabetes and BMI more than 30 was significantly associated with arthritis and hypertension (Oster, & Maskides, 2005). Thus, with more people surviving in later life, more obese will be living and having certain morbidities as the effect of obesity.

WORLD SCENARIO

Prevalence of obesity is increasing in both developed and developing countries (Prentice & Jebb, 1995). It is considered the fifth leading risk factor for deaths all over the world as about 2.8 million people die due to obesity each year directly or indirectly. Obesity in elderly is considered one of the most serious public health challenges for all over the world. The prevalence of obesity in different countries varies from 10%-40%. It was estimated that the prevalence of obesity in elderly Americans, aged 60 years and older is 37.4%. While 25% of Australians aged 65–74 years and 14.4% over 75 years were obese. In the United Kingdom, nearly 25% of women and 18% of men aged 65–75 years and 22% of women and 12% of men aged 75 years or older suffering from overweight or obesity (Elisabeth, Vliegen, Basdevant, & Finer 2012; Dutra et al., 2013). In general, Prevalence of obesity in the Middle Eastern countries has reached to an alarming rate among all age groups as Prevalence of obesity in Bahrain 37.9%, Jordan 37.9% and Lebanon 27.4%. While, In Saudi 15.75% of elderly aged 60 years and more are obese. On the other hand, In Egypt 2006, the prevalence of Overweight and obesity among elderly in rural population is 62.3%. (Mahfouz, Sameh, & Areny, 2006; Musaiger, 2011).

INDIAN SCENARIO

India has 76.6 million people at or over the age of 60, constituting above 7.7% of total population. According to a 2001 census and the projection made by the United Nations (1996 revision), the elderly constitute 7.5% of the Indian population, and by all indications 21% of the Indian population will be 60 years and above by 2050. In India, the proportion of the population in the working age group, i.e., 15–59 years, and the retired age group of 60 years and above are both increasing, whereas the age group of 0–14 years is decreasing. The elderly population (≥60 years), which accounted for 6.7% of the total population in 1991, is expected to increase to more than 10% by the year 2021 (Amarya, Singh, & Sabharwal, 2014). In the twenty-first century, obesity has reached epidemic proportions in India, with morbid obesity affecting 5% of the country's population (Chintala, Krishna, & Reddy, 2015). According to National Family Health Survey (NFHS-3), the overall prevalence of overweight/obesity in India was 12.1% in men and 16% in women. There was a large difference in the prevalence of overweight or obese across various states. Punjab had the highest prevalence (men, 30.3%; women, 37.5%), and Tripura had the lowest prevalence (men 5.2%; women, 5.3%) (Rajkamal, Singh, Stalin, & Muthurajesh, 2015). Central obesity in an elderly population of India is a major health problem. In India, the study conducted by Swami et al. (2005) in Chandigarh estimated that prevalence of overweight and obesity among elderly in an urban area was 33%.

ASSESSMENT

Obesity in an older adult is addressed by the following key measures.

A Comprehensive Health History

History consideration is important for assessment it includes cognitive and physical functions, food access and preparation, physical activity patterns, and medications that may adverse side-effects such as fatigue that limit physical activity and promote weight gain(Valerie & Molloy, 2015).

A Nutritional Evaluation

Assessment of food shopping behavior and the individual's approach to food preparation are important in determining the older person's capabilities for improving nutrition. It helps in improving intake of calories and composition of fats. For obese adults 65 years or older, assuming a low level of physical activity. The 2010 Dietary Guidelines recommend a total calorie intake of 1800-2200 kcal/day. / Fat intake is aimed at limiting saturated and trans-fat intake(Valerie & Molloy, 2015).

A Physical Examination

Level of physical activities is important to asses. As physical inactivity can be profound effects on skeletal muscle metabolism. The clinician should first assess the older patient's level of fitness (for example with the timed "up-and-go" test or with cardiac stress testing for those being considered for more aggressive exercise programs). A physical activity program should then be recommended. The program should include a prescription for cardiovascular exercise, along with flexibility, balance, and strength-building exercises that address the sarcopenic changes of aging. Initiating an exercise program in older patients should emphasize not just weight reduction, but also the goals of improving physical function and lessening symptoms of co-morbidities such as the joint pain of arthritis or the dyspnea and fatigue of chronic lung disease, all of which are worsened by poor fitness and overweight/obesity. An excellent resource for clinicians that includes information on exercise prescriptions is "Exercise is Medicine, "an initiative of the American College of Sports Medicine in collaboration with the American Medical Association (Valerie & Molloy, 2015). Goals of assessment include being able to characterize obesity status and determine the level of health risk. Additionally, assessment of comorbid conditions that may be caused or exacerbated by overweight and obesity may help target weight management strategies and impact patient motivation to improve these associated conditions.

PATHOGENESIS

Obesity directly caused by a mismatch between energy expenditure and excessive energy intake, and the process is accentuated in the elderly, as sarcopenia and ageing result in lower basal metabolic rate. It usually develops slowly, e.g. 1 kg/year, through very small (undetectable) energy imbalance, generated by complex rafts of behavioral, psychological, social and metabolic factors. Fat distribution changes with age such that there is an increase in visceral fat, which is more marked in women than in men. The higher visceral fat is the main determinant of impaired glucose tolerance in the elderly. Increased intramuscular and intrahepatic fat contribute to impaired insulin action through locally released adipokines and free fatty acids. Increased pancreatic fat with declining β-cell function also plays a role. The rapid rise in WC of older people probably relates most strongly to lower physical activity at work and in household activities. The decrease in energy expenditure, particularly in the 50- to 65-year-old age group, contributes to the increase in body fat as we age. In those 65 years of age and older, hormonal changes that occur during aging may cause the accumulation of fat. Aging is associated with a decrease in growth hormone secretions, reduced responsiveness to thyroid hormone, decline in serum testosterone, and resistance to leptin (Corpas, Harman, & Blackman, 1993). Various other factors are discussed in the following order.

Genetic Factors

Obesity tends to run in families may lead us to believe that obesity is related to the genes a person has inherited; and science does show a link between obesity and heredity (NIH, 2006). Recent studies show the role of biological inheritance in fat variations. Researchers used structural equation modeling to identify the specific relationship between genetic loci that affect adiposity and those that affect muscle growth (Brockman, Tsaih, Neuschi, Churchill, & Li, 2008).

Environmental and Sociological Factors

The environment includes the world around us; it influences access to healthy food and safe places to walk. Our environment can prevent us from eating healthy foods and/or getting adequate exercise in a number of ways. What we eat, our level of physical activity and our lifestyle behaviors are influenced by our environment. The main dietary driver to obesity is a high-fat intake, with sugars also contributing to energy-dense foods and high-energy drinks. These issues tend to come together, since an energy-dense obesogenic diet usually tends to include excess saturated fats, excess salt and insufficient fruits and vegetables (Newman, 2009).

Other Causes of Obesity

Co-morbidities such as metabolic/endocrine disorders and a number of drugs commonly used in the elderly including steroids, antipsychotics, antidepressants and antileptics and anti-hyperglycemic agents, are known to promote weight gain (Han, Tajar, & Lean, 2011). The older adults who are obese are more likely than those who are not obese to report symptoms of depression, such as feelings of sadness, worthlessness, and hopelessness (Center on an Aging Society, 2003). Lack of sleep may also contribute to obesity as it may stimulate the appetite, cause water retention, or slow the metabolism rate (NIH, 2008). Finally, the complex relationship between functional ability and lifestyle patterns merits attention as a contributor to obesity (Center on an Aging Society, 2003). Joint pain decreased mobility, and activity intolerance may lead to weight gain because of decreased activity. Older adults are more likely than younger adults to experience functional limitations associated with chronic illnesses that may begin a stress-pain-depression cycle that can result in lifestyle patterns leading obesity (Lorig, Sobel, Laurent, Gonzalez, & Minor, 2006).

CONSEQUENCES OF OBESITY IN OLDER ADULTS

In 2005, World Health Organization (WHO) classified Health problems associated with obesity either nonfatal or life threatening (WHO, 2005).

Nonfatal Health Problems Related to Obesity

Debilitating conditions, such as those associated with respiratory, chronic musculoskeletal, Urinary incontinence and skin problems are classified as nonfatal.

Respiratory Problems

Obesity plays a key role in the development of obstructive sleep apnea and obesity hypoventilation syndrome. In a 5-year prospective study, older heavier men had the greatest increase in the respiratory disturbance index, which is the number of apneas and hypopneas divided by the estimated hours of sleep. Increased weight on the chest wall decreases respiratory compliance, increases the work of breathing, and restricts ventilation. Older obese men may be particularly predisposed to developing weight-related sleep apnea (Amarya, Singh, & Sabharwal, 2014). The natural decrease in respiratory function in older patients exacerbates the decrease caused by obesity which may in turn lead to an increase in the sleep apnea syndrome, which, in these patients, is related to a greater risk of developing hallucinatory and cognitive disorders caused by hypoxia during sleep (Donini, Chumlea, Vellas, delBalzo, & Cannalla, 2006).

Arthritis and Osteoarthritis

Arthritis is the leading cause of disability in older adults. It is one big cause of physical immobility in older adults, resulting in reduced energy expenditure and high risk of weight gain (Amarya, Singh, & Sabharwal, 2014). Obese older people above the age of 50 who have arthritis are more likely to say their condition limits their activities than non-obese adults in this age group (Center on an Aging Society, 2003). By 65 years of age the prevalence of osteoarthritis is 68% in women and 58% in men. This age-related increase in the prevalence of osteoarthritis may reflect bodily changes as a result of a lifetime of being overweight which results in strain on weight-bearing joints (Villareal, Apovian, Kushner, & Klein, 2005). Obesity, or even being overweight, increases the load placed on joints, especially the knee and hip joints. A breakdown in cartilage, resulting from the increased weight on joints, may result in pain and further functional disability (Lorig & Fries, 2006). People with arthritis are particularly vulnerable to the stress-pain-depression cycle, in which the pain and stiffness caused by the disease lead to decreased mobility, thereby increasing stress, pain, and depression and likely decreasing the quality of life (Newman, 2009).

Urinary Incontinence

Whilst obesity is a well-known risk factor for urinary incontinence in women (Subak et al., 2009), little information is available in men. In women, the prevalence of all types of urinary incontinence (urge, stress or mixed) increase with increasing BMI (Hunskaar, 2008), as this problem persists into the older age to aggravate an already-common problem (Brown et al., 1996; Larrieu et al., 2004). In obese individuals, it is often thought that urinary incontinence is due to the effects of excessive weight exerting strain and stretch and eventual weakening of the neuromuscular structures. The obese diabetic is at particularly high risk of incontinence if autonomic neuropathy and/or osmotic effects are present.

Impaired Cognitive Function

Obesity has been shown to associate with impaired cognitive function. In the elderly, the obesity-related gene *FTO* has also been linked to Alzheimer's disease (Ho et al., 2010) but an excess of cerebral vascular insufficiency and long-term hypoxia through sleep apnoea probably play major roles. A decline in cognitive function has also been observed to associate with vascular risk factors including dyslipidaemia and hyperglycaemia (Nooyens, Baan, Spijkerman, & Verschuren, 2010) and the metabolic syndrome in the presence of inflammation (Yaffe et al., 2004).

Skin Conditions

75% of the obese population found skin problems, including itching, skin breakdown, redness, and rashes (Brown, Wimpenny, & Maughan, 2004). The two main causes of the reported skin problems were perspiration and friction. Groin, limbs, and under breasts were identified as the most troubling areas. This combination of older age, fragile skin and obesity increases the risk for pressure sores (Flood & Newman, 2007). Older adults who are obese and have skin problems face additional complications because their skin naturally loses about 20% of its dermal thickness with age (Baranoski, 2001).

Life-Threatening Illnesses Related to Obesity

The World Health Organization has noted that life-threatening illnesses related to obesity include cardiovascular disease; conditions associated with insulin resistance, such as type 2 diabetes; certain types of cancers, especially hormonally related and large-bowel cancer; and gallbladder disease.

Cardiovascular Disease

Coronary artery diseases (CADs) are the major cause of disability, thus limiting the activity and eroding the quality of life of millions of elderly people each year. In recent years, the incidence of coronary artery diseases (CADs) has shown an increasing trend in India (Lopez, 1993). Various studies suggest that obesity can raise the risk of cardiovascular disease in older adults. Data from longitudinal population studies suggest that obesity increases the risk of cardiovascular disease in older men, but not necessarily in older women (Harris, 1997). Increased BMI in older men was associated with an increase in new cases of coronary heart disease, fatal and nonfatal infarction, and cardiovascular disease mortality during 12–15 years of subsequent observation. Grundy (2004) has described obesity as a major underlying factor contributing to atherosclerotic cardiovascular disease (ASCVD) and a factor associated with multiple other ASCVD risk factors, including elevated blood pressure, hypertriglyceridemia, low high-density lipoproteins, high cholesterol, and high fasting plasma glucose. Even though there is a strong association between obesity and ASCVD, the relationship underlying the mechanism is not well understood. The fact that obesity acts on so many metabolic pathways, producing so many potential risk factors, makes it challenging to delineate the specific mechanism by which obesity contributes to ASCVD.

Diabetes

"Type 2 diabetes is highly prevalent in older adults due to the physical inactivity associated with advancing age as well as the obesity epidemic" (The Endocrine Society, 2016). It results from an interplay between genetic factors and environmental factors that contribute to obesity. Even a 15-pound weight gain can increase a person's risk of diabetes by 50% (Daniels, 2006). Coronary disease is the most common and lethal sequel to type 2 diabetes. Lean-muscle mass begins to diminish after the age of 65. This decrease may be related to decreasing physical activity, disability, anabolic hormone production, or increased cytokine activity. If calorie intake continues at the same rate while the muscle mass decreases, the older person will most likely experience fat weight gain (Newman A., 2009). The effect of sedentary behavior, particularly television watching, in relation to risk of type 2 diabetes was positively associated with risk of obesity and type 2 diabetes (Hu, Li, Colditz, Willett, & Manson, 2003).

Nonalcoholic Fatty Liver Disease

Nonalcoholic fatty liver disease (NAFLD) includes steatosis (an accumulation of extra fat in the liver), nonalcoholic steatohepatitis (NASH) accompanied by inflammation resulting from damaged hepatic cells, liver fibrosis, and liver cirrhosis. According to a Rotterdam study of 2811 elderly people aged more than 65 years, the overall prevalence rate of NAFLD was 35.1% (Koehler, Schouten, & Hansen, 2012). Insulin resistance, which is known to be a primary cause of the NAFLD, is a major component of the metabolic syndrome, which is often observed in elderly people. Current treatments for NAFLD are to control body weight by changing lifestyle and improve insulin resistance. If body weight is decreased through a medium level of dietary restrictions and increased body activity by 5–10%, it can reduce the fat accumulated inside the liver by approximately 40% (Mahrouf-Yorgov, de L'hortet, & Cosson, 2011). Also, exercise and diet therapy for the elderly can reduce the fat accumulation in the liver and improve hyperlipidemia, hypertension, and insulin resistance (Shah, Stufflebam, & Hilton, 2009; Villareal, Chode, & Parim, 2011).

Cancer

Obesity is associated with an increased risk of several types of cancer that occur more commonly in older than in young adults, including breast, colon, gallbladder, pancreas, renal, bladder, uterine, cervical, and prostate cancers (Wolk et al., 2001; Bergstrom, Pisani, Tenet, Wolk, & Adami, 2001). Breast cancer in older women is increasingly being linked to obesity (Sweeney, Blair, Anderson, Lazovich, & Folsom, 2004). Twenty-five to 30% of several major cancers, including breast (postmenopausal), colon, kidney, and esophageal, have been linked to obesity and physical inactivity (Bianchini, Kaaks, &Vainio, 2002). Men who are obese are more likely to develop cancer of the colon, rectum, or prostate than men who are not obese. Cancer of the gallbladder, uterus, cervix, or ovaries is more common in women who are obese compared with women who are not obese (NIH, 2006).

Renal Disease

The prevalence of renal failure increases with age, and obesity is a significant risk factor for end-stage renal disease (Hsu, Iribarren, McCulloch, Darbinian & Go, 2009). A recent report indicated that increased waist-to-hip ratio was a significant and independent predictor of chronic renal disease in elderly Taiwanese (Chou et al., 2008). In a cross-sectional study of African Americans, increasing age and waist circumference were associated with increased chronic kidney disease (Flessner et al., 2009). Collectively, this information suggests that obesity, particularly abdominal adiposity, imparts a negative effect on renal disease in the older population.

BENEFICIAL EFFECTS OF OBESITY

Obesity is associated with increased bone mineral density (BMD) and decreased osteoporosis and hip fracture in older men and women. In obese person's hormonal factors that are increased such as circulating estrogens, insulin, and leptin, might contribute to the beneficial effects of obesity on BMD, by stimulating bone growth and inhibiting bone remodeling. Both body fat mass and FFM are directly correlated with BMD; the relation between fat mass and BMD is stronger in women than in men. In addition, high BMI values are associated with a slower rate of bone loss induced by estrogen deficiency after menopause, presumably because of increased conversion of adrenal precursors to estrogen in adipose tissue (Villareal, Apovian, Kushner, & Klein, 2005).

MANAGEMENT OF OBESITY AND RECOMMENDATIONS

The study of geriatric obesity and its management is a relatively new area of research and is especially true for groups of obese elders with important additional risk factors for malnutrition, including poverty, isolation, healing challenges due to surgery and/or hospitalization, institutionalization, and advanced mental or physical disabilities. The primary purpose for weight-loss therapy may differ across age groups. Preventing and treating the medical complications of obesity may be the most important goal of therapy in young and middle-aged adults, whereas improving physical function and quality of life may be the most important goal of therapy in older adults. In addition, the therapeutic approach may differ between younger and older adults, because of the increased importance of preventing loss of muscle and bone mass that occurs with weight loss in older persons. Weight-loss therapy that minimizes muscle and bone losses is recommended for older persons who are obese and who have functional impairments or metabolic complications that can benefit from weight loss. A thorough medical history, physical examination, appropriate laboratory tests, review of medications, and assessment of readiness to lose weight are essential before weight-loss therapy is initiated (Villareal, Apovian, Kushner, & Klein, 2005).

LIFESTYLE INTERVENTION

The primary approach is to achieve a sustained lifestyle change. Lifestyle modification includes strategies that aid older individual combinations of an energy-deficit diet, increased physical activity, and behavior therapy, including self-monitoring, goal setting, social support, and stimulus control, cause moderate weight loss. Regular exercise is not essential for achieving initial weight loss, but it can help maintain weight loss and prevent weight regain (National Institutes of Health, 1998; Wing, & hill, 2001). Nonetheless, the introduction of an exercise component early in the treatment course, including aerobic and resistance training, may be particularly beneficial for older persons because endurance and resistance exercises improve physical function and can ameliorate frailty (Banks, Klein, Sinacore, Siener, &Villareal, 2005; Fiatarone et al., 2002). Lifestyle and behavior modification can be facilitated by counseling from a dietitian, exercise specialist, or behavioral therapist who has weight-management experience.

Common geriatric situations, such as dependency on others, cognitive impairment, institutionalization, widowhood, loneliness, isolation, and depression should be addressed because these factors can make it more difficult to lose weight. Because dependency may be common, lifestyle-change programs must include participation by family members and care providers. Consideration must also be given to obstacles to learning faced by older adults, such as impaired vision and hearing, multiple co-morbidities, and limited financial resources. Regular physical activity is particularly important in obese older persons to improve physical function and help preserve muscle and bone mass. The goals of regular exercise in obese older persons are to increase flexibility, endurance, and strength; therefore, a multi component exercise program that includes stretching, aerobic activity, and strength exercises are recommended. Older population has the highest risk of medication-related problems. So, all medications should be carefully reviewed, particularly because some may cause weight gain (e.g., steroids, anticonvulsants, antidepressants, and antipsychotics).

PHARMACOTHERAPY

Pharmacotherapy in obese older persons is limited. Of the currently available medications, or list at may be the safest for older persons. Orlistat therapy in a selected group of obese older persons, particularly those with constipation, might be a useful adjunct to lifestyle modification. It is a lipase inhibitor, blocks the digestion and absorption of fat up to one-third of the ingested amount, thereby causing an energy deficit of approximately 300 kcal/ d (1260 kJ). The weight loss by Orlistat is 2 to 3 kg more than with placebo and results in improvement in glucose tolerance and blood pressure dependent on the rate of weight loss (Padwal & Majumdar, 2007).

SURGERY

Bariatric surgery should be considered in selected older subjects who have disabling obesity that can be ameliorated with weight loss and who meet the criteria for surgery. Bariatric surgery for older patients has been shown to be safe and effective for Excess Weight Loss and in an improvement of obesity co-morbidities, especially type II diabetes and blood pressure with trends in greater improvement for older patients than younger patients after Roux-en-Y gastric bypass (Dunkle-Blatter et al., 2007). Individuals who underwent bariatric surgery had a significantly reduced number of total and fatal cardiovascular events compared with matched obese controls that did not undergo surgery. Furthermore, cancer rates have been reduced to nearly 50% in post-surgical bariatric patients (Sjostrom et al., 2012). The specific bariatric surgical procedure that is performed will depend on the skill and experience of the surgeon.

Opportunities to improve both body weight and nutritional status in the community are hampered by programs that are inadequate at identifying and treating obesity in older adults who would benefit from intervention. Such programs have the potential to promote better health for these elders on dramatic public health scale. Thus, increased efforts to improve the management of geriatric obesity in the community at all levels, clinical practice, medical research, implementation practices, programmatic policies, and the built environment, are strongly encouraged.

FUTURE RESEARCH DIRECTIONS

Future research might focus more on determining behavioral treatment how these behavioral techniques can be best applied in a real-world setting. Behavioral treatment is an approach used to help individuals develop a set of skills to achieve a healthier weight. It is more than helping people to decide what to change; it is helping them identify how to change. The behavior change process is facilitated through the use of self-monitoring, goal setting, and problem solving. Telemedicine potentially can address gaps in primary care service coverage in rural areas to overcome the hurdles of reduced widespread implementation of the Medicare Obesity Benefit (MOB).

REFERENCES

Amarya, S., Singh, K., & Sabharwal, M. (2014). Health consequences of obesity in the elderly. *Journal of Clinical Gerontology and Geriatrics*, *5*(3), 63–67. doi:10.1016/j.jcgg.2014.01.004

Banks, M., Klein, S., Sinacore, D. R., Siener, C., & Villareal, D. (2005). Effects of weight loss and exercise on frailty in obese elderly subjects. *Journal of the American Geriatrics Society*, *53*, S16.

Baranoski, S. (2001). Skin tears. *Nursing Management*, *32*(8), 25–31. doi:10.1097/00006247-200108000-00010 PMID:15129526

Bergström, A., Pisani, P., Tenet, V., Wolk, A., & Adami, H. O. (2001). Overweight as an avoidable cause of cancer in Europe. *International Journal of Cancer*, *91*(3), 421–430. doi:10.1002/1097-0215(200002)9999:9999<::AID-IJC1053>3.0.CO;2-T PMID:11169969

Bianchini, F., Kaaks, R., & Vainio, H. (2002). Overweight, obesity, and cancer risk. *The Lancet Oncology*, *3*(9), 565–574. doi:10.1016/S1470-2045(02)00849-5 PMID:12217794

Binder, E. F., Schechtman, K. B., Ehsani, A. A., Steger-May, K., Brown, M., Sinacore, D. R., ... Holloszy, J. O. (2002). Effects of exercise training on frailty in community-dwelling older adults: Results of a randomized, controlled trial. *Journal of the American Geriatrics Society*, *50*(12), 1921–1928. doi:10.1046/j.1532-5415.2002.50601.x PMID:12473001

Brockman, G., Tsaih, S., Neuschi, C., Churchill, G., & Li, R. (2008). Genetic factors contributing to obesity and body weight can act through mechanisms affecting muscle weight, fat weight or both. *Physiological Genomics*, *10*, 1152. PMID:18984673

Brown, J. S., Seeley, D. G., Fong, J., Black, D. M., Ensrud, K. E., & Grady, D.Study of Osteoporotic Fractures Research Group. (1996). Urinary incontinence in older women: Who is at risk? *Obstetrics and Gynecology*, *87*(5), 715–721. doi:10.1016/0029-7844(96)00013-0 PMID:8677073

Brown, J., Wimpenny, P., & Maughan, H. (2004). Skin problems in people with obesity. *Nursing Standard*, *18*(35), 38–42. doi:10.7748/ns2004.05.18.35.38.c3609 PMID:15160455

Center on an Aging Society (2003). *Obesity among older Americans.* Retrieved July 23, 2008, from http://ihcrp.georgetown.edu/agingsociety/pdfs/obesity2.pdf

Chintala, K. K., Krishna, B. H., & Reddy, M. (2015). Heart rate variability in overweight health care students: Correlation with visceral fat. *Journal of Clinical and Diagnostic Research: JCDR*, *9*(1), CC06. PMID:25737980

Chou, C. Y., Lin, C. H., Lin, C. C., Huang, C. C., Liu, C. S., & Lai, S. W. (2008). Association between waist-to-hip ratio and chronic kidney disease in the elderly. *Internal Medicine Journal*, *38*(6a), 402–406. doi:10.1111/j.1445-5994.2007.01587.x PMID:18336543

Corpas, E., Harman, S., & Blackman, M. (1993). Human growth hormone and human aging. *Endocrinology Review*, *14*(1), 20–39. doi:10.1210/edrv-14-1-20 PMID:8491152

Daniels, J. (2006). Obesity: America's epidemic. *The American Journal of Nursing*, *106*(1), 40–49. doi:10.1097/00000446-200601000-00028 PMID:16481779

Donini, L., Chumlea, W., Vellas, B., delBalzo, V., & Cannalla, C. (2006). In preparation for the International Symposium on 'Obesity in the Elderly'. *Aging Health, 2*(1), 47–51. Retrieved August 12, 2008 from www.futuremedicine.com.doi/abs/ doi:10.2217/1745509X.2.1.47

Dunkle-Blatter, S. E., Jean, M. R. S., Whitehead, C., Strodel, W., Bennotti, P. N., Still, C., & Petrick, A. T. (2007). Outcomes among elderly bariatric patients at a high-volume center. *Surgery for Obesity and Related Diseases, 3*(2), 163–169. doi:10.1016/j.soard.2006.12.004 PMID:17331804

Dutra, M., Uliano, E., Machado, D., Martins, T., Vinholes, D., Trevisol, F., & Trevisol, D. (2013). Obesity prevalence among elderly people using different measurement methods: A population-base study. *International Journal of Diseases and Disorders, 1*(2), 24–32.

Elisabeth, M. H., Vliegen, M., Basdevant, A., & Finer, N. (2012). Prevalence, Pathophysiology, Health Consequences and Treatment Options of Obesity in the Elderly: A Guideline. *Obesity Facts, 5*(3), 460–483. doi:10.1159/000341193 PMID:22797374

Farooqi, S., Bochukova, E., Huang, N., Keogh, J., Henning, E., Purmann, C., & Blaszczyk, K. (2010). Large, rare chromosomal deletions associated with severe early-onset obesity. *Nature Journal, 463*(7281), 666–670. doi:10.1038/nature08689 PMID:19966786

Fiatarone, M. A., O'Neill, E. F., Ryan, N. D., Clements, K. M., Solares, G. R., Nelson, M. E., ... Evans, W. J. (1994). Exercise training and nutritional supplementation for physical frailty in very elderly people. *The New England Journal of Medicine, 330*(25), 1769–1775. doi:10.1056/NEJM199406233302501 PMID:8190152

Flessner, M. F., Wyatt, S. B., Akylbekova, E. L., Coady, S., Fulop, T., Lee, F., ... Crook, E. (2009). Prevalence and awareness of CKD among African Americans: The Jackson heart study. *American Journal of Kidney Diseases, 53*(2), 238–247. doi:10.1053/j.ajkd.2008.08.035 PMID:19166799

Flood, M., & Newman, A. (2007). Obesity in older adults: Synthesis of findings and recommendations for clinical practice. *Journal of Gerontological Nursing, 33*, 19–35. PMID:18183745

Grundy, S. M. (2004). Obesity, metabolic syndrome, and cardiovascular disease. *The Journal of Clinical Endocrinology and Metabolism, 89*(6), 2595–2600. doi:10.1210/jc.2004-0372 PMID:15181029

Han, T., & Bchir, M. (2013). Obesity and weight management in the elderly: A focus on men. *Best Practice & Research. Clinical Endocrinology & Metabolism, 27*(4), 509–525. doi:10.1016/j.beem.2013.04.012 PMID:24054928

Han, T. S., Tajar, A., & Lean, M. E. J. (2011). Obesity and weight management in the elderly. *British Medical Bulletin, 97*(1), 169–196. doi:10.1093/bmb/ldr002 PMID:21325341

Harris, T. B., Launer, L. J., Madans, J., & Feldman, J. J. (1997). Cohort study of effect of being overweight and change in weight on risk of coronary heart disease in old age. *BMJ (Clinical Research Ed.), 314*(7097), 1791. doi:10.1136/bmj.314.7097.1791 PMID:9224080

Ho, A. J., Stein, J. L., Hua, X., Lee, S., Hibar, D. P., Leow, A. D., & Foroud, T. (2010). A commonly carried allele of the obesity-related FTO gene is associated with reduced brain volume in the healthy elderly. *Proceedings of the National Academy of Sciences of the United States of America, 107*(18), 8404–8409. doi:10.1073/pnas.0910878107 PMID:20404173

Hsu, C. Y., Iribarren, C., McCulloch, C. E., Darbinian, J., & Go, A. S. (2009). Risk factors for end-stage renal disease: 25-year follow-up. *Archives of Internal Medicine*, *169*(4), 342–350. Retrieved from http://win.niddk.gov/publications/understanding.htm doi:10.1001/archinternmed.2008.605 PMID:19237717

Hu, F., Li, T., Colditz, G., Willett, W., & Manson, J. (2003). Television watching and other Sedentary

Hunskaar, S. (2008). A systematic review of overweight and obesity as risk factors and targets for clinical intervention for urinary incontinence in women. *Neurourology and Urodynamics*, *27*(8), 749–757. doi:10.1002/nau.20635 PMID:18951445

Koehler, E. M., Schouten, J. N., Hansen, B. E., van Rooij, F. J., Hofman, A., Stricker, B. H., & Janssen, H. L. (2012). Prevalence and risk factors of non-alcoholic fatty liver disease in the elderly: Results from the Rotterdam study. *Journal of Hepatology*, *57*(6), 1305–1311. doi:10.1016/j.jhep.2012.07.028 PMID:22871499

Larrieu, S., Peres, K., Letenneur, L., Berr, C., Dartigues, J. F., Ritchie, K., & Barberger-Gateau, P. (2004). Relationship between body mass index and different domains of disability in older persons: The 3C study. *International Journal of Obesity*, *28*(12), 1555–1560. doi:10.1038/sj.ijo.0802755 PMID:15314627

Lopez, A. D. (1993). Assessing the burden of mortality from cardiovascular diseases. *World Health Statistics Quarterly. Rapport Trimestriel de Statistiquess Anitairesmondiales*, *46*(2), 91–96.

Lorig, K., & Fries, J. (2006). *The arthritis helpbook* (6th ed.). Reading, MA: Perseus.

Lorig, K., Holman, H., Sobel, D., Laurent, D., Gonzalez, V., & Minor, M. (2006). *Living a healthy life with chronic conditions* (3rd ed.). Boulder, CO: Bull.

Mahfouz, E., Sameh, E., & Areny, T. (2006). Prevalence and correlates of overweight and obesity among elderly population residing a rural community, Minia, Egypt. Faculty of medicine, Minia University.

Mahrouf-Yorgov, M., De L'Hortet, A. C., Cosson, C., Slama, A., Abdoun, E., Guidotti, J. E., & Gilgenkrantz, H. (2011). Increased susceptibility to liver fibrosis with age is correlated with an altered inflammatory response. *Rejuvenation Research*, *14*(4), 353–363. doi:10.1089/rej.2010.1146 PMID:21548759

Musalakis, K., Mintziori, G., Kaprara, A., Tarlatzis, B., & Goulis, D. (2013). The complex interaction between obesity, metabolic syndrome and reproductive axis: A narrative review. *Metabolism: Clinical and Experimental*, *62*(4), 457–478. doi:10.1016/j.metabol.2012.08.012 PMID:22999785

Musaiger, A. (2011). Overweight and obesity in eastern mediterranean region: prevalence and possible causes. Retrieved 3 June 2015 from http://www.hindawi.com/journals/jobe/2011/407237/

National Institutes of Health. (1998). Clinical guidelines on the identification, evaluation, and treatment of overweight and obesity in adults: The evidence report. *Obesity Research*, *6*(2), 51S–209S. PMID:9813653

Newman, A. (2009). Obesity in older adults. *Online Journal of Issues in Nursing*, *14*(1).

NIH Publication No. 01-3680 (2006). *Understanding adult obesity.*

NIH Publication No. 01-3680 (2006). *Understanding adult obesity.* Retrieved July 23, 2008 from, http://win.niddk.gov/publications/understanding.htm

Nooyens, A. C., Baan, C. A., Spijkerman, A. M., & Verschuren, W. M. (2010). Type 2 diabetes and cognitive decline in middle-aged men and women. *Diabetes Care*, *33*(9), 1964–1969. doi:10.2337/dc09-2038 PMID:20519662

Oster, G.V., & Maskides, K.S (2005). Obesity & health conditions in elderly Mexican Americans. the Hisposic EPSESE, Established populator epidemiological studies of elderly. Ethn D's, 10(1), 318.

Padwal, R.S., & Majumdar, S.R. (2007). Drug treatments for obesity: orlistat, sibutramine, and rimonabant. *Lancet, 369,* 71–77. 104.

Prentice, A. M., & Jebb, S. A. (1995). Obesity in Britain: Gluttony or sloth? *BMJ: British Medical Journal*, *311*(7002), 437–439. doi:10.1136/bmj.311.7002.437 PMID:7640595

Rajkamal, R., Singh, Z., Stalin, P., & Muthurajesh, E. (2015). Prevalence and determinants of overweight and obesity among elderly population in an urban area of Puducherry. *International Journal of Medical Science and Public Health*, *4*(3), 369–372. doi:10.5455/ijmsph.2015.3110201477

Salihu, H. M., Bonnema, S. M., & Alio, A. P. (2009). Obesity: What is an elderly population growing into? *Maturitas*, *63*(1), 7–12. doi:10.1016/j.maturitas.2009.02.010 PMID:19328637

Shah, K., Stufflebam, A., Hilton, T. N., Sinacore, D. R., Klein, S., & Villareal, D. T. (2009). Diet and exercise interventions reduce intrahepatic fat content and improve insulin sensitivity in obese older adults. *Obesity (Silver Spring, Md.)*, *17*(12), 2162–2168. doi:10.1038/oby.2009.126 PMID:19390517

Sjöström, L., Peltonen, M., Jacobson, P., Sjöström, C. D., Karason, K., Wedel, H., & Bouchard, C. (2012). Bariatric surgery and long-term cardiovascular events. *Journal of the American Medical Association*, *307*(1), 56–65. doi:10.1001/jama.2011.1914 PMID:22215166

Stevens, J. (2000). Impact of age on association between weight & mortality. *Nutrition Reviews*, *58*(5), 129–137. doi:10.1111/j.1753-4887.2000.tb01847.x PMID:10860392

Subak, L. L., Wing, R., West, D. S., Franklin, F., Vittinghoff, E., Creasman, J. M., ... Macer, J. (2009). Weight loss to treat urinary incontinence in overweight and obese women. *The New England Journal of Medicine*, *360*(5), 481–490. doi:10.1056/NEJMoa0806375 PMID:19179316

Swami, H. M., Bhatia, V., Gupta, A. K., & Bhatia, S. P. S. (2005). An epidemiological study of obesity among elderly in Chandigarh. *Indian Journal of Community Medicine*, *30*(3), 255–258.

Sweeney, C., Blair, C. K., Anderson, K. E., Lazovich, D., & Folsom, A. R. (2004). Risk factors for breast cancer in elderly women. *American Journal of Epidemiology*, *160*(9), 868–875. doi:10.1093/aje/kwh276 PMID:15496539

ScienceDaily. (2016). The Endocrine Society: Older overweight and obese adults with diabetes benefit from better diet and exercise. Retrieved July 11, 2017 from www.sciencedaily.com/releases/2016/04/160401130616.htm

United Nation Population Assessment. (1992). In: WHO Technical Report Series 853. Geneva, p. 4.

Valerie, K. S., & Margory, A. M. (2015). Aging and obesity: General assessment and management considerations. *Geriatric Nursing*, *36*(5), 407–409. doi:10.1016/j.gerinurse.2015.08.008 PMID:26734699

Villareal, D. T., Apovian, C. M., Kushner, R. F., & Klein, S. (2005). Obesity in older adults: Technical review and position statement of the American Society for Nutrition and NAASO, The Obesity Society. *Obesity (Silver Spring, Md.)*, *13*(11), 1849–1863. PMID:16339115

Villareal, D. T., Apovian, C. M., Kushner, R. F., & Klein, S. (2005). American Society for Nutrition; NAASO, The Obesity Society. Obesity in older adults: Technical review and position statement of the American Society for Nutrition and NAASO, The Obesity Society. *The American Journal of Clinical Nutrition*, *82*(5), 923–934. PMID:16280421

Villareal, D. T., Chode, S., Parimi, N., Sinacore, D. R., Hilton, T., Armamento-Villareal, R., & Shah, K. (2011). Weight loss, exercise, or both and physical function in obese older adults. *The New England Journal of Medicine*, *364*(13), 1218–1229. doi:10.1056/NEJMoa1008234 PMID:21449785

Westendorp, R. (2006). What is healthy aging in the 21st century? *The American Journal of Clinical Nutrition*, *83*(2), 404–409. PMID:16470003

Wing, R. R., & Hill, J. O. (2001). Successful weight loss maintenance. *Annual Review of Nutrition*, *21*(1), 323–341. doi:10.1146/annurev.nutr.21.1.323 PMID:11375440

Wolk, A., Gridley, G., Svensson, M., Nyrén, O., McLaughlin, J. K., Fraumeni, J. F., & Adami, H. O. (2001). A prospective study of obesity and cancer risk (Sweden). *Cancer Causes & Control*, *12*(1), 13–21. doi:10.1023/A:1008995217664 PMID:11227921

World Health Organization [WHO]. (2005). *Global strategy on diet, physical activity, and health.* Retrieved July 24, 2008, from www.who.int/dietphysicalactivity/publications/facts/obesity/en/

WHO. (2000). Obesity: Preventing and managing the global epidemic. Report of a WHO Consultation. WHO Technical Report.

Yaffe, K., Kanaya, A., Lindquist, K., Simonsick, E. M., Harris, T., Shorr, R. I., ... Newman, A. B. (2004). The metabolic syndrome, inflammation, and risk of cognitive decline. *Journal of the American Medical Association*, *292*(18), 2237–2242.

KEY TERMS AND DEFINITIONS

Ageing: The process of growing old or developing the appearance and characteristics of old age

Assessment: The term assessment refers to the wide variety of methods or tools that educators use to evaluate, measure, and document the academic readiness, learning progress, skill acquisition, or educational needs of students.

Consequences: A consequence is a "result" or "conclusion," and the Latin sequi, "to follow," is part of its history.

Obesity: A condition characterized by the excessive accumulation and storage of fat in the body

Physical and Mental Health: Health as a state of complete physical, mental and social well-being and not merely the absence of disease or infirmity.

Chapter 17
Sleep and Sleep Disorders in Old Age:
Assessment and Non-Pharmacological Management

Garima Srivastava
Allahabad University, India

Rakesh Kumar Tripathi
King George's Medical University, India

ABSTRACT

Sleep complaints are prevalent among older adults. Sleep quality and quantity changes with advancing age. There are changes in sleep patterns that are normal with ageing but many changes are the sign of disordered sleep. Sleep can be divided into rapid eye movement (REM) sleep and non-rapid eye movement sleep (NREM). Each has unique characteristics that are differentiated by their waveforms on the electroencephalogram (EEG) and by other physiological signals; several physiological age-related changes are thought to produce alterations in circadian rhythms. While there are numerous psychological and social factors contributing to quality and quantity of sleep, specific sleep disorders more prevalent in old age are insomnia, sleep apnea, and rapid eye movement disorder. Non-pharmacological treatment is effective in management of sleep disorders. Cognitive behaviour therapy is most effective to tackle insomnia. Cognitive behavior therapy along with meditation is beneficial for other sleep disorders and a new technique is also emerging: mindfulness.

INTRODUCTION

Sleep is a process in which important physiological changes (i.e. shift in brain activity, slowing of basic bodily functions) are accompanied by major shifts in consciousness (Barron, 2001). The pattern of sleep progression is called sleep architecture. Markov and Goldman (2006) reported two types of sleep architecture, rapid eye movement (REM) sleep and non-rapid eye movement (NREM) sleep. NREM sleep is

DOI: 10.4018/978-1-5225-3480-8.ch017

characterized by a reduction in physiological activity. As sleep gets deeper, the brain waves measured by electroencephalogram (EEG) gets slower and have greater amplitude, breathing and heart rate slow down, and blood pressure drops. The NREM phase consists of four stages. When an individual is awake and alert, EEG contains many beta waves, relatively high frequency (14-30 cycles per second or Hz) low voltage activity. During the transitions between wakefulness and sleep, beta waves are replaced by low-voltage(amplitude) rhythmic alpha activity(8-13Hz). As the individual fall asleep and enter into stage 1 sleep, these alpha waves are replaced by low voltage mixed frequency (4-8Hz) theta waves. In stage 1, muscle activity is diminished from that of wakefulness, asynchronous eye movements are present for the first few minutes and the individual may be easily aroused as this is the most "shallow" of all aspects of sleep (Erwin et al, 1984). After spending about 10 minutes in stage 1, individual enters into stage 2 sleep, which is marked by sleep spindles and K complexes. Sleep spindles are short bursts of 12 to14 Hz wave forms for the duration of 1.5 seconds occurring 2 to 5 times per minute. They reduce brain sensitivity to sensory input which helps to enter deeper stages of sleep. K complexes are sudden, sharp waveforms that occur once in a minute and it may help in remaining asleep. The arousal threshold is increased in stage 2 sleep, muscle tone declines and no eye movements are seen. After that sleep enter into slow wave stage 3 followed by stage 4 which is marked by EEG pattern consisting of synchronized high amplitude (>75μV) and slow (0.5-2 Hz) delta waves.EEG activity during stage 4 is characterized by a greater amount ((>50%) of delta waves compared to stage 3 (20-50%). Slow wave sleep (SWS) is considered the deepest stage of sleep as it has a much higher arousal threshold, eye movements are not observed and muscle tone continues to decline.

After the ninety minutes of process in different stages of sleep, individual enters into REM sleep. During this phase electrical activity of brain changes rapidly, delta activity disappears and becomes nearly similar to the wakefulness state of brain activity which is characterized by low voltage high frequency alpha activity(8-14 Hz) waves. Along with the activated periods of REM sleep, rapid eye movements and muscle atonia are seen (Vaughn, 2008). Tonic (Persistent) REM sleep is continuous throughout this stage and is characterized by muscle atonia and desynchronized EEG. Intermittent phasic (Episodic) events of rapid eye movements and irregular respiration and heart rate are present during REM sleep (Hirshnowitz, 2004). REM sleep has also been termed paradoxical sleep. Pulse, respiration and blood pressure in humans are all high during REM sleep- much higher than during NREM sleep and often higher than during the awake state. There is near total paralysis of the skeletal (Postural) muscles so the body movement is absent during REM sleep. The most distinctive feature of REM sleep is dreaming. (Graphical representation of EEG brains waves is shown in Figure 1. The periods of REM and NREM stages of sleep continues to alternate by one another throughout the night, the duration of which is vari-

Table 1. Stages of sleep pattern in the EEG wave forms

Wakefulness	Low voltage, mixed frequency activity Alpha (8-13cps) activity with eye closed.
Stage 1	Low voltage, mixed frequency activity Theta (3-7) Activity vertex sharp waves
Stage 2	Voltage mix frequency background with sleep spindles (10-14 cps bursts) and K Complexes (negative sharp waves followed by positive slow waves)
Stage 3	High-amplitude (≥75μV) slow waves (≤ 2 cps) occupying 20 to 50 percent of epoch
Stage 4	High amplitude slow wave occupy > 50% of epoch
REM sleep	Low- voltage mixed frequency activity, saw tooth waves, theta activity and slow alpha activity

Figure 1. EEG brain waves of NREM and REM sleep
Source: Retrieved from Nielsen, 2012

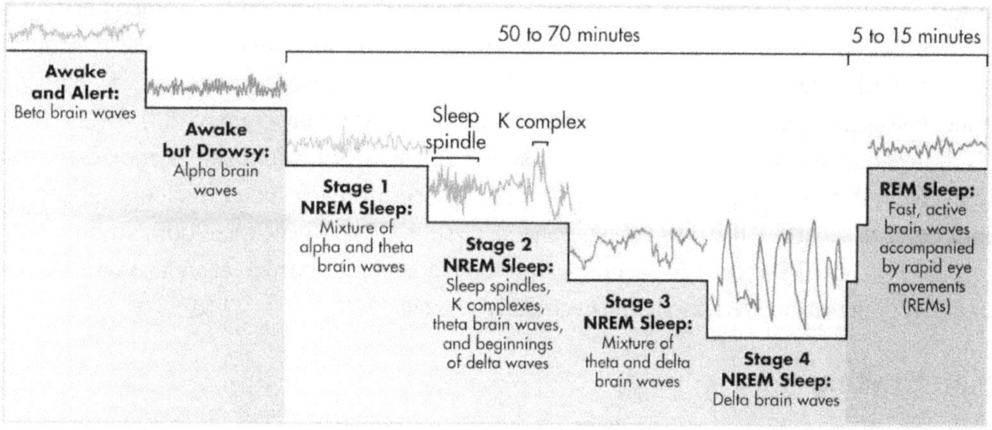

able.REM periods tend to increase in length towards morning as the first REM period reported lasts only 5 to 10 minutes, the final one lasts up to 30 minutes and periods of Non REM sleep contain an increasing portion of stage 2 sleep and gradually less of stage 3 and 4.

Sleep Wake Cycle

Sleep is regulated by two body systems sleep – awake homeostasis and the circadian biological clock. Sleep wake homeostasis adjust the sleep wake function. When an individual stays awake longer, the greater the readiness to sleep and the circadian rhythm is responsible for the change in sleep propensity that is tied to the time of day. Sleep is based on the interaction between these two processes.

Figure 2. Changes of hours of NREM and REM sleep with ageing process
The human brain: From neurons to nervous system (n.d)

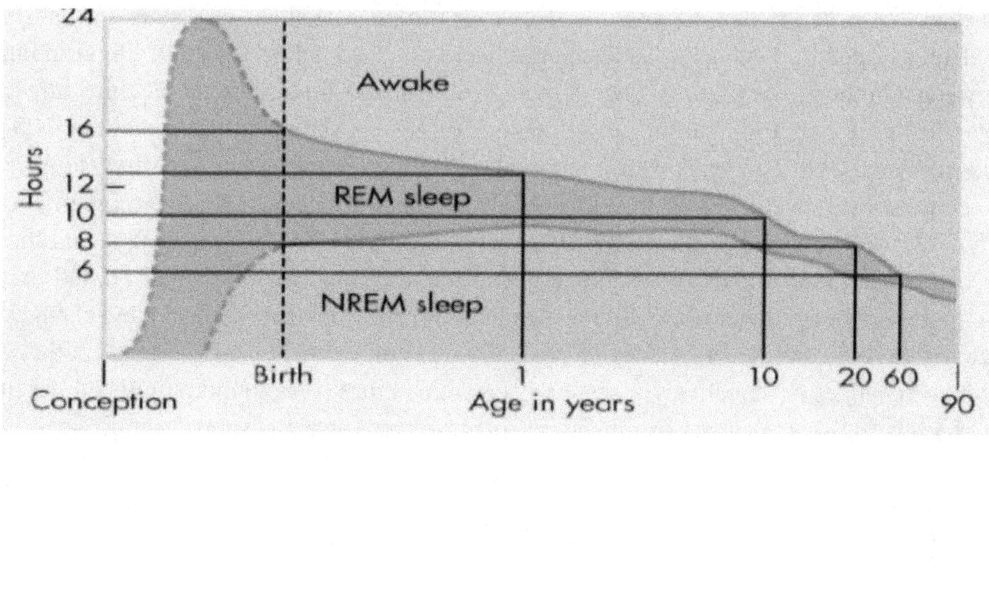

Homeostasis

Homoeostasis regulation of sleep has a restorative effect on the brain like other homeostasis system such as that body temperature. Sleep deprivation is followed by extra recovery sleep that is proportional to the sleep loss. An influential model of sleep regulation, proposed by Borbely and colleagues includes both homeostasis and circadian drives for sleep (Borbely, 1985; Achermann, 2003). The homeostatic process is thought to be due to some structure or substance possibly Adenosine (neucleoside that occurs naturally in the cell body). The adenosine proposed as 'accumulates 'need to sleep' during prolonged wakefulness and discharges this homeostasis need during sleep (Strecker, 2000; Radulovacki, 1984, Benington, 1995). NREM and REM sleep probably have separate homeostasis mechanism and after a period of sleep deprivation NREM sleep is typically replete first.

Circadian Rhythm

The Circadian Rhythm is a daily cycle of biological activity influenced by variation in the environment such as the alteration of day and night. In humans, circadian rhythm oscillates approximately every 90 minutes. Individuals often feel high level of energy and alertness during the morning hours and energy declining by the end of the day. Several factors may affect the circadian rhythm like, light, temperature, thermoregulation (the body's ability to regulate its own temperature) food, drug, physical activity etc. (Circadian Rhythm, 2007). Thus the homeostasis system tend to make us sleepier as the time goes throughout the waking period whether its night or day while the circadian system tends to keep us awake as long as there is day light prompting us to sleep as soon as it becomes dark. Due to complexity of this interaction it is generally agreed that sleep quality and restlessness are best when the sleep schedule is regularly synchronized to the internal circadian rhythm and that of the external light dark cycle.

Sleep With Ageing

In the researches (Foely, 1995; Ohayon, 2004; Vitiell, 2009) it was clear that the changes occur in sleep with advancing age, along with it was presumed that the change start in sleep architecture continues with the same pace across life span, for instance the sleep of the typical 75 year old was presumed to be worse than that of the typical 65 year old. However the meta-analysis measures across the human life span demonstrated that the age related changes were not seen across the adult life span but rather, occur between adulthood. Beginning at age 19 to age 60, changes in sleep macroarchitecture becomes asymptote, declining only minimally from age 60 to age 102. In the study (Ohayon et al.,2004) when the adults from ages19 to 102 years were examined on components of sleep measures, four most consistently reported age related changes in studies of sleep macroarchitecture was decrease in Total Sleep Time (TST), decreases in Sleep Efficiency(SE), decrease in Slow Wave Sleep (SWS) and increase in Waking After Sleep Onset (WASO). Studies also reported less consistently that age related changes increase in stage 1 and stage 2 sleep, and decrease in REM sleep. Conversely, age related changes in both Sleep Latency (SLAT) and REM Latency (REMLAT) were minimal. It is also important that all these significant age changes in objectively assessed sleep architecture were found only when the full adult life span of 19 to 102 years age was examined. Further the meta-analysis shows that no sleep measures showed any significant age-related change within the older adult with the single exception of SE which declined significantly with the rate of 3% per decade. This finding suggests that there are normative age related changes in sleep architecture however average sleep duration does not change in entire aging population. There are various medical and psychiatric comorbidities with aging which might exacerbate the sleep related complain in general ageing population.

Circadian Rhythms in Old Age

With the advancing age there are not only changes of quality of sleep across the life span but also the timing of sleep onset with ageing. As the individuals age, their circadian rhythms becomes weaker, de-synchronized and of low amplitude. It was considered that the circadian amplitude is reduced, circadian rhythm moves earlier relative to the environment and the ability to tolerate rapid phase shifts due to travel (Jet lag) declines. However the evidence only supports the two assumptions that the older people tend to have earlier circadian phases, with a corresponding tendency to go to bed and arise from bed earlier than younger adults and facing more trouble than younger adults adjusting to the rapid phase shifts due to shift work and jet lag at least in terms of sleep quality, subjective complaint and performance measures. It was hypothesized that the deterioration of the suprachiasmatic nucleus and its subsequent weakened functioning contribute to the disruption of circadian rhythms in older adults. The external cues that are necessary to entrain the circadian rhythm of sleep- wake cycles may be weak or missing in older adults.

So the changes in sleep structure among persons over 65 years of age involve both REM sleep and NREM sleep. The changes of the REM sleep includes decrease in the percentage time of rapid eye movement while the percentage of light sleep (stage 1 and stage 2) increases. Furthermore slow wave sleep had no significant change after age sixty.

SLEEP DISORDERS

There are several sleep disorders as classified under Diagnostic and Statistical Manual of Mental Disorders (DSM V-TR, 2013) and International Classification of Mental and Behavior disorder (ICD-10, 1994). DSM-V classifies sleep disorder under the heading of Sleep-Wake Disorders. This encompasses ten disorders and disorder groups. The typical presentation of these disorders is the sleep wake complaint and satisfaction with the quality, timing and amount of the sleep which results in day time distress. ICD-10 includes sleep disorders under the heads of Non-Organic Sleep Disorder which deals with only those disorders in which emotional causes are considered to be primary factor. This includes the Dyssomnia and Parasomnias. *Dyssomnia* is considered as primarily psychogenic conditions in which the pre-dominant disturbance is in the amount, quality or timing of sleep due to emotional causes, i.e. Insomnia, hypersomnia and disorder of sleep wake schedule. *Parasomnia*is characterized as abnormal episodic event occurring during sleep as sleepwalking, sleep terrors and nightmares. In adulthood they are predominantly psychogenic. The sleep disorder of organic origin such as Kleine-Levin Syndrome, Non psychogenic disorders including narcolepsy and cataplexy disorder of sleep wake schedule and sleep apnea are coded elsewhere in ICD. Classification of sleep disorders according to both diagnostic guidelines (DSM-V & ICD-10) with symptom characteristics is given in Table 2.

Sleep Disorders in Old Age

Advanced age is the most important factor associated with the increased prevalence of sleep disorder in comparison to younger adults. Sleep related complaints by older adults are day time sleepiness, day time napping and the use of hypnotic drugs. Clinically older adults experience higher rates of breathing –related sleep disorder than younger adults. Among dyssomnias most complaints are related to insomnias, nocturnal myclonous, restless leg syndrome and sleep apnea while among the parasomnias, rapid eye movement (REM) sleep behavior disorder occurs almost exclusively among elderly men.

Insomnia

Insomnia means disorder of Initiation and/or maintenance of sleep. It is characterized by difficulty in initiating sleep and/or difficulty in maintaining sleep. This may include frequent awakening during night and early morning awakening. Individuals suffering from insomnia get poor quality of sleep or non refreshing sleep.

As suggested by DSM-V, these complaints continue for at least three month however according to ICD-10, the disturbance must occur at least three times a week for a month. When insomnia is repeatedly experienced it can lead to an increased fear of sleepiness and preoccupation with its consequences. It is not necessary that all individuals having night time disturbance also suffer from functional impairment in old age. Although they are suffering from sleep discontinuity, they identify themselves as good sleeper. Day time sleepiness due to insomnia is more common in old age and this may lead to stress.

Although in older adults insomnia may be a primary sleep disorder and it is often co-morbid with chronic medical and psychiatric conditions. Insomnia is the most prevalent of all sleep disorders. Commonly the first episode of onset of insomnia is in young adulthood, late life onset is generally occurring with co- morbid medical conditions and other mental disorders. New onset insomnia may occur during menopause in females and persists till the other symptoms (e.g. hot flashes) have resolved. Insomnia complaints are more common in middle-age and older man. The type of insomnia symptoms changes as a function of age, difficulty in initiating sleep is more prevalent in young adults but problem in maintaining sleep is more prevalent in middle –age and older adults. The increased prevalence of insomnia in older adults is partly explained by the higher incidence of physical health problem in ageing.

CLASSIFICATION OF INSOMNIA

There are various ways of classifying Insomnia. Existing classification system of mental disorders i.e., DSM-V TR and ICD-10 along with ICSD 3 are classified slightly different from one another. One way to classify insomnia is on the basis of its course (Galimi, 2010). It includes

Transient Insomnia (TI)

TI lasts only a few days before or during a stressful experience. Transient insomnia may occur in those who normally sleep well and may be due to an alteration in the conditions that surround sleeping (e g noise, secondary to work patterns changing, travel) It usually lasts no longer than 7 days.

Table 2. Classification of sleep disorders (DSM V-TR and ICD-10)

DSM V Sleep Wake Disorders	ICD-10 Non-Organic Disorders	Cardinal Symptoms
	Dyssomnias	
Insomnia Disorder	**Non- Organic Insomnia**	Difficulty in Initiation and/or maintenance of sleep
Hypersommolence Disorder -Narcolepsy	**Non-Organic Hypersomnia**	Excessive sleepiness
CircadiumRythym Sleep Wake Disorder Delayed sleep phase type Advance sleep phase type Irregular sleep wake type Non- 24 hour sleep wake type Shift work type	**Non- Organic Disorder of Sleep Wake Schedule**	Disturbance in timing of sleep
Breathing Related Sleep Disorder Obstructive sleep apnea Central sleep apnea Sleep related hypoventilation		Pause in breath, Snoring and day time sleepiness
	PARASOMNIAS	
Non- rapid Eye Movement Sleep Arousal Disorder -Sleep walking -Sleep terrors	**Sleep Walking** (Somnambulism)	Rising from nocturnal sleep and walking
	Sleep Terrors (night Terrors)	Nocturnal episode of extreme terror, amnesia about incident
Nightmares	**Nightmares**	Awakening after intensive frightening dreams,vivid recall
Rapid Eye Movement Sleep Behavior Disorder		Repeated episode of arousal with vocalization and complex motor behavior
Restless Leg Syndrome		Urge to move the legs unpleasant sensation in the legs at the time of rest
Substance /Medication induced Sleep Disorder		Disturbance in sleep due to use of substance/ Medication, warrant independent clinical attention
Other Sleep Disorder -Other specified insomnia disorder -Unspecified insomnia disorder -Unspecified hypersommloence disorder -Other specified sleep wake disorder	**Other Non-organic Sleep disorders, Non-organic Sleep disorder, unspecified**	Where the disorder not fill the criteria for diagnosis but have significant impairment in socio-occupational functioning

Short Term Insomnia (STI)

STI is an abrupt onset of difficulty in initiating and maintaining sleep that is associated with an identifiable trigger. This type of insomnia is arbitrarily defined as less than four weeks in duration. Short term insomnia is most commonly the result of stressful events or environmental disturbances.

Chronic Insomnia (CI)

CI lasts longer than 3 weeks. Chronic insomnia can be related to another sickness but more often, it is caused by so called perpetuating factors which cause insomnia to remain even when the primary causation of it is gone(NIMH,1984). One most practical and popular way to classify insomnia is *Primary*

Insomnia: Which is characterized by trouble initiating or maintaining sleep or by non-restful sleep that causes impaired daytime functioning and is not attributable to a general medical condition, medication, another sleep disorder or a mental disorder. *Secondary insomnia*: Refers to the difficulty in initiating and/ or maintaining sleep that occurs as a result of co-morbidity in conjunction with a medical, psychiatric or psychological process. National Institute of Health [NIH] (2005) recommends the term "comorbid insomnia'' in place of "secondary insomnia".

Classification of Insomnia According to Diagnostic Classification

The two major classification systems Diagnostic and Statistical Manual of Mental Disorders and International Classification of Diseases of mental health along with International classification of Sleep Disorders classified insomnia differently.

Diagnostic and Statistical Manual of Mental Disorders

DSM was revised in 2013 and its 5th revision came into existence. DSM 5 acknowledges the bidirectional and interactive effects between sleep disorder and co-existing medical and mental disorders. Two previous diagnosis, primary and secondary insomnia have been eliminated and sleep disorder related to another mental disorder and sleep classification for diagnosis of primary insomnia disorder was replaced for single "insomnia disorder" (Neikrug & Ancoli, 2010).

International Classification of Sleep Disorders

Last update of ICSD occurred in 2014 and its content revision was in line with the DSM. One of the major changes includes a single entry for the disorder of insomnia. Formal revision ICSD -2 listed several subtypes of primary insomnia (psychophysiological insomnia, idiopatheic insomnia, inadequate sleep hygiene and paradoxical insomnia. Due to the difficulties in clinical practice because single patient meet diagnostic criteria more subtypes. Therefore new classification ICSD -3 includes only one diagnosis of chronic insomnia disorder, encompassing all forms of chronic insomnia (Zuconni & Ferri, 2014). There are two other diagnostic categories for insomnia disorder i.e., disorder of short term insomnia and another insomnia disorder. Chronic insomnia disorder is characterized by difficulty falling asleep and/or complaints of sleep maintenance associated with day time impairment for at least 3 months. In condition of sleep difficulties exceed frequency limits (at least three times per week) are according to former criteria. This change in insomnia diagnostic criteria in ICSD-3 and DSM-V implies a paradigm shift according to the editor of ICSD -3, Michael Sateia, (2014) recommended that insomnia is a disorder in itself that needs independent clinical attention.

International Classification of Diseases

In ICD-10 Insomnia divided into two forms "non-organic insomnia" F51.0 and "organic insomnia" under neurological condition (disorder of initiating sleep and maintaining sleep- insomnia) ICD-10 G47.0, the next revision of ICD classification is due in 2017. Non-organic insomnia includes difficulty in falling asleep, difficulty staying asleep or early final waking with any organic reason and problem should persist at least for a month. Insomnia is common symptom of many mental disorders. If it dominates the clinical picture then it can be diagnosed as basic disorder in addition with other disorder. Organic insomnia is another coding under neurological condition.

CAUSES OF INSOMNIA

There are many factors determining the initiation and maintenance of insomnia.

Concept of Hyperarousal

Insomnia is considered as disorder of hyperarousal. Hyperarousal have negatively correlated with sleep continuity (Perlis et al, 2005). Different theoretical model explain arousal in different perspective. Physiological model studies show that poor sleeper exhibit increases physiological arousal. This arousal was particularly evident at sleep onset. (Monroe, 1967; Haynes, 1981). Cognitive model suggests that arousal in the form of worry and rumination interfere with the sleep continuity and may serve as predisposing factor for insomnia, precipitating cause for acute phase and perpetuating factor for chronic insomnia. Behavioural model of insomnia suggests chronic insomnia results from maladaptive behavior that disrupts sleep. This instrumentally conditioned arousal as a possible perpetuating factor for chronic insomnia. Behavioural pattern like poor sleep hygiene and maladaptive coping behavior may cause insomnia. Neurocognitive Model of insomnia claims that the arousal is an outcome of three intersecting dimensions (somatic, cognitive and cortical) and focuses on the measurement and the consequences of conditioned cortical arousal. Cortical arousal, it is argued, occurs as a result of classical conditioning and may be observed in patients with primary insomnia

Inhibition of Wakefulness

Espie (2002) has given an alternative point of view. This psychobiologic inhibition model suggests that in the early stages of chronic insomnia problem of sleep initiation and sleep maintenance may occur because of dysfunction in the neurobiological mechanism that inhibits wakefulness and permit sleep to occur. The failure of wakefulness is thought to result from two cognitive phenomenon i.e., Inability to sleep which may hinder in preventing attention from automatic process and this will make sleep initiation difficult. Another explanation is that when people are unable to sleep, they consciously effort for sleep to occur but this effort enhances attention and results in sustained wakefulness. Merica and colleagues, proposed that cortical arousal may occur in insomnia patient as a failure to down regulate normal level cerebral activity before and during NREM sleep (Merica, 1997).

Homeostasis

Impaired sleep homeostasis may be an important etiological factor in insomnia (Stepanski, 2002; Besset, 1998; Smith, 2002). Homeostasis has been moderator and/or mediator effect on somatic, cognitive and cortical arousal which causes interference in sleep pattern.

Circadian Rhythm

Circadian rhythmsare implicated in the development of insomnia when there is mismatch between an individual's internal circadian rhythm and the timing of their sleep wake cycle (Taylor, 2014).

Age

Ageing itself is an important factor for insomnia. Older age is associated with insomnia and is, in part, due to the increased prevalence of other medical problems that disrupt sleep. In addition there are normal, age related changes in sleep that predispose older individuals to insomnia (Anacoli-Isareal & Ayalon, 2006).

Psycho-Social Factors

Insomnia initiation and maintenance are affected by several psychosocial factors like social isolation, loneliness, inactivity, retirement, life style changes, poor sleep hygiene, burden of care giving and bereavement etc.

Environmental Factors

Several environmental factors can-contribute to the development and maintenance of insomnia are noise, light, temperature, and presence of electronic and communication devices in the bedroom.

Secondary Causes of Insomnia

There are several secondary causes which are responsible for insomnia. Psychiatric illness- depression is a significant factor for development of insomnia especially early morning insomnia. Medical Illness- Arthritis, chronic pain and pulmonary disease may cause insomnia. Drug induced-old age people are surrounded by many physical and mental complaints and consequently more often than not they are on medication. Many medications (e.g., anti-hypertensives, inhale steroids) used in the old age because of hypertension and chronic obstructive pulmonary disease causes sleep difficulties in older adults.

(Spielman, 1987) proposed most accepted 3P model which describe predisposing conditions, precipitating circumstances and perpetuating factors for predisposing to chronic insomnia. Predisposing conditions like hyperarousal and familial or genetic tendency may have a role in development of insomnia. Precipitating factors such as illness, family, work and other stressors may adversely influence sleep. Maladaptive sleep habits (eg, extended time in bed, irregular sleep wake schedules, irregular napping, sleep incompatible activities in bed, dysfunctional cognitions (e.g. worry, unrealistic expectations, misattributions) are the perpetuating factors of insomnia(Bootzin & Epstien, 2011).

Breathing Related Sleep Disorder

Breathing related sleep disorder encompasses three relative distinct disorders- obstructive sleep apnea/hyonea, central sleep apnea and sleep related hypoventilation. Obstructive sleep apnea/hyonea, is the most common among them. The prevalence of sleep apnea increases 2 to 15percent in middle-aged and more than 20 percent in old age individuals. Prevalence is high in males but gender differences decline in old age because of tendency to increased prevalence in female after menopause. Insomnia and obstructive sleep apnea/hyponea may co-exit. Central sleep apnea is also prevalent with age and most patients are older than 60 years. Other breathing related sleep disorder like hypoventilation does not occur in old age.

Sleep Apnea

Sleep Apnea is a condition in which patients periodically stop breathing while asleep. The most common cause of sleep apnea is due to temporary obstruction of the upper airway. The extreme changes in the concentration of oxygen and carbon dioxide in the blood that develop after 1 minute and a few noisy, choking gasps refill the lungs. Obstructive sleep apnea is the most common medical cause of excessive day time somnolence. Usually the patients are not aware of the episodes because there are partial arousals for a brief time. A common symptom includes snoring and pauses in breathing. The number of instances of apnea hyponea per hour of sleep is called Apnea Hyponea Index (AHI). Diagnosis of SDB is made when a Patient has an AHI > 5-10 (Susan & Israel, 2010).

Circadian Rhythm Sleep Disorder

It is disruption in sleep pattern primarily in the circadian rhythm or misalignment between the circadian rhythm and sleep wake schedule. This disruption of sleep may cause insomnia or excessive sleepiness or both. Advance sleep phase type and Irregular sleep- wake type is prevalent in old age. *Advance sleep phase* type is characterized by sleep wake times that are several hours earlier than desired or conventional time. Excessive sleepiness associated with advance sleep phase can have negative effect on cognitive performance, social interaction and safety. *Irregular sleep wake type* is characterized by lack of discernable sleep wake circadian rhythm. There is no major sleep period and sleep is fragmented into at least three periods in 24 hrs a day. Irregular sleep wake cycle is commonly associated with neurodegenerative disorder such as Alzheimer disease, Parkinson disease and Huntington disease

Restless Leg Syndrome

It is characterized by dysesthesia in legs (uncomfortable itching, tingling sensation) in legs which relived only after movement of leg. It usually occurs when the person is in resting or relaxing state. The prevalence increases with age and most often twice more prevalent in females than in males. Restless Leg Syndrome (RLS) are common in older adults. The prevalence of RLS increases significantly with age (Ancoli et al., 1991).

Rapid Eye Movement Sleep Behavior Disorder (RBD)

The skeletal muscle tonia is absent. Patients are often described as 'acting out their dreams'. This disorder is characterized by the display of elaborate movements during REM sleep. These can include kicking, punching, running and/or yelling. The patients's uncontrolled movements are sometimes aggressive and/or violent and might result in injuries either to the patient himself and/or the patient's bed partner. The etiology of chronic RBD is currently unknown, yet it appears to be strongly related to a number of underlying neurological or neurodegenerative disorders. Approximately40% of RBD cases are related to such conditions. Some data suggests that RBD may be the first manifestation and/or indication of a neurodegenerative disease. One study reported 50% of those diagnosed with RBD developed Parkinson's disease or Multiple System Atrophy within 3-4 years (Olson, 2000). Prevalence rate range from 2 to7 percent. Females are 1.5 to 2 times more likely facing problem of RBD than males. In late onset RBD, rapid progression is typical and aggravating factors are common.

Etiology of Sleep Disorder in Old Age

While there are numerous psychological and social factors contributing to quality and quantity of sleep, certain physiological conditions can be disruptive to sleep. In ageing men, melatonin secretion decreases and the circadian periodicity of melatonin is gradually disrupted. Sleep in older men can be shallow and fragmented and these alterations influence growth hormone secretion which occurs with deeper stages of sleep. The disruptions of normal sleep patterns in ageing may have important health consequences, especially on mood and cognitive functions. Some factors of etiology of sleep disorder were discussed in heading of causes of insomnia in this chapter. A series of other factors contributing to sleep disorders include:

Medical Conditions

Many Physical and Mental Health conditions in late life may cause for sleep disorder like Dementia, Parkinson disease, chronic pain, cardiovascular disease etc. Sleep disorders are frequent symptoms of depression or dementia and may disappear when the underlying cause is treated.

Institutionalization

Persons living in nursing homes are required to go to bed according to Personnel shift changes and are often awakened for checks or medication throughout the night. Noise, lack of privacy and rooms either too warm or too cold further contribute to sleep disturbance.

The Ageing Process

Older people, whether living at home or in care facilities, experience sleep disorders with greater frequency than their younger counterparts. Consequently, sleep efficiency (the ratio of time spent sleeping to total time spent in bed) decreases from 95% in adolescence to less than 80% in old age.

Risk factors for sleep disturbance in older adults, described by Achermann in 2003 (Achermann & Borbely, 2003).

- Age related changes in sleep architecture
- Comorbidities cardiovascular disease, diabetes, Pulmonary disease, muscoletal disorder, CNS Disorder (Parkinson disease, seizure disorder, dementia), urinary incontinence)
- Pain
- Depression, anxiety, delirium, psychosis
- Polypharmacy
- Life stressor/ response to stress
- Sleep habit (daily, activity, cycle, napping)

- Limited exposure to sun light, environmental noises, institutional routines
- Poor sleep hygiene, lack of exercise

ASSESSMENT OF SLEEP DISORDER

Assessment of sleep disturbance requires a holistic approach. A full psychiatric and medical history like Screening Questions, sleep history and other Investigations like video recording, wrist scintigraphy and polysomnography EEG, EMG etc should be done.

Sleep History

The history should include details about sleep habits; history of sleep complaints, history of current or previous medical, neurological and psychiatric illnesses; drug and alcohol consumption as well as family history. The entire 24 hour sleep –wake cycle must be included in brief history. Symptoms occurring in the early evening when the patient is lying in bed or at sleep onset may suggest a diagnosis of Restless Legs Syndrome (RLS). Repeated awakenings throughout the night, snoring, cessation of breathing during sleep, fatigue may suggest a diagnosis of obstructive sleep apnea syndrome (OSAS). Additionally, excessive sleepiness in the daytime and irresistible desire to fall asleep and the feeling of being refreshed following daytime sleep are characteristic symptoms of narcolepsy. If the patient shows abnormal movements and behavior during the first third of the night, a diagnosis of arousal disorder (sleep walking, sleep terror, confusional arousal) is strongly suggested. In contrast the occurrence of complex motor activities and behavior with or without injury. It is important to conduct an interview with the patient's bed partner or care giver for diagnosis of abnormal movements and behavior as well as breathing disorders during sleep. The bed partner or caregiver of the patient is trained to observe and note the sleeping habits, history of drug use, and history of stress at home, work and changes in sleep habits. Completing a sleep questionnaire or keeping a sleep log or diary over a 2 week period may give important indications of sleep habits and sleep hygiene. History must be followed by careful physical examination to document evidence of various medical disorders such as respiratory, cardiovascular, endocriological or neurological disorders, especially those that affect the brain stem region or the neuromuscularsystem.

Laboratory Test

Laboratory assessment must be considered an extension of the history and physical examination. The two most important laboratory tests are Overnight Polysomnography (PSG) and Multiple Sleep Latency Test (MSLT).

Polysomnography

All night PSG studies simultaneously record several physiological variables (EEG, EMG, EOG, EKG, airflow at the nose and mouth, respiratory effort and oxygen saturation) and are important in confirming the diagnosis of Obstructive sleep apnea as well as documenting the severity of sleep apnoea, hypoxaemia and sleep fragmentation. The PSG recording should also include body position monitoring and snoring recording. Overnight PSG with simultaneous video recording can confirm REM sleep behavior.

Multiple Sleep Latency Test

It is an essential test to record pathological sleepiness (e.g. sleep onset latency less than 8 minute). The time needed to fall asleep for brief naps during the day is measured.

SLEEP QUESTIONNAIRES

Sleep questionnaires offer a very cost-effective way to obtain extensive information on sleep patterns and sleep problems. Epworth Sleepiness Scale (ESS), Insomnia Severity Scale, Pittsburg Sleep Quality Index (PSQI), and scale of dysfunctional beliefs and attitudes about sleep.

Epworth Sleepiness Scale (ESS)

It is a self-administered scale with eight item questions. Respondents are asked to rate on a4 point scale (0-3). Scale item includes usual chances of falling asleep while engaging in eight different activities. The ESS score ranges from 0-24, the higher ESS score, the higher that person's average sleep propensity in daily life. The cut off score is 0-5 lower day time sleepiness, 6-10 higher day time sleepiness, 11-12 mild excessive day time sleepiness, 13-15 moderate excessive day time sleepiness,16- 24 severe excessive day time sleepiness and reliability of the scale is 0.88 (Johns, 1997).

Insomnia Severity Index (ISI)

The Insomnia Severity Index (ISI) is a seven-item scale, a brief screening measure of insomnia. Scale content measures the subject's current (within the past 2 weeks) perception of symptom severity, distress and daytime impairment. Items include the severity of sleep onset and maintenance (middle and early morning awakening) difficulties, satisfaction with current sleep pattern, interference with daily functioning, appearance of impairment attributed to the sleep problem and the degree of concern caused by insomnia. The ISI has also been validated on samples of young adults (mean age 20 years) and older adults (mean age 65 years) with primary insomnia. It is a five-point Likert scale (0 not at all to 4 extremely). Score range is 0-28. 0 - 7 no clinically significant insomnia; 8 –14 sub-threshold insomnia; 15–21 clinical insomnia of moderate severity; 21–28 severe clinical insomnia. Reliability of the scale is 0.74 to 0.78(Morin, 1999).

Medical Outcomes Study (MOS) Sleep Scale

The sleep scale is one subscale of the Medical Outcomes Study (MOS) health status measure. It consists of 12 items to measure six sleep dimensions: Initiation (time to fall asleep), quantity (hours of sleep each night), maintenance, respiratory problems, perceived adequacy, and somnolence (the last 4 items reported using a 6- item likert scale ranging from "All of the time" to "None of the time"). The time frame for the responses is "the past 4 weeks". The score range is 12–71. Reliability ranges from 0.75 to 0.88 (Hays, 1992).

Pittsburgh Sleep Diary

The Pittsburgh Sleep Diary is designed to quantify subjectively reported sleep and waking behaviors. The scale is organized into 2 daily questionnaires completed at "bedtime" and "wake time." The wake time questionnaire is comprised of eleven general items. The bedtime questionnaire is comprised of six general items The bedtime questionnaire gathers data on the timing of meals, consumption of caffeine, alcohol and tobacco products, medication use, the timing and duration of exercise and nap periods. The wake time questionnaire gathers data on bedtime, "lights out time", sleep latency, final wake time, method of final awakening, frequency of nightly awakenings, wake after sleep onset time, and reason for nightly awakenings, sleep quality, mood on final wakening and alertness on final wakening. The night-time questionnaire is to be completed immediately before retiring to bed. The morning questionnaire is to be completed shortly after waking. Instruction is required on properly estimating wake after sleep onset time and the use of visual analog scales. Individuals complete both questionnaires each day for a period of 1 to 2 weeks or longer." Frequency of nightly awakenings is indicated using a 6-point likert scale: 0–5 or more. Frequency of awakenings to use the bathroom, awakenings by noise/bed partner, awakenings due to physical discomfort and spontaneous awakenings are indicated on the same 6-point likert scale. Ratings of sleep quality, mood on final wakening and alertness are made on 100- mm visual analog scales. Monk et al reported significant (*P*_ 0.001) long-term test-retest correlation coefficients (r) for select wake time questionnaire variables with a mean interest interval of 22 months (range 12–30 months): FNA 0.67, WASO 0.56, Sleep Quality 0.59, Mood on waking 0.61, Alertness on waking 0.65, bedtime 0.81, Lights out 0.80 and Final wake time 0.66 (Monk, 1994)

NONPHARMACOLOGICAL MANAGEMENT OF SLEEP DISORDERS

Treatment of Insomnia in Older Adults

Behavioral therapy is considered as a very effective treatment protocol for treatment of insomnia. The most effective behavioral therapy for insomnia is Cognitive Behavior Therapy. The cognitive portions of sleep deal with the misconceptions or unrealistic combination of sleep. While the behavioral combination involves a combination of sleep restriction therapy, stimulus control therapy, relaxation techniques and good sleep hygiene practices, cognitive strategies such as paradoxical intervention and cognitive restructuring.

Sleep Education and Sleep Hygiene

Sleep hygiene education primarily focuses on identifying and modifying lifestyle behaviors and environmental factors that affect sleep. Sleep hygiene education should be incorporated into all treatment modalities when treating an elderly patient (Morin, 1999). In a process of sleep education inaccurate attribution are challenged and misunderstanding challenged by giving the information about what sleep is measured, how the sleep changes with age, probable reason about sleep loss and educating about good hygiene practices. This is useful in insomnia with combination of other techniques. Good sleep hygiene measures are:

Sleep Hygiene Measures:

- Going to bed and arise at the same time daily.
- Not taking caffeine, nicotine, alcohol, stimulants before bed time.
- Avoid day time naps.
- Regular exercise but avoid late night exercise.
- Avoid television before bed time.
- Eat at regular time daily, avoid large food near bed time.
- Practice evening relaxation routines.
- Maintain comfortable sleeping conditions.

Stimulus Control Therapy

Stimulus control therapy is based on the assumption that it is a conditioned response to temporal and environmental cues usually associated with sleep by removing all the stimuli from the bedroom which may hinder the sleep onset or/and maintenance and associate the bed and bedroom with rapid sleep onset and restrict the use of bed for sleeping only and not for other activities such as reading and watching television.

Stimulus control therapy includes:

- Going to bed only when sleepy.
- Leaving the bed and going to another room when unable to fall asleep within the 20 min and returning only when sleep is imminent.
- Arising at the same time every morning regardless of the amount of sleep obtained.
- Reserving the bed and bedroom for sleep and sexual activities.
- Minimizing daytime napping.

Elderly patients may be reluctant to follow all the instructions involved in stimulus control therapy. For example, a patient may worry about falling when getting out of bed. Participating in an activity after they get out of bed (e.g. reading) will help patients take their mind off their sleep problem.

Sleep Restriction Therapy

Sleep restriction therapy may help insomniacs by consolidating sleep and creating sleep efficiency (the ratio of time asleep to time in bed). Individuals are instructed to decrease the amount of time they spend in bed. Initially, the time allowed for sleeping is obtained by averaging the amount of time spent sleeping for 1 week. Weekly adjustments are made in 15 to 20 minute increments depending on the sleep efficiency for that week. If the patient exceeds 90% efficiency, the time spent in bed is increased. If the patient falls below 80% efficiency, the time spent in bed is decreased. One study demonstrated that sleep restriction therapy improved sleep efficiency in as little as 1 week in some patients (Morin, 1995). Fatigue and sleepiness is likely seen in early treatment; however, changes in sleep are well maintained in the future.

Cognitive Control

This technique is used to restrict the thought during bed to give the chance of 'thought session' in advance. The individual with insomnia is asked to set aside 15-20 minutes in early evening to rehearse the day and plan for tomorrow. It is a technique of dealing with incomplete work and rehearsal planning for next day and self evaluative thought which may intrude during the sleep onset period.

Thought Stopping

Thought stopping is a technique to suppress the ruminating thought to interfere the flow of thought by vocally saying the word 'the' for every 3 sec because the vocal suppression of thought influence the information processing in short term memory. This technique may be effective during the night to rapid return to sleep.

Relaxation Therapy

Relaxation therapy is an approach to treating insomnia based on the observation that hyperarousal interferes with sleep. It is the most common nonpharmacologic treatment for insomnia. Progressive muscle relaxation, autogenic training and imagery training or meditations are examples of methods used. Stimulus control and sleep restriction therapy may be more effective than relaxation therapy (Morin, 1994). Older adults may find relaxation therapy difficult. Although not a good candidate for first-line therapy in this population, it may serve as a useful adjunct.

Exercise

Regular aerobic exercise has been shown to deepen sleep. In a study of older adults with moderate sleep complaints regular moderate-intensity exercise was beneficial for improving subjective quality of sleep.

Light Therapy

Light therapy is also recommended for elderly patients with insomnia because bright light exposure is associated with individual circadian rhythm. Various studies indicate light therapy may improve sleep efficacy, sleep quality, insomnia due to delayed sleep phase syndrome (difficulty falling asleep and difficulty waking at desired times) and insomnia due to advanced sleep phase syndrome (difficult staying awake and waking too early). However more research is needed to establish their effectiveness.

Paradoxical Intention

Paradoxical Intention is to allow sleep to occur naturally through passively attempting to remain quietly wakeful rather than attempting to fall asleep. This technique is useful in situations where performance anxiety has developed and where efforts to produce a response itself inhibit that response. Paradoxical Intention is to work initially by focusing on and enhancing the anxious and interfering thoughts and then subjecting it to appraisal through rationalization and experience.

NON PHARMACOLOGICAL TREATMENT FOR OTHER SLEEP DISORDERS

Little is known about therapeutic intervention of sleep disorders other than insomnia. The prevalence of Insomnia is higher in comparison to other sleep disorders is also present in co-morbidity with other sleep disorders. Although the distress and negative emotionality is common in all sleep disorders. Non-pharmacological treatments in association with other specific treatment modalities work better in treating insomnia. Multiple modality approach may include medication for restless leg syndrome, wake promoting treatment for narcolepsy and positive airway pressure for obstructive sleep apnea. The emerging researches show that cognitive behavior therapy is useful in management of other sleep disorders (restless leg syndrome and parasomnia). Hyper arousal and distress accompanied in other sleep disorders can be rational for developing psychological treatment modalities which take care of hyperarousal. Mindfulness can be an option for reducing hyperarousal and provide indirect way of reducing worry and rumination about sleep (Ong et al., 2012) Mindfulness can be defined as nonjudgmental, present-focused awareness (Kabat et al., 1998). There is Mindfulness based stress reduction program(MBSR) by (Cincotta et al., 2011) is emerging clinical modality for wellness. MBSR programs focus on the active development of conscious awareness and self regulation of attention via techniques such as focused breathing, sitting meditation, 'body scanning' and walking meditation as well as cognitive treatment elements (Heidenreich et al., 2006). Results have suggested that MBSR in combination with the behavioral component of CBT is a promising treatment for reducing symptoms of insomnia and sleep-related arousal recently, mindfulness has been suggested as a psychological treatment for restless legs syndrome (Bablas, 2015). Meta cognition is another one way of reducing hyperarousal. The two-level model of arousal devised by Ong and colleagues (2012) distinguishes primary arousal (the cognitive activity directly related to sleep difficulty) from secondary arousal (how one relates to thoughts about sleep). Essentially this model differentiates cognitive from meta cognitive processes. In a theoretical paper by Lundh (2005) the target of treatment is the relationship with cognition, rather than the thoughts themselves, which is in turn likely to reduce overall (cognitive, cortical and physical) arousal.

PREVENTION

Old age people are more prone to sleep disturbances. Changes in sleep pattern along with many physical and medical conditions contribute towards sleep disturbances in old age. Therefore preventive steps are needed to be adapted for wellbeing at least in terms of sleep. The establishment and maintenance of regular tight routine in both pre bed time and sleep schedule may be an important preventive factor. Proper management of jet lag, management of change in any daily routine, lifestyle and appropriate management of life during retirement period and if the emotionally and aroused thought managed efficiently then distress associated with sleep loss can be properly handle. Try to make sleep inductive environment rather than thinking about reason of sleep disturbance. An unrealistic expectation about sleep requirement in old age also needs to be tackled.

REFERENCES

Achermann, P., & Borbely, A. A. (2003). Mathematical models of sleep regulation. *Frontiers in Bioscience*, *8*(6), S683–S693. doi:10.2741/1064 PMID:12700054

American Academy of Sleep Medicine. (2005). *International Classification of Sleep Disorders. Diagnostic and Coding Manual* (2nd ed.). Westchester, IL: American Academy of Sleep Medicine.

American Academy of Sleep Medicine. (2014). *International classification of Sleep Disorders* (3rd ed.). Darien, IL: American Academy of Sleep Medicine.

American Psychiatric association. (2012). *Diagnostic and statistical mannual of mental disorder* (5th edn, revised). Washington, DC: American Psychiatric Association.

Ancoli-I, S., Kripke, D. F., Klauber, M. R., Mason, W. J., Fell, R., & Kaplan, O. (1991). Periodic limb movements in sleep in community-dwelling elderly. *Sleep*, *14*(6), 496–500. doi:10.1093/sleep/14.6.496 PMID:1798881

Ancoli-Israel, S., & Ayalon, L. (2006). Diagnosis and treatment of sleep disorders in older adults. *The American Journal of Geriatric Psychiatry*, *14*(2), 95–103.

Bablas, V., Yap, K., Cunnington, D., Swieca, J., & Greenwood, K. M. (2015). Mindfulness-based stress reduction for restless legs syndrome: A proof of concept trial. *Mindfulness*, *7*(2), 396–408. doi:10.1007/s12671-015-0457-9

Baron, R. A. (2001) States of consciousness: Psychology, 5th eds, Pearson education, New work.

Benington, J. H., & Heller, H. C. (1995). Brain energy metabolism as the function of sleep. *Progress in Neurobiology*, *45*(4), 347–360. doi:10.1016/0301-0082(94)00057-O PMID:7624482

Besset, A., Villemin, E., Tafti, M., & Billiard, M. (1998). Homeostatic process and sleep spindles in patients with sleep-maintenance insomnia:Effect of partial sleep deprivation. *Electroencephalography and Clinical Neurophysiology*, *107*(2), 122–132. doi:10.1016/S0013-4694(98)00048-0 PMID:9751283

Bootzin, R., & Epstein, D. (2011). Understanding and Treating Insomnia. *Annual Review of Clinical Psychology*, *7*, 435–458.

Borbely, A. A., & Tobler, I. (1985). Brain Mechanisms of Sleep. Academic Press.

Cincotta, A. L., Gehrman, P., Gooneratne, N. S., & Baime, M. J. (2011). The effects of amindfulness-based stress reduction programme on pre-sleep cognitive arousal and insomnia symptoms: A pilot study. *Stress and Health*, *27*(3), E299–E305. doi:10.1002/smi.1370

Circadian Rhythm. (2007). *American Heritage Science Dictnarary*. Houghton Mifflin.

Erwin, C. W., Somerville, E. R., & Radtke, R. A. (1984). A review of electroencephalographic features of normal sleep. *Journal of Clinical Neurophysiology*, *1*(3), 253–274. doi:10.1097/00004691-198407000-00001 PMID:6399909

Espie, C. A. (2002). Insomnia: Conceptual issues in the development, persistence, and treatment of sleep disorder in adults. *Annual Review of Psychology*, *53*(1), 215–243. doi:10.1146/annurev.psych.53.100901.135243 PMID:11752485

Foley, D. J., Monjan, A. A., Brown, S. L., Simonsick, E. M., Wallace, R. B., & Blazer, D. G. (1995). Sleep complaints among elderly persons: An epidemiologic study of three communities. *Sleep*, *18*, 425–432.

Galmi, R. (2010). Insomnia in the elderly: An update and future challenges. *Journal of Gerontology*, *58*, 231–247.

Harvey, A. G. (2002). A cognitive model of insomnia. *Behaviour Research and Therapy*, *40*, 869–893.

Haynes, S. N., Adams, A., & Franzen, M. (1981). The effects of pre-sleep stress on sleep-onset insomnia. *Journal of Abnormal Psychology*, *90*, 601–606.

Hays, R. D., & Stewart, A. L. (1992). Sleep measures. In A. L. Stewart & J. E. Ware (Eds.), *Measuring functioning and wellbeing:the Medical Outcomes Study Approach*. Durham, NC: Duke University.

Heidenreich, T., Strohle, G., & Michalak, J. (2006). Mindfulness: Conceptual aspects and results of the Freiburg mindfulness inventory. *Verhaltenstherapie*, *16*, 33–40. doi:10.1159/000091521

Hirshkowitz, M. (2004). Normal human sleep: An overview. *The Medical Clinics of North America*, 88.

Johns, M. W. (1991). A new method for measuring daytime sleepiness: The Epworth Sleepiness Scale. *Sleep*, 50–55. PMID:1798888

Kabat-Z, J., Wheeler, E., Light, T., Skillings, A., Scharf, M. J., & Cropley, T. G. (1998). Influence of a mindfulness meditation based stress reduction intervention on rates of skin clearing in patients with moderate to severe psoriasis undergoing phototherapy (UVB) and photochemotherapy (PUVA). *Psychosomatic Medicine*, *60*(5), 625–632. doi:10.1097/00006842-199809000-00020 PMID:9773769

Lundh, L. G. (2005). The Role of Acceptance and mindfulness in the treatment of insomnia. *Journal of Cognitive Psychotherapy*, *19*(1), 29–39. doi:10.1891/jcop.19.1.29.66331

Markov, D., & Goldman, M. (2006). Normal sleep and circadian rhythms: Neurobiologic mechanisms underlying sleep and wakefulness. *The Psychiatric Clinics of North America*, *29*(4), 841–853. doi:10.1016/j.psc.2006.09.008 PMID:17118271

Merica, H., & Fortune, R. D. (1997). A neuronal transition probability model for the evolution of power in the sigma and delta frequency bands of sleep EEG. *Physiology & Behavior*, *62*(3), 585–589. doi:10.1016/S0031-9384(97)00165-0 PMID:9272668

Monk, T. H., Reynolds, C. F. III, Kupfer, D. J., Buysse, D. J., Coble, P. A., Hayes, A. J., ... Ritenour, A. M. (1994). The Pittsburgh Sleep Diary. *Journal of Sleep Research*, *3*(2), 111–120. doi:10.1111/j.1365-2869.1994.tb00114.x

Monroe, L. J. (1967). Psychological and physiological differences between good and poor sleepers. *Journal of Abnormal Psychology*, *72*(3), 255–264. doi:10.1037/h0024563 PMID:6045597

Morin, C. M., Colecchi, C., Stone, J., Sood, R., & Brink, D. (1999). Behavioral and pharmacological therapies for late life insomnia. *Journal of the American Medical Association*, *281*(11), 991–999. doi:10.1001/jama.281.11.991 PMID:10086433

Morin, C. M., Colecchi, C. A., Stone, J., Sood, R. D., & Brink, D. (1995). Cognitive-behavior therapy and pharmacotherapy for insomnia: Update of a placebo-controlled clinical trial. *Sleep Research*, *24*, 303.

Morin, C. M., Culbert, J. P., & Schwartz, S. M. (1994). Nonpharmacological interventions for insomnia: A meta-analysis of treatment efficacy. *The American Journal of Psychiatry*, *151*(8), 1172–1180. doi:10.1176/ajp.151.8.1172 PMID:8037252

National Institutes of Health (NIH). (2017). Manifestations and management of chronic insomnia in adults. *NIH Consensus and State-of-the-Science Statements*, *22*, 5–17. Retrieved from http:// consensus.nih.gov

Neikrug, A. B., & Ancoli-Israel, S. (2010). Sleep Disorders in the Older Adults- A Mini- Review. *Gerontology*, *56*(2), 181–189. doi:10.1159/000236900 PMID:19738366

Nielsen, J. (2012) Exploring the sleep deprivation. (online image) Retrived August8, 2017from https;// jordannielson.blogspot.in/2012/an- introduction to – sleep.html

Ohayon, M. M., Carskadon, M. A., Guilleminault, C., & Vitiello, M. V. (2004). Meta-analysis of quantitative sleep parameters from childhood to old age in healthy individuals: Developing normative sleep values across the human lifespan. *Sleep*, *27*(7), 1255–1273. doi:10.1093/sleep/27.7.1255 PMID:15586779

Olson, E. J., Boeve, B. F., & Silber, M. H. (2000). Rapid eye movement sleep behaviour disorder: Demographic, clinical and laboratory findings in93 cases. *Brain*, *123*, 331–339.

Ong, J., Ulmer, C. S., & Manber, R. (2012). Improving sleep with mindfulness andacceptance: A metacognitive model of insomnia. *Behaviour Research and Therapy*, *50*(11), 651–660. doi:10.1016/j.brat.2012.08.001 PMID:22975073

Perlis, M. L., & Smith, M. T. (2005). Etiology and Pathophysiology of insomnia. In Principles and practice of sleep medicine. Elsevier. doi:10.1016/B0-72-160797-7/50067-7

Radulovacki, M., Virus, R. M., Djuricic-Nedelson, M., & Green, R. D. (1984). Adenosine analogs and sleep in rats. *The Journal of Pharmacology and Experimental Therapeutics*, *228*, 268–274. PMID:6694111

Roepke, S. K., & Ancoli-Israel, S. (2010). Sleep disorders in the elderly. *The Indian Journal of Medical Research*, *131*, 302–310.

Sateia, M. J. (2014). International Classification of Sleep Disorders-third edition: Highlights and modifications. *Chest*, *146*(5), 1387–1394. doi:10.1378/chest.14-0970 PMID:25367475

Smith, M. T., Perlis, M. L., & Chengazi, V. U. (2002). Neuroimaging of NREM sleep in primary insomnia: A Tc-99-HMPAO single photon emission computed tomography study. *Sleep*, *25*, 325–335. PMID:12003163

Spielman, A., Caruso, L., & Glovinsky, P. (1987). A behavioral perspective on insomnia treatment. *The Psychiatric Clinics of North America, 10*, 541–553. PMID:3332317

Stepanski, E. J. (2000). Behavioral therapy for insomnia. In M. H. Kryger, T. G. Roth, & W. C. Dement (Eds.), *Principles and Practice of Sleep Medicine* (pp. 647–656). Philadelphia: WB Saunders.

Strecker, R. E., Morairty, S., Thakkar, M. M., Porkka-Heiskanen, T., Basheer, R., Dauphin, L. J., ... McCarley, R. W. (2000). Adenosinergic modulation of basal forebrain and preoptic/anterior hypothalamic neuronal activity in the control of behavioral state. *Behavioural Brain Research, 115*(2), 183–204. doi:10.1016/S0166-4328(00)00258-8 PMID:11000420

Susan, K. R., & Israel, S. A. (2010). Sleep Disorders in the Elderly. *The Indian Journal of Medical Research, 131*, 302–310. PMID:20308755

Taylor, D., Gehrman, P., Dautovich, N. D., Lichstein, K. L., & McCrae, C. S. (2014). Causes of Insomnia. In Handbook of insomnia. Springer Healthcare Communitation. DOI. doi:10.1007/978-1-907673-73-3-2

The human brain: From neurons to nervous system (n.d) Sleep Disorder (online image) Retrived 27 August, 2017 from neurons co.uk/Neurosciences/Chapter/%206/P.6%20Sleep%20 Disorders.html.

Vaughn, B. V., & Giallanza, P. (2008). Technical review of polysomnography. *Chest, 134*, 1310–1319.

Vitiello, M. V. (2009). *Sleep and Circadian rhythms disorders in human ageing and dementia. University of Washington*. Seattle, WA, USA: Elsevier Ltd.

World Health Organization. (1992). *The ICD-10 Classification of mental and behavioral disorders: clinical descriptions and diagnostic guidelines*. Geneva: World Health Organization.

Zucconi, M., & Ferri, R. (2014) Assessment of sleep disorders and diagnostic procedure, sleep medicine Textbook. *Europian Sleep Research Society*. Reterived from www.esrs.eu/fileadmin/user... /ESRS_Sleep_Medicine_Textbook_cChapter_b1.pdf Acesseed on 20,August,2017,95-109

KEY TERMS AND DEFINITIONS

Cognitive Behaviour Therapy: A form of cognitive therapy that focuses on changing illogical pattern of thoughts. It is useful in many mental and physical health problems.

Circadian Rhythms: Refers to the daily rhythms in physiology and behavior that oscillate once approximately every 24 hours. The rhythms are generated by neural structure in hypothalamus; those functions work like a biological clock. The sleep wake cycle is one of these rhythms.

EEG Brain Waves (Electroencephalogram): A record of electrical activity within the brain. EEG plays an important role in the scientific study of sleep.

Insomnia: Has been historically defined by patterns of inappropriate wakefulness that occur during the sleep period. It is a disorder involving the inability to fall asleep or maintain sleep.

Sleep Apnea: A sleep disorder characterized by repetitive collapse of the pharyngeal airway (interrupted breathing) during sleep due to which the patient wakes up many times.

Sleep Architecture: Represents the predictable cyclical pattern of sleep, alternating between non-rapid eye movement (NREM) and rapid eye movement (REM) sleep. It occurs throughout the night consisting of four NREM phases and one REM phase.

Sleep-Wake Cycle: Refers to the biological pattern of alternating sleep and wakefulness. The sleep-wake system is thought to be regulated by the interplay of two major processes, one that promotes sleep and one that maintains wakefulness. This cycle is roughly 8 hours of nocturnal sleep and 16 hours of daytime activity in humans in a single day.

Chapter 18
Impact of Tuberculosis in Elderly Population

Gagan Chooramani
King George's Medical University, India

Pooja Singh
Indian Institute of Technology Delhi, India

ABSTRACT

The World Health Organization has declared that the spread of tuberculosis is a global emergency. Despite the implementation of strong tuberculosis-control initiatives by WHO, this highly infectious disease continues to affect all vulnerable populations, including the elderly population. Adverse social factors and poor living conditions also affect the elderly much more than the young. The clinical characteristics of tuberculosis in older adults can be unusual and may be confused with age-related illnesses. Various factors related to old age can also cause complications in the diagnosis, treatment, and disease outcomes for tuberculosis patients. The contributory factors may be poor memory, deafness, mental confusion, or impairment of speech. In addition, therapy for tuberculosis in elderly individuals is challenging because of the increased incidence of adverse drug reactions. Hence, understanding the impact of these substantial aspects will help to overcome the problem of tuberculosis in the elderly population.

INTRODUCTION

Tuberculosis is emerging as a significant health problem in the elderly. It is a classic example of a disease that can have a long latent period between infection and clinically evident disease. After the infection, the disease can be quiescent and remain dormant for a variable period of time, sometimes forever. Because of this behavior, most individuals who have become infected can be at a risk for clinical disease at any time, particularly if debilitated or immunosuppressed. Previously TB is known to be a disease of poor, now affecting people of all age and social status. But still the major effect of disease is seen on elder peoples. In recent years, there has been increased focus on active case finding among groups considered to be vulnerable to develop tuberculosis, including people living with HIV (Raviglione, Narain, & Kochi, 1992), people with diabetes (Van Crevel & Dockrell, 2014) and children (Marais, Schaaf, & Graham,

DOI: 10.4018/978-1-5225-3480-8.ch018

2014). In low and middle-income countries attention is given to vulnerable groups but older adults are still neglected. While in high income countries older people are vulnerable and acknowledged. With increasing life expectancy, the number of people who are 60 years and more (the defined age for senior citizen according to Indian legislation) is increasing in India. Due to the presence of drug-resistant strains of tuberculosis older adults in India, which has the highest proportion of tuberculosis cases globally, face further complications (Udwadia & Vendoti, 2013; Babu & Laxminarayan, 2012).Clinical presentation and spectrum of disease make its diagnosis difficult in older adults TB (Chan-Yeung, Noertjojo, Tan, Chan, & Tam 2002; Morris, 1990).

WORLD SCENARIO

Tuberculosis continues to be a world-leading cause of disease and death, particularly in low- and middle-income countries, which carry the bulk (>95%) of the global tuberculosis disease burden (WHO Global Tuberculosis Report 2013). Worldwide, the number of people > 60 years is expected to increase by more than double, from 841 million people in 2013 to more than two billion people in 2050. It is projected that in 2047, older persons will exceed the number of children for the first time. Currently older people live in the developed world, but the older population is also growing rapidly in less developed regions such that projections for 2050 predict nearly 80% of the world's older population will be living in less developed countries. (WHO, 2013). The 2010 Global Burden of Disease estimates shows that 57% of all tuberculosis deaths globally occurred among people older than 50, with more than half of these deaths in those aged 65 and above (Negin, Abimbola, & Marais, 2015).

INDIAN SCENARIO

India is the highest tuberculosis (TB) burden country in the world accounting for nearly 25% of the global TB. The Revised National Tuberculosis Control Programme (RNTCP), implemented throughout the country, has been successful in achieving the global targets of 70% case detection and 85% treatment success rates in new smear positive TB patients since 2007. Over the next 5 years (2012–17), the program aims to achieve universal access to TB services with a treatment success rate of at least 90% (CTD, 2012). Previous studies were done in India, Hong-King, Ethiopia have shown that TB patients aged 60 years and above are one such sub-group with poor treatment success owing to poor treatment adherence, poor tolerance to therapy, higher mortality rates and co-morbidities (Mukherjee, Saha, & Paul, 2008). In May 2012, Tuberculosis was declared as a notifiable disease by Indian government because of its increased prevalence. In some regions of India older adults are estimated to make up 14% of all tuberculosis patients and have a higher likelihood of unfavorable outcomes due to drug-related adverse events, increased co-morbidity, and a higher rate of poverty than younger adults (Ananthakrishnan et al., 2013; Velayutham et al., 2014).

TUBERCULOSIS AND BIOPSYCHOSOCIAL FACTORS IN AGEING

Many risk factors such as age, sex, malnutrition, diabetes, human immunodeficiency virus (HIV) infection (biological factors), tobacco smoking, alcoholism (behavioral factors), poverty, overcrowding and poor housing (socio-economic factors) are known to be associated with the development of pulmonary TB. Most of these factors contribute to the risk of infection rather than to progression to disease, while others are mostly responsible for progression from infection to disease.

Comorbidity

Comorbidity results in reduced innate immunity. Various Comorbid conditions-include Diabetes, renal failure, chronic pulmonary disease, edema, immobility. These conditions can increase the incidence of infection and mortality in the elderly individuals. Perhaps the best clinical example in which comorbidity contributes heavily to infection risk is Chronic Pulmonary disease (COPD). This disease, most often caused by prolonged exposure to tobacco smoke, has a high prevalence in older adults (Schaaf, Collins, Bekker., & Davies, 2010).

Ageing

Ageing is a major risk factor for any disease. The effects of aging have been attributed to a decline in numerous macrophage functions which figure prominently in host defense in pulmonary TB (Meyer, 2005).

Gender

The immune response is different in the two sexes, indicating sexual dimorphism. This sexual dimorphism in immune response may explain the higher risk among males of developing TB. Evidence suggests that at physiological levels, estrogen is beneficial to the immune system, (Markovic, 2004).Whereas the male sex hormone, testosterone, is immunosuppressive (Cutol et al., 2004).

Smokers/Nonsmokers

Smokers have a 2.1 times higher risk of developing TB than non-smokers after controlling for the effects of other factors. Recent work on the physiological effects of nicotine, the major toxic compound in tobacco smoke, showed that nicotine turns off the production of tumor necrosis factor-alpha by lung macrophages, thereby rendering smokers more susceptible to the progression of latent infection to active disease (Sopori, Kozak, Savage, Geng, & Kluger, 1998).

Alcohol Abuse

Alcoholics have a 1.5 times higher risk of developing TB than non-alcoholics, after controlling for the effects of age, sex and smoking on alcoholism. Buskin et al. reported a relative risk of 2.0 for heavy alcohol consumers (Buskin, Gale, & Weiss, 1994).

Nutrition

The poor dietary intake particularly consumption of uncooked meat, unpasteurized milk and elevated serum iron were risk factors for TB infection. Intake of uncooked meat and drinking unpasteurized cow milk was statistically significant in the increased likelihood of TB infection compared to those who consumed boil cow milk and goat milk (Mfinanga et al., 2003).

TB With Co-Infection

Co-infection is associated with poorer treatment outcomes. For example, individuals co-infected with tuberculosis and diabetes in China was 4.5 times more likely to fail treatment than those with tuberculosis only. Diabetes triples the risk for active tuberculosis, so with rates of diabetes rapidly rising in many tuberculosis endemic areas, it is likely that the present tuberculosis epidemic will be sustained – in particular among older people most affected by diabetes. Glycemic control, necessary to address diabetes and also to improve tuberculosis outcomes, is particularly challenging in the context of multi-morbidity.

PATHOGENISIS

Mainly tuberculosis transmitted almost by inhalation of an aerosol containing viable members of the species called as *Mycobacterium tuberculosis* (*M.tb*). *M. tuberculosis* is carried in airborne particles, called droplet nuclei, of 1– 5 microns in diameter. These droplet nuclei are generated when persons having pulmonary TB disease cough, sneeze, shout or sing. Depending on the environment, these tiny particles can remain suspended in the air for several hours. Transmission occurs when a person inhales droplet nuclei containing *M. tuberculosis*, and the droplet nuclei travel through mouth or nasal passages, upper respiratory tract, and bronchi to reach the alveoli of the lungs.

Here in alveoli, these bacilli are ingested by alveolar macrophages; and these macrophages destroy or inhibit majority of bacilli. These macrophages having TB bacilli are presented to other white blood cells. This triggers the immune response in which white blood cells kill or encapsulate most of the bacilli, leading to the formation of a granuloma. At this point, Latent Tuberculosis Infection (LTBI) has been established. Within weeks after infection, the immune system is usually able to halt the multiplication of the tubercle bacilli, preventing further progression. Persons with LTBI have *M. tuberculosis* in their bodies, but do not have TB disease and cannot spread the infection to other people. A person with LTBI is not regarded as having a case of TB.

In some people, due to weak immunity, the immune system cannot keep the tubercle bacilli under control, and bacilli began to multiply rapidly, resulting in progression from LTBI to TB disease. A small number of tubercle bacilli enter the bloodstream and spread throughout the body. The tubercle bacilli may reach any part of the body, including areas where TB disease is more likely to develop (such as the brain, larynx, lymph node, lung, spine, bone. Persons who have TB disease are usually infectious and may spread the bacteria to other people. Without treatment, approximately 5% of persons who have been infected *with M. tuberculosis* will develop the disease in the first year or 2 after infection, and another 5% will develop disease sometime later in life. Thus, without treatment, approximately 10% of persons with normal immune systems who are infected with *M. tuberculosis* will develop TB disease at some point in their lives (CDC, 2013).

WHY ELDER POPULATION IS AT MORE RISK OF TUBERCULOSIS

Aging has significant effects on both the innate and adaptive immune system-and contribute to the increased risk of infection. Primarily immune protection against tuberculosis infection can be achieved by cell mediated immunity, through the coordinated action of phagocytic cells and adaptive immune T cell responses that serve to kill or contain the bacteria. The principal route of entry of *M. tuberculosis,* as well as the major organ of disease, is the lung. Elderly people have an increased susceptibility to infectious diseases, particularly of the respiratory tract, and suffer greater morbidity and mortality compared to younger individuals (Byang-Maddick & Noursadeghi, 2016). In older adults, tuberculosis may be either exogenous or endogenous in origin. Over 90% of cases in the elderly represent endogenous tuberculosis, i.e., reactivation of dormant infection in the lungs or elsewhere in the body. In the remainder, it may be exogenous, i.e., acquired from an outside source, usually a sputum positive case. It is well known that age related decline in the cell-mediated immunity influences reactivation of latent infection in the elderly (Sood, 2000). Due to the prolonged life expectancy in the elders increased the use of drugs that suppress cellular immunity, and may further increase the incidence of pulmonary TB among them. In individual cases, the presence of intercurrent illnesses like diabetes mellitus, chronic renal failure, malnutrition, alcohol abuse, certain malignancies and use of immunosuppressive drugs like corticosteroids further impair cell mediated immunity. These can thereby increase the risk of reactivation of the disease.

Age-related changes in the phenotype and function of macrophages are also reported, which might be expected to compromise their role in protection against TB. These include reduced expression of innate immune receptors, reduced production of tumor necrosis factor (TNF) and reduced phagocytosis (Shaw, Goldstein, & Montgomer, 2013). Clear evidence for how these may impact the host-pathogen interactions between macrophages and Mtb is lacking (Guerra-Laso et al., 2013). Approximately 90% of cases of tuberculosis disease that involve elderly persons are caused by reactivation of primary Infection (Yoshikawa, 1992). Tuberculosis infection without disease may occur in 30%–50% of individuals. Rarely, previously infected older persons may experience elimination of the viable tubercle bacilli and revert to a tuberculin-negative state and a “naive” immunologic status; these persons are at risk for new infection (re-infection) with *M. tuberculosis*. Thus, older persons potentially at risk for tuberculosis include individuals never exposed to *M. tuberculosis* those with latent and dormant primary infection that may reactivate, and those who are no longer infected and thus are at risk for re-infection (Thomas & Rajagopalan, 2001).

Adverse social factors and poor living conditions also affect the elderly much more than the young. Relatively large proportions of the elderly population of certain countries in Latin America live in urban or peri-urban slums; with a lack of adequate sanitation and overcrowding creating a perfect environment for the propagation of tuberculosis. Social marginalization, reduced mobility and financial dependency often discourage health care seeking. This may delay diagnosis, leading to worse outcomes and potentially prolonged transmission (Bushan, Kajal, Maske, & Singh, 2012). Older careers with tuberculosis also pose a risk to vulnerable young children in settings where grandparents often perform child-care duties (Negin, Abimbola, & Marais, 2015).

CLINICAL PRESENTATION AND SYMPTOMS

Clinical presentation of active TB in elderly adults is different occurring in younger people. Its symptoms mainly depend upon the site of infection. However some classical symptoms remain same but their severity can vary.

Pulmonary Tuberculosis

Pulmonary tuberculosis is by far most common form of TB in elders accounting for approximately 75% of elderly TB cases. Although aging patients with pulmonary tuberculosis can present with typical respiratory as well as systemic symptoms (e.g., sputum production, hemoptysis, fever, night sweats, weight loss, and anorexia), a significant number of such patients may manifest atypical complaints or may exhibit minimal pulmonary symptoms. Dysponea is more common and haemoptysis is less common in elderly. These symptoms can mimic age related illness such as reduced functional capacity, chronic fatigue, cognitive impairment, anorexia or pyrexia of unknown origin. An accurate history may be difficult to obtain due to poor memory, impaired hearing, sight or speech (Yoshikawa, 1992).

Miliary Tuberculosis

Miliary, or disseminated, tuberculosis occurs with greater frequency among aging patients; many cases are detected only at autopsy. Miliary tuberculosis is typically associated with an acute or subacute pattern of high, intermittent fever and clinical evidence of meningeal or serosal involvement. Clinical features include unexplained fever, weight loss, and hepatosplenomegaly, without other focal signs; this form of tuberculosis should be considered in the differential diagnosis of fever of unknown origin (Thomas & Rajagopalan, 2001).

Tuberculous Meningitis

TB meningitis in elderly patients results from reactivation of a primary dormant focus or is associated with miliary seeding of infection and generally present with a subacute onset of fever, headache, and confusion, with concomitant or preceding systemic symptoms of weakness, anorexia, and fatigue. Tuberculous meningitis is associated with exceedingly high mortality among elderly persons; neurological deficits are common among survivors (Thomas & Rajagopalan, 2001). However, some older patients can also manifest unexplained dementia or obtundation without fever or nuchal rigidity; for such patients, a high index of suspicion for tuberculous meningitis must be maintained until the suspicion is disproven.

Skeletal Tuberculosis

In elderly persons, the involvement of bone in *M. tuberculosis* infection commonly affects the spine. The thoracic and lumbar spines are commonly involved; cervical disease is unusual. Para-vertebral abscesses, or cold abscesses, are often associated with spinal infection. Primary symptoms of spinal tuberculosis include pain over the involved vertebrae. With the advancement of disease neurological deficits and sinus tracts may also include with Low-grade fever, weight loss, fatigue, and anorexia. In elderly persons tuberculosis arthritis commonly involves the large, weight-bearing joints, peripheral joints (i.e., the knees, wrists, ankles). Pain and swelling of the involved joints and loss of range of motion can occur sometimes. Because older patients often have the degenerative joint disease or other arthritis, the diagnosis of coexisting tuberculosis arthritis may easily be overlooked (Thomas & Rajagopalan, 2001).

Genitourinary Tuberculosis

Although genitourinary tuberculosis occurs more often in persons in the third, fourth, and fifth decades of life, this form of the disease is also seen in elderly persons. The kidney is the major site of involvement, and as many as 20%–30% of patients are asymptomatic. Genitourinary tuberculosis may involve the ureters, bladder, prostate, epididymis, and seminal vesicles. It includes symptoms, dysuria, urinary frequency, flank pain, and hematuria. The diagnosis is often considered when an abnormal urinary sediment, pyuria without bacteruria, or hematuria is noted (Thomas & Rajagopalan, 2001).

DIAGNOSIS OF TUBERCULOSIS

AFB Smear

World Health Organization (WHO) recommended two sputum smears for diagnosis of pulmonary tuberculosis. One on spot and second brought in the following morning. Diagnosis of TB primarily relies on the identification of AFB in sputum smears using a conventional light microscope. The sputum specimens are smeared directly on to the slides and subjected to Ziel-Neelsen (ZN) staining. Now WHO, recommended-fluorescence microscopy as an alternative for conventional ZN microscopy as it takes less time to examine smears stained with ZN and have higher sensitivity and similar specificity. This microscopic examination of two sputum samples decrease time of patient's diagnosis and initiation of treatment and decreased number of patients dropping out of diagnostic pathway

TB Culture

Culture is more sensitive than AFB smear microscopy for the detection of *M. tuberculosis*. It detects as few as 10 to 100 viable bacteria/ml before culture, sputum requires decontamination to kills all the normal flora of the respiratory tract capable of overgrowing in the culture. Culture is used for drug sensitivity testing, and for characterization of species. Specimen from sterile sites does not require decontamination. The main problem with culture is it takes long time to grow. To reduce the turnaround time WHO recommended liquid culture and DST. This is a rapid and affordable method of species identification and can yield the result within few weeks. Although culture is not routinely performed in resource poor settings except for purposes of surveillance, treatment failure, or detection of drug resistance. Culture is critically important in detecting TB in HIV-positive individuals who often have low bacillary loads in sputum specimens (Getahun, Harrington, O'Brien, & Nunn, 2007).

Molecular Line Probe Assays

This is PCR-based reverse-hybridization line probe assay (LPA) developed for the rapid detection of RIF resistance. This is highly sensitive and specific for the detection of Rif. Resistance alone or in combination with Inh. In *M. tuberculosis* isolates in smear positive sputum specimens. The direct use of LPA on smear negative specimen not recommended. Ministry of Health (MOH) within the context of country plans for the appropriate management of MDR-TB patients adopted of LPAs for the rapid detection of MDR-TB patients. It includes the development of country-specific screening algorithms and timely access to quality-assured second-line anti-TB drugs. The adoption of LPAs does not eliminate the need for conventional culture DST capability; culture remains necessary for the definitive diagnosis of TB in smear negative patients, and conventional DST is required to diagnose XDR-TB (WHO, 2008).

Direct Detection of TB in Patient Specimens

Nucleic Acid Amplification (NAA) /Xpert MTB/RIF (Xpert) assay (Cepheid Inc., Sunnyvale, CA, USA) is a cartridge-based, semi-automated, rapid molecular assay, which permits rapid TB diagnosis through detection of the DNA of *Mycobacterium tuberculosis* and simultaneous identification of a majority of the mutations that confer rifampicin resistance (which is highly predictive of multi-drug resistant TB [MDR-TB]). Testing of diagnostic specimens can reduce the overall turnaround time for the laboratory of diagnosis of tuberculosis. NAA testing performed on pulmonary as well as extrapulmonary specimens from patients with sign and symptoms of tuberculosis, independent of smear microscopy results (Lawn et al, 2013).

DIAGNOSTIC DIFFICULTIES IN ELDERS

The biggest problem in diagnosis of TB in older adults is an inability to give an accurate account of their symptoms. The contributory factors may be poor memory, deafness, mental confusion or impairment of speech. Old people, and sometimes also their family members wrongly attribute their symptoms to the effect of old age. A delay in TB diagnosis increases the severity of the disease. The presence of other chronic diseases may confuse the clinical picture, both for the patient and the doctor. In particular, the concomitant malignant disease can mask the symptoms of tuberculosis since the two conditions may coexist at this age. The basis of this problem is that in old age the body's reaction to tuberculosis as also to other infections is often diminished. The likely reasons for failure of recognition of pulmonary tuberculosis are a paucity of respiratory symptoms, the presence of significant underlying diseases like chronic obstructive airway disease (COAD) and inability to produce sputum and above all, atypical radiographic findings like solitary nodules, mass like densities, extensive broncho-pneumonia and lower lobe infiltrates (Sood, 2000). Age-related changes in the tuberculin skin reaction and a high incidence of underlying illnesses also play a role in prolonging the final diagnosis (Lee, Haan, Jae, Woe, & Chung, 2005). Difficulties in diagnosis tuberculosis in older adults has been assessed in a meta-analysis of studies focusing on tuberculosis in older adults, which found that common symptoms used to identify tuberculosis such as dyspnoea, haemoptysis and fever are less prominent in older than in younger adults. Older adults also have a reduced ability to produce a high quality sputum specimen. Furthermore, one of the most common tests that assist a diagnosis of sputum smear-negative tuberculosis, the Mantoux skin test, tends to produce false negative results in older patients (Negin, Abimola, & Marais, 2015).

CHALLENGES FOR TREATING TB IN ELDERS

Treatment of tuberculosis does not vary by age but toxicities of anti-tuberculosis therapy may be more prevalent with advanced age, and drug interactions are common. Treatment failure among geriatric patients can occur due to decreased absorption of drugs associated with age-related physiological changes such as gastric pH, modified gastric emptying rate and slower intestinal transmit time and drug intolerance associated with the likelihood of polytherapy.

Tuberculosis treatment outcomes in older adults are often poorer due to delayed diagnosis, increased rates of drug-related adverse events, frequent co-morbidity and overarching poverty (Lee, Han, Song, & Chung, 2005). Targeted efforts to improve case detection and treatment outcomes in this population are needed to achieve global tuberculosis targets. Focused outreach services to places where older adults congregate are the temples, social clubs or old-age homes are needed along with clinical training to assist diagnosis and optimal case management. Caring for increasing numbers of older adults with tuberculosis may prove difficult in regions where health resources are already constrained, but health systems will have to confront the challenge of an aging population and the integrated services required to address their health needs. This also emphasizes the need to include older people in the assessment of new tuberculosis drugs. (Negin, Abimola, & Marais, 2015).

SOLUTIONS AND RECOMMENDATIONS

Older adults provide society's careers, community leaders and mentors, and play an important role in educating the younger generation. Including them as a key population in tuberculosis prevention, active case finding, and treatment interventions will have positive cascading effects on families, communities and societies.

Socio-Demographic

Based on socio-demographic factors associated with the occurrence of TB, public health practice should liaise with other programmes. As these programmes have gender issue and TB prevention as part of their agenda and empower females through job and skill acquisition schemes, increase girl-child education, and encourage improvement in family cohesion and this will reduce the social inequalities thereby preventing the TB transmission. The importance of social reform could be observed which has helped significantly in decreasing infectious diseases such as TB, malaria, and HIV prevalence including the reduction in social and health inequalities across the population.

Socioeconomic Status

Poverty, low income, low educational status, and unskilled occupation were associated with increased risk for TB infection. Deteriorated healthcare system and the poor working condition have been attributed to increased risk of TB transmission. Development of poverty reduction policy document and related procedure which will guarantee that the TB prevention and control strategy promotes fairness in access and financial protection for the low socioeconomic gradient and the poor should be tackled by in national strategies. Public health through its TB initiatives should also use social support for TB cases and families, microfinance system and vocational training to empower the less privileged population which in long run will reduce TB transmission.

Social Behavior

Tobacco smoking and alcohol abuse were associated with increased risk for TB infection. The integration of public health initiatives such as tobacco smoking cessation and alcohol harm reduction programme into the present TB control and prevention strategy may help strengthen TB control and prevention efforts. Public health should liaise with the legislature to enforce tobacco companies to not only smoking causes lung cancer but to include TB infection as the harmful effect of tobacco smoking and this may help to decrease TB transmission. Public awareness regarding the causal link between TB infection and smoking and alcohol should be increased through the use of radio, poster, fliers and billboard especially in local languages for better understanding.

Nutrition

Poor dietary intake particularly consumption of uncooked meat, unpasteurized milk and elevated serum iron were reported as risk factors for TB infection. The collaboration of public health authorities with government will improve food security to reduce malnutrition and unhealthy dietary intake which will reduce the TB transmission. Therefore, TB control programme should coordinate with food safety agencies including legislature to emphasise the food process industries to determine the average daily dietary iron requirement and label it on the food package to avoid iron overload which will prevent TB transmission as being done for diabetes and yielded a good outcome. The public should be informed of the harmful effect of consumption of uncooked meat, fresh cow blood, and unpasteurized milk and avoid such practice as it causes TB transmission. In addition, consumption of properly cook the meat, boil the cow blood and milk should be encouraged which will help to prevent TB transmission among this population. Also the public health should link with the agricultural department to engage in routine and active latent TB screening of the cow for quarantine and treatment so that human-animal TB transmission will be prevented.

Living/Working Condition and Physical Environment

From the historical background, TB is known as a disease of poverty and is associated with poor housing environments. On average, people with low socioeconomic status are likely to be in overcrowded and poorly ventilated living environments, have more frequent contact with active TB cases, more food insecurities, low levels of awareness about healthy behavior and limited access to health care. In addition, lack of housing ownership may lead to poor building hygiene maintenance. In such kind of environment there is an increased probability of inhaling droplets expelled by infectious individuals in overcrowded and poorly ventilated place. Living conditions of people, should be improved so that the chance of the infection could be reduced to stop TB. It is also important that people should be educated and facilitated with proper health care and medical facility.

REFERENCES

Ananthakrishnan, R., Kumar, K., Ganesh, M., Kumar, A. M., Krishnan, N., Swaminathan, S., ... Gupta, D. (2013). The profile and treatment outcomes of the older (aged 60 years and above) tuberculosis patients in Tamilnadu, South India. *PLoS One*, *8*(7), e67288. doi:10.1371/journal.pone.0067288 PMID:23861755

Bhushan, B., Kajal, N. C., Maske, A., & Singh, S. P. (2012). Manifestations of tuberculosis in elderly versus young hospitalised patients in Amritsar, India. *The International Journal of Tuberculosis and Lung Disease*, *16*(9), 1210–1213. doi:10.5588/ijtld.11.0778 PMID:22794086

Buskin, S. E., Gale, J. L., Weiss, N. S., & Nolan, C. M. (1994). Tuberculosis risk factors in adults in King County, Washington, 1988 through 1990. *American Journal of Public Health*, *84*(11), 1750–1756. doi:10.2105/AJPH.84.11.1750 PMID:7977912

Byng-Maddick, R., & Noursadeghi, M. (2016). Does tuberculosis threaten our ageing populations? *BMC Infectious Diseases*, *16*(1), 119. doi:10.1186/s12879-016-1451-0 PMID:26968654

CDC Manual. (2013). *Introduction to the core curriculum on tuberculosis: what the clinician should know*. Retrieved from www.cdc.gov/tb

Central Tuberculosis Division. (2012). *Tuberculosis India. Annual Report of the Revised National Tuberculosis Control Programme*. Directorate General of Health Services, Ministry of Health and Family Welfare, Government of India.

Cutolo, M., Sulli, A., Capellino, S., Villaggio, B., Montagna, P., Seriolo, B., & Straub, R. H. (2004). Sex hormones influence on the immune system: Basic and clinical aspects in autoimmunity. *Lupus*, *13*(9), 635–638. doi:10.1191/0961203304lu1094oa PMID:15485092

Getahun, H., Harrington, M., O'Brien, R., & Nunn, P. (2007). Diagnosis of smear-negative pulmonary tuberculosis in people with HIV infection or AIDS in resource-constrained settings: Informing urgent policy changes. *Lancet*, *369*(9578), 2042–2049. doi:10.1016/S0140-6736(07)60284-0 PMID:17574096

Guerra-Laso, J. M., González-García, S., González-Cortés, C., Diez-Tascón, C., López-Medrano, R., & Rivero-Lezcano, O. M. (2013). Macrophages from elders are more permissive to intracellular multiplication of Mycobacterium tuberculosis. *Age*, 1–16. PMID:22791369

Jacobson, J. M. (1992). Alcoholism and tuberculosis. *Alcohol Research & Health*, *16*(1), 39.

Lawn, S. D., Mwaba, P., Bates, M., Piatek, A., Alexander, H., Marais, B. J., & Abubakar, I. (2013). Advances in tuberculosis diagnostics: The Xpert MTB/RIF assay and future prospects for a point-of-care test. *The Lancet Infectious Diseases*, *13*(4), 349–361. doi:10.1016/S1473-3099(13)70008-2 PMID:23531388

Marais, B. J., Schaaf, H. S., & Graham, S. M. (2014). Child health and tuberculosis. *The Lancet. Respiratory Medicine*, *2*(4), 254–256. doi:10.1016/S2213-2600(14)70009-8 PMID:24717618

Marković, L. (2004). Interaction involving the thymus and the hypothalamus-pituitary axis, immunomodulation by hormones. *Srpski Arhiv za Celokupno Lekarstvo*, *132*(5-6), 187–193. doi:10.2298/SARH0406187M PMID:15493593

Meyer, K. C. (2005). Aging. *Proceedings of the American Thoracic Society*, *2*(5), 433–439. doi:10.1513/pats.200508-081JS PMID:16322596

Mfinanga, S. G., Mørkve, O., Kazwala, R. R., Cleaveland, S., Sharp, J. M., Shirima, G., & Nilsen, R. (2003). The role of livestock keeping in tuberculosis trends in Arusha, Tanzania. *The International Journal of Tuberculosis and Lung Disease*, *7*(7), 695–704. PMID:12870693

Mukherjee, A., Saha, I., & Paul, B. (2008). Tuberculosis in Patients Below and Above 60 years and Their Treatment Outcome Under RNTCP–A study in Rural West Bengal, India. *Journal Indian Academy of Geriatric*, *4*, 60–63.

Negin, J., Abimbola, S., & Marais, B. J. (2015). Tuberculosis among older adults–time to take notice. *International Journal of Infectious Diseases*, *32*, 135–137. doi:10.1016/j.ijid.2014.11.018 PMID:25809769

Raviglione, M. C., Narain, J. P., & Kochi, A. (1992). HIV-associated tuberculosis in developing countries: Clinical features, diagnosis, and treatment. *Bulletin of the World Health Organization*, *70*(4), 515. PMID:1394786

Shaw, A. C., Goldstein, D. R., & Montgomery, R. R. (2013). Age-dependent dysregulation of innate immunity. *Nature Reviews. Immunology*, *13*(12), 875–887. doi:10.1038/nri3547 PMID:24157572

Sood, R. (2000). The problem of geriatric tuberculosis. *Journal of Indian Academy of Clinical Medicine*, *5*, 157.

Sopori, M. L., Kozak, W., Savage, S. M., Geng, Y., & Kluger, M. J. (1998). Nicotine-induced modulation of T Cell function. Implications for inflammation and infection. *Advances in Experimental Medicine and Biology*, *437*, 279–289. doi:10.1007/978-1-4615-5347-2_31 PMID:9666281

Thomas, T. Y., & Rajagopalan, S. (2001). Tuberculosis and aging: A global health problem. *Clinical Infectious Diseases*, *33*(7), 1034–1039. doi:10.1086/322671 PMID:11528577

Van Crevel, R., & Dockrell, H. M. (2014). TANDEM: Understanding diabetes and tuberculosis. *The Lancet. Diabetes & Endocrinology*, *2*(4), 270–272. doi:10.1016/S2213-8587(14)70011-7 PMID:24703039

Velayutham, B. R. V., Nair, D., Chandrasekaran, V., Raman, B., Sekar, G., Watson, B., & Swaminathan, S. (2014). Profile and response to anti-tuberculosis treatment among elderly tuberculosis patients treated under the TB Control programme in South India. *PLoS One*, *9*(3), e88045. doi:10.1371/journal.pone.0088045 PMID:24618888

World Health Organization. (2008). Molecular line probe assays for rapid screening of patients at risk of multidrug-resistant tuberculosis (MDR-TB). *Policy Statement, 27.*

World Health Organization. (2011). Same-day diagnosis of tuberculosis by microscopy. *Policy statement. World Health Organization Document WHO/HTM/TB/2011.7, 1*(11).

World Health Organization. (Ed.). (2013). *Global tuberculosis report 2013*. World Health Organization.

World Health Organization. (2013). *United Nations. World Population Aging*. WHO.

Yoshikawa, T. T. (1992). Tuberculosis in aging adults. *Journal of the American Geriatrics Society*, *40*(2), 178–187. doi:10.1111/j.1532-5415.1992.tb01941.x PMID:1740604

KEY TERMS AND DEFINITIONS

Diagnosis: The identification of the nature of an illness or other problem by examination of the symptoms.

Elderly Population: The elderly population is defined as people aged 65 and over. The elderly dependency rate is defined as the ratio between the elderly population and the working age (15-64 years) population.

Tuberculosis (TB): Is an infectious disease caused by the bacterium *Mycobacterium tuberculosis* (MTB). Tuberculosis generally affects the lungs, but can also affect other parts of the body.

Chapter 19
Thyroid Disease in Ageing and Risk Factors

Shamsi Akbar
King George's Medical University, India

Barre Vijaya Prasad
Dharwad Institute of Mental Health and Neurosciences (DIMHANS), India

ABSTRACT

Thyroid disorders are highly prevalent, most frequently afflicting aging women. It is crucial to advance the means of diagnosing thyroid diseases, especially overt and subclinical hypothyroidism in elderly people, because thyroid-associated symptoms are very similar to symptoms of the normal aging process. Thyroid hormone production, metabolism, and action change with aging. The reference ranges for serum thyrotropin and thyroid hormones are derived mainly from younger populations. Thus, the prevalence of subclinical thyroid dysfunction is increased greatly in the elderly. There has been increasing interest in thyroid function in the elderly because of association of thyroid status with disability, cognitive function, cardiovascular disease risk, and longevity.

INTRODUCTION

Thyroid gland hormone production is directly stimulated by TSH, which is synthesized and secreted in the anterior pituitary under stimulation of thyrotropin- releasing hormone produced in the hypothalamus. In patients with an intact hypothalamic- pituitary- thyroid axis, a negative feedback regulatory mechanism controls thyroid gland metabolism. The pituitary serves as a biosensor of thyroid hormone levels and regulates TSH levels according to the feedback of free-thyroxine (FT4) and free-triiodothyronine (FT3) levels. Decreases in thyroid hormone production stimulate more TSH secretion. The control system has a relatively slow response time and during periods of non-equilibrium, as occurs in the beginning of hypothyroidism, it is possible to find some discordance between the plasma thyroid hormone concentrations and the levels of TSH.TSH measurement is considered to be the main test for detecting thyroid disease, specifically overt and subclinical hypothyroidism, for three main reasons. Firstly, there is an inverse log-linear relationship between the concentrations of TSH and FT4. Consequently, small linear

DOI: 10.4018/978-1-5225-3480-8.ch019

reductions in FT4 concentrations are associated with an exponential increase in TSH concentrations. Secondly, most cases of hypothyroidism in clinical practice are due to primary disease of the thyroid gland. Thirdly, immunometric assays for TSH present greater than 99% sensitivity and specificity (Glenn, 1996; Ain et al., 2000). Epidemiological studies have revealed that several changes in thyroid hormone concentrations occur with aging. The Whickham Survey undertaken in Britain provided data showing that TSH levels did not vary with age among males, but increased markedly among females after the age of 45 years. Furthermore, this rise in TSH with age among women was virtually abolished when persons with antithyroid antibodies were excluded from the sample.1 Data from the National Health and Nutrition Survey (NHANES III) confirmed that both TSH levels and the presence of antithyroid antibodies are greater in women, increase with age, and are more common in whites than in blacks (Hollowell et al., 2002).

THYROID DISEASES IN ELDERLY

Thyroid diseases regardless of age can be classified as functional disorders (hypothyroidism and hyperthyroidism), inflammatory conditions (thyroiditis) and neoplastic conditions (nodules and carcinomas). Overt hypothyroidism occurs in 2–5% of the patients older than 60 years. (Mariotti, Franceschi, Cossarizza., & Pinchera, 1995). Hyperthyroidism, on the other hand, is more common in the younger population. The prevalence in the elderly is approximately 0.5–3%, but 10–15% of the patients with hyperthyroidism are older than 60 years. (1998. US department of health and human services (Hollowell et al., 2002; Kennedy, & Caro, 1996). Different thyroid problems cause different symptoms and are treated differently. Common thyroid disorders and problems include:

Hypothyroidism

A number of large surveys reported a high incidence of hypothyroidism in elderly patients (Sawin, Chopra., & Azizi, 1979). Again, gender appears to be a factor: high TSH levels were found among more women than men older than 75 (17.4% of women older than 75, compared with 7.5% of women overall; 3.5% among men older than 75, compared with 2.8% of men overall). The clinical manifestations of hypothyroidism in elderly patients may differ greatly from those encountered in younger persons. In an older patient, the following clinical features should heighten your index of suspicion for hypothyroidism

Causes of Hypothyroidism

Hypothyroidism, by contrast, stems from an underproduction of thyroid hormones. Since our body's energy systems require certain amounts of thyroid hormones, a drop in hormone production leads to lower energy levels. Causes of hypothyroidism include:

- **Hashimoto's Disease:** In this autoimmune disorder, the body's own immune system attacks thyroid tissue, leading to reduced thyroid hormone.
- **Removal of the Thyroid Gland:** The thyroid may be surgically removed or chemically destroyed as a treatment for hyperthyroidism. Exposure to excessive amounts of iodide. Cold and sinus medicines, the heart medicine amiodarone or certain contrast dyes given before X-rays may expose too

much iodine. Who exposed they then be at greater risk of developing hypothyroidism, especially if anyone have had thyroid problem in the past.

- **Lithium:** This drug has also been linked to hypothyroidism.

Hypothyroidism and Other Risk Factors

- **Cognitive Impairment:** Overt adult onset hypothyroidism, which is marked by elevated thyroid stimulating hormone (TSH) levels and reduced levels of circulating thyroid hormones, has been associated with increased risk of deficits in specific cognitive domains including attention, concentration, memory, perceptual function, language, executive function, and psychomotor speed (Constant et al., 2005; Correia et al., 2009). However, controversies persist as to whether subclinical hypothyroidism (SCH), defined as mild elevation of TSH in the presence of normal free thyroxine (fT4), is associated with declines in these specific cognitive domains. This is especially relevant in the older adults, as the prevalence of subclinical hypothyroidism increases with age and is estimated to be up to 22% in women aged more than 60 years and somewhat lower in men (Sawin et al., 1985; Canaris, Manowitz, Mayor., & Ridgway, 2000).
- **Cardiovascular Effects:** The general clinical impression that patients with overt Hypothyroidisms have increased cardiac morbidity and mortality, real evidence is scarce. More controversial is the morbidity and mortality when considering mild or subclinical hypothyroidism. Most available evidence is based on surrogate markers such as adverse lipid profile, endothelial dysfunction, increased arterial stiffness and cardiac performance (Fazio, et al., 2004). However, some population studies have provided a reasonable level of evidence for the mortality and cardiovascular morbidity rates in hypothyroidism (Rasmussen, 2011)
- **Myxedema Coma:** Myxedema coma occurs almost exclusively in older adults with longstanding primary hypothyroidism. It is usually precipitated by a concomitant medical illness. Patients may present with a rapid development of stupor, seizures, or coma along with respiratory depression. Hallmark signs of myxedema coma include localized neurological signs, hypothermia, bradycardia, hyponatremia and hypoglycemia (Li, 2002).). Myxedema coma is a severe and life-threatening clinical state in older adults with a mortality rate as high as 40% (Jordan, R.M. (1995)
- **Management Issues:** Management of subclinical hypothyroidism in older adults is controversial and guidelines have been published both for (Gharib, Tuttle., & Baskin, 2005) and against (Surks, Ortiz., & Daniels, 2004; Chu, & Crapo, 2001) routine treatment in older adults. The treatment goals for hypothyroidism are to reverse clinical progression and correct metabolic derangements, as evidenced by normal blood levels of thyroid-stimulating hormone (TSH) and free thyroxine (T4). Thyroid hormone is administered to supplement or replace endogenous production. In general, hypothyroidism can be adequately treated with a constant daily dose of levothyroxine (LT4). Thyroid hormone can be started at anticipated full replacement doses in individuals who are young and otherwise healthy. In elderly patients and those with known ischemic heart disease, treatment should begin with one fourth to one half the expected dosage, and the dosage should be adjusted in small increments after no less than 4-6 weeks. For most cases of mild to moderate hypothyroidism, a starting levothyroxine dosage of 50-75 µg/day will suffice. Clinical benefits begin in 3-5 days and level off after 4-6 weeks. Achieving a TSH level within the reference range may take several months because of delayed readaptation of the hypothalamic-pituitary axis. In patients receiving treatment with LT4, dosing changes should be made every 6-8 weeks until the patient's TSH is in target range (Arthur, 2017)

In patients with central (ie, pituitary or hypothalamic) hypothyroidism, T4 levels rather than TSH levels are used to guide treatment. In most cases, the free T4 level should be kept in the upper third of the reference range. After dosage stabilization, patients can be monitored with annual or semiannual clinical evaluations and TSH monitoring. Patients should be monitored for symptoms and signs of overtreatment, which include the following:

- Tachycardia
- Palpitations
- Atrial fibrillation
- Nervousness
- Tiredness
- Headache
- Increased excitability
- Sleeplessness
- Tremors
- Possible angina

The updated guidelines on hypothyroidism issued by the American Thyroid Association in 2014 maintain the recommendation of levothyroxine as the preparation of choice for hypothyroidism, with the following considerations (Jonklaas, 2014):

- If levothyroxine dose requirements are much higher than expected, consider evaluating for gastrointestinal disorders such as *Helicobacter pylori* –related gastritis, atrophic gastritis, or celiac disease; if such disorders are detected and effectively treated, re-evaluation of thyroid function and levothyroxine dosage is recommended.
- Initiation or discontinuation of estrogen and androgens should be followed by reassessment of serum TSH at steady state, since such medications may alter levothyroxine requirement.
- Serum TSH should be reassessed upon initiation of agents such as tyrosine kinase inhibitors that affect thyroxine metabolism and thyroxine or triiodothyroninedeiodination.
- Serum TSH monitoring is advisable when medications such as phenobarbital, phenytoin, carbamazepine, rifampin, and sertraline are started.
- When deciding on a starting dose of levothyroxine, the patient's weight, lean body mass, pregnancy status, etiology of hypothyroidism, degree of TSH elevation, age, and general clinical context, including the presence of cardiac disease, should be considered. The serum TSH goal appropriate for the clinical situation should also be considered.
- Thyroid hormone therapy should be initiated as an initial full replacement or as partial replacement with gradual increments in the dose titrated upward using serum TSH as the goal.
- Dose adjustments should be made upon significant changes in body weight, with aging, and with pregnancy; TSH assessment should be performed 4-6 weeks after any dosage change.
- Reference ranges of serum TSH levels are higher in older populations (eg, >65 years), so higher serum TSH targets may be appropriate.
- A meta-analysis of randomized, controlled trials of T4-triiodothyronine (T3) combination therapy versus T4 monotherapy for treatment of clinical hypothyroidism found no difference in effectiveness between combination therapy and monotherapy with respect to side effects such as bodily

pain, depression, fatigue, body weight, anxiety, quality of life, and total low-density lipoprotein (LDL) and high-density lipoprotein (HDL) cholesterol and triglyceride levels. (Grozinsky-Glasberg, Fraser, Nahshoni, Weizman., & Leibovici, 2006).

- A study of athyrotic patients found a high heterogeneity in these patients' ability to produce T3 when treated with levothyroxine. Approximately 20% of these athyrotic patients did not maintain normal free T4 or free T3 values despite a normal TSH. (Gullo et al., 2011). However, it is unclear whether more physiologic treatments offer any benefit, even in subgroups of hypothyroid patients.
- In patients who continue to have symptoms (eg, weight gain and fatigue) despite normalization of the TSH level, one should consider causes other than hypothyroidism, rather than simply increasing the thyroid hormone dose on the basis of symptoms alone (see DDx). In some cases, however, symptom persistence is the result of a polymorphism of the deiodinase 2 enzyme, which converts T4 to T3 in the brain; these patients may benefit from combined LT4-liothyronine (LT3) therapy, using a physiologic LT4-to-LT3 ratio in the range of 10-14:1.
- Most patients with hypothyroidism can be treated in an ambulatory care setting. Patients who require long-term continuous tube feeding routinely require intravenous (IV) LT4 replacement because the absorption of oral agents is impaired by the contents of tube feeds. Alternatively, tube feeds can be withheld for 1 hour while the patient receives an oral preparation of LT4. It should be noted that oral and IV preparations of LT4 are not equivalent; consequently, great care must be taken in switching between these formulations.
- Patients with severe hypothyroidism requiring hospitalization (eg, myxedema) may require aggressive management. Overreplacement or aggressive replacement with any thyroid hormone may precipitate tachyarrhythmias or, very rarely, thyroid storm and should be balanced against the need for urgent replacement. Risk is higher with T3 therapy.
- Surgery is rarely needed in patients with hypothyroidism; it is more commonly required in the treatment of hyperthyroidism. However, surgery is indicated for large goiters that compromise tracheoesophageal function.

Hyperthyroidism

In general, the signs and symptoms of hyperthyroidism or thyrotoxicosis, which often are striking in younger patients, are muted in the elderly. The hyperthyroid state, however, imposes such a burden on the heart that in an elderly patient, the most prominent symptoms may be those of congestive heart failure. This phenomenon was first described in 1924 by Levine and Sturgis, who used the term "masked hyperthyroidism" to designate elderly hyperthyroid patients who presented with congestive heart failure. In these patients, the cardiac symptoms so predominated that the diagnosis of hyperthyroidism, which was the underlying cause of the heart failure, was initially overlooked.

Among younger hyperthyroid patients, such symptoms as weight loss, increased appetite, muscle weakness, palpitations, rapid pulse, and exophthalmos often are prominent, but according to what may be the definitive report in this area, these are far less often found among elderly hyperthyroid patients (Davis, & Davis, 1974). Some of the specific findings from this and the Bartels and Kingsley study are detailed in the Box.

An elderly patient with thyrotoxicosis is much more likely than a younger one to present with apathy and depression. Although weight loss may be a prominent symptom in an elderly hyperthyroid patient, it is as likely to reflect reduced food intake as increased catabolism resulting from the excess thyroid hormone. Such elderly, depressed hyperthyroid patients often appear sad and lethargic and have little interest in either themselves or their surroundings. Be sure, therefore, to consider the possibility of hyperthyroidism in any elderly patient who exhibits such symptoms. A recent change in mental status thus can be an important sign. (Thomas, Mazzaferri, & Skillman, 1970)

Causes of Hyperthyroidism

All types of hyperthyroidism are due to overproduction of thyroid hormones, but the condition can be caused in several ways:

- **Graves' Disease:** This is an auto-immune condition and is the commonest cause of an overactive thyroid gland.
- **Toxic Adenomas:** Nodules develop in the thyroid gland and begin to secrete thyroid hormones, upsetting the body's chemical balance. Some goitres may contain several of these nodules.
- **Subacute Thyroiditis:** This is where inflammation of the thyroid causes the gland to 'leak' excess hormones, resulting in temporary hyperthyroidism. The condition generally lasts a few weeks, but it may persist for months.

Pituitary gland malfunctions or cancerous growths in the thyroid gland. In rare cases, hyperthyroidism can also be due to these causes.

Hyperthyroidism and Other Risks Factors

- **Atrial Fibrillation:** Atrial fibrillation (AF) is the most common cardiac arrhythmia other than sinus tachycardia encountered in hyperthyroidism. Atrial fibrillation occurs in 10-15% of patients with hyperthyroidism (Sawin et al., 1994). It may be the presenting problem in some of them. Higher prevalence occurs in elderly and in those with other coexisting risk factors for atrial fibrillation. Low serum thyroid stimulating hormone is an independent risk factor for development of atrial fibrillation (Forfar, Miller., &Toft, 1979). AF in thyrotoxicosis is associated with significant mortality and morbidity resulting from embolic events (Staffurth, Gibberd., & Tang, 1977). Thyroid hormones exert their cardiovascular effects either directly through nuclear thyroid receptors or indirectly by influencing sympathoadrenergic system and altering peripheral vascular resistance. Binding of thyroid hormones to nuclear receptors result in increased gene transcription of cardiac myocyte proteins (Lazer, 1993). Thyroid hormones upregulate sarcoplasmic Calcium ATPase, myosin heavy chain alfa, voltage gated K+ channels, Na+ channels and beta1 adrenergic receptors (Shimoni, & Severson, 1995). These effects result in increased heart rate, systolic hypertension, increased ventricular contractility and cardiac hypertrophy. Changes in electrophysiological characteristics of atria result in dysrhythmias, especially atrial fibrillation, in patients with hyperthyroidism (Klein, &Ojamaa, 2001).
- **Cardiovascular Mortality:** Overt hyperthyroidism induces a hyperdynamic cardiovascular state (high cardiac output with low systemic vascular resistance), which is associated with a faster heart rate, enhanced left ventricular systolic and diastolic function, and increased prevalence of supraventricular tachyarrhythmias *(Fazio, Palmieri, Lombardi., &Biondi, 2004).* Several cross-sectional and case-control studies have found that decreased levels of serum TSH are associated

with increased cardiovascular mortality in older adults (Rodondi, Bauer, & Cappola, 2008). In addition, subclinical hyperthyroidism has been shown to be associated with left ventricular hypertrophy, which is a predictor of cardiovascular mortality (Dorr, Wolff., & Robinson, 2005)

- **Osteoporosis:** Osteoporosis is a uniform feature of untreated and sustained thyrotoxicosis. Numerous reports have described a consistent decrease in BMD and increase in fracture (especially in older women) risk in untreated overt hyperthyroidism (Vestergaard, & Mosekilde, 2003). This effect on Thyrotoxicosis on Bone Density (BMD) is evident in both pre- and postmenopausal women (Chen, Chen, & Yang, 2004). Hyperthyroidism differentially influences trabecular and cortical bone metabolism, with the latter more predominantly affected (Greenspan, & Greenspan, 1999). An early study demonstrated up to 40% increase in osteoclast resorption in cortical bone, compared to 2.7% reduction in trabecular bone volume (Bianchi et al., 1972). Recently, a cross-sectional, population-based study of euthyroid and hyperthyroid women over 40 years of age evaluated the correlation between serum TSH levels and BMD of the distal and ultradistal forearm (Svare et al., 2009). This is the site most profoundly affected by parathyroid hormone dysregulation (Kosowicz, Baszko-Błaszyh, Horst-Sikorska, & Baumann-Antczak, 1999). The study, which reported a statistically higher risk of osteoporosis at the radius in hyperthyroidism, found a stronger association between low TSH and low BMD in distal (cortical) bone in comparison to the ultradistal (trabecular) bone of the radius, complementing previous publications recommending distal forearm BMD measurements as appropriate for studying thyroid effects on bone (Greenspan, & Greenspan, 1999; Svare et al., 2009). Other areas of the skeleton that have demonstrated significant BMD decreases associated with hyperthyroidism include the lumbar spine, total hip and femoral neck. The severity of hyperthyroidism appears to influence the degree of bone loss and increase the probability of osteoporosis when looking at the relative degree of TSH suppression, rather than looking at free T4 and free T3 levels.
- **Ophthalmopathy:** Contradicting studies exist regarding the association of symptoms and signs of ophthalmopathy in Graves' disease with increasing age. Most studies published on this subject demonstrated a positive correlation between prevalence and severity of ophthalmopathy with increasing age (Lin, Hsu., & Bee, 2008). Graves' eye disease is an eye condition that occurs in about 50% of patients who currently have, or have had Graves' hyperthyroidism if eyelid changes are included. The percentage is slightly higher if sensitive techniques such as orbital computed tomography are used. Such an approach is however not warranted in most patients. Approximately 10% of patients who have this eye disorder never develop hyperthyroidism. The reasons for the association of hyperthyroidism with the eye disease are not completely understood. Fortunately, only 5% of patients will have a severe form. Graves' eye disease, like Graves' hyperthyroidism and Hashimoto's thyroiditis, is an autoimmune disorder. It is caused by the reaction of antibodies and certain white blood cells called lymphocytes, with proteins in eye muscle, the connective tissue and fat around the eyeball. This condition must be distinguished from the mild eye signs of "poppy" eyes and spasm of the eye lids which occur in most hyperthyroid patients due to an effect of excessive thyroid hormones (Health Guides on Thyroid Disease (2017).

Treatment modalities that may be used for the hyperthyroidism include radioactive iodine ablation therapy, antithyroid medications or thyroidectomy.

NORMAL THYROID FUNCTION IN THE ELDERLY

Several studies have investigated the role of thyroid function in the aging process. Study reports have shown increased serum TSH levels with increasing age, independent of antithyroid antibody presence (Surks & Hollowell, 2007), while in contrast, others have demonstrated decreased serum TSH in older adults (Mariotti, Franceschi., &Cossarizza, 1995; Mariotti, Barbesino., & Caturegli, 1993). Populations in which the dominant thyroid pathology is thyroid deficiency secondary to Hashimotos' thyroiditis display a trend for the TSH upper limit to increase with age (Hollowell, Staehling.,& Flanders, 2002; Bjoro, Holmen., & Kruger, 2000). On the contrary, an inverse relationship between TSH and age is seen in iodine-deficient populations in which the dominant thyroid pathology is nodularity and increasing thyroid autonomy with age (Volzke, Alte.,& Kohlmann, 2005). In regards to free T3 levels, most studies have demonstrated an age-dependent decline, while free T4 levels remain relatively unchanged (Mariotti et al., 1995; Mariotti et al., 1993) and rT3 levels increase with increasing age. However, interpretation of thyroid function tests in older adults is often complicated by the presence of chronic illness (where free T3 can be low and rT3 high) and polypharmacy (Peeters, Debaveye, & Fliers, 2006). Furthermore, differences in iodine intake and the presence of autoimmune thyroid disease make the distinction between age-related and disease-related thyroid function abnormalities even more challenging (Chiovato, Mariotti., &Pinchera, 1997).

There is convincing evidence that higher levels of TSH are associated with longevity, Atzmon et al. (2009), concluded that serum TSH levels were significantly higher in centenarians (mean age=98 years) as compared to controls ($p<0.001$) (Atzmon, Barzilai., & Hollowell, 2009). Several other studies have also shown increased TSH levels (mean age=85 years) and low to low-normal FT4 levels (mean age=78 years) to be associated with a better survival in older adults (Gussekloo, van Exel, de Craen, 2006; Van Den Beld, Visser., & Feelders, 2000). It is hypothesized that the association of a higher TSH level with longevity may be due to a correlated lower bioactivity of thyroid hormone, which in turn leads to a lower basal metabolic rate and thus potentially may serve as an adaptive mechanism to prevent catabolism in older adults (Van Den Beld et al, 2000).Moreover, the offspring of individuals with longevity were also shown to have higher TSH levels than age-matched controls without familial longevity (mean age=70 years), indicating a genetic predisposition (Atzmon, Barzilai, & Surks, 2009).

THYROID DYSFUNCTION WITH AGING

The process of aging affects both the prevalence and clinical presentation of hypo- and hyperthyroidism. Importantly, subclinical disturbances of thyroid function are more frequent than overt diseases in general population, as well as in elderly people (Cooper, 2004; Surks, Ortiz,Daniels.,&Sawin., 2004). Although it is known that overt thyroid disorders negatively affect physical and cognitive function in elderly people – for example, overt hypothyroidism is associated with the impairment of attention, concentration, memory, perceptual functions, language, and executive functions (Kramer, von Muhlen, Kritz-Silverstein., & Barrett-Connor, 2009) subclinical hypothyroidism is not associated with impairment of physical and cognitive function or depression in individuals aged 65 years and older, as compared to euthyroidism (deJongh et al., 2011) and Park et al. (2009) have demonstrated that subclinical hypothyroidism in elderly subjects is neither associated with cognitive impairment, depression, poor quality of life nor with metabolic disturbances. On the other hand, other studies demonstrated the presence of

– at least – mild cognitive impairment in people with subclinical hypothyroidism at mean age under 65 years (reviewed in(Begin, Langlois, Lorrain, & Cunnane, 2008). Furthermore, as reported by de Jongh et al. (2011), subclinical hypothyroidism was also not associated with the increased overall mortality risk. Similar findings were shown by (Rodondi et al., 2010).who analyzed data from numerous large prospective cohorts and demonstrated that total mortality was not increased in subjects with subclinical hypothyroidism, although the risk of coronary heart disease (CHD) events and of CHD mortality increased with TSH levels 10 mIU/l or higher. Nevertheless, it should be emphasized that this analysis regarded numerous different populations (cohorts) which consisted of not only elderly people and that the effect in question, i.e. of increasing TSH level on CHD incidents was not influenced by age (Rodondi et al.,2010).

Most recent results indicate that even in euthyroid older men with normal levels of TSH, differences in FT_4levels within the normal range predict specific health outcomes relevant to aging. For example, higher FT_4within the normal range was independently associated with frailty in euthyroid men aged ≥70 years. Yeap (2012). Moreover, higher FT_4 levels within the normal range were associated with lower hip bone mineral density, increasing bone loss and fracture risk in postmenopausal women (Murphy et al., 2010). Therefore, it seems that further studies are required to explain whether higher FT_4 levels contribute causally (or not) to the above mentioned poorer health outcomes. Moreover, it is of interest to clarify whether FT_4 levels in the low-normal range could be considered as potential biomarkers for healthy aging (Yeap, 2012).

Although numerous studies demonstrate that the increased TSH level resulting from subclinical hypothyroidism further rises with aging. Yeap BB (2012), other findings suggest that aging is associated – in the absence of any thyroid disease – with lower TSH levels (Over, Mannan, Nsouli-Marktabi, Burman, & Jonklaas, 2010). It has been known that TSH secretion in response to thyrotropin-releasing hormone (TRH) is reduced in aging individuals, and serum TSH level is usually lower in older than in young people in response to decreased thyroid hormone concentrations, suggesting a certain level of insensitivity of thyrotrophic cells in anterior pituitary, occurring with age; moreover, nocturnal surge of TSH is – to various degree – lost in the elderly. On the other hand, Bremner et al. (2012) have recently reported that the TSH increase – observed by other authors during aging – seems to be a consequence of age-related alteration in the TSH set point or reduced TSH bioactivity. Interestingly, the largest TSH increase is observed in people with the lowest TSH at baseline, and, in turn, people with higher baseline TSH levels had proportionally smaller increases in TSH concentrations (Bremner et al., 2012). It is worth adding that TRH and FT_4 serum levels do not differ between young, middle-aged and elderly

Thyroidism and Other Risk Factors

Thyroid Nodules

It is known that the prevalence of thyroid nodules increases with age (Gupta, K. L. (1995). By age of 65 years, nearly 50% of individuals in iodine-sufficient areas have thyroid nodules when evaluated with ultrasound (Mazzaferri, 1993). A survey by Cavaliere and his colleagues (2002) showed that the prevalence of multinodular goiter in older adults in an iodine-deficient area was 74% in patients aged 55–75 years and 54% in patients aged 76–84 years (Cavaliere, et al., 2002). Thyroid nodules may be benign adenomas, cysts, cancer or inflammation.

Management

The approach to the management of a solitary thyroid nodule in an older adult is the same as that in a younger patient. With the discovery of a new thyroid nodule, a complete history and physical examination should be performed. Pertinent questions should include history of head and neck or whole body irradiation, exposure to ionizing radiation, and family history of thyroid cancer or syndromes such as multiple endocrine neoplasia. Physical findings such as palpable cervical lymphadenopathy, voice hoarseness or fixation of the nodule to surrounding tissue raise suspicion for malignancy (Maria & Megan, 2012).

Thyroid Cancer

The prevalence of thyroid nodules and thyroid neoplasms is increased in the elderly. Among elderly people, males are at higher risk of cancer and thyroid cancer is more aggressive in men than in women (Rukhman & Silverberg, 2011). Papillary thyroid carcinoma (PTC) is the most common endocrine malignant neoplasm in the older individuals. Women are affected by PTC two to three times more often than men (Kilfoy et al., 2009). Nevertheless, female-to-male ratio seems to decline with the process of aging. Importantly, the mortality rate of PTC is usually higher in the elderly (Toniato, Bernardi, Piotto, Rubello, &Pelizzo, 2011). Presumably, it is a consequence of increased mitotic activity of these tumors and increased likelihood of distant metastases (Toniato, 2011). It is known that in general population patients with aggressive variants of PTC have higher risk for the metastatic disease development (Chrisoulidou et al., 2011). Follicular thyroid carcinoma (FTC) occurs also often in older people and is the second most common and the second least aggressive thyroid cancer. This cancer is more likely to metastasize hematogenously to distant sites, resulting in a worse prognosis in comparison with PTC (Rukhman, & Silverberg, 2011). Medullary thyroid carcinoma (MTC), which derives from the parafollicular cells (C cells) of the thyroid gland, constitutes up to 5% of all thyroid malignancies. Its sporadic form, more frequent than is familial MTC, occurs more commonly in the older population (Habra, & Sarlis, 2005). Rapidly growing and typically very aggressive anaplastic (undifferentiated) thyroid carcinoma (ATC) is rare. However, one should strongly emphasize that its prevalence is considerably higher in older than in younger people. By the time of diagnosis, most patients have widespread local invasion and distant metastases. Age appears to be a strong predictor of poor prognosis in ATC (Rukhman, & Silverberg, 2011).

Management

The treatment of choice for patients diagnosed with thyroid cancer is surgery, when possible. Usually, surgery is followed by treatment with radioiodine and thyroxine therapy. Generally, radiation therapy and chemotherapy do not have a prominent role in the treatment of thyroid cancer. Usually under the consideration of age and cancer, palliative care is a best option. End-of-life issues comfort, and care options are essential considerations during initial treatment planning.

Thyroid Cancer and Gender Differences

However, the incidence of thyroid cancer is significantly higher in women compared with men. The 2002 GLOBOCAN database reports 103,589 female thyroid cancer cases worldwide compared with only 37,424 male thyroid cancer cases, representing a female to male (F:M) ratio of greater than 2:1.

However, this incidence pattern is not observed across all thyroid cancer types. When categorized by histology, the incidence of differentiated thyroid cancer (DTC; papillary thyroid carcinoma [PTC] or follicular thyroid carcinoma [FTC]) is three-times higher in women than in men, while that of anaplastic thyroid carcinoma (ATC) is twice as common in women as men. There is no significant difference in the incidence of medullary carcinomas (MTC) between men and women (Grubbs, Rich., & LiGetal, 2008), While the only currently established causative risk factor for thyroid cancer is exposure to ionizing radiation, (Grubbs et al., 2008) the discrepancy between male and female disease incidence has led to the suggestion that female gender is a possible epidemiologic risk factor. A prospective cohort study by Iribarren, Haselkorn, Tekawa and Friedam (2001) of 204,964 individuals living in San Francisco (CA, USA) reported a relative risk of 1.56 for the development of thyroid cancer for female gender by multivariate Cox proportional hazard models ((Iribarre, Haselkorn, Tekawa, & Friedman, 2001). No other studies have analyzed female gender as a risk factor for thyroid cancer in the general population. Regardless, the marked variation in thyroid cancer incidence between females and males has long led to speculation about possible underlying biological theories in the development and progression of thyroid cancer. In reference to historical trends, thyroid cancer incidence has steadily increased overall. Over the period 1973–2002, there was a 2.4-fold increase in age-adjusted rate of incidence of thyroid cancer (Zheng, Holford., & Chen., 1996; Liu, Semeciw, Ugnat., & Mao, 2001).

CONCLUSION

The process of aging strongly affects entire endocrine system. Consistently, thyroid gland is also impacted by aging. One should emphasize that thyroid diseases-associated symptoms in the elderly people are very similar to symptoms of the normal aging. Therefore, broadening the knowledge on alterations in thyroid function, which may be observed during aging, appears to be very important and constitutes a challenge for thyroid researchers, given that some specific thyroid dysfunctions may contribute to lifespan extension. Thyroid disorders have no age limits; indeed, hypothyroidism is clearly more common in older than in younger adults. Despite the increased frequency of thyroid problems in older individuals, physicians need a high index of suspicion to make the diagnosis since thyroid disorders often manifest as a disorder of another system in the body. Older patients with thyroid disorders require special attention to gradual and careful treatment, and, as always, require lifelong follow-up.

REFERENCES

Atzmon, G., Barzilai, N., Hollowell, J. G., Surks, M. I., & Gabriely, I. (2009). Extreme longevity is associated with increased serum thyrotropin. *The Journal of Clinical Endocrinology and Metabolism*, *94*(4), 1251–1254. doi:10.1210/jc.2008-2325 PMID:19158193

Atzmon, G., Barzilai, N., Surks, M. I., & Gabriely, I. (2009). Genetic predisposition to elevated serum thyrotropin is associated with exceptional longevity. *The Journal of Clinical Endocrinology and Metabolism*, *94*(12), 4768–4775. doi:10.1210/jc.2009-0808 PMID:19837933

Begin, M. E., Langlois, M. F., Lorrain, D., & Cunnanem, S. C. (2008). Thyroid function and cognition during aging. *Current Gerontology and Geriatrics Research*, *2008*, 1–11. doi:10.1155/2008/474868 PMID:19415145

Bianchi, G. S., Meunier, P., Courpron, P., Edouard, E., Bernard, J., & Vignon, G. (1972). Osseous effects of hyperthyroidism. *Revue du Rhumatisme et des Maladies Osteo-Articulaires*, *39*(1), 19–32. PMID:4342875

Biondi, B., Palmieri, E. A., & Fazio, S. (2004). Endogenous subclinical hyperthyroidism affects quality of life and cardiac morphology and function in young and middle-aged patients. *The Journal of Clinical Endocrinology and Metabolism*, *85*(12), 4701–4705. PMID:11134131

Bjoro, T., Holmen, J., Kruger, O., Midthjell, K., Hunstad, K., Schreiner, T., ... Brochmann, H. (2000). Prevalence of thyroid disease, thyroid dysfunction and thyroid peroxidase antibodies in a large, unselected population. The Health Study of Nord-Trondelag (HUNT). *European Journal of Endocrinology*, *143*(5), 639–647. doi:10.1530/eje.0.1430639 PMID:11078988

Bremner, A. P., Feddema, P., Leedman, P. J., Brown, S. J., Beilby, J. P., Lim, E. M., ... Walsh, J. P. (2012). Age-related changes in thyroid function: A longitudinal study of a community-based cohort. *The Journal of Clinical Endocrinology and Metabolism*, *97*(5), 1554–1562. doi:10.1210/jc.2011-3020 PMID:22344200

Canaris, G. J., Manowitz, N. R., Mayor, G., & Ridgway, E. C. (2000). The Colorado thyroid disease prevalence study. *Archives of Internal Medicine*, *160*(4), 526–534. doi:10.1001/archinte.160.4.526 PMID:10695693

Cavaliere, R., Antonangeil, L., & Vitti, P. (2002). The aging thyroid in a mild to moderate iodine deficient area of Italy. *Journal of Endocrinological Investigation*, *25*(101), 66–68. Retrieved from https://www.ncbi.nlm.nih.gov/pubmed/12508922 PMID:12508922

Chen, C. H., Chen, J. F., & Yang, B. Y. (2004). Bone mineral density in women receiving thyroxine suppressive therapy for differentiated thyroid carcinoma. *Journal of the Formosan Medical Association*, *103*(6), 442–447. PMID:15278189

Chiovato, L., Mariotti, S., & Pinchera, A. (1997). Thyroid diseases in the elderly. *Baillieres Clinical Endocrinology Metabolism*, *11*(2), 251–70. Retrieved from https://www.ncbi.nlm.nih.gov/pubmed/9403122

Chrisoulidou, A., Boudina, M., Tzemailas, A., Doumala, E., Iliadou, P. K., Patakiouta, F., & Pazaitou-Panayiotou, K. (2011). Histological subtype is the most important determinant of survival in metastatic papillary thyroid cancer. *Thyroid Research*, *4*(1), 12. doi:10.1186/1756-6614-4-12 PMID:21771294

Chu, J. W., & Crapo, L. M. (2001). The treatment of subclinical hypothyroidism is seldom necessary. *The Journal of Clinical Endocrinology and Metabolism*, *86*(10), 4591–4599. doi:10.1210/jcem.86.10.7961 PMID:11600508

Collet, T.H., Gussekloo, J., Bauer, D.C., den Elzen, W.P., & Cappola, A.R., Balmer, P., … Rodondi, N. (2012). Thyroid Studies Collaboration: Subclinical hyperthyroidism and the risk of coronary heart disease and mortality. *Archieves International Medcine*, *172*, 799–809. doi:10.1001/archinternmed.2012.402 PMID:22529182

Constant, E. L., Adam, S., Seron, X., Bruyer, R., Seghers, A., & Daumerie, C. (2005). Anxiety and depression, attention, and executive functions in hypothyroidism. *Journal of the International Neuropsychological Society, 11*(05), 535–544. doi:10.1017/S1355617705050642 PMID:16212680

Cooper, D. S. (2004). Thyroid disease in the oldest old: The exception to the rule. *Journal of the American Medical Association, 292*(21), 2651–2654. doi:10.1001/jama.292.21.2651 PMID:15572724

Correia, N., Mullally, S., Cooke, G., Tun, T. K., Phelan, N., Feeney, J., ... Gibney, J. (2009). Evidence for a specific defect in hippocampal memory in overt and subclinical hypothyroidism. *The Journal of Clinical Endocrinology and Metabolism, 94*(10), 3789–3797. doi:10.1210/jc.2008-2702 PMID:19584178

Davis, P. J., & Davis, F. B. (1974). Hyperthyroidism in patients over the age of 60 years. Clinical features in 85 patients. *Medicine; Analytical Reviews of General Medicine, Neurology, Psychiatry, Dermatology, and Pediatries, 53*(3), 161–181. doi:10.1097/00005792-197405000-00001 PMID:4133091

deJongh, R. T., Lips, P., van Schoor, N. M., Rijs, K. J., Deeg, D. J. H., Comijs, H. C., ... Dekkers, O. M. (2011). Endogenous subclinical thyroid disorders, physical and cognitive function, depression, and mortality in older individuals. *European Journal of Endocrinology, 165*(4), 545–554. doi:10.1530/EJE-11-0430 PMID:21768248

Dorr, M., Wolff, B., Robinson, D. M., John, U., Lüdemann, J., Meng, W., ... Völzke, H. (2005). The associations of thyroid function with cardiac mass and left ventricular hypertrophy. *The Journal of Clinical Endocrinology and Metabolism, 90*(2), 673–677. doi:10.1210/jc.2004-1554 PMID:15522926

Fazio, S., Palmieri, E. A., Lombardi, G., & Biondi, B. (2004). Effects of Thyroid Hormone on the Cardiovascular System. *Recent Progress in Hormone Research, 59*(1), 31–50. doi:10.1210/rp.59.1.31 PMID:14749496

Forfar, J. C., Miller, H. C., & Toft, A. D. (1979). Occult thyrotoxicosis: A reversible cause of "idiopathic" atrial fibrillation. *The American Journal of Cardiology, 44*(1), 9–12. doi:10.1016/0002-9149(79)90243-1 PMID:110126

Gharib, H., Tuttle, R. M., Baskin, H. J., Fish, L. H., Singer, P. A., & McDermott, M. T. (2005). Subclinical thyroid dysfunction: A joint statement on management from the American Association of Clinical Endocrinologists, the American Thyroid Association, and the Endocrine Society. *The Journal of Clinical Endocrinology and Metabolism, 90*(1), 581–585. doi:10.1210/jc.2004-1231 PMID:15643019

Glenn, G. C. (1996). Practice parameter on laboratory panel testing for screening and case finding in asymptomatic adults.Laboratory Testing Task Force of the College of the American Pathologists. *Archives of Pathology & Laboratory Medicine, 120*(10), 929–943. PMID:12049072

Greenspan, S. L., & Greenspan, F. S. (1999). The effect of thyroid hormone on skeletal integrity. *Annals of Internal Medicine, 130*(9), 750–758. doi:10.7326/0003-4819-130-9-199905040-00016 PMID:10357695

Grozinsky-Glasberg, S., Fraser, A., Nahshoni, E., Weizman, A., & Leibovici, L. (2006). Thyroxine-triiodothyronine combination therapy versus thyroxinemonotherapy for clinical hypothyroidism: Meta-analysis of randomized controlled trials. *The Journal of Clinical Endocrinology and Metabolism, 91*(7), 2592–2599. doi:10.1210/jc.2006-0448 PMID:16670166

Grubbs, E. G., Rich, T. A., Li, G., Sturgis, E. M., Younes, M. N., Myers, J. N., ... Evans, D. B. (2008). Recent advances in thyroid cancer. *Current Problems in Surgery*, *45*(3), 156–250. doi:10.1067/j.cpsurg.2007.12.010 PMID:18346477

Gullo, D., Latina, A., Frasca, F., Le Moli, R., Pellegriti, G., & Vigneri, R. (2011). Levothyroxine monotherapy cannot guarantee euthyroidism in all athyreotic patients. *PLoS One*, *6*(8), e22552. doi:10.1371/journal.pone.0022552 PMID:21829633

Gupta, K. L. (1995). Neoplasm of the thyroid gland. *Clinical Geriatric Medicine*, *11*, 271–90. Retrieved from https://www.ncbi.nlm.nih.gov/pubmed/16440564

Gussekloo, J., van Exel, E., & de Craen, A. J. (2006). Thyroid function, activities of daily living and survival in extreme old age: The 'Leiden 85-plus Study'. *Nederlands Tijdschrift voor Geneeskunde*, *150*(2), 90–96. Retrieved from https://www.ncbi.nlm.nih.gov/pubmed/16440564 PMID:16440564

Gussekloo, J., van Exel, E., de Craen, A. J. M., & Meinders, A. E. M. (2004). Thyroid status, disability and cognitive function, and survival in old age. *Journal of the American Medical Association*, *292*(21), 2591–2599. doi:10.1001/jama.292.21.2591 PMID:15572717

Habra, M., & Sarlis, N. J. (2005). Thyroid and aging. *Reviews in Endocrine & Metabolic Disorders*, *6*(2), 145–154. doi:10.1007/s11154-005-1494-9 PMID:15843886

Health Guides on Thyroid Disease. (2017). *Graves' Eye Disease (Ophthalmopathy).* Retrieved from http://www.thyroid.ca/ophthalmopathy.php

Hollowell, J. G., Staehling, N. W., Flanders, W. D., Hannon, W. H., & Gunter, E. W. (2001). Cohort study of thyroid cancer in a San Francisco Bay area population. *International Journal of Cancer*, *93*(5), 745–750. doi:10.1002/ijc.1377 PMID:11477590

Hollowell, J. G., Staehling, N. W., Flanders, W. D., Hannon, W. H., Gunter, E. W., Spencer, C. A., & Braverman, L. E. (2002). Serum TSH, T(4), and thyroid antibodies in the United States population (1988 to 1994): National Health and Nutrition Examination Survey (NHANES III). *The Journal of Clinical Endocrinology and Metabolism*, *87*(2), 489–499. doi:10.1210/jcem.87.2.8182 PMID:11836274

Iribarren, C., Haselkorn, T., Tekawa, I. S., & Friedman, G. D. (2001). Cohort study of thyroid cancer in a San Francisco Bay area population. *International Journal of Cancer*, *93*, 745–750.

Jonklaas, J., Bianco, A. C., Bauer, A. J., Burman, K. D., Cappola, A. R., Celi, F. S., ... Sawka, A. M. (2014). Guidelines for the treatment of hypothyroidism: Prepared by the American Thyroid Association task force on thyroid hormone replacement. *Thyroid*, *24*(12), 1670–1751. doi:10.1089/thy.2014.0028 PMID:25266247

Jordan, R. M. (1995). Myxedema coma. Pathophysiology, therapy, and factors affecting prognosis. *The Medical Clinics of North America*, *79*(1), 185–194. doi:10.1016/S0025-7125(16)30091-8 PMID:7808091

Kennedy, J. W., & Caro, J. F. (1996). The ABC of managing hyperthyroidism in the older patient. *Geriatric, 51*, 22–32. Retrieved from https://www.ncbi.nlm.nih.gov/pubmed/8621100

Kilfoy, B. A., Devesa, S. S., Ward, M. H., Zhang, Y., Rosenberg, P. S., Holford, T. R., & Anderson, W. F. (2009). Gender is an age-specific effect modifier for papillary cancers of the thyroid gland. *Cancer Epidemiology, Biomarkers & Prevention, 18*(4), 1092–1100. doi:10.1158/1055-9965.EPI-08-0976 PMID:19293311

Klein, I., & Ojamaa, K. (2001). Thyroid hormone and the cardiovascular system. *The New England Journal of Medicine, 344*(7), 501–509. doi:10.1056/NEJM200102153440707 PMID:11172193

Kosowicz, J., Baszko-Błaszyh, D., Horst-Sikorska, W., & Baumann-Antczak, A. (1999). Bone mineral density in primary hyperparathyroidism. Polskie Archiwum Medycyny Wewnetrznej, 101(2), 133–138.

Kramer, C., Von Muhlen, D., Kritz-Silverstein, D., & Barrett-Connor, E. (2009). Treated hypothyroidism, cognitive function, and depressed mood in old age: The Rancho Bernardo Study. European. *The Journal of Endocrinology, 161*, 917–921. doi:10.1530/EJE-09-0606 PMID:19755406

Lazar, M. A. (1993). Thyroid hormone receptors: Multiple forms, multiple possibilities. *Endocrinology Review, 24*, 184–193. PMID:8325251

Levine, S. A., & Sturgis, C. C. (1924). Hyperthyroidism masked as heart disease. *Boston Medical and Surgical Journal, 190*(7), 23–237. doi:10.1056/NEJM192402141900703

Li, T. M. (2002). Hypothyroidism in elderly people. *Geriatric Nursing, 23*(2), 88–93. doi:10.1067/mgn.2002.124325 PMID:11956521

Lin, M. C., Hsu, F. M., Bee, Y. S., & Ger, L.-P. (2008). Age influences the severity of Graves' ophthalmopathy. *The Kaohsiung Journal of Medical Sciences, 24*(6), 283–288. doi:10.1016/S1607-551X(08)70154-2 PMID:18635413

Liu, S., Semeciw, R., Ugnat, A. M., & Mao, Y. (2001). Increasing thyroid cancer incidence in Canada, 1970–1996: Time trends and age-period-cohort effects. *British Journal of Cancer, 86*(9), 1335–1339. doi:10.1054/bjoc.2001.2061 PMID:11720471

Mariotti, S., Barbesino, G., & Caturegli, P. (1993). Complex alteration of thyroid function in healthy centenarians. *The Journal of Clinical Endocrinology and Metabolism, 77*, 1130–1134. Retrieved from https://www.ncbi.nlm.nih.gov/pubmed/8077303 PMID:8077303

Mariotti, S., Franceschi, C., & Cossarizza, A. (1995). The aging thyroid. *Endocrinology Review, 16*, 686–715. Retrieved from https://www.ncbi.nlm.nih.gov/pubmed/8747831

Mariotti, S., Franceschi, C., Cossarizza, A., & Pinchera, A. (1995). The aging thyroid. *Endocrinology Review, 16*(6), 686–715. doi:10.1210/edrv-16-6-686 PMID:8747831

Mazzaferri, E. L. (1993). Management of a solitary thyroid nodule. *New England Journal of Medicnie, 25*, 553–9. Retrieved from https://www.ncbi.nlm.nih.gov/pubmed/16399019

Murphy, E., Gluer, C. C., Reid, D. M., Felsenberg, D., Roux, C., Eastell, R., & Williams, G. R. (2010). Thyroid function within the upper normal range is associated with reduced bone mineral density and an increased risk of non-vertebral fractures in healthy euthyroid postmenopausal women. *The Journal of Clinical Endocrinology and Metabolism, 95*(7), 3173–3181. doi:10.1210/jc.2009-2630 PMID:20410228

Over, R., Mannan, S., Nsouli-Marktabi, H., Burman, K. D., & Jonklaas, J. (2010). Age and the thyrotropin response to hypothyroxinemia. *The Journal of Clinical Endocrinology and Metabolism*, *95*(8), 3675–3683. doi:10.1210/jc.2010-0281 PMID:20484476

Park, Y. J., Lee, E. J., Choi, S. H., Park, J. H., Lee, S. B., Lim, S., ... Kim, K. W. (2010). Subclinical hypothyroidism (SCH) is not associated with metabolic derangement, cognitive impairment, depression or poor quality of life (QoL) in elderly subjects. *Achieves of Gerontololgical Geriatric*, *50*(3), e68–e73. doi:10.1016/j.archger.2009.05.015 PMID:19545916

Peeters, R. P., Debaveye, Y., Fliers, E., & Visser, T. J. (2006). Changes within the thyroid axis during critical illness. *Critical Care Clinics*, *22*(1), 41–55. doi:10.1016/j.ccc.2005.08.006 PMID:16399019

Rasmussen, U. F. (2011). Subclinical Hypothyroidism and Cardiovascular Risk –An Overview of Current Understanding: Thyroid disorder. *European Endocrinology*, *27*(1), 53–57.

Rodondi, N., Bauer, D.C., & Cappola, A.R. (2008). Subclinical thyroid dysfunction, cardiac function, and the risk of heart failure. The Cardiovascular Health study. *Journal of American College of Cardiology, 30*, 1152–9.

Rodondi, N., den Elzen, W. P., Bauer, D. C., Cappola, A. R., Razvi, S., Walsh, J. P., ... Gussekloo, J. (2010). Thyroid Studies Collaboration: Subclinical hypothyroidism and the risk of coronary heart disease and mortality. *Journal of the American Medical Association*, *304*(12), 1365–1374. doi:10.1001/jama.2010.1361 PMID:20858880

Rukhman, N., & Silverberg, A. (2011). Thyroid cancer in older men. *The Aging Male*, *14*(2), 91–98. doi:10.3109/13685538.2010.529195 PMID:21087173

Sawin, C. T., Castelli, W. P., Hershman, J. M., McNamara, P., & Bacharach, P. (1985). The aging thyroid. Thyroid deficiency in the Framingham study. *Archieves International Medicinie*, *145*(8), 1386–1388. doi:10.1001/archinte.1985.00360080056006 PMID:4026469

Sawin, C. T., Chopra, D., & Azizi, F. (1979). The aging thyroid. Increased prevalence of elevated serum thyrotropin levels in the elderly. *Journal of the American Medical Association*, *242*(3), 247–250. doi:10.1001/jama.1979.03300030019013 PMID:448912

Sawin, C. T., Geller, A., Wolf, P., Belanger, A., Baker, E., Bacharach, P., ... D'agostino, R. B. (1994). Low serum thyrotropin concentrations as a risk factor for atrial fibrillation inolder persons. *The New England Journal of Medicine*, *331*(19), 1249–1252. doi:10.1056/NEJM199411103311901 PMID:7935681

Shimoni, Y., & Severson, D. L. (1995). Thyroid status and potassium currents in rat ventricular myocytes. *The American Journal of Physiology*, *268*, H576–H583. PMID:7864182

Staffurth, J. S., Gibberd, J. S., & Tang, F. S. (1977). Arterial embolism in thyrotoxicosis with atrial fibrillation. *British Medical Journal*, *2*(6088), 688–690. doi:10.1136/bmj.2.6088.688 PMID:902055

Surks, M. I., & Boucai, L. (2010). Age- and race-based serum thyrotropin reference limits. *The Journal of Clinical Endocrinology and Metabolism*, *95*(2), 496–502. doi:10.1210/jc.2009-1845 PMID:19965925

Surks, M. I., & Hollowell, J. G. (2007). Age-specific distribution of serum thyrotropin and antithyroid antibodies in the US population: Implications for the prevalence of subclinical hypothyroidism. *The Journal of Clinical Endocrinology and Metabolism*, *92*(12), 4575–4582. doi:10.1210/jc.2007-1499 PMID:17911171

Surks, M. I., Ortiz, E., Daniels, G. H., Sawin, C. T., Col, N. F., Cobin, R. H., ... Weissman, N. J. (2004). Subclinical thyroid disease: Scientific review and guidelines for diagnosis and management. *Journal of the American Medical Association*, *291*(2), 228–238. doi:10.1001/jama.291.2.228 PMID:14722150

Svare, S., Nilsen, T. I. L., Bjoro, T., Forsmo, S., Schei, B., & Langhammer, A. (2009). Hyperthyroid levels of TSH correlate with low bone mineral density: The HUNT 2 study. *European Journal of Endocrinology*, *161*(5), 779–786. doi:10.1530/EJE-09-0139 PMID:19671706

Thomas, F. B., Mazzaferri, E. L., & Skillman, T. G. (1970). Apathetic thyrotoxicosis: A distinctive clinical and laboratory entity. *Annals of Internal Medicine*, *72*(5), 679–685. doi:10.7326/0003-4819-72-5-679 PMID:4194420

Toniato, A., Bernardi, C., Piotto, A., Rubello, D., & Pelizzo, M. R. (2011). Features of papillary thyroid carcinoma in patients older than 75 years. *Updates in Surgery*, *63*(2), 115–118. doi:10.1007/s13304-011-0060-0 PMID:21416286

Van Den Beld, A. W., Visser, T. J., Feelders, R. A., Grobbee, D. E., & Lamberts, S. W. J. (2000). Thyroid hormone concentrations, disease, physical function and mortality in elderly men. *The Journal of Clinical Endocrinology and Metabolism*, *90*(12), 6403–6409. Retrieved from https://www.ncbi.nlm.nih.gov/pubmed/16174720. doi:10.1210/jc.2005-0872 PMID:16174720

Vestergaard, P., & Mosekilde, L. (2003). Hyperthyroidism, bone mineral, fracture risk-a meta-analysis. *Thyroid*, *13*(6), 585–593. doi:10.1089/105072503322238854 PMID:12930603

Volzke, H., Alte, D., Kohlmann, T., Lüdemann, J., Nauck, M., John, U., & Meng, W. (2005). Reference intervals of serum thyroid function tests in a previously iodine-deficient area. *Thyroid*, *15*(3), 279–285. doi:10.1089/thy.2005.15.279 PMID:15785248

Yeap, B. B. (2012). (in press). Hormones and health outcomes in aging men. *Experimental Gerontology*. doi:10.1016/j.exger.2012.07.012 PMID:22884846

Zheng, T., Holford, T. R., Chen, Y., Ma, J. Z., Flannery, J., Liu, W., ... Boyle, P. (1996). Time trend and age-period-cohort effect on incidence of thyroid cancer in Connecticut, 1935–1992. *International Journal of Cancer*, *67*(4), 504–509. doi:10.1002/(SICI)1097-0215(19960807)67:4<504::AID-IJC7>3.0.CO;2-W PMID:8759608

KEY TERMS AND DEFINITIONS

Ageing: "Aging" refers to the biological process of growing older in a deleterious sense and one of the most complex biological processes.

Hyperthyroidism: Hyperthyroidism is the overproduction of thyroid hormones by an overactive thyroid.

Hypothyroidism: Hypothyroidism, or underactive thyroid, develops when the thyroid gland fails to produce or secrete as much thyroxine (T_4) as the body needs.

Management: Management is the way people control different parts of their lives.

Thyroid: Thyroid is the gland responsible for body growth and metabolism.

Chapter 20
Music Therapy:
An Intervention in Alzheimer's Disease

Manjunath R. Bajantri
Dharwad Institute of Mental Health and Neurosciences (DIMHANS), India

Barre Vijaya Prasad
Dharwad Institute of Mental Health and Neurosciences (DIMHANS), India

Ashok Kori
Dharwad Institute of Mental Health and Neurosciences (DIMHANS), India

ABSTRACT

Alzheimer's disease (AD) is a worldwide epidemic. Multiple domains including memory, cognitive abilities, language, behaviour, and emotions are affected, resulting in significant disability and distress both for patients and caregivers. The management of patients with Alzheimer's disease is a significant public health problem. Different strategies have been applied to prevent/delay onset of Alzheimer's disease or at least to improve quality of life and health conditions of Alzheimer's disease patients and their caregivers. Given the limited effectiveness of pharmacological therapies combined with iatrogenic effects of drug treatments, the development of nondrug care has become a necessity. This chapter focuses on music therapy as an advanced intervention strategy for this population. Music therapy has evolved from a social science model to a neuroscience model of clinical practice and research. This paradigm shift has resulted in the formation of a new theory known as neurologic music therapy (NMT).

INTRODUCTION

Alzheimer's disease (AD) is a progressive neurodegenerative disorder (Chengxuan, Miia., & Eva von, 2009) with characteristic neuropathological and neurochemical features characterised by symptom complex in which there is disturbance of multiple higher cortical functions, including memory, thinking, orientation, comprehension, calculation, learning capacity, language and judgement. These neurocognitive disturbances are occasionally preceded or often accompanied by deterioration in emotional control, social behaviour or motivation (ICD -10). Noncognitive neuropsychiatric symptoms (NPS) commonly

DOI: 10.4018/978-1-5225-3480-8.ch020

occur in AD and are associated with adverse outcomes for patients and their caregivers (McClam, & Marano, 2015). These Behavioural and psychological symptoms in dementia (BPSD) are defined as signs and symptoms of disturbed behaviour, mood, thought or perception. These disturbances, namely agitation, depression, elation, delusions and hallucinations, are strongly correlated with each other. In addition, at least 50% of patients with dementia present with significant BPSD on a monthly basis (Ryu, Katona., & Rive, 2005). Agitation, together with depression, hinder activities and relationships, cause feelings of helplessness and distress in families and formal caregivers and are strong predictors for poor quality of life, as well as nursing home admission (Gaugler, Yu., & Krichbaum, 2009). First-line treatment options often involve drug therapies aimed at slowing down the progression of the illness and antipsychotic medication to address challenging behaviours. To date, research into non-pharmacological interventions has been limited. There is however growing interest in identifying non-pharmacological therapies effective in improving quality of life and reducing challenging behaviours (Yu-Shiun et al., 2015). Significant reduction in symptom severity has been reported with nearly all the nonpharmacologic interventions. Given the anticipated increase in the population aged 65 and over, the prevalence of persons with AD is expected to increase exponentially during the next 30 years (McClam et al., 2015). The burden is enormous and challenging to Health care systems to meet the needs of patients and their care givers. Research is actively underway to develop interventions, both to delay disease onset and to slow the progression. Among the innovative interventions evidence for Music Therapy a form of non-pharmacological therapies, is promising as an intervention for even late cases of Alzheimer's disease. The music as a hierarchical, compound language of time, with its unique ability to access affective/motivational systems in the brain, provides time structures enhancing perception processes, mainly in the range of cognition, language and motor learning. It allows for emotional expression and improvement of the motivation for rehabilitation activities. Music regulates attention and arousal in the brain in a complex, bilaterally distributed fashion. Learning verbal material through song accesses different neural network configurations than learning through verbal presentation. Clinical outcome studies with music therapy points towards superiority of music than without music in the management of patients with Dementia. It is of paramount importance to know the epidemiology, burden of the disease, the determinants and the various innovative interventions available, with focus on evidence of research for Music Therapy in the management of the disorder.

Epidemiology

Data on the prevalence of Alzheimer's indicate increasing prevalence. By 2050, one new case of AD is expected to develop every 33 seconds with an estimated prevalence to range from 11 million to 16 million (Alzheimer's disease facts and figures[ADFF], 2015). It is now a worldwide epidemic. Research estimates reveal that 48% of cases worldwide are in Asia, and that the percentage in Asia will grow to 59% by 2050 described in table 1.

Burden of the Disease

AD significantly shortens life expectancy and is one of the principal causes of physical disability, institutionalization, and decreased quality of life among the elderly (Chengxuan et al., 2009). The Management of the patients with Alzheimer's disease is a significant public health problem. Total payments in 2016 for health care, long-term care and hospice services for people age $\geq$ 65 years with dementia are estimated to be $236 billion (ADFF, 2016). Average per-person Medicare payments for services to beneficiaries age 65 years with AD and other dementias are more than two and a half times as great as payments for all beneficiaries without these conditions (ADFF, 2015) As the costs of Alzheimer's care places a substantial financial burden on families, such findings highlight the need for solutions to prevent dementia-related costs from jeopardizing the health and financial security of the families of people with Alzheimer's (ADFF, 2016). Interventions that both delay disease onset and delay progression by even a modest amount would result in significant reduction of the global burden of disease (Sloane et al., 2002).

INTERVENTIONAL STRATEGIES

Alzheimer's dementia with Core symptoms of Cognitive decline, Functional decline and Social decline and Associated symptoms of Agitation, Aggression, Depression, Psychosis, Repetitive vocalisation, Sleep disturbance and Non-specific behaviour disturbance evolves over a period of time which, including the preclinical period, may extend over three decades (Masters et al., 1994). It is a multifactorial disease reflecting the cumulative effect of protective and risk factors with moderate to strong evidence supporting the role of genetic, vascular, and psychosocial factors. Research evidence tends to support the notion that dementia onset may be postponed by implementing interventions. The appropriateness of different treatment and management strategies for AD varies according to the sequential processes of this disease, the earliest critical period the primary prevention is aimed at potential etiologic factors (both risk and protective factors)followed by early detection (secondary prevention),and finally the tertiary prevention with appropriate care, pharmacotherapy and nonpharmacological interventions to stabilize cognitive functions, reduce agitation, control neuropsychiatric symptoms, and improve the quality of life (Larson, & Kukull, 1996) Non-pharmacological interventions for the behavioural and psychological symptoms(neuropsychiatric symptoms) of dementia are used to ensure that underlying causes of behavioural disturbance are explored and to provide personalised approaches to presenting problems.

*Table 1. Projections of Alzheimer's disease prevalence (in millions) in 2006 and 2050, by regions and stage of disease**

	Prevalence (in millions)					
	2006			2050		
	Overall	Early stage	Late stage	Overall	Early stage	Late stage
Africa	1.33	0.76	0.57	6.33	3.58	2.75
Asia	12.65	7.19	5.56	62.85	34.84	28.01
Europe	7.21	4.04	3.17	16.51	9.04	7.47
Latin America and Caribbean	2.03	1.14	0.89	10.85	5.99	4.86
North America	3.10	1.73	1.37	8.85	4.84	4.01
Oceania	0.23	0.13	0.10	0.84	0.46	0.38
Total	26.55	14.99	11.56	106.23	58.75	47.48

* Regions defined according to the United Nations Population Division (4). Oceania includes Australia, New Zealand, Melanesia, Micronesia, and Polynesia (Ron, Elizabeth, Kathryn, & Michael, 2007)

PHARMACOLOGICAL INTERVENTIONS

Current medications widely used for AD and dementia, include cholinesterase inhibitors (donepezil, rivastigmine, and galantamine) the N-methyl-D-aspartate-receptor antagonist (memantine), Ginkgo, antidepressants, Antipsychotics which are designed to target clinical symptoms of the disease such as cognitive and neuropsychiatric disturbances.

Advances in Pharmacological Interventions

Effective pharmacological interventions for prevention and treatment of AD, that is, the disease-modifying therapies, are lacking. Review of the potential disease-modifying therapies and some compounds that are currently undergoing preclinical and clinical evaluations focus on Cholinesterase inhibitors, Aβ-targeting strategies, β-secretase inhibitors, γ-secretase inhibitors/modulators, α-secretase activators/modulators, M1 muscarinic agonists, Aβ-aggregation inhibitors, Immunotherapy, Aβ-degrading enzymes, Apolipoprotein E (ApoE) promotes Aβ clearance, Drugs influencing Aβ blood–brain barrier transport, Drugs development based on the metals hypothesis, HMG-CoA reductase inhibitors (the "statins"), Monoamine oxidase inhibitors, Treatments based on tau pathology, N-methyl-D-aspartate receptor (NMDA) antagonist, Non-steroidal anti-inflammatory drugs (NSAIDs), Estrogens, Nicotine, Melatonin, Cell transplantation and gene therapy(Yang Hong -Qi, Sun Zhi-Kun (2012)

Non- Pharmacological Interventions

- Music Therapy
- Reality orientation therapy,
- Recreational activities,
- simulated presence,
- validation therapy,
- Multisensory stimulation (MSS),
- Physical activities,
- Light Therapy

MUSIC THERAPY AND ALZHEIMER'S

Music Therapy is an established health profession in which music is used within a therapeutic relationship to address physical, emotional, cognitive, and social needs of individuals. It is a goal directed process in which the therapist helps the patients to improve, maintain or restore a state of well-being. Music therapy is defined by world federation of music therapy as the use of music and or its musical elements (sound, rhythm, melody and harmony) by a qualified music therapist, with a client or group, in a process designed to facilitate and promote communication, relationships, learning, mobilization, expression, organization and other relevant therapeutic objectives in order to meet physical, emotional, mental, social and cognitive needs.

Working Factors

The mechanisms of the effects of music therapy are not well understood. A heuristic model consisting of five working factors has been presented by Hillecke and his colleague which include:

- Attention modulation
- Emotion modulation
- Cognition modulation
- Behaviour modulation
- Communication modulation (Hillecke, & Nickle, 2005)

Altered musical processing is a common feature in AD. AD subjects show partially spared abilities for temporal organization of music, though not for melodic perception and musical memory. This peculiar dysfunctional pattern could depend on the neurodegenerative involvement of some specific areas for music perception and memory in the brains of AD patients (Campanelli et al., 2016). Various types of music memory exist and are differentially impaired in the different types of dementia. Accumulating evidence shows that persons with dementia enjoy music, and their ability to respond to music is potentially preserved even in the late or severe stages of dementia when verbal communication may have ceased (Baird & Samson, 2014). People with AD tend to speak less as the disease progresses and their speech becomes confused. However, the ability to sing old tunes sometimes remains intact throughout the disease. Analysis revealed that songs from the participants' past-elicited memories, especially songs related to their social and national identity (Dassa, & Amir, 2014). Familiar music from the past can assist memory recall and elicit memories associated with positive feelings (Baker, 2002) studies regarding music perception in Dementia reveal that Patients with dementia had group-level deficits of global pitch (melody contour) processing. The findings suggest that particular aspects of music perception such as pitch pattern analysis may open a window on the processing of information streams in major dementia syndromes. The potential selectivity of musical deficits for particular dementia syndromes and particular dimensions of processing warrants further systematic investigation (Golden & Clark, 2016). Multidomain interventions, aimed at affecting several risk factors simultaneously, offer a versatility that may attain improved outcomes in comparison with single-domain prevention trials. These multidomain interventions involve diet, physical exercise, cognitive training and social activities, while music therapy, improving self-consciousness and reducing neurofibrils, may contribute to deceleration/delay onset of Alzheimer's disease progression (Corsi et al., 2016). Music is unique in its powerful ability to elicit both memories and emotions. This can provide an important link to individual's past and a means of nonverbal communication with carers, which make it an ideal stimulus for persons with dementia (Baird et al., 2015). Music therapy acts mainly through emotional and psycho-physiological pathways. It includes a series of techniques that can respond to targeted therapeutic objectives. Some studies have shown that music therapy reduces anxiety, alleviates periods of depression and aggressive behaviour and thus significantly improves mood, communication and autonomy of patients. Psychosocial interventions, such as music therapy, can contribute to maintain or rehabilitate functional cognitive and sensory abilities, as well as emotional and social skills and to reduce the severity of some behavioural disorders (Guetin et al., 2013). Music/music therapy is an effective intervention for maintaining and improving active involvement, social, emotional and cognitive skills, and for decreasing behavioural problems of individuals with dementias (Koger, Chapin., & Brotons 1999). Twenty-one empirical studies, with a total of 336 subjects suffering from symptoms of dementia, were included in the meta-analysis. Overall, the effect of music/music therapy was found to be highly significant (Koger, & Chapin, 1999). The 2011 Cochrane Review of 10 randomized controlled trials on music therapy for people with dementia determined that, because of the poor methodologies used in the reported literature, it was impossible to do a meta-analysis and draw any solid conclusions about its efficacy (Vink, Bruinsma., & Scholten, 2011).

Delirium is common among patients with Dementia in acute care settings. The prevalence of delirium superimposed on dementia has been reported in 22% of hospitalized patients more than 65 years of age. Physical and chemical restraints used in management of delirium and or dementia particularly the disruptive behaviours unfortunately carry the risk of adverse effects. Consequently, music therapy a non-pharmacological alternative approach has been researched and increasingly accepted as an effective intervention in improving engagement and reduce agitated behaviours in individuals with dementia, mostly in long term hospital care settings (Young, 2008; Bradley, Siddique, & Dufron 1995, Cohen-Mansfield, & Werner, 1997). Evidence from a series of small under powered studies suggests that exposure to music, tailored to the individual's taste, can relieve agitation but not aggressive behaviour in people with dementia. It is not possible to determine whether the beneficial effect seen is the result of music therapy itself or other factors, such as the presence of the researcher. Music therapy is a safe and low-cost intervention that could potentially be offered by mental health nurses and other carers working in residential settings. Three studies (Narme & Clément, 2014, Sakamoto & Ando, 2013; Svansdottir & Snaedal, 2006) provided evidence of the effectiveness of music therapy for reducing agitation in institutionalized patients with moderately severe and severe AD. This result was particularly strong when the intervention included individualized (related to special positive memories of the participants) and interactive (including clapping, singing, and dancing) music (Sakamoto & Ando, 2013). A study comparing resident outcomes before and after implementation of an individualized music program, MUSIC & MEMORY (M&M), offered the first evidence that the M&M individualized music program is associated with reductions in antipsychotic medication use, anxiolytic medication use, and behavioural and psychological symptoms associated with dementia (BPSD) symptoms among long-stay nursing home residents with Alzheimer's disease and related dementias (ADRD) (Thomas et al., 2017). A study performed music therapy using singing training with Alzheimer's disease for 6 months by means of karaoke and a unique vocal training (the YUBA Method). After the intervention period, patients showed a significant improvement in psychomotor speed and BPSD. The analysis with fMRI showed a reduction in the size of activated brain regions during the task performance, which suggested the organization of a new cognitive strategy in the brain. Singing is an easy and joyful activity, and the introduction of singing training with karaoke as well as the voice training (the YUBA Method) may provide a valuable tool for the care. (Masayuki et a., 2015)

Variables in Music Therapy

- Active or Passive; Active intervention requiring active participation in activities like singing and playing instruments or games versus passive involvement such as listening to music, studies using live versus taped music. Active intervention appears to be more effective than passive involvement.
- Music live or taped: Live music appears to be more effective than taped sessions.
- Therapist's training (trained music therapist vs. other professional).

Forms of Music Therapy: Recent Advances

Creative Music Therapy (CMT)

CMT may exert its benefits in engagement and mood due to the effects of music on attention (Sung & Chang, 2005), general well-being, and quality of life. It may also redirect patient's attention from confusing stimuli and consequently ameliorate anxiety and agitation. Success in singing, playing instruments, moving to music, or sharing memories related to music, may also fulfil a person's unmet needs for self-expression, achievement, meaning, and purpose. Studies on CMT mention the limitations of not supporting the long-lasting effects beyond the sessions.

Neurologic Music Therapy

The neurologic music therapy is a new scope of music therapy. Music can be used as an alternative modality to access functions unavailable through non-musical stimulus. The music as a hierarchical, compound language of time, with its unique ability to access affective/motivational systems in the brain, provides time structures enhancing perception processes, mainly in the range of cognition, language and motor learning. It allows for emotional expression and improvement of the motivation for rehabilitation activities. A possibility of the brain monitoring during the processing of musical information and musical production has contributed to better understanding of how music "works" in therapy and to elaborate more precisely the scientific foundation of music therapy. With the advent of modern research techniques, since 1990s, in cognitive neuroscience, such as brain imaging, brain-wave recordings and kinematic motor analysis have provided a greater understanding of the neural processes involved in the perception and production of music (de l'Etoile, 2011). Consequently, music therapy has evolved from a social science model to a neuroscience model. This paradigm shift has resulted in the formation of a new theory known as Neurologic Music Therapy (NMT) (Thaut, 2005). Neurologic Music Therapy (NMT) has dominated other ranges of music therapy in the United States, because it provides evidence that long-term music training and the associated sensimotor skill learning can be a strong stimulant for neuroplastic changes in the developing as well as in the adult brain. It also increases a motivation for treatment through the activation of reward system in the patient.

Mechanisms of Music in Neurologic Music Therapy

Thaut (2005), in the USA presumed as the creator of neurological music therapy, identifies four mechanisms of music in neurological rehabilitation

1. Rhythmic stimulation and entrainment.
2. Patterned information processing.
3. Differential neurological processing of musical components by means of different, not only auditory (described above), brain structures.
4. Affective-aesthetic response: arousal, motivation, emotions (Elzbieta, 2015).

- **Binaural Beat Stimulation:** Rhythmic sensory stimulation or rhythmic music in combination with rhythmic light therapy where multimodal forms of stimulation are used in the treatment of stroke, brain injury, dementia and other cognitive deficits.
- **Multisensory Stimulation:** Music as a component of multisensory stimulation and combined therapies uses relaxing music, recorded sounds and a variety of equipment such as lighting effects, massage cushions, tactile surfaces and fragrances to create a multisensory environment. Other studies have used combinations of massage, aromatherapy with essential oils, such as lavender and lemon balm, and music (A National Clinical guideline, 2006).

Reviews suggest that music therapy has strong evidence as an effective non-pharmacological intervention compared to other non-pharmacological interventions such as bright light therapy, simulated therapeutic touch or aroma therapy for reducing agitation in institutionalized AD patients. However, more evidence with better methodologies to overcome the past limitations regarding the long-term effects of Music therapy itself is needed in future.

CONCLUSION

Although the published literature demonstrates that music/music therapy is an effective method overall for treating symptoms of dementia, systematic variation of treatment protocols is necessary to identify the underlying mechanisms and delineate the most effective techniques. Studies with meta-analysis also suggest music/music therapy is an effective intervention when dealing with patients with dementia. However, it is crucial to systematically address the methodological issues currently limiting interpretation of these literatures.

FUTURE RESEARCH DIRECTIONS

Although majority of the studies on music therapy as a non-pharmacological intervention in patients with dementia endorse the beneficial effects, methodological issues currently limit the interpretation of the results. Hence future research should meticulously address the issues of:

- Experimenter expectancy biases.
- Direct experimental comparisons of potential moderating variables would provide clarification of the most effective approach to administer music therapy
- Future investigations to correlate severity of dementia with responsiveness to intervention is needed.
- Long term follow-up studies are necessary to determine if the effects are lasting.

REFERENCES

A National Clinical guideline. (2006). *Management of Patients with Dementia SIGN*. Scottish Intercollegiate Guidelines Network.

Alzheimer's disease facts and figures. (2015). *Alzheimer's & Dementia, The Journal of Alzheimer Association, 11*(3), 332-84.

Alzheimer's disease facts and figures. (2016). *Alzheimer's & Dementia, The Journal of Alzheimer Association, 12*(4), 459-509.

Baird, A., & Samson, S. (2015). Music and dementia. *Programme Brain Research, 217*, 207–235. doi:10.1016/bs.pbr.2014.11.028 PMID:25725917

Baker, F. (2002). The effects of live, taped and no music on people experiencing posttraumatic amnesia. *Journal of Music Therapy, 38*, 82–104. PMID:11570931

Bradley, L., Siddique, C. M., & Dufron, B. (1995). Reducing the use of physical restraints in long-term care facilities. *Journal of Gerontological Nursing, 21*(9), 21–34. doi:10.3928/0098-9134-19950901-07 PMID:7560818

Campanelli, A., Rendace, L., Parisi, F., D'Antonio, F., Imbriano, L., de Lena, C., & Trebbastoni, A. (2016). Musical cognition in Alzheimer's disease: Application of the Montreal Battery of Evaluation of Amusia. *Annals of the New York Academy of Sciences, 1375*(1), 28–37. doi:10.1111/nyas.13155 PMID:27447536

Chengxuan, Q., & Miia, K., & Eva von S. (2009). Epidemiology of Alzheimer's disease: Occurrence, determinants, and strategies toward intervention Dialogues. *Clinical Neuroscience (New York, N.Y.), 11*(2), 111–128.

Cohen-Mansfield, J., & Werner, P. (1997). Management of verbally disruptive behaviours in the nursing home. *Journal of Gerantology Nursing, 24*, 10–17.

Corsi, M., Di Raimo, T., Di Lorenzo, C., Rapp-Ricciardi, M., Archer, T., & Ricci, S. B. (2016). Cognitive disability in Alzheimer's disease and its management. *Research in Clinical Therapy, 167*(5), e123–e126. doi:10.7417/CT.2016.1955 PMID:27845490

Dassa, A., & Amir, D. (2014). The role of singing familiar songs in encouraging conversation among people with middle to late stage Alzheimer's disease. *Journal of Music Therapy, 51*(2), 131–153. doi:10.1093/jmt/thu007 PMID:25013944

de l'Etoile, S. (2011). Processes of music therapy: clinical and scientific rationales and models. In S. Hallam, I. Cross, & M. Thaut (Eds.), *The Oxford handbook of music psychology* (pp. 493–502). Oxford, UK: Oxford University Press.

Elżbieta, G. (2015). Music therapy in neurological rehabilitation settings. *Psychiatria Polska*, *49*(4), 835–846. PMID:26488358

Gaugler, J. E., Yu, F., Krichbaum, K., & Wyman, J. F. (2009). Predictors of nursing home admission for persons with dementia. *Medical Care*, *47*(2), 191–198. doi:10.1097/MLR.0b013e31818457ce PMID:19169120

Golden, H.L., Clark, C.N., Nicholas, J.M., Cohen, M.H., Slattery, C.F., Paterson, R.W., ... Warren, J.D. (2016). Music Perception in Dementia. *Journal Alzheimer's Disorder, 11*.

Guetin, S., Charras, K., Berard, A., Arbus, C., Berthelon, P., & Leger, J. M. (2013). An overview of the use of music therapy in the context of Alzheimer's disease: A report of a French expert group. *Dementia (London)*, *12*(5), 619–634. doi:10.1177/1471301212438290 PMID:24337333

Hillecke, T., Nickle, A., & Bolay, H.V. (2005). Scientific perspectives on music therapy *Annals of New York Academy of Science*, *1060*, 271-282.

Koger, S. M., Chapin, K., & Brotons, M. (1999). Is Music Therapy an Effective Intervention for Dementia? A Meta-Analytic Review of Literature. *Journal of Music Therapy*, *36*(1), 2–15. doi:10.1093/jmt/36.1.2 PMID:10519841

Larson, E. B., & Kukull, W. A. (1996). Prevention of Alzheimer disease: A perspective based on successes in the prevention of other chronic diseases. *Alzheimer Disease and Associated Disorders*, *10*(1), 9–12. doi:10.1097/00002093-199601031-00003 PMID:8876781

Masayuki, S. T., Ken-ichi, T., Yukari, O., Hirotaka, K., Hajime, S., & Hidekazu, T. (2015). Music Therapy Using Singing Training Improves Psychomotor Speed in Patients with Alzheimer's disease: A Neuropsychological and fMRI Study Dementia. *Geriatric Cognition Disorder Extra*, *5*(3), 296–308. doi:10.1159/000436960

Masters, C. L., & Beyreuther, K. (1994). Alzheimer's disease: A clever definition of the genetic components, Alzheimer's Association Australia. *4th Natl. Conf.* Sydney: Alzheimer's Association.

McClam, T. D., Marano, C. M., Rosenberg, P. B., & Lyketsos, C. G. (2015). Interventions for Neuropsychiatric Symptoms in Neurocognitive Impairment Due to Alzheimer's Disease: A Review of the Literature. *Harvard Review of Psychiatry*, *23*(5), 377–393. doi:10.1097/HRP.0000000000000097 PMID:26332220

Narme, P., Clément, S., & Ehrlé, N. (2014). Efficacy of musical interventions in dementia: Evidence from a randomized controlled trial. *Journal of Alzheimer's Disease*, *38*, 359–369. PMID:23969994

Ron, B., Elizabeth, J., Kathryn, Z., & Michael, A. H. (2007). Forecasting the global burden of Alzheimer's disease ELSEVIER. *Alzheimer's & Dementia*, 3186–3191.

Ryu, S. H., Katona, C., & Rive, B. (2005). Persistence of and changes in neuropsychiatric symptoms in Alzheimer disease over 6 months: The LASER-AD study. *The American Journal of Geriatric Psychiatry*, *13*, 976–983. PMID:16286441

Sakamoto, A., & Tsutou, A. (2013). Comparing the effects of different individualized music interventions for elderly individuals with severe dementia. *International Psychogeriatric, 25,* 775–784.

Sloane, P. D., Zimmermanm, S. Z., Suchindran, C., Reed, P., Wang, L., & Boustani, M. (2002). The public health impact of Alzheimer's disease, implication of treatment advances. *Annual Review of Public Health, 23*, 213–231. doi:10.1146/annurev.publhealth.23.100901.140525 PMID:11910061

Svansdottir, H. B., & Snaedal, J. (2006). Music therapy in moderate and severe dementia of Alzheimer's type: A case-control study. *International Psychogeriatrics, 18*(04), 613–621. doi:10.1017/S1041610206003206 PMID:16618375

Thaut, M. H. (2005). *Rhythm, music and the brain: scientific foundations and clinical applications*. New York: Routledge.

The ICD-10 Classification of Mental and Behavioural Disorders. (n.d.). *Clinical descriptions and diagnostic guidelines*. World Health Organization.

Thomas, K. S., Baier, R., Kosar, C., Ogarek, J., Trepman, A., & Mor, V. (2017). Individualized Music Program is Associated with Improved Outcomes for U.S. Nursing Home Residents with Dementia. *The American Journal of Geriatric Psychiatry, 25*(9), 931–938. doi:10.1016/j.jagp.2017.04.008 PMID:28483436

Vink, A. C., Bruinsma, M. S., & Scholten, R. J. (2011). Music therapy for people with dementia. *Cochrane Database of Systematic Reviews, 3*, CD003477. PMID:15266489

Young, J. (2008). Supporting health and physical well-being. In M. Downs & B. Bowers (Eds.), *Excellence in Dementia Care: Research into Practice* (pp. 256–257). Berkshire, UK: Open University Press.

Yu-Shiun, C. H., Chyn-Yng, C., Yang Jui-Chen, T., Min-Huey, C., Yuan-Mei, L., Mei-ju, C., & Liu Kuei-Ru, C. (2015). The efficacy of music therapy for people with dementia: A meta-analysis of randomised controlled trials. *Journal of Clinical Nursing*. PMID:26299594

KEY TERMS AND DEFINITIONS

Dementia: Is a loss of mental ability severe enough to interfere with normal activities of daily living, lasting more than six months, not present since birth, and not associated with a loss or alteration of consciousness.

Intervention: An intervention is the act of inserting one thing between others, like a person trying to help.

Music Therapy: Music therapy is the clinical and evidence-based use of music interventions to accomplish individualized goals within a therapeutic relationship by a credentialed professional who has completed an approved music therapy program.

Section 4

Medical and Psychiatric Comorbidities in Ageing

Chapter 21
Ageing and Mental Health: A Psychological Aspect of Later Life

Neelam Verma
Talk to Cure, India

ABSTRACT

Estimated research findings suggest that almost two-thirds of adults with psychiatric conditions do not receive the required treatment services. This chapter enables readers to understand various aspects of ageing, how physical and mental health aspects are correlated, and which mental health conditions are most common in later life. The chapter also discusses major models of mental health in the context of ageing. Major psychiatric and psychological conditions that are most common in old age are outlined along with a major milestone of old age (i.e., retirement: a major lifestyle change that pushes older people towards psychological problems and adjustment issues with a new phase of life). A brief description is presented on the current status of psychiatric and psychological services for mental health issues of the elderly. The chapter concludes by summarizing the contents of discussed areas. Studies are presented throughout the chapter to accompany and enrich the discussion and validate the chapter content.

INTRODUCTION

When we talk about ageing and mental health it undoubtedly involves studying geriatrics. Geriatrics involves medical paradigms of old age such as clinical conditions and strategies to treat them. In psychology, a branch especially devoted to study ageing and provision of clinical services for older adults is *Geropsychology*. The field expands knowledge of normal ageing process and develop treatment modalities to address problems that occur when people age. Most individuals enjoy a good time in later life; however, American Psychological Association says that it is anticipated that the number of older adults with mental and behavioural health problems will almost quadruple from 4 million in 1970 to 15 million in 2030. Mental health conditions adversely affect the ability to function especially in later ages. World Health Organization (1948) defines health as "a state of complete physical, mental and social wellbeing and not merely the absence of disease or infirmity." Since the description of health includes mental health and wellbeing, it must be taken into account that psychological health is an important paradigm of

DOI: 10.4018/978-1-5225-3480-8.ch021

one's overall health including older adults, and need to be recognized and treated with equal urgency as required for other physical illnesses. A conceptual definition given by Baltes and Baltes (1990a) explains normal ageing as" ageing without biological or mental pathology". It thus concerns the ageing process that is dominant within a society for persons who are not suffering from a manifest illness. Further in their conceptual framework optimal ageing has been referred as a kind of utopia; namely, "ageing under development-enhancing and age friendly environmental conditions" and pathological ageing characterizes an "ageing process determined by medical aetiology and syndromes of illness".

If we see the above definition of normal ageing which says that "normal ageing does not include manifestation of illness" it will be difficult to justify the fact presented by Centres for Disease Control and Prevention and the Merck Company Foundation [CDC & MCF](2007) which advocates that "chronic disease is typical of the experience of ageing". According to their database, in United States more than 80% older have at least one chronic medical illness and 65% older have at least two chronic medical illnesses. For example, Arthritis is considered to be an age-related illness but old age does not manifest its occurrence because every older does not suffer from this condition. Also, the functional ability or disability which is an important part of old age which affects the ageing process. Functional disability could be present physically (weakness, deterioration in physical health, inability to walk properly or slow walking etc.) or mentally (stress, irritability, and deterioration in cognitive skills). These functional manifestations of ageing are commonly seen in our own family members who are getting aged. Often, presence of physical illnesses leads to psychological issues or vice versa. According to Cohen (1992):

- Psychogenic stress (or stress that has psychogenic basis) may lead to health issues.
- Medical illnesses or other health problems may lead to emergence of psychiatric conditions.
- Interaction of coexisting mental and physical health problems may lead to occurrence of other psychological or physical health issues.
- Social and psychosocial resources may affect the course of psychological or physical health problems.

Plethora of literature talks about conceptual, statistical and functional aspects of ageing and mental health but there is lot more to explore. Further contents of the chapter will unfold other aspects of ageing and related mental health issues.

MAJOR MODELS OF MENTAL HEALTH IN CONTEXT OF AGEING

Psychodynamic Model

Psychodynamic model of psychological functioning is considered to be the oldest, yet most comprehensive model in context of psychological wellbeing and disorders. Its contribution as mental health model in later life was relatively late but the presented facts turned out to be as good as presented in the very first theory of this school proposed by Sigmund Freud; originally called psychoanalytic model. Journey from psychoanalytic model to psychodynamic model involved contribution of many legends of the field. Explanation of psychodynamic theory revolves around basic personality structure, developmental process and interpersonal relationships. This school of thought emphasizes on the complex interrelation among cognitive, emotional and motivational forces that work on formation of personality. As psychoanalytic explanation of personality development emphasizes a linkage between childhood experiences and development of adult personality, the theory in context of later life advocates strong correlation between adult personality and old age. Precisely, the theory says that elderly come to their latter part of lives extremely influenced not only by their childhood experiences, but also by their adult episodes and adaptations made during that phase of life. According to Newton and his colleagues (1986) the individual enters later life with a personality structure that reflects a long history of life experiences. In later life the adult confronts age correlated events (retirement, physical changes and illness, loss through death of friends and family) and the internal psychological changes can re-evoke unresolved conflicts. Despite of external events being important for adjustment with ageing process, individuals' basic personality has been found to be the mediator of adaptation in old age. Hildebrand (1982) explained that how difficulties in later life affect the mental health of elderly. these difficulties included fear of diminution/loss of sexual potency, threat of redundancy in work roles or being replaced by younger people, the need to reconsider and perhaps remake the marital relationship after children left, awareness of one's own ageing, illness and possible dependence, awareness that what one can achieve now is limited, the feeling of having failed as a parent, loss of partner and of intimacy, and the fact of one's own death in terms of narcissistic loss and pain. Mental health in later life demands overcoming all these fears and threats, and those who are able to negotiate them are said to have a good mental health. Cohler (1993); Schiff and Cohler (2001) emphasized the importance of '*deriving meaning*' as a major component of mental health in old age. According to their perspective, meaning must be worked out for the entire life cycle in the form of a coherent '*narrative*' that explains the continuity of an individual's life in the face of interruptions and adverse events, and those who fail to establish this integrity and unable to preserve or build a coherent narrative suffer from mental health issues in later life. Psychodynamic theory explains the nature of old age mental health issues with following assumptions or causal factors:

- **Childhood Losses Re-Enact as Losses in Old Age:** The model emphasizes importance of childhood trauma or loss and its impact on intra-psychic structures. Adaptive capacity is affected especially in cases of loss of attachment figure in childhood and grief caused by that evokes the anxiety of living in an unprotected world (due to loss of attachment figure). Wounds of childhood trauma or bad experiences definitely leave their scars that affect an individual for the whole life. Significant losses in old age evoke re-experience of negative feelings or grief experienced in childhood and increase vulnerability to get affected easily in similar situations.
- **Underdeveloped Self or Immature Defences Cause Insufficient Strength to Deal with Psychological Challenges of Later Life:** As discussed earlier about Erikson's developmental tasks in different ages, it is important to note that developmental tasks keep changing in every stage of development and those who have not mastered the earlier stage face difficulty while facing the current developmental task. It affects the ability to adapt in new situations. Gutman (1987) establishes a relationship between personality defences and loss using immune system analogy. He advocates that loss is dominated only when one's personality is vulnerable to the loss and those are affected most with losses of old age who adapted to early losses in immature ways. Precisely saying, an underdeveloped self, exaggerates the capacity of loss to induce or provoke pathology in later life.

- **Decline or Loss of Physical, Emotional and Cognitive Strengths Weakens the Functioning of Ego:** Self psychologists have pointed out the negative impact of physical and functional decline on self-esteem and balancing it by finding restitution for loss. If the surroundings of an older adult are not supportive enough or they fail to maintain the ego functioning they might use compensatory mechanisms (possibly pathological in nature) like putting the blame on others for their losses or remembering or recounting past achievements and glories.
- **Personal Narratives Cannot Integrate with Events and Transitions of Later Life:** Life constructs of earlier adulthood may be inadequate or insufficient to integrate experiences and expectations of old age into personal narratives requiring a developmental shift or transition and inability to make the transition may lead to develop vulnerability towards personal fragmentation.

Psychodynamic model focuses on the transitions of inner processes over the life span of an individual. It emphasizes the development of strategies to cope with the imbalance between inner life and outer world and how interpersonal dynamics in old age continue to have a great impact on quality of life.

Eriksonian Psychosocial Development Model

Erik Erikson's model is an epigenetic model of psychosocial development which describes human development across life. It comprises of a series of eight developmental challenges from infancy to old age where every stage is a foundation for the next stage. The theory emphasizes that not meeting the developmental challenges adequately in midlife results in stagnation and emotional despair in later life (Erikson, 1984; Erikson & Erikson, 1998). The eight stages of development comprise of two opposing statements representing the challenges faced by a person at a particular stage. Following description provides a glimpse of eight stages and their significance for later life and associated mental health aspects.

1. **Trust vs. Mistrust:** This stage belongs to infancy in which infants receive care from their primary care givers. If the care is consistent, predictable and reliable they develop a sense of trust and virtue of hope. Failure to meet the needs of this stage leads to mistrust in all other relationships made in future. This may also result in anxiety and insecurity in later life.
2. **Autonomy vs. Shame and Doubt:** This is the stage of discovering skills by learning to do self tasks such as walking, buttoning, putting on clothes etc. children allowed and encouraged to learn with trial and error are thought to be more confidant and develop the virtue of will. on the contrary, children who are not given ample opportunity to learn or consistently criticized for accidents made during this learning begin to feel inadequate in their skills and suffer from low self esteem and a sense of failure in later stages of life.
3. **Initiative vs. Guilt:** At this stage, individuals begin to plan and initiate activities with playmates. If given opportunity, they develop skills to lead others and make decisions. Conversely, if they are excessively controlled or criticised in their decisions or initiatives they develop a sense of guilt. This leads to control them always and they lack in self initiatives throughout their lives. If a healthy balance is maintained between initiative and guilt it leads to the virtue of purpose which helps them in retaining a good psychological health in later stages of life.
4. **Industry vs. Inferiority:** Teachers play an important role at this stage of development as the child learns to read, write, perform sums etc. Peer group has a greater significance at this stage and a major source of child's self esteem. Encouragement and reinforcement to take initiatives and per-

form tasks successfully develops a sense of pride in the children and they feel confident to achieve goals later in life. Conversely, if they are restricted to initiate tasks by teachers and parents they begin to feel inferior and start doubting their potentials. If a healthy balance is maintained between competence and modesty, it leads to the virtue of competence which is one of the major aspects of life satisfaction and sense of achievement. Subsequently, it helps in carrying out all tasks of personal and professional life confidently and developing a sense of fulfilment in late life.

5. **Identity vs. Role Confusion:** This stage belongs to the search of self and personal identity by exploring personal values, beliefs and goals. The person learns and explores about what role he or she will occupy as an adult. Also, it involves exploration of two identities i.e. sexual and occupational. Accepting the body image and understanding the physiological changes during adolescence leads to the virtue of fidelity which is important to accept others and maintain relationships in further stages or adulthood. Failure to establish an understanding of self may cause role confusion and identity crisis which results in rebellion tendencies, negative identity and feelings of unhappiness with self. Such feelings result in poor mental health in later life when a person goes to other physiological changes and loss of physiological and cognitive skills.
6. **Intimacy vs. Isolation:** This stage belongs to formation of relationships with others and commitments for long term with people other than family. Successful completion of this stage results in healthy relationships, fulfilment of commitments, a sense of security and safety and care in other relationships. On the contrary, avoiding intimacy, fear from committing to others and hesitation to form intimate relationships leads to isolation and loneliness. Successful completion of this stage leads to the virtue of love that helps in maintaining close and intimate relationships.
7. **Generativity vs. Stagnation:** This stage belongs to the establishment of career, settlement in personal and professional life, beginning and raising family/children and a sense of being responsible. Successful completion of this stage leads to the virtue of care; however, those who fail to succeed at this stage suffer from stagnation and feel unproductive.
8. **Ego Integrity vs. Despair:** In context of ageing, this is the most important stage of this model. Individuals are considered senior citizens at this stage as the productivity goes low and they explore life as a retired person. This is the time where an individual cherishes accomplishments of life and develops a sense of integrity through what has been achieved in life. Successful completion of this stage leads to the virtue of wisdom which provides a sense of completeness and develop acceptance of death as a natural process without fear and regrets. If an individual at this stage sees his or her life unproductive and regrets for the decisions made in earlier stages, it leads to dissatisfaction, despair and often depression characterized by hopelessness.

The theory advocates that if the challenges of one stage are not resolved they are likely to affect further stages and stay as a problem in later life. Each and every stage has a major contribution in an individual's life; however, Generativity may have particular significance in context of ageing as it is linked with emotional and cognitive capacities; an important functional aspect of later life (Mc. Adams, 2001; Slater, 2003). Erikson; 1950, proposed a series of developmental tasks in adult life such as forming intimate relationships, being productive and committing to guide younger generation (experiencing generativity), and coming to terms with past and future in the face of upcoming death with wisdom (experiencing ego integrity). According to him, those who failed to meet these developmental challenges successfully in their adulthood were thought to be more vulnerable to emotional distress as they aged. Other sources indicate that integrity versus despair and disgust are more often associated with later life as mature forms of psychological achievements in adulthood are integrated into a comprehensive sense of wisdom in old age (Erikson et al., 1986, pp. 55-56). Consistent with Erikson's model, a wide range of research findings suggests that relationships, work and identity formed in social contexts have important implication for healthy ageing (Cohen, 2004; Everard, Lach, Fisher, & Baum, 2000; Sato et al., 2008; Thomas, 2011). However, more researches are needed to establish links between Erikson's developmental model and cognitive and psychological functioning of people ageing.

Cognitive Behavioural Model

Cognitive behavioural model is an integration of two distinct approaches i.e. *cognitive* and *behavioural* which turned out great together. Cognitive model emphasizes the importance of thoughts and belief system to maladaptive behaviours and negative emotions. Dobson and Dozois(2001); Dozois, Frewen and Covin (2006)suggested that all cognitive theories share three fundamental hypotheses i.e. 1. Cognition affects emotion and behaviour 2. Cognition can be monitored and changed 3. Cognitive alteration can bring desired emotional and behavioural changes. The behavioural model focuses on behaviour rather than emotion, motives or biological factors. This model suggests that an individual's behaviour is the result of interaction between the person and environment and according to the principles of learning theory it supports the notion that environmental cues influence the acquisition, performance rate and termination of certain behaviours. The model supports primarily observable behaviours; however, some internal behaviour like feelings and thoughts are equally covered under the basic learning principles that are possible to modify through behavioural management techniques. In behavioural approach, the term "mentally healthy" has an alternative term called "adaptation" which denotes capacity to effectively meet one's own needs within the environment. Individuals unable to adapt to their environment are said to have mental health issues due to certain factors such as 1. Learning maladaptive behaviours or frameworks, 2. Inability to learn appropriate behaviours due to poor or unsupportive learning environment, and 3. Poor self-regulation or responding to wrong environmental contingencies. Cognitive behavioural paradigm of mental health for older adults (similar for other population as well) focuses on patterns of thoughts, values, belief system and behaviours leading to adaptation and adjustment in the current environment or impairment in one's functioning. Here, especially with elderly, the process of adjustment might be challenging because of some common challenges associated with age and decline in overall functioning. This limited functional ability restricts them to respond appropriately to environmental contingencies. Conversely, freedom from responsibilities (Looking after family, career, education of children etc.) makes them more responsive towards social situations or stimuli. Baltes and Baltes (1990b) advocate that older adults show high rates of adaptability or "behavioural plasticity" to modify their behaviour and adjust to the changing capacities and environment. This adaptation takes place through selective optimization and compensation for the lost skills. Some research findings suggest that the life in nursing homes is highly challenging for older adults in reference to their mental health as it limits the environmental stimulation (all work is done by the hospital staff), thus their responsiveness towards environmental changes fails to adapt and adjust (Molinary, 2000; Rosowsky, Casciani, & Arnold, 2008; Snowden, Sato, & Roy-Byrne, 2003).

The cognitive behavioural model enables to understand a framework in which problem behaviour is easily identified and treated. Knight and Satre (1999); Satre, Knight and David (2006) emphasized the significance of this model for cognitively intact elderly to treat conditions like depression, anxiety, insomnia etc. Some other treatments, especially more behaviourally focused (for example, incontinence program, improving activities of daily living, self-care etc.) have been found to be successful even on cognitively impaired older adults.

Stress and Coping Model

This model presents a stress and coping perspective especially to work with elderly. Research work done by Aldwin (2007) suggested that it is useful to see stress and coping mechanisms as a process with three major elements i.e. 1. Strain an internal state of an individual, 2. Stressors; external events, and 3. Transactions: an experience derived from the interaction between an individual and his/her environment.

Strain encompasses physiological reactions of an individual such as sympathetic activation, parasympathetic suppression, neuroendocrine changes, and changes in immune functions, and emotional reactions such as positive or negative feelings, emotional numbness etc. Studies on mind body relationship are not new in the field but such researches have worked behind studying a relatively new field i.e. psychoneuroimmunology (PNI) that studies the interaction between physiological processes, nervous system and immune system of human body. Gruenewald and Kemeny (2007) studied and suggested substantial link between clinical depression and adverse immune response and geriatric population has been found to be most affected by this condition. Penedo and Dahn (2005) studied a similar line and established a correlation among stress caused by being diagnosed with cancer and its treatment, other stressors of life and subsequent health status. It thus clarifies that the stress does affect the immune system and there is an established link between the two.

Stressors are the events or conditions that cause stress or strain in an individual. Having problems in marriage, being victimized in a crime, death of a loved one are few examples of traumatic experiences that cause stress. Similarly, there could be other types of stressors like physical environment (weather), stress related to individual role (daughter to care for ageing parents, single parent to give healthy upbringing to children), and stress related to routine hazards such as traffic, conveyance etc. stress and stressors are distinct from each other in terms of their occurrence as stress is generally chronic but stressors are mostly acute. An individual faces stress in various contexts in a life span and when it comes to older adults it is even important. In cases of older adults social, historical and physical/non-normative contexts play a very important role in generating stress and it all concerns a series of events for them as being in a later age makes them see these things throughout their life span. An older would be a witness of all three contexts thus would be influenced by all three categories. Age graded influences cover entering school or passing out from college, history graded influences cover a particular historic period in which the individual has lived such as world war, terrorist attacks in country or a natural disaster. Non-normative influences are usually unexpected and may occur at any point of life such as loss of a loved one at a time when it is unlikely to happen or a big financial loss in business. Krause (1995a) suggested significant influence of financial strain on social and mental wellbeing of older adults. Its significance was found to be prominent for depressive symptoms and physical illness as well.

Transactions are the third important element as well as highlighting a cognitive dimension of the stress process. It summarizes the interaction between person and environment with a basic assumption that a person's perception of the stressor affects his or her coping response. Performance in final exams may have a different dimension for different students. Some may take it as a challenge for their intellectual skills; some may see it as a threat to their mental health and wellbeing, while others may take it as an opportunity to enhance their knowledge in the course topics. The perception of performance for final exams would influence the action of the students. In this process, appraisal of the intensity of stressor also plays an important role and it is said that stressors appraised with stronger intensity generate stronger emotional and physiological responses. Lazarus and colleagues explained coping based on perception of stress as problem focused and emotion focused coping. Problem focused coping focuses on altering the problem whereas emotion focused coping focuses on regulating the stress causing emotions. According to Lazarus and Folkman (1984) problem focused coping is implemented where there is an amenability to change the situation and emotion focused coping is used where nothing can be done to alter the situation. A person's style of coping depends on how a person perceives the stressful event and in many cases individual's use the combination of both styles to cope with a problem. Skaff (2007) presented perception in terms of 'Sense of control' over the event as a central element and a classic study done by Zautra, Reich and Newsome (1995) found links between sense of control, loss of autonomy and mental health amongst elderly. Their study focused on mental health of elderly in view of adapting to a phase of loss of autonomy caused by either decline in physical or mental abilities or due to loss or bereavement. Results showed high association between sense of personal control over events and positive mental health. Review of the results and literature by Skaff (2007) suggested that entering into old age with a strong sense of control is highly adaptive and promotes wellbeing of elderly.

Although the researches have been synthesized well in this field but the findings may not be implemented on every older adult. Thus, according to Gatz, Kasl-Godley, & Karel (1996) the approach needs to be more pragmatic as coping with stress involves an individual factor and said to be a function of three major elements i.e. 1. Level of vulnerability (includes genetic effect, acquired biological vulnerabilities and physiological factors affecting adaptation of the individual such as pessimistic tendency, poor problem solving and communication skills), 2. Stress being encountered (includes psychosocial and environmental elements and individual's way of perceiving the stress), and 3. Protective factors (include biological, social and psychological elements that help to moderate the stress by being physically active, having effective coping strategies or having a good social support network).

This model helps to understand that how the interaction between person and environment (i.e. individual capacities and environmental characteristics) affect the development and course of psychological disorder and influence the mental health and well-being of elderly. This area of work is highly progressive; however, caution needs to be taken while implementing this model in research work as we are still in process of learning about stress, coping and ageing altogether. Despite of limited knowledge this framework could be utilized while working with elderly and challenges of their life.

Family Systems Model

A family systems model focuses on interrelatedness of elderly with their families. It explores importance of considering ways in which their positive mental health is enhanced by supporting and smoothening the family functioning. Also, the model assesses the possibility of family dysfunctions that might be causing deterioration in mental health of elderly. In today's world where we have made communications limited to texting and phone calls, it is a positive fact that despite of isolation and abandonment of elderly from their families, they have been found to have regular contact with their children. In a research done by Troll & Bengtson (1993) it was found that even very old parents around the age of 85 years managed to have weekly face to face meetings and high frequency of phone calls/letters/greeting cards or gifts with at least one of their children. In this context, technology has been found to have a positive impact on parent- child relationship in old age when children are mostly far from their parents either for education or for occupation. According to Pruchno, Blow, and Smyer (1984) families are primary components of the "life event web" in which the ripple effects of major life changes are felt. Parent-child ties are very important yet crucial to understand. In early years parents provide care to their children and as ageing takes place the role reverses and children are expected to be the caregiver of their parents; however, the latter one is not guaranteed. Still, the care giving process from parents goes on for their children throughout their lives as they grow and need assistance from their parents for career, marriage, nurturance of their own children, marital conflicts, and divorce, physical or psychological illness and so on. According to Fingerman et al. (2009) an older adult being taken care by their children and great grandchildren is a common image in society and accurate as well because care giving and care receiving are important functions of families and later-life families. Indeed, families serve plenty of other functions for older adults other than just providing needed care such as providing mutual support in times of stress, help indecision making, sharing views on family tasks, celebrating individual developmental milestones etc. There are changes in the quality of relationship with family members and older adults that take place with time and as the person ages. Qualls (1995a) advocates that in a lifetime there are three major life transitions that cause restructuring of family relationships namely 1. Emptying and re-emptying of the nest, 2. Retirement, and 3. Onset of chronic physical illness. These life transitions affect various aspects of family relationships like time structure, individual roles, communication among family members, power balance, gap between generations and nurturance. Despite of such changes families often find an organization in new relationship patterns and familial structure.

The systems model also emphasizes on social context and conceptualizes family as a social unit. Thus, the problems are acknowledged to reside in the social unit (family) rather than an individual (family members facing the problem). Although the problems are particularly faced by one single individual, it is more distressing if the social unit is unable to manage it effectively. An elderly in the family suffering from Alzheimer's diseases would be a concern for everyone and if the problem is not being managed well by the family members it will worsen the wellbeing of the elderly and caregivers as well. Systems approach advocates that social units promoting fulfilment of family members needs are considered to be functional and those who are unable to do so or inhibit the process are considered problematic. Hence, mental health of elderly in systems model is not conceptualized on individual level, it is rather a mutual concept as everyone affects others and vice-versa. Families with poor functional structure are likely to face problems and unable to meet demands of family members throughout the life span including later life. However, many times even well-functioning families are stuck in problems and unable to adapt to the situation. Family with a demented family member would definitely face problems while taking care of the individual if they are unaware of basic issues related to that condition. Inability to provide appropriate care causes stress among family members and also affects the quality of relationship. The model also emphasizes on examining the interpersonal environment of family as mental health of older adults is highly influenced by the family characteristics and dynamics. The basis to demonstrate impact and utility of systems model for elderly's mental health is limited but the research works done by Qualls and Noecker (2009); Shields, King and Wynne (1995); Gaugler et al. (2008) and Mittelman et al.(1996) are promising. More empirical work is needed to establish the importance of systems model in context of elderly's mental health; however, available researches and their outcomes cannot be discarded.

MAJOR PSYCHIATRIC AND PSYCHOLOGICAL CONDITIONS OF LATER LIFE

As our loved ones grow old they are likely to have changes in their life that are common in old age such as normal forgetfulness, decreased attention, physical illnesses etc. According to National Institute of Mental Health, about 20% of individuals aged 55 years or older face mental health issues, but unfortunately around one in three of them do not receive required clinical attention. A major problem to detect psychiatric condition in older adults concerns physiological disorders that usually lead to secondary psychological or psychiatric disorders and overlap while diagnosing the problem. Many times even the common physical and emotional stressors in old age might be a cause of concern and put elderly at risk of developing major psychiatric conditions. The Geriatric Mental Health Foundation has proposed some conditions that may trigger the onset or development of psychiatric disorders in elderly such as physical disability, long term illness (like cancer or CVDs), Alzheimer's disease causing dementia, medical conditions affecting cognitive processing such as thyroid or adrenal disease, change of environment, illness and death of loved ones, interactions of medication, substance/alcohol abuse, and malnutrition or poor diet pattern. Gatz and her colleagues (1996) suggested three types of influential factors causing development of mental health conditions i.e. 1. Individual's level of vulnerability (biological and physiological factors affecting the risk of developing such conditions), 2. Stress (both kind of stressors like environmental and social stressors could cause development of psychiatric conditions in elderly), and 3. Protective factors (psychological, biological and social buffers for development of psychiatric conditions in old age). They suggest that risk factors and protective factors together make the individual susceptible to develop mental disorders.

There are some other demographic factors also that contribute to the psychiatric conditions among elderly. A study done by Singh, Kumar and Reddy (2012) suggested depression to be the most common problem amongst elderly. Other conditions included anxiety disorder, substance abuse, organic disorder and alcohol dependence respectively. Prevalence of psychiatric disorders was reported to be high in the illiterate population as compared to the literate population and females were reported to be more affected by psychiatric conditions as compared to males. Usually it is thought that older living in the old age homes have poor mental health, but results of this study turned out to be surprising as elderly living in community were found to have high rates of psychiatric disorders as compared to those living in old age homes. Based on empirical work following are some of the major psychiatric and psychological conditions seen in later life including conditions related to cognitive impairments:

Delirium

Delirium is a common condition causing cognitive impairment in older adults. Inouye et al. (2014b) defines Delirium as a state of acute and sudden change in attention and overall cognitive function is a serious medical problem for older persons which are often fatal. It is found to be the most frequent concern of older persons aged 65 years needing hospitalization. The condition is often unrecognized despite of its increased rate of incidence and prevalence, and poor prognosis put patients at risk of developing long term cognitive impairments (Pandharipande et al., 2013; Rudolph et al., 2010, Saczynski et al., 2012). Delirium is a potent risk factor for increased rate of mortality and illness among elderly along with long term care placement (Saxena & Lawley, 2009).

Dementia

According to American Psychiatric Association (2000) Dementias are a class of brain disorder characterized by irreversible declines in cognitive functioning that interfere with social and occupational functioning of an individual. It is most commonly seen in older adults because of its high prevalence in old age. It is estimated that approximately 35.6 million people had dementia worldwide in the year 2010. In this account, the population with dementia is expected to be 65.7 million in the year 2030 and 115.4 million in the year 2050 (Prince et al. 2013). According to the Alzheimer's Association, approximately 5.2 million Americans have Alzheimer's disease (most common cause of dementia) and it is estimated as the sixth leading cause of death in United States (Theis et al., 2013). Major risk factor for dementia is ageing and gender has been identified as another risk factor for development of this condition as females being at higher side of the risk (Sheshadri et al., 2008).

Depression

Depressive disorder is believed to be normative with ageing; however, the rate of this condition is relatively lower in older adults as compared to younger adults. Despite of its lower rate among older adults many studies based on the epidemiological framework consistently report presence of clinically significant depression among around 15-25% elderly. Thus, the condition must be taken seriously especially if encountered in later life. Many times the symptoms might be so minor that they do not meet the diagnostic criteria of any of the category specified for depression in the classification system; however, the impact of even minor symptoms of depression on physical and mental health cannot be denied. A review study done by Fiske et al. (2009) indicated that institutionalization could be a risk factor for depression in later life as nursing home residents reported an increase in symptoms. Old age is a phase of life where people go through so many changes in their own life and their surroundings. Loss of a loved one, limited resources for enjoyment, and poor social and familial support along with poor coping mechanisms may contribute to the development of depressive symptoms (Zarit&Zarit, 2007). Another study highlighted Depression being a prevalent and disabling condition in elderly increasing the rate of mortality and negatively influencing quality of life (Sivertsen, Bjorklof, Engedal, Salbaek & Helvik, 2015).

Schizophrenia

Views on schizophrenia were first presented by Kraepelin (1971) as Dementia Praecox because the condition resulted in progressive deterioration in an individual's cognitive and functional ability. Initiation of this condition was believed to be in young adulthood; however, studies on schizophrenia and ageing possess strong challenge to this belief. Studies conducted by Reeves and Brister (2008) on older population have resulted in initiation of the disorder in middle and old age. Although the studies vary on the onset of schizophrenia but it's clear that it could be early-onset schizophrenia (occur in late life as lifelong disorder) or late-onset schizophrenia (first occur in old age). While some studies indicate worsening of the cognitive and functional decline symptoms of schizophrenia in old age, other indicate substantial improvement in the symptoms with growing age (Folsom et al., 2009 and Jeste et al., 2003) and rest show elderly struggling with the persistent symptoms throughout the life span (Palmer, Heaton, & Jeste, 1999). Schizophrenia in old age is a challenging situation even for the health practitioners as there are many comorbid situations that complicate the condition. Common factors include medical comorbidity such as hypertension, diabetes, cardio vascular diseases, obesity etc. other factors include substance abuse, cognitive decline and premature institutionalization for elderly (Andrews, Bartels, Xie, & Peacock, 2009; Bartels, 2004; Rystedt & Bartels, 2008). Many times negative symptoms of schizophrenia overlap with the neurological cases having traumatic brain injury (TBI) involving frontal lobe functioning (Jackson, 1984).

Anxiety Disorders

Epidemiology for anxiety disorder suggests its occurrence in older adults more than the depressive disorder. Studies conducted in the United States (Kessler, Berglund, Demler, Jin, & Walters, 2005) and in Canada (Streiner, Cairney, &Veldhuizen, 2006) have signified elderly reporting symptoms sufficiently prominent to be diagnosed under the category of anxiety disorder. Among various categories of anxiety, phobias (Cairney, et.al., 2007) are most commonly reported. Since old age brings so many associated medical conditions it is difficult to establish a clear-cut diagnosis because the symptoms subjectively reported by elderly might be overlapping with symptoms of their medical conditions like heart diseases, hypertension etc. Also, there are various psychiatric disorders that overlap anxiety symptoms, and depression is commonest amongst them (Beekman et al., 2000; Mehta et al., 2003). Depression is also believed to have a neurological and psychological linkage to anxiety (Teachman, Siedlecki, & Magee, 2007). Apart from depression personality disorders (Coolidge, Segal, hook, & Stewart, 2000) and dementia (Twelftree & Qazi, 2006; Fisher & Noll, 1996) are also found to be comorbid with anxiety.

Sexual Disorders

It is believed that older adults are not interested neither capable of sexual activities; however, the recent pharmaceutical advances have made a remarkable impact on sexual functioning of men (Potts, Grace, Vares, &Gavey, 2006). Reduced rate of sexual activities in old age relates largely to the physiological changes among men and women and also it is normative in this age which may not necessarily be a sexual disorder. The rate of sexual activities dramatically drops in persons aged 75-85 years (Lindau et al., 2007). Reason for the same, apart from sexual disorder could be loss of partner, medical conditions and disabilities which affect the access as well as opportunity of sexual activities. Diagnostic criteria for sexual disorder remains same for individuals of all age group (including old age) and most common conditions are erectile dysfunction (genital erection during the sexual activity) and dyspareunia (pain during sexual activity) among men and women respectively and both men and women are vulnerable to sexual dysfunctions due to medical illnesses that interfere with sexual response. Attitude towards sexual activities and sexual response also influences the rate of being sexually active in old age and the findings vary across cultures as well as across gender. It is found that intensity of physical & emotional pleasure and satisfaction is reported to be low by women as compared to men, and western countries reporting higher satisfaction with sexual activities as compared to Asian countries (Laumann et al., 2005). Sexual functioning also has a linkage to cognitive impairments in old age and especially in cases where one partner is a victim and other is the caregiver. It is found that affection and sexual functioning, both declines in couples if any of the partners is diagnosed with dementia (Wright, 1998). Despite of changes in individual's sexual response many would report their sexual functioning satisfying as they are able to cope with the changes caused by ageing without identifying or may be without focusing on them. Another study pointed erectile dysfunction being most common among men and arousal disorder among women; in addition, the study also highlighted that biology plays an important role in male sexual dysfunction whereas psychology plays an important role in female sexual dysfunction (Sathyanarayana, Shajahan, Darshan & Abhinav, 2015).

Sleep Disorders

Sleep disturbances are commoner among elderly than any other age group. Almost half of all older adults experience or reports sleep difficulties at some point of life. Insomnias are most commonly reported by elderly and the pattern of difficulties may involve difficulty initiating or falling asleep, difficulty falling back to sleep after awakening in night-time or early morning awakening. In a study, approximately 15-45% reported difficulty initiating sleep, 20-65% reported interrupted sleep, 15-54% reported terminal insomnia and 10% reported non-restorative insomnia (Ohayon, 2002). Bio-psychosocial model is best to describe the sleep disorders amongst elderly as their condition may be caused by physiological (medication induced insomnia), psychological (due to depression), and social factors (interference due to house hold responsibilities). Chronic illnesses and their treatment drugs have adverse effect on sleep and they may significantly contribute to sleep disorders in old age (Ancoli-Israel & Ayalon, 2006). Psychological causes of sleep disturbances usually involve anxiety, depression, loneliness, worrying etc. (Quan et al., 2005). Social causes behind sleep disturbances may include looking after a cognitively impaired partner who has the tendency to roam around the house during night or due to institutionalization because most day time is spent in bed which decreases or disrupts the sleep during night.

Substance Use/Abuse

Substance use and abuse among elderly is a complicated issue as it is difficult to understand the presentation of effect of substances due to their medical illnesses and drugs being taken for treatment of the same. Also, the misuse of prescribed drugs or medication by elderly is another issue and its use among elderly is common and higher than marijuana. In figures it would lay approximately 0.8% vs. 0.4% (as found in National Survey on Drug Use and Health, 2007). Apart from alcohol, use of prescribed benzodiazepine and opioids has been found to be in frequent use in later age. It is estimated that approximately 20-25% elderly (aged between 50-65 years) have substance abuse problems and consumption of alcohol by them is more than the standard set by National Institute of Health (NIH); however, only 3-5% have diagnosable substance use disorder (Behavioural Health News 2015). It is estimated that by the year 2030 the number of elderly with substance use issues would double especially for prescribed and illegal drugs. A systematic review done by National Survey on Drug and Health (NSDUH) in the United States suggested that more than 2/3rd men and half of women (aged 50 years and above) consume alcohol. Amongst them, the percentage of heavy drinkers was noted as 12.2% and binge drinkers as 3.2%. Approximately 6.7% elderly aged 65 years and above were found as heavy or binge drinkers (Blazer et al., 2009). It is found that women drinkers under 65 years of age are at higher risk of social isolation and economic deprivation (Choi & Dinitto, 2011). Use of other illicit drugs among elderly is rare and there is scarcity in the researches and literature. Initial epidemiological researches reported 11.3% prevalence of alcohol misuse among Indian population aged 55-64 years and 16.8% population aged 65-74 years (Sethi & Trivedi, 1979). One community based study reported 10% prevalence of alcohol use in the population aged below 60 years of age (Gupta et al., 1995). Prevalence of alcohol use disorders is found to be high in urban elderly population as compared to the rural elderly population of India (Nadkarni, Murthy, Crome& Rao, 2013 and Srinivasan, Vaz, & Thomas, 2010).

Personality Disorders

There is little known about the Personality Disorders (PDs) in later life probably because of the difficulty to carry out long term researches with elderly. Reason for the same could be medical conditions of elderly, high dropout rate, and unwillingness to participate in studies. DSM-V (Diagnostic and Statistical Manual of Mental Disorders) defines a personality disorder (PD) as "an enduring pattern of inner experience and behaviour that deviates markedly from the expectations of the individual's culture" (p. 646). This definition implies that maladaptive personality traits occurred during the adolescence or early adulthood may persist in later life; thus have a chronic course of illness. Despite of this assumed chronicity of PDs in later age there are limited resources of knowledge available focusing on PDs in adults aged 65 years or older. An integrative literature review suggested 3-13% of prevalence rate of PDs among elderly (Van Alphen, Derksen, Sadavoy & Rosowsky, 2012). A study conducted by National Epidemiological Survey on Alcohol and Related Conditions (NESARC), which is the largest study on prevalence of PDs in later life suggested that the prevalence of at least one PD in old age was 8% and among various categories of PDs, Obsessive Compulsive PDs covered most of the sample. Along with this, disability, medical and mental conditions of elderly were found to be highly associated with PDs in old age (Schuster, Hoertel, Le Start, Manetti & Limoson, 2013). Despite of limited literature at least recent findings indicate towards an optimistic future of researches to know more about PDs in old age. Having more knowledge about this area would definitely help in developing better assessment tools and treatment plan for elderly with PDs.

Elderly Abuse

Elderly abuse is a community based problem instead of an individual concern. Abuse might be physical, psychological, sexual, verbal, financial, intentional or unintentional. Definition of elderly abuse developed by Action on Elder Abuse in the United States (Action on Elder Abuse Bulletin, 1995) and further adopted by the International Network for Prevention of Elder Abuse says that "Elder abuse is a single or repeated act, or lack of appropriate action, occurring within any relationship where there is an expectation of trust which causes harm or distress to an older person." This definition holds a greater impact of outcomes of researches conducted in various countries like Canada, the United States, China, Finland, India, Greece, Ireland, Norway, Israel, Poland and South Africa (Koseberg & Garcia, 1995). Research works focusing on identification of factors for elderly abuse have identified several factors contributing to abusive and neglecting behaviour of family members towards the elderly living in home. Some studies identified cognitive impairment as one of the reason for such abuse (Pillermer, 1988), whereas others denied the fact (Paveza, 1992, and Cooney & Mortimer, 1995). Female elderly have been identified to be at greater risk for abuse due to economical disadvantages (Aitken & Griffin, 1996), on the contrary, male elderly in community based studies were identified to be abused more by their spouses, children and other relatives (Pillermer & Finkelhor, 1988 and Podnieks, 1992). As result of such neglectful and abusive behaviour elderly suffer from depression and psychological distress as compared to their non-abused peers (Bristowe & Collins, 1989; Phillips, 1983). Not only depression, but alienation, guilt, shame, fear, anxiety, denial and post-traumatic stress are also found to have a link with elderly abuse (Booth, Bruno & Marin, 1996 and Goldstein, 1996). Elderly abuse is a sensitive issue and must be taken care of. There is a need for awareness about human rights and prevention of abuse of older people. People working in institutional and community settings must receive a basic training for detection of elderly abuse and offering primary help to them. There is a wide literature available on psychiatric and psychological conditions among elderly; however, only the most common conditions are presented here in this chapter. Apart from the above mentioned conditions there is one paradigm of old age that every employed person faces at a particular time in life. With a time which technically says goodbye to one's career and profession i.e. "Retirement". We will discuss here, how this phase of life affects one's life and how it connects to one's psychological wellbeing.

RETIREMENT: A PHASE OF TRANSITION

Retirement is one of the biggest transition phases of an individual's life as it brings a drastic change in regular life style; however, for some, retirement may be stressing; for others, it may be a relaxing moment. In the literature of psychology retirement has been found to be a potentially stressful factor for retirees (Salami & Samuel, 2010) and researchers have been able to find out causal relationship between retirement and stress caused by that (Hammen & Constance, 2005). Since retirement leads to decrease in financial status it has been found to be linked with decreased subjective wellbeing and lower life satisfaction (Diener et al., 1993). Retirement may also cause decreased social networking which leads to social isolation and further leads to psychological distress (Sugisawa et al., 1997). Many research findings suggest mixed results on retirement and its impact on one's wellbeing. Dave et al. (2006) suggested that retirement causes 6-9% decline in mental health. Another study was conducted by Bonsang, Erik and Klein(2012) on two different samples including people with voluntary and involuntary retirement which indicated that there is no significant effect of voluntary retirement on one's wellbeing, however, the impact was found to be significant in case of involuntary retirement. Although there is less availability of literature on gender differences related to this concern of retirement and mental health as most research work has been done including the male sample. Some available researches suggest that men are found to be more affected by the retirement as compared to women as men report a greater degree of loss of social status after retirement (Barnes, Helen & Parry, 2004). No doubt retirement could be a great source of stress but it could be seen as a reward after long years of consistent work. Many people live even better life after retirement by being physically active and involving themselves in activities they could not participate during their career. They see this phase as exploration of themselves and devote time to their young age passions and hobbies. Staying physically active, being connected to social groups, spending time with spouse, volunteering for social services are some very good examples of healthy retirement.

CURRENT SCENARIO OF ELDERLY MENTAL HEALTH: THE FACT SHEET

It is well recognized that mental health of elderly is a globally neglected issue; however, it has been able to draw attention of mental health care providers in recent times. Required concern and appropriate actions in this direction have made the situation far better and commendable for elderly mental health as elderly are expected to be more active in family and community activities. Concerns of mental health professionals have been able to identify several issues important in elderly mental health such as abuse and maltreatment in old age, stereotypes against active ageing called ageism, poverty in later life, institutionalization etc. Involvement of civil societies, non-government and non-profitable organizations, and mutual efforts of community and mental health care providers are expected to gain good results for promotion of mental health of older persons. In the year 2015, WHO organized the first ministerial conference on global action against dementia that focused on public health and economic challenges posed by Dementia that has been identified as a public health challenge and need action at national and international levels. Dementia and depression have been included in the WHO mental health gap action programme (mhGAP) which aims at improving concerns and care for mental, neurological and substance use disorders by providing guidance and health care services to the elderly. The Institute of Medicine (IOM, 2012) and The Substance Abuse and Mental Health Services Administration (SAMHSA) reported lack of trained professionals working in the field of elderly mental health care and this shortage is likely to increase as the older population grows year by year. It has been confirmed by the researchers that older adults are less likely to receive mental health care services as compared to young adults and even if they receive some amount of care it is least likely to be delivered by a trained geropsychologist (Karel, Gatz & Smyer, 2012). Due to coexisting physical symptoms they are most likely to receive treatment in primary health care centres rather than particular mental health care centres (IOM, 2012). Also, medications are the first line treatment offered to elderly; however, they are rarely offered counselling and psychotherapy as an alternative treatment modality (Koh et al., 2010; Arean et al., 2002).

Mental health care issues of elderly are crucial and need prompt response of mental health care providers. Not only professionals, even family members and social network can modify current scenario of old age problems. They may work as a dignity booster for older adults and play a protective role in treatment outcomes of elderly's mental health and related interventions. Mental health in later age can be tackled well by promoting healthy ageing. Encouraging older people to participate more in meaningful and fruitful activities, bonding with family and peers and being physically active are very good sources of maintaining a good later life. Promoting healthy lifestyle among older adults can bring drastic changes in the current scenario of elderly mental health which requires contribution of mental health care professionals, authorities behind making provisions and policies about elderly mental health care, community and most importantly care givers.

REFERENCES

Aitken, L., & Griffin, G. (1996). *Gender issues in elder abuse*. London: Sage Publication.

Aldwin, C. M. (2007). *Stress, coping and development: An integrative perspective* (2nd ed.). New York: Guilford.

American Psychiatric Association. (2000). *Diagnostic and Statistical Manual of Mental Disorders, Text Revision* (4th ed.). Washington, DC: American Psychiatric Association.

Ancoli-Israel, S., & Ayalon, L. (2006). Diagnosis and treatment of sleep disorders in older adults. *The American Journal of Geriatric Psychiatry*, *14*(2), 95–103. doi:10.1097/01.JGP.0000196627.12010.d1 PMID:16473973

Andrews, A. O., Bartels, S. J., Sie, H., & Peacock, W. J. (2009). Increased risk of nursing home admission among middle aged and older adults with schizophrenia. *The American Journal of Geriatric Psychiatry, 17*(8), 697–705. doi:10.1097/JGP.0b013e3181aad59d PMID:19625787

Arean, P. A., Alviderz, J., Barrera, A., Robinson, G. S., & Hicks, S. (2002). Would older medical patients use psychological services? *The Gerontologist, 42*(3), 392–398. doi:10.1093/geront/42.3.392 PMID:12040142

Baltes, P. B., & Baltes, M. M. (1990a). Selective optimization with compensation. In P. B. Baltes & M. M. Baltes (Eds.), *Successful aging: Perspectives from the behavioural sciences* (pp. 1–34). New York: Cambridge University Press. doi:10.1017/CBO9780511665684.003

P. B. Baltes, & M. M. Baltes (Eds.). (1990b). *Successful aging: Perspectives from the behavioural sciences.* Cambridge, UK: Cambridge University Press. doi:10.1017/CBO9780511665684

Barnes, H., & Parry, J. (2004). Renegotiating identity and relationships: Men and women's adjustment to retirement. *Ageing and Society, 24*(2), 213–233. doi:10.1017/S0144686X0300148X

Bartels, S. J. (2004). Caring for the whole person: Integrated health care for older adults with severe mental illness and medical comorbidity. *Journal of the American Geriatrics Society, 52*, 249–257. doi:10.1111/j.1532-5415.2004.52601.x PMID:15541165

Beekman, A. T. F., De Beurs, E., van Balkom, A. J. L. M., Deeg, D. J. H., Van Dyck, R., & Van Tilburg, W. (2000). Anxiety and depression in later life: Co-occurrence and communality of risk factors. *The American Journal of Psychiatry, 157*(1), 89–95. doi:10.1176/ajp.157.1.89 PMID:10618018

Blazer, D. G., & Wu, L. T. (2009). The epidemiology of substance use and disorders among middle aged and elderly community adults: National Survey on drug use and health. *The American Journal of Geriatric Psychiatry, 17*(3), 237–245. doi:10.1097/JGP.0b013e318190b8ef PMID:19454850

Bonsang, E., & Klein, T. (2012). Retirement and subjective wellbeing. *Journal of Economic Behavior & Organization, 45*, 251–278.

Booth, B. K., Bruno, A. A., & Marin, R. (1996). Psychological therapy with abused and neglected patients. In Abuse, neglect and exploitation of older patients: Strategies for assessment and intervention (pp. 185-206). Baltimore, MD: Health Professions Press.

Bristowe, E., & Collins, J. B. (1989). Family mediated abuse of non-institutionalized elder men and women living in British Columbia. *Journal of Elder Abuse & Neglect, 1*(1), 45–54. doi:10.1300/J084v01n01_05

Cairney, J., McCabe, L., Veldhuizen, S., Corna, L. M., Streiner, D., & Herrmann, N. (2007). Epidemiology of social phobia in later life. *The American Journal of Geriatric Psychiatry, 15*(3), 224–233. doi:10.1097/01.JGP.0000235702.77245.46 PMID:17213375

Centers for Disease Control and Prevention and the Merck Company Foundation. (2007). *The state of ageing and health in America 2007.* Whitehouse Station, NJ: The Merck Company Foundation. Retrieved from http://www.cdc.gov/ageing/pdf/saha_2007.pdf

Choi, N. G., & Dinitto, D. M. (2011). Heavy/binge drinking and depressive symptoms in older adults: Gender differences. *International Journal of Geriatric Psychiatry*, *26*(8), 860–868. doi:10.1002/gps.2616 PMID:20886659

Cohen, G. D. (1992). The future of mental health and aging. In J. E. Birren, R. B. Sloane, & G. D. Cohen (Eds.), *Handbook of mental health and aging* (2nd ed.; pp. 893–914). San Diego, CA: Academic Press. doi:10.1016/B978-0-12-101277-9.50037-1

Cohen, S. (2004). Social relationships and health. *The American Psychologist*, *59*(8), 676–684. doi:10.1037/0003-066X.59.8.676 PMID:15554821

Cohler, B. J. (1993). Aging, morale, and meaning: The nexus of narrative. In T. R. Cole, W. A. Achenbaum, P. L. Jakobi, & R. Kastenbaum (Eds.), *Voices and visions of aging: Toward a critical gerontology* (pp. 107–133). New York: Springer.

Coolidge, F. L., Segal, D. L., Hook, J. N., & Stewart, S. (2000). Personality disorders and coping among anxious older adults. *Journal of Anxiety Disorders*, *14*(2), 157–172. doi:10.1016/S0887-6185(99)00046-8 PMID:10864383

Cooney, C., & Mortimer, A. (1995). Elder abuse and dementia: A pilot study. *The International Journal of Social Psychiatry*, *41*(4), 276–283. doi:10.1177/002076409504100405 PMID:8815051

Dhaval, D., Inas, R., & Spasojevic, J. (2006). The effects of retirement on physical and mental health outcomes. *National Bureau of Economic Research*, w12123.

Diener, E. D., Sandvik, E., Seidlitz, L., & Diener, M. (1993). The relationship between income and wellbeing. Relative or absolute? *Social Indicators Research*, *28*(3), 195–223. doi:10.1007/BF01079018

Dobson, K. S., & Dozois, D. J. A. (2001). Historical and philosophical bases of the cognitive behavioural therapies. In K. S. Dobson (Ed.), *Handbook of cognitive-behavioral therapies* (2nd ed.; pp. 3–39). New York: Guilford.

Dozois, D. J. A., Frewen, P. A., & Covin, R. (2006). Cognitive theories. In J. C. Thomas & D. L. Segal (Eds.), Personality and everyday functioning. Hoboken, NJ: John Wiley & Sons, Inc.

Erikson, E. H. (1950). *Childhood and society*. New York: Norton.

Erikson, E. H. (1984). Reflections on the last stage-and the first. *The Psychoanalytic Study of the Child*, *39*(1), 155–165. doi:10.1080/00797308.1984.11823424 PMID:6514889

Erikson, E. H., & Erikson, J. M. (1998). *The life cycle completed (extended version)*. New York: WW Norton & Company.

Erikson, E. H., Erikson, J. M., & Kivnick, H. Q. (1986). *Vital involvement in old age*. New York: W. W. Norton & Co.

Everard, K. M., Lach, H. W., Fisher, E. B., & Baum, M. C. (2000). Relationship of activity and social support to the functional health of older *adults. The Journals of Gerontology. Series B, Psychological Sciences and Social Sciences*, *55*(4), 208–212. doi:10.1093/geronb/55.4.S208 PMID:11584883

Fingerman, K. L., Miller, L. M., & Seidel, A. J. (2009). Functions families serve in old age. In S. H. Qualls & S. H. Zarit (Eds.), *Aging families and caregiving* (pp. 19–44). Hoboken, NJ: John Wiley & Sons, Inc.

Fisher, J. E., & Noll, J. P. (1996). Anxiety disorders. In L. L. Carstensen, B. A. Edelstein, & L. Dornobrand (Eds.), The practical handbook of clinical gerontology (pp. 304-323). Thousand Oaks, CA: Sage.

Fiske, A., Wetherell, J. L., & Gatz, M. (2009). Depression in older adults. *Annual Review of Clinical Psychology*, *5*(1), 363–389. doi:10.1146/annurev.clinpsy.032408.153621 PMID:19327033

Folsom, D. P., Depp, C., Palmer, B. W., Mausbach, B. T., Golshan, S., Fellows, I., ... Jeste, D. V. (2009). Physical and mental health related quality of life among older people with schizophrenia. *Schizophrenia Research*, *108*(1-3), 207–213. doi:10.1016/j.schres.2008.12.008 PMID:19168328

Gatz, M., Kasl-Godley, J. E., & Karel, M. J. (1996). Aging and mental disorders. In J. E. Birren & K. W. Schaie (Eds.), *Handbook of the psychology of aging* (4th ed.; pp. 365–382). San Diego, CA: Academic Press.

Gaugler, J., Roth, D., Haley, W., & Mitterlman, M. (2008). Can counselling and support reduce burden and depressive symptoms in caregivers of people with Alzheimer's disease during the transition to institutionalization. Results from the New York University Caregiver Intervention Study. *Journal of the American Geriatrics Society*, *56*(3), 421–428. doi:10.1111/j.1532-5415.2007.01593.x PMID:18179495

Goldstein, M. (1996). Elder mistreatment and PTSD. In Ageing and post-traumatic stress disorder (pp. 126-135). American Psychiatric Association.

Gruenewald, T. L., & Kemeny, M. E. (2007). Psychoneuroimmunological process in aging and health. In C. M. Aldwin, C. L. Park, & A. Spiro (Eds.), *Handbook of health psychology and aging* (pp. 97–118). New York: Guilford.

Gupta, R., Sharma, S., Gupta, V. P., & Gupta, K. D. (1995). Smoking and alcohol intake in a rural Indian population and correlation with hypertension and coronary heart disease prevalence. *The Journal of the Association of Physicians of India*, *43*, 243–248. PMID:8713264

Gutmann, D. L. (1987). *Reclaimed powers: Toward a new psychology of men and women in later life.* New York: Basic Books.

Hammen & Constance. (2005). Stress and depression. *Annual Review of Clinical Psychology, 1,* 293-319.

Hildebrand, H. P. (1982). Psychotherapy with older patients. *The British Journal of Medical Psychology*, *55*(1), 19–28. doi:10.1111/j.2044-8341.1982.tb01477.x PMID:7059528

Inouye, S. K., Westendorp, R. G., & Saczynski, J. S. (2014b). Delirium in elderly people. *Lancet*, *383*(9920), 911–922. doi:10.1016/S0140-6736(13)60688-1 PMID:23992774

Institute of Medicine. (2012). *The Mental Health and Substance Use Workforce for Older Adults: In Whose Hands?* Retrieved from: http://www.iom.edu/reports/2012/The-Mental-Health-and-Substance-Use-Workforce-for-Older-Adults.aspx

Jackson, J. H. (1984). Remarks on the evolution and dissolution of the nervous system. *The Journal of Mental Science*, *33*, 25–48.

Jeste, D. V., Twamley, E. W., Eyler Zorrilla, L. T., Golshan, S., Patterson, T. L., & Palmer, B. W. (2003). Aging and outcome in schizophrenia. *Acta Psychiatrica Scandinavica, 107*(5), 336–343. doi:10.1034/j.1600-0447.2003.01434.x PMID:12752029

Karel, M. J., Gatz, M., & Smyer, M. (2012). Ageing and mental health in the decade ahead: What psychologists need to know. *The American Psychologist, 67*(3), 184–198. doi:10.1037/a0025393 PMID:21942364

Kessler, R. C., Berglund, P. A., Demler, O., Jin, R., & Walters, E. E. (2005). Lifetime prevalence and age of onset distributions of DSM-IV disorders in the National Comorbidity Survey Replication (NCS-R). *Archives of General Psychiatry, 62*(6), 593–602. doi:10.1001/archpsyc.62.6.593 PMID:15939837

Knight, B. G., & Satre, D. D. (1999). Cognitive behavioural psychotherapy with older adults. *Clinical Psychology: Science and Practice, 6*(2), 188–203. doi:10.1093/clipsy.6.2.188

Koh, S., Blank, K., Cohen, C. I., Cohen, G., Faison, W., Kennedy, G., ... Streim, J. (2010). Public's view of mental health services for the elderly: Responses to dea Abby. *Psychiatric Services (Washington, D.C.), 61*(11), 1146–1149. doi:10.1176/ps.2010.61.11.1146 PMID:21041356

Koseberg, J. I., & Garcia, J. L. (1995). Common and unique themes on elder abuse from a worldwide perspective. In J. I. Kosberg & J. L. Garcia (Eds.), *Elder abuse: International and cross-cultural perspectives*. Binghamton, NY: Haworth Press.

Kraepelin, E. (1971). *Dementia praecox and paraphrenia* (R. M. Barclay, Trans.). Huntington, NY: Rovert E. Kreiger. (Original work published 1919)

Krause, N. (1995a). Stress and well-being in later life: *Using research findings to inform intervention design*. In L. A. Bond, S. J. Cutler, & A. Grams (Eds.), *Promoting successful and productive aging* (pp. 203–219). Thousand Oaks, CA: Sage.

Laumann, E. O., Nicolosi, A., Glasser, D. B., Paik, A., Gingell, C., Moreira, E., & Wang, T. (2005). Sexual problems among women and men aged 40-80 years: Prevalence and correlates identified in the Global Study of Sexual Attitudes and Behaviours. *International Journal of Impotence Research, 17*(1), 39–57. doi:10.1038/sj.ijir.3901250 PMID:15215881

Lazarus, R. S., & Folkman, S. (1984). *Stress, appraisal and coping*. New York: Springer.

Lindau, S. T., Schumm, L. P., Laumann, E. O., Levinson, W., O'Muircheartaigh, C. A., & Waiter, L. J. (2007). A study of sexuality and health among older adults in the United States. *The New England Journal of Medicine, 357*(8), 762–774. doi:10.1056/NEJMoa067423 PMID:17715410

McAdams, D. P. (2001). Generativity in midlife. In M. Lachman (Ed.), *Handbook of midlife deveopment* (pp. 395–443). New York: Wiley.

Mehta, K. M., Simonsick, E. M., Penninx, B. W. J. H., Schulz, R., Rubin, S. M., Satterfield, S., & Yaffe, K. (2003). Prevalence and correlates of anxiety symptoms in well-functioning older adults: Findings from the Healthy Aging and Body Composition Study. *Journal of the American Geriatrics Society, 51*(4), 499–504. doi:10.1046/j.1532-5415.2003.51158.x PMID:12657069

Mittelman, M. S., Ferris, S. H., Shulman, E., Steinberg, G., & Lvin, B. (1996). A family intervention to delay nursing home placement of patients with Alzheimer's disease: A randomized controlled trial. *Journal of the American Medical Association, 276*, 1725–1731. doi:10.1001/jama.1996.03540210033030 PMID:8940320

V. Molinary (Ed.). (2000). *Professional psychology in long term care: A comprehensive guide*. New York: Hatherleigh Press.

Nadkarni, A., Murthy, P., Crome, I. B., & Rao, R. (2013). Alcohol use and alcohol use disorders among older adults in India: A literature review. *Aging & Mental Health, 17*(8), 979–991. doi:10.1080/13607863.2013.793653 PMID:23659339

Newton, N., Brauer, D., Gutmann, D. L., & Grunes, J. (1986). Psychodynamic therapy with the aged: A review. *Clinical Gerontologist, 5*(3-4), 205–229. doi:10.1300/J018v05n03_01

Ohayon, M. M. (2002). Epidemiology of insomnia: What we know and what we still need to learn. *Sleep Medicine Reviews, 6*(2), 97–111. doi:10.1053/smrv.2002.0186 PMID:12531146

Palmer, B. W., Heaton, S. C., & Jeste, D. V. (1999). Older patients with schizophrenia: Challenges in the coming decades. *Psychiatric Services (Washington, D.C.), 50*(9), 1178–1183. doi:10.1176/ps.50.9.1178 PMID:10478904

Pandharipande, P. P., Girard, T. D., Jackson, J. C., Morandi, A., Thompson, J. L., Pun, B. T., ... Ely, E. W. (2013). Brain ICU study investigators: Long term cognitive impairment after critical illness. *The New England Journal of Medicine, 369*(14), 1306–1316. doi:10.1056/NEJMoa1301372 PMID:24088092

Paveza, G. J., Cohen, D., Eisdorfer, C., Freels, S., Semla, T., Ashford, J. W., ... Levy, P. (1992). Severe family violence and Alzheimer's disease: Prevalence and risk factors. *The Gerontologist, 32*(4), 493–497. doi:10.1093/geront/32.4.493 PMID:1427252

Penedo, F. J., & Dahn, J. R. (2005). Psychoneuroimmunology and aging. In K. Vedhara & M. Irwin (Eds.), Human psychoneuroimmunology (pp. 81-106). New York: Oxford University Press.

Phillips, L. R. (1983). Theoretical explanations of elder abuse. In *Elder abuse: Conflict in the family* (pp. 197–217). Dover, UK: Auburn House.

Pillermer, K., & Finkelhor, D. (1988). Prevalence of elder abuse: A random sample survey. *The Gerontologist, 28*(1), 51–57. doi:10.1093/geront/28.1.51 PMID:3342992

Podnieks, E. (1992). National survey on abuse of the elderly in Canada. *Journal of Elder Abuse & Neglect, 4*(1-2), 5–58. doi:10.1300/J084v04n01_02

Potts, A., Grace, V. M., Vares, T., & Gavey, N. (2006). Sex for life"?Men's counter-stories on "erectile dysfunction", male sexuality and ageing. *Sociology of Health & Illness, 28*(3), 306–329. doi:10.1111/j.1467-9566.2006.00494.x PMID:16573718

Prince, M., Bryce, R., Albanese, E., Wimo, A., Ribeiro, W., & Ferri, C. P. (2013). The global prevalence of dementia: A systematic review and meta-analysis. *Alzheimer's & Dementia, 9*(1), 63–75. doi:10.1016/j.jalz.2012.11.007 PMID:23305823

Pruchno, R. A., Blow, F. C., & Smyer, M. A. (1984). Life events and interdependent lives: Implications for research and intervention. *Human Development*, *27*(1), 31–41. doi:10.1159/000272901 PMID:6698531

Qualls, S. H., & Noecker, T. L. (2009). Caregiver family therapy for conflicted families. In S. H. Qualls & S. H. Zarit (Eds.), *Aging families and caregiving: A clinician's guide to research, practice, and technology* (pp. 155–188). Hoboken, NJ: John Wiley & Sons, Inc.

Qualls, S. H., & Smyer, M. A. (1995a). Mental health. In G. L. Maddox (Ed.), *The encyclopaedia of aging* (2nd ed.; pp. 629–631). New York: Springer.

Quan, S. F., Katz, R., Olson, J., Bonekat, W., Enright, P. L., Young, T., & Newman, A. (2005). Factors associated with incidence and persistence of symptoms of disturbed sleep in an elderly cohort: The Cardiovascular Health Study. *The American Journal of the Medical Sciences*, *329*(4), 163–172. doi:10.1097/00000441-200504000-00001 PMID:15832098

Reeves, R. R., & Brister, J. C. (2008). Psychosis in late life: Emerging issues. *Journal of Psychosocial Nursing and Mental Health Services*, *46*(11), 45–52. doi:10.3928/02793695-20081101-09 PMID:19051578

E. Rosowsky, J. Casciani, & M. Arnold (Eds.). (2008). *Geropsychology and long-term care: A practitioner's guide*. New York: Springer.

Rudolph, J. L., Inouye, S. K., Jones, R. N., Yang, F. M., Fong, T. G., Levkoff, S. E., & Marcantonio, E. R. (2010). Delirium: An independent predictor of functional decline after cardiac surgery. *Journal of the American Geriatrics Society*, *58*(4), 643–649. doi:10.1111/j.1532-5415.2010.02762.x PMID:20345866

Rystedt, I. B., & Bartels, S. J. (2008). Medical comorbidity. In K. T. Mueser & D. V. Jeste (Eds.), *Clinical handbook of schizophrenia* (pp. 424–436). New York: Guilford.

Saczynski, J., Marcantonio, E. R., Quach, L., Fong, T. G., Gross, A., Inouye, S. K., & Jones, R. N. (2012). Cognitive trajectories after postoperative delirium. *The New England Journal of Medicine*, *367*(1), 30–39. doi:10.1056/NEJMoa1112923 PMID:22762316

Salami, & Samuel, O. (2010). Retirement context and psychological factors as predictors of wellbeing among retired teachers. *Europe's Journal of Psychology, 6*(2), 47-64.

Sathyanarayana Rao, T. S. (2015). Sexual disorder among elderly: An epidemiological study in South Indian rural population. *Indian Journal of Psychiatry*, *57*(3), 236–241. doi:10.4103/0019-5545.166618 PMID:26600575

Sato, T., Kishi, R., Suzukawa, A., Horikawa, N., Saijo, Y., & Yoshioka, E. (2008). Effects of social relationships on mortality of the elderly: How do the influences change with the passage of time? *Archives of Gerontology and Geriatrics*, *47*(3), 327–339. doi:10.1016/j.archger.2007.08.015 PMID:17936379

Satre, D., Knight, B. G., & David, S. (2006). Cognitive behavioural interventions with older adults: Integrating clinical and gerontological research. *Professional Psychology, Research and Practice*, *37*(5), 489–498. doi:10.1037/0735-7028.37.5.489

Saxena, S., & Lawley, D. (2009). Delirium in the elderly: A clinical review. *Postgraduate Medical Journal*, *85*(1006), 405–413. doi:10.1136/pgmj.2008.072025 PMID:19633006

Schiff, B., & Cohler, B. J. (2001). Telling survival backwards: Holocaust survivors narrate the past. In G. M. Kenyon, P. G. Clark, & B. de Vries (Eds.), *Narrative gerontology: Theory research, and practice* (pp. 113–136). New York: Springer.

Schuster, J. P., Hoertel, N., Le Start, Y., Manetti, A., & Limoson, F. (2013). Personality disorders in older adults: Findings from the National Epidemiological Survey on Alcohol and Related Conditions. *The American Journal of Geriatric Psychiatry*, *21*(8), 757–768. doi:10.1016/j.jagp.2013.01.055 PMID:23567365

Sethi, B. B., & Trivedi, J. K. (1979). Drug abuse in rural population. *Indian Journal of Psychiatry*, *21*, 211–216.

Sheshadri, S., Beiser, A., Kelly-Hayes, M., Kase, C. S., Au, R., Kannel, W. B., & Wolf, P. A. (2008). The lifetime risk of stroke: Estimates from the Framingham Study. *Stroke*, *37*(2), 345–350. doi:10.1161/01.STR.0000199613.38911.b2 PMID:16397184

Shields, G. C., King, D. A., & Wynne, L. C. (1995). Interventions with later life families. In R. H. Mikesell, D. Lusterman, & S. H. McDaniel (Eds.), *Integrating family therapy: Handbook of family psychology and systems theory* (pp. 141–158). Washington, DC: American Psychological Association. doi:10.1037/10172-008

Singh, A. P., Kumar, K. L., & Reddy, C. P. (2012). Psychiatric morbidity in geriatric population in old age homes and community: A comparative study. *Indian Journal of Psychological Medicine*, *34*(1), 39–43. doi:10.4103/0253-7176.96157 PMID:22661806

Sivertsen, H., Bjorklof, G. H., Engedal, K., Selbaek, G., & Helvik, A. S. (2015). Depression and quality of life in older persons: A review. *Dementia Gereatria Cognition Disorder*, *40*, 5–6. PMID:26360014

Skaff, M. M. (2007). Sense of control and health: A dynamic duo in the aging process. In C. M. Aldwin, C. L. Park, & A. Spiro (Eds.), *Handbook of health psychology and aging* (pp. 186–209). New York: Guilford.

Slater, C. L. (2003). Generativity versus stagnation: An elaboration of Erikson's adult stage of human development. *Journal of Adult Development*, *10*(1), 53–65. doi:10.1023/A:1020790820868

Srinivasan, K., Vaz, M., & Thomas, T. (2010). Prevalence of health related disability among community dwelling urban elderly from middle socioeconomic strata in Bangaluru, India. *The Indian Journal of Medical Research*, *131*, 515–521. PMID:20424302

Streiner, D. L., Chairney, J., & Veldhuizen, S. (2006). The epidemiology of psychological problems in the elderly. *Canadian Journal of Psychiatry*, *51*(3), 185–191. doi:10.1177/070674370605100309 PMID:16618010

Sugisawa, A., Hidehiro, S., Yomeni, N., & Hiroshi, S. (1997). Effect of retirement on mental health and social wellbeing among elderly Japanese. *Japanese Journal of Public Health*, *44*(2), 123–130. PMID:9130849

Teachman, B. A., Siedlecki, K. L., & Magee, J. C. (2007). Aging and symptoms of anxiety and depression: Structural invariance of the tripartite model. *Psychology and Aging*, *22*(1), 160–170. doi:10.1037/0882-7974.22.1.160 PMID:17385992

Theis, W., & Bleiler, L. (2013). Alzheimer's association: Alzheimer's disease facts and figures. *Alzheimer's & Dementia, 9*(2), 208–245. PMID:23507120

Thomas, P. A. (2011). Trajectories of social engagement and limitations in late life. *Journal of Health and Social Behavior, 52*(4), 430–443. doi:10.1177/0022146511411922 PMID:22144732

Troll, L. E., & Bengtson, V. L. (1993). The oldest-old in families: An intergenerational perspective. In L. Burton (Ed.), *Families and ageing* (pp. 70–89). Amityville, NY: Baywood Press.

Twelfree, H., & Qazi, A. (2006). Relationship between anxiety and agitation in dementia. *Aging & Mental Health, 10*(4), 362–367. doi:10.1080/13607860600638511 PMID:16798628

Van Alphen, S. P. J., Derksen, J. J., Sadavoy, J. J., & Rosowsky, E. E. (2012). Features and challenges of personality disorders in late life. *Aging & Mental Health, 16*(7), 805–810. doi:10.1080/13607863.2012.667781 PMID:22417221

World Health Organization. (1948). *Constitution of the World Health Organization*. Available at: http//www.who.int/governance/eb/who_constitution_en.pdf

Wright, L. K. (1998). Affection and sexuality in the presence of Alzheimer's disease: A longitudinal study. *Sexuality and Disability, 16*(3), 167–179. doi:10.1023/A:1023042924997

Zarit, S. H., & Zarit, J. M. (2007). *Mental disorders in older adults (2nd ed.)*. Guilford.

Zautra, A. J., Reich, J. W., & Newsom, J. T. (1995). Autonomy and sense of control among older adults: An examination of their effects on mental health. In L. A. Bond, S. J. Cutler, & A. Grams (Eds.), *Promoting successful and productive aging* (pp. 153–170). Thousand Oaks, CA: Sage.

KEY TERMS AND DEFINITIONS

Elderly Mental Health: Elderly mental health refers to conditions affecting mental health aspects of individuals who are ageing.

Geropsychology: A branch of psychology that deals with the process of ageing and related mental health issues. It is also known as geriatric psychology or gerontology.

Mental Healthcare Services: A group or government, private or lay organizations operating at a community/state/national/international level to aid in the prevention and treatment of mental disorders.

Old Age: Old age refers to ages nearing or surpassing the expectancy of human beings, and is thus the end of human life cycle.

Psychological Conditions: A state of mind of an individual with emotional and behavioural problems that need intervention by a mental health professional.

Psychological Wellbeing: It refers to overall satisfaction with one's life characterized by self-acceptance, sense of autonomy, establishment of quality ties to others, pursuit of meaningful goals, continued growth, and ability to manage complex environment to meet personal needs and values.

Chapter 22
Factors Contributing of Ageing:
Factors in Ageing

Smita Pandey
Gujarat Forensic Sciences University, India

ABSTRACT

Ageing is related to problems in physical, emotional, and mental health. If we can delay the ageing process, we may be able to live more happily and successfully. Several factors are responsible for ageing: age, sleep, dietary habits, nutrition, physical activity, general health condition, emotional well-being, physical impairment, cultural factors, life events, social support, family well-being, financial resources, cognitive functioning, and diseases. The chapter is based on the above views and mainly focuses on the various factors that contribute to ageing.

INTRODUCTION

Ageing is the process of growing old, with a number of transitions in the journey of life. As they grow old their physical and mental capacities decline and they are not able to manage their life as good as they were doing it earlier. The transitions may include retirement, relocation, death of spouse or friends, geriatric syndromes such as frailty, decline in physical activity, problems with memory and so on. World Health Organization (WHO) states: "Active Ageing is the process of optimizing opportunities for health, participation and security in order to enhance quality of life as people age" (WHO, 2002). Susan and Andrew (2016) defined ageing as "the process during which structural and functional changes accumulate in an organism as a result of the passage of time. The changes manifest as a decline in peak fertility and physiological functions, until death." Ageing is challenging and at the same time full of opportunities. If the elderly is active, he can enjoy his life without perceiving himself as aged. The elderly can enjoy going out and meeting people more frequently, that he was not able to do it earlier, because of the preoccupation with his work. He can focus more on his hobbies or he can spend time with his grandchildren. It is to be specified here that there are factors that contributes to ageing and there are factors that delays ageing. In this chapter we will be focusing on the factors that contribute to ageing.

DOI: 10.4018/978-1-5225-3480-8.ch022

Senescence and Ageing

Senescence is the progressive deterioration of cellular growth and decline in metabolic processes, through the passage of time. Senscence starts at the end of reproductive age and is also called as old age. Senescence is defined as reducing fertility and increasing the mortality (Monaco & Silveria, 2009). The concepts of aging is simply defined as the unavoidable passage of time, senescence the progressive physiologic impairment, and senility the pathological development of diseases (Monaco & Silveria, 2009).

There are several factors that contribute to ageing. These factors may be biological, life style, social, psychological, spiritual, and cognitive and the diseases in the old age. These factors may not only lead to ageing but also to several diseases in the ageing process.

BIOLOGICAL FACTORS

Several biological factors like genetics, temperature, glycation, metabolism and oxidation affects the ageing process of humans.

Genetics

The genes of humans are genetically programmed for ageing. The human genes consist of a protein called rapamycin that has been responsible for regulation in ageing and growth (Rogers et al., 2016). There is genetic theory that longevity of life is determined by the longevity of their parents and grandparents and that identical twins have similar age span than fraternal twins (Rogers et al., 2016).

Metabolism and Oxidation

The metabolism plays an important role in the regulation of ageing and growth. Metabolism produces reactive chemicals or oxidizing agents that may increase the ageing process due to the damage in cells. (Bratic&Trifunovic,2010).

Wear and Tear

The cells of an organism are always getting damaged and worn out on daily basis. But, sometimes, permanent damage occurs to more or less permanent basis that these cannot be repaired easily, leading to ageing (Rogers et al., 2016).

OTHER PSYCHOPSYCHOLOGICAL FACTORS

Lifestyle Factors

Lifestyle reflects the individual's attitude, way of living, values, how to take care of self and how to view the world around him. Many of the lifestyles are the choices by individuals, but few others have physical or technical constraints to be followed (Spaargaren & VanVliet, 2000). Several lifestyle factors including smoking, consuming alcohol, sedentary lifestyle, low physical exercise, unhealthy eating habits, being overweight or underweight, lack of nutrition and poor sleep hygiene, affect the ageing process in the geriatric population. In a study it was found that the hazard ratio was higher in men with low lifestyle scores (based upon smoking, alcohol consumption, diet, body mass index and physical activity) than in men with high lifestyle scores (Spencer et al., 2005). In another study researchers stated that, the possibility of living up to 90 years of age is 54% in those living in healthy lifestyle including no smoking, had normal blood pressure and weight and normally physically active (Yates et al., 2008).

Smoking

Smoking is a habit that affects health of the geriatric population in different aspects. In a study it was depicted that the median age of the non-smokers with normal weight was one year longer than those with smokers who had been underweight (Rizzuto et al., 2012). In a review, LaCroix and Omenn (1992) stated that the individuals who stopped smoking improved in various aspects of health-related diseases, including the reduced risk of death by one to two years, lesser rate of cardiac arrests, low cancer related diseases, lesser respiratory problems, lower rates of osteoporosis and hip fractures, better mobility and physical health. Smoking has also been related to cognitive decline and dementia in the elderly (Ansteyetal, 2007). Smokers are also reported to have poorer memory and decline in reasoning than non smokers (Sabia et al., 2008). Current smokers have 10 year decline in global cognitive functioning and executive functions (Sabia, et al., 2012).

Dietary Habits

As the individual grows with age, their dietary habits also start changing. There is decline in their energy intake and shifts in dietary and eating habits. The deficits in taste or smell may cause less interest in food (Morley, 2001; Rolls & Drewnowski, 1996). Sometimes, their habits involve eating monotonous food. Inadequate intakes of proteins minerals and vitamins are of prime concern in geriatric population (Blumberg, 1997). There may be risk of diseases like post menopausal osteorporosis in women and fractures in the elderly (Blumberg, 1997). Also, due to imbalanced nutrition, there may be chances of impaired muscle function, decreased bone density, anemia, reduced cognitive function, poor wound healing and increased visit and admissions to the hospital (Chapman, 2006). The factors related to nutrition as stated above may accelerate the ageing process.

Alcohol

The consumption of alcohol is sometimes overlooked in the elderly and mistaken for age related problems. However, alcohol consumption may lead to premature and exaggerated ageing. (Seeman & Robbins, 1994). The excessive use of alcohol may lead to some types of cancers, liver damage, immune system disorders and brain damage. It may worsen the high blood pressure, diabetes, osteoporosis and ulcers. Also, it may increase the risk for heart attacks and forgetfulness that may further lead to Alzheimer's disease (National Institute of Ageing, 2012).

Physical Exercise

The growing population is living a sedentary style for the older generation as well. The definition of sedentary, in a summary literature, has been considered from < 20 minutes exercise per week to < 150 minutes exercise per week (Bennet et al., 2006). The most specified is < 60 minutes per week in about 12 studies out of 43 trials, while rest of the studies had a varied definition of sedentary (Bennet et al., 2006).In a way sedentary lifestyle is causing lot of physical hazards in older adults. Joyner and Pederson (2011) stated that failure of regulation at multiple levels may cause several diseases. Pederson (2009) in an article summarized 35 chronic diseases that may cause accelerates ageing and premature death. These may include metabolic syndrome, low cardiorespiratory fitness, obesity, insulin resistance and type diabetes, deep vein thrombosis, bone fracture, osteorporosis, cognitive dysfunction, depression and anxiety, rheumatoid arthritis, colon cancer, breast cancer, polycystic ovaries, erectile dysfunction, constipation and gall bladder diseases (Boothetal., 2012).It has also been stated that Alzheimer's and dementias have a large component of inactivity(Boothetal.,2012).

Sleep Disorders

The older adults have more prevalence of sleep disorders than the other age groups. Nearly, half of the older adults complaints of sleep disorder. The reasons may be many like the medications, changes in circadian rhythms, restless leg syndrome, sleep behavior disorder and insomnia etc.(Roepke & Anconi-Israel, 2010).In a study it was found that about 62% elderly were having sleep apnea index above 10 indicating sleep breathing disorders(Young et al. 2002). In another study it was found to be more substantial (33%-70%) in older adults dwelling in old age homes than those living in the community (Gehrman, Martin, Shochat Nolan, Corey-Bloom, & Ancoli-Israel, 2003).The restless leg syndrome increases with age and is about twice as prevalent in women than with males (Phillips et al., 2000). Rapid eye movement disorder is characterized by complex motor movements and is most prevalent among older adult males (Oksenberg et al., 2002). Insomnia is one of the most common sleep disorders reported in older adults (Roepke & Anconi-Israel, 2010). About 40-50% of the elderly population has difficult in initiating or maintaining sleep (Ancoli-Israel, 2000).

Incidence of increased circadian rhythm disturbance (Touitou, 2001) causes increased night awakenings in elderly (Vitiello, 1996). The changes related with menopause also affect the sleep and causes disturbances in sleep (Roepke & Anconi-Israel, 2010).

The social factors affecting the old age include the socioeconomic factors, socio-physical environment and life events and social support etc.

Socio-Economic Factors

The persons with lower socio-economic status have fewer facilities for health checkups and hospital visits have poor socio-physical environments that could be age friendly for them and they have not the capacity to have proper nutrition. Few of them have to work constantly, to meet their daily needs. This factor is very important in old age especially when they lose their ability to work efficiently. Each component of socio economic status -education, occupation and income have an independent influence on the individual (Bunker et.al., 1989; Williams, 1990). Individuals with greater education appears to have better sense of control (Mirowsky, 1995) and are more likely to engage in active problem solving (Pearlin

& Schooler, 1978). Similarly, lower occupational status, also reduces the sense of control, reducing the complexity the work, more supervision and highly routine tasks. This reduces problem solving ability, promotes conformity and increases resistance to change (Kohn & Schooler, 1983). Lower income group have more undesirable life events, due to their lesser efficiency to buy good, materials and services (McLeod & Kessler, 1990; Ross & Mirowsky, 1989).

LIFE EVENTS AND SOCIAL SUPPORT

The older adults may be vulnerable to life events and stressors. Vulnerability may be external -risks, shocks, and stress to an individual and internal - a lack of means to cope with the stress. (Chambers, 1989). The older adults may also be vulnerable to losses like becoming or being physically weaker, economically impoverished, socially dependent, and humiliated or psychologically harmed (Chambers, 1989). There may be various negative life events like death of significant others, severe illness of significant others negative socioeconomic circumstances, sudden unexpected events negative events with relationships, daily hassles and abuse (Kraaij et al., 2002).

In geriatric population, loneliness, daily and chronic stress, lack of social support and mourning may be the cause of distress. Also, economical aspects such as retirement and job loss are major risk factors that may cause depression. A number of stressful psychosocial factors, like chronic distress, anxiety, marital status and bereavement may lead to depression. The other individual stressors like illness, loss of job, economic conditions and important life events that created transitions in their routines may lead to some emotional impact. Negative life events were reported to result in poorer mental health conditions in advanced age. It caused cumulative stressful events or traumas and many of these were left untreated too. Furthermore, cognitive functions may be negatively affected by lifelong chronic stressors. The consequences of these events also depend on the duration of the stressor, or the time of life span it has occurred (Gameiro et al., 2014).

In a meta-analysis it was found that the illness to an individual was a major factor causing depression in the old aged. Also, the illness of significant other was also distressing. Experiencing negative events in the relationships was contributing to higher depression scores. Also, it was found that the illness to oneself and to their significant other was causing more depression than the problems with socio economic status. The experiences of many of daily hassles also led to distress. The emotional abuse resulted in higher depression scores (Kraaij et al., 2002).

Social Support

The various factors that lead to deficiency in social network and other resources may lead to loneliness and lack of social support. Besides the external factors of social networking, the inner factors like psychological resources, personality and coping are also responsible for feelings of loneliness in older adults. These feelings of loneliness may bring more age-related complications and further deterioration of their wellbeing, in old aged. The older adults may experience loneliness because, they may be living alone, have poor family ties, may lack participation in the activities of their own culture and may have problems with sharing the local programs (Heikkinen et al., 1995). The death of a spouse and social disengagements due to retirement or other physical causes may lead to lack of perceived social support. The lack of perceived social support makes the older adults prone to depression, leading to early mortality (Max et al., 2005).

Having few social contacts or living alone does not itself indicate loneliness. In fact, some older adults are happier with the people living outside their families and get more perceived support from them (Mullins et.al., 1988). Also, it has been seen that older people prefer to be friendly with the people of their own age cohort. Those who have more intellectual, physical and material resources are found to have more social capital (Posner, 1995).

PSYCHOLOGICAL FACTORS

The psychological factors mainly include the inner resources that the person has to cope with the problems or handle day to day hassles. Personality is one of the major factors besides that include optimism, happiness, attitude towards life, motivation, meaningfulness etc.

Personality

Every individual has a different personality. The well-being of an older adult depends upon the personality they have. Personality is related to how individuals usually behave, have experiences, believe and feel toward themselves, others and the world (Neri, 2005). It has been found that the low levels of dominance and high levels of neuroticism has been found to be exhibiting more depressive symptoms in the elderly (Steunenberg et al., 2006). It has been seen that individuals who have higher extroversion and lower levels of neuroticism have reduced risk of mortality rates (Wilson et al., 2005). Also, it has been found that the individuals who are more optimistic are healthier, have more positive mood and more successful than the pessimistic individuals. The pessimistic individuals were more inclined towards ill health and depression (Hoyer & Roodin, 2003).

Optimism

Optimism is about hoping for the positive outcome in future. It is the expectation of the best results in the coming time. There are several studies that indicate that optimism contributes to the healthy ageing. Vijayshri (2015) studied 300 participants from Delhi, India, between the age group of 60 to 85 years and found that the pessimism was the major predictor of depression in older adults. Also, the optimism was found to be a predictor of healthy ageing. Velden et al. (2007) found that the pessimistic had little hope for future and they developed more symptoms of anxiety and depression. The living status of spouse was a major predictor of pessimism in older adults (Vijayshri, 2015). Marshall et al. (1992) reported that pessimism was more related with neuroticism and negative affect and optimism was more related with extraversion and positive affect.

Subjective Well Being

Chida and Steptoe (2008) in a meta-analysis found that there was an association between positive well-being and mortality in both healthy and diseased population. The positive psychological well-being was related to lower mortality in both healthy and diseased population. The feelings of joy, happiness, greater satisfaction with life and sense of humor predicted longevity in older adults (Chida & Steptoe, 2008). Rugulies (2002) in a meta- analysis, reported that the coronary heart disease was found to be greater in healthy individuals, when they become depressed and they would be more likely to have clinical depression than depressed mood. Williams and Schneiderman (2002) argued that there subjective well-being is the predictor of cardiovascular diseases in healthy populations.

Pressman and Cohen (2005) in a review reported that there is evidence that the positive affect is associated with longevity in normal populations while they found the mixed results for those who are diseased. Blazer and Hybels (2004) found in a study that the positive affect was related with longevity. Brummet et al. (2006) reported from their study that pessimistic individuals have lower rate of longevity. Fitsgerald et al. (2000) and Davidson et al. (2010) found that the increased positive affect was the protector of coronary heart disease and have reduced risk of angina and other heart diseases.

Spirituality

Spirituality is an essential component of the older adults. Spirituality refers to the way individuals seek and express meaning and purpose and the way they experience their connectedness to the moment, to self, to others, to nature, and to the significant or sacred. (Puchalski et al., 2014). It is found in the integration of several deep connections: the connection with one's true and higher self; the connection with society and especially with the poor, the deprived and underprivileged; the connection with the world of nature and other life forms; and for some, a connectedness with the transcendent (National Health Service Scotland, 2009). Spiritual reminiscence was also considered an element of spiritual care and an important component of seeking meaning in later life and in navigating the latter stages of life's journey (MacKinlay & Trevitt, 2010).

The various researches demonstrated the positive impact of spiritual well-being, existential well-being and spiritual outlook, when the individual is thinking negatively (Zinnbauer et al., 1997). It has been seen as a coping style to combat stress. Spirituality deals effectively with the life's problems and sufferings and can be seen as enhancing mental health. (Bergin, 1983; Koenig, 1989; Koenig, 1998). It exerts positive impact on the disabilities and depressive outcomes of older adults (Idler & Kasl, 1997a; Lavretsky, 2010). A few studies suggest that religiosity can moderate the association between physical health conditions and depression through various coping mechanisms and spiritual individual make faster recovery from a number of health disorders (Koenig et al., 1992). It has been noticed that cognition also improves and enhances with spirituality (Corsentino et al., 2009).

Spirituality induces sense of hope, peace, love, joy, meaning and purpose in life, awareness and acceptance of mortality. It increases the sense of well-being and heightens the emotional well-being of older adults (Boehnlein, 2008; Poloma & Pendleton, 1989; Poloma & Pendleton, 1991). Spirituality prolongs the age by facilitating good physical and mental health (Crimmins et al., 1994; Jagger, 2006).

COGNITIVE FACTORS

It has been experienced that the size of the brain shrinks due to the changes in neurotransmitters and hormones. It has been reported that the incidence of stroke, white matter lesions and chances of dementia increases in old age (Peters, 2006). There is a decline in memory in old age. Episodic memory declines with old age. It affects recall rather than recognition (Parkin, 1997). Semantic memory increased from middle age to young elderly but it starts declining in the late elderly (Nyberg & Backman, 2004). Elderly are reported to have slower reaction times, lower attentional levels, slower processing speeds, detriments in sensory and or perceptual functions, or potentially a lesser ability to use strategies (Cabeza, 2004; Lustig & Buckner, 2004; Cabeza et al., 2004).

DISEASES

Over 60% of the individuals over 65 have multiple diseases (Vogeli et al., 2007). The older adults with one disease are more likely to develop other diseases than those who are not having any diseases (Meliset al., 2014). Fabri et al. (2015) suggested that the ageing brings dysregulation in the system and when certain threshold is reached it causes the diseases (Fabbri et al., 2015).

Musculoskeletal Diseases

Musculoskeletal conditions cause functional limitations and are the major causes of disability and back pain are the three leading musculoskeletal diseases in the older adults (Woolf & Pfleger, 2003).

Cardiovascular Diseases

Cardiovascular diseases like coronary artery disease, stroke, heart failure are 10 fold higher in old age than at the age of 45 years (Mozaffarian et al., 2015). Ageing leads to arterial stiffening and impaired vasodilatory responses, that has the onset from about 40-50 years of age and may lead to hypertension (Harvey et.al., 2015; Sun, 2015). Hypertension is a major risk for atherosclerosis and cardiac failure. The ageing associated major contributor to cardiovascular morbidity and mortality is arthrosclerosis. It is responsible for myocardial infarction, angina, ischaemic stroke and peripheral vascular disease (Mozaffarian et al., 2015).

Diabetes Mellitus

Diabetes Mellitus Type 2 is a chronic metabolic disorder with a prevalence of 8.5% in 2014 (WHO diabetes fact sheet, 2016). The diabetes brings changes in blood glucose levels termed as hyperglycemia (Mahler & Adler, 1999; Scheen, 2003). Hyperglycemia can cause widespread damage to blood vessels causing neuropathy, retinopathy and significant increase in chances of stroke, coronary heart disease, peripheral and arterial disease (Adler et al., 2003; Cade, 2008). Insulin resistance can increase the risk of non-alcoholic fatty liver disease (Wild et al., 2016). This may be the cause of various cancers, including colon, liver, pancreatic and breast cancers (Tsugane & Inoue, 2010; O' Neil & O' Driscoll, 2015). In addition, patients suffering from type 2 diabetes mellitus have significant incidence of mild cognitive impairment (Barbagallo & Dominguex, 2014). Also, they have significantly higher risk of developing Alzheimer's disease.

Neurodegenerative Diseases

Neurodegenerative disorders, such as Alzheimer's disease and Parkinson's disease increases with age (Szewczyl-Krolikowskietet.al., 2016). As the neurons age, the oxidative stress increases and their disturbance in mitochondrial function and accumulation of misfolded proteins, that are exacerbated in Alzheimer's disease and Parkinson's disease. Alzheimer's disease is a etiologically multifactorial disease (Talwar et al., 2015). Histologically, Alzheimer's disease is characterized by extensive neurodegeneration, extra cellular disposition of amyloid-peptide forming senile plaques and intraneuronal accumulations of hyperphosphorelated microtubule associated protein tau, and the neurofibrillary tangles Dickson et al., 1988).Parkinson's disease is a chronic disorder that is incurable. Its incidence increases with age and affects 1-3% of population world-wide (Szewczyk-Krolikowski et al., 2014; Johnson & Bobrovskaya, 2015). It is characterized by the loss of dopaminergic neurons of substantianigra and locus coerleusin parallel with astrocytosis and microgliosis (Syme et al., 2002).

AGEING AND HEALTH CARE

In accordance with a recent World Health Resolution (67/13), a comprehensive Global Strategy and Action Plan on Ageing and Health is being developed by WHO in consultation with Member States and other partners. The Strategy and Action Plan draws on the evidence of the World report on ageing and health (2017) and builds on existing activities to address 5 priority areas for action.

Commitment to Healthy Ageing

It requires making the individuals aware of the value of the concept of Healthy Ageing. It involves the sustained commitment and action to formulate evidence-based policies that strengthen the abilities of older persons (WHO, 2017).

Aligning Health Systems With the Needs of Older Populations

Health systems need to be better organized around older people's needs and preferences. It needs to be designed to enhance older people's intrinsic capacity, and integrated across settings and care providers. The actions in this area must be closely aligned with other work to strengthen the universal health care and people-centered and integrated health services (WHO, 2017).

Developing Systems for Providing Long-Term Care

The systems of long-term care are needed in all countries to meet the needs of older people. This requires developing, sometimes from nothing, governance systems, infrastructure and workforce capacity. WHO's work on long-term care (including palliative care) aligns closely with efforts to enhance universal health coverage, address non-communicable diseases, and develop people-centered and integrated health services (WHO, 2017).

Creating Age-Friendly Environments

This will require actions to combat ageism, enable autonomy and support healthy ageing in all policies and at all levels of government. These activities build on and complement WHO's work during the past decade to develop age-friendly cities and communities including the development of the Global Network of Age Friendly Cities and Communities and an interactive information sharing platform Age-friendly World (WHO, 2017).

Improving Measurement, Monitoring and Understanding

Focused research, new metrics and analytical methods are needed for a wide range of ageing issues (WHO, 2017). Several of the above studies have suggested about the factors that contributes to ageing. It is evident that the ageing is affected by genetics, nutrition, sleep, work activity, stress and social support. The healthy ageing is the product of resilience to stress, personality factors, like optimism, positivity and spirituality and cognitive factors, as well as absence of diseases. Ageing is the natural process and it is evident in all living beings.

CONCLUSION

Although, we cannot avoid ageing, but we can delay it by taking into account certain life style changes, developing social skills, personality changes and cognitive enhancement. Also, we can be ageing in a healthy manner if we keep on track of our healthy life style, good nutritive diet, good amount of exercise, being independent and autonomous, having a good social support and being positive, flexible and adaptive in life. In a nut shell, we can age by body, but our mind can remain young if we are proactive towards it.

REFERENCES

Adler, A. I., Stevens, R. J., Manley, S. E., Bilous, R. W., Cull, C. A., Holman, R. R., & Ukpds, G. (2003). Development and progression of nephropathy in type 2 diabetes: theUnited Kingdom prospective diabetes study (UKPDS 64). *Kidney International*, *63*(1), 225–232. doi:10.1046/j.1523-1755.2003.00712.x PMID:12472787

Ancoli-Israel, S. (2000). Insomnia in the elderly: A review for the primary care practitioner. *Sleep*, *23*, S23–S30. PMID:10755805

Barbagallo, M., & Dominguez, L. J. (2014). Type 2 diabetes mellitus and Alzheimer'sdisease. *World Journal of Diabetes*, *5*(6), 889–893. doi:10.4239/wjd.v5.i6.889 PMID:25512792

Bennet, J. A., Winters-Stone, K., Nail, L. M., & Scherer, J. (2006). Definitions of Sedentary in physical-activity-intervention trials: A summary of the literature. *Journal of Aging and Physical Activity*, *14*(4), 456–477. doi:10.1123/japa.14.4.456 PMID:17215562

Bergin, A.E. (1983). *Religiosity and mental health: A critical reevaluation and meta-analysis*. Academic Press.

Blumberg, J. (1997). Nutritional needs of seniors. *Journal of the American College of Nutrition, 16*, 517–523. PMID:9430078

Boehnlein, J. K. (2008). *Psychiatry and religion: The convergence of mind and spirit.* Washington, DC: American Psychiatric Publishing.

Booth, F. W., Roberts, C. K., & Laye, J. (2012). Lack of exercise is a major cause of chronic diseases. *Comprehensive Physiology*, *2*(2), 1143–1211. doi:10.1002/cphy.c110025 PMID:23798298

Bratic, I., & Trifunovic, A. (2010). Mitochondrial energy metabolism and ageing. *BiochimicaetBiophysica Acta (BBA) – Bioenergetics*, *1797*(6-7), 961–967. doi:10.1016/j.bbabio.2010.01.004

Brummett, B. H., Helms, M. J., Dahlstrom, W. G., & Siegler, I. C. (2006). Prediction of all-cause mortality by the Minnesota Multiphasic Personality Inventory Optimism-Pessimism Scale scores: Study of a college sample during a 40-year follow-up period. *Mayo Clinic Proceedings*, *81*(12), 1541–1544. doi:10.4065/81.12.1541 PMID:17165632

Bunker, P., Gomby, D. S., & Kehrer, B. H. (1989). *Pathways to health: the role of social factors.* Menlo Park, CA: Kaiser Family Foundation.

Cabeza, R. (2004). Commentary: neuroscience frontiers of cognitive ageing: approaches to cognitive neuroscience of ageing. In R. Dixon, L. Bäckman, & L. Nilsson (Eds.), *New frontiers in cognitive ageing* (pp. 179–198). Oxford, UK: Oxford University Press. doi:10.1093/acprof:oso/9780198525691.003.0009

Cabeza, R., Daselaar, S., Dolcos, F., Prince, S. E., Budde, M., & Nyberg, L. (2004). Task-independent and task-specific age effects on brain activity during working memory, visual attention and episodic retrieval. *Cerebral Cortex*, 14364–14375. PMID:15028641

Cade, W. T. (2008). Diabetes-related microvascular and macrovascular diseases inthe physical therapy setting. *Physical Therapy*, *88*(11), 1322–1335. doi:10.2522/ptj.20080008 PMID:18801863

Chambers, R. (1989). Vulnerability, Coping and Policy. *Institute of Development Studies-Bulletin*, *20*(2), 1–7. doi:10.1111/j.1759-5436.1989.mp20002001.x

Chapman, I. M. (2006). Nutritional disorders in the elderly. *The Medical Clinics of North America*, *90*(5), 887–907. doi:10.1016/j.mcna.2006.05.010 PMID:16962848

Chida, Y., & Steptoe, A. (2008). Positive psychological well-being and mortality: A quantitative review of prospective observational studies. *Psychosomatic Medicine*, *70*(7), 741–756. doi:10.1097/PSY.0b013e31818105ba PMID:18725425

Corsentino, E. A., Collins, N., Sachs-Ericsson, N., & Blazer, D. G. (2009). Religious attendance reduces cognitive decline among older women with high levels of depressive symptoms. *The Journals of Gerontology. Series A, Biological Sciences and Medical Sciences*, *64*(12), 1283–1289. doi:10.1093/gerona/glp116 PMID:19675176

Crimmins, E. M., Hayward, M. D., & Saito, Y. (1994). Changing mortality and morbidity rates and health status and life expectancy of the older population. *Demography*, *31*(1), 159–175. doi:10.2307/2061913 PMID:8005340

Davidson, K. W., Mostofsky, E., & Whang, W. (2010). Don't worry, be happy: Positive affect and reduced 10-year incident coronary heart disease: *The Canadian Nova Scotia Health Survey. European Heart Journal, 31*(9), 1065–1070. doi:10.1093/eurheartj/ehp603 PMID:20164244

Dickson, D. W., Farlo, J., Davies, P., Crystal, H., Fuld, P., & Yen, S. H. (1988). Alzheimer'sdisease. A double-labeling immunohistochemical study of senile plaques. *American Journal of Pathology, 132*, 86–101. PMID:2456021

Fabbri, E., An, Y., Zoli, M., Simonsick, E. M., Guralnik, J. M., Bandinelli, S., ... Ferrucci, L. (2015). Aging and the burden of multimorbidity: Associations within flammatory and anabolic hormonal biomarkers. *The Journals of Gerontology. Series A, Biological Sciences and Medical Sciences, 70*(1), 63–70. doi:10.1093/gerona/glu127 PMID:25104822

Gameiro, G.R., & Minguini, P. I., & FerrazAlves, T.C. (2014). The role of stress and life events in the onset of depression in the elderly. *Review of Medicine, 93*(1), 31–40.

Gehrman, P. R., Martin, J. L., Shochat, T., Nolan, S., Corey-Bloom, J., & Ancoli-Israel, S. (2003). Sleep disordered breathing and agitation in institutionalized adults with Alzheimer's disease. *The American Journal of Geriatric Psychiatry, 11*(4), 426–433. doi:10.1097/00019442-200307000-00005 PMID:12837671

Harvey, A., Montezano, A. C., & Touyz, R. M. (2015). Vascular biology ofageing-implications in hypertension. *Journal of Molecular and Cellular Cardiology, 83*, 112–121. doi:10.1016/j.yjmcc.2015.04.011 PMID:25896391

Heikkinen, R., Berg, S., & Avland, K. (1995). Depressive symptoms in late life. *Journal of Cross-Cultural Gerontology, 10*(4), 315–330. doi:10.1007/BF00972332 PMID:24389881

Hoyer, W. J., & Roodin, P. A. (2003). *Adult development and aging* (5th ed.). New York: McGraw-Hill.

Idler, E. L., & Kasl, S. V. (1997). Religion among disabled and nondisabled persons I: Cross-sectional patterns in health practices, social activities, and well-being. *The Journals of Gerontology. Series B, Psychological Sciences and Social Sciences, 52*(6), S294–S305. doi:10.1093/geronb/52B.6.S294 PMID:9403523

Jagger, C. (2006). Can we live longer, healthier lives? In Y. Zeng (Ed.), Longer life and healthy aging. Springer.

Joyner, M., & Pedersen, B. (2011). Ten Questions about Systems Biology. *The Journal of Physiology, 589*(5), 1017–1030. doi:10.1113/jphysiol.2010.201509 PMID:21224238

Koenig, H. G. (1989). Research on religion and mental health in later life: A review and commentary. *Journal of Geriatric Psychiatry, 23*, 23–53. PMID:2212522

Koenig, H. G. (1998). *Handbook of religion and mentaldisorders*. San Diego, CA: Elsevier.

Koenig, H. J., Cohen, D. G., Blazer, C., Pieper, K. G., & Meador, F. S. (1992). Religious coping and depression among elderly, hospitalized medically ill men. *The American Journal of Psychiatry, 149*(12), 1693–1700. doi:10.1176/ajp.149.12.1693 PMID:1443246

Kohn, M. L., & Schooler, C. (1983). *Work and personality: An inquiry into the impact of social stratification*. Norwood, NJ: Ablex.

Kraaij, V., Arensman,E., & Spinhoven, P. (2002). Negative Life Events and Depression in Elderly Persons: A Meta-Analysis. *Journal of Gerontology*, *57B*(1), 87–94.

Lavretsky, H. (2010). Spirituality and aging. *Aging Health*, *6*(6), 749–769. doi:10.2217/ahe.10.70

Lustig, C., & Buckner, R. (2004). Preserved neural correlates of priming in old age and dementia. *Neuron*, 42865–42875. PMID:15182724

Mahler, R. J., & Adler, M. L. (1999). Type 2 diabetes mellitus: Update on diagnosispathophysiology, and treatment. *The Journal of Clinical Endocrinology and Metabolism*, *84*(4), 1165–1171. doi:10.1210/jcem.84.4.5612 PMID:10199747

Marshall, G. N., Wortman, C. B., Kusulas, J. W., Hervig, L. K., & Vickers, R. R. Jr. (1992). Distinguishing optimism from pessimism: Relations to fundamental dimensions of mood and personality. *Journal of Personality and Social Psychology*, *62*(6), 1067–1074. doi:10.1037/0022-3514.62.6.1067

Max, L. S., David, J. V., Jacobijn, G., & Aartjan, T. F. (2015). Is depression in old age fatal only when people feel lonely? *The American Journal of Psychiatry*, *162*, 178–180.

McLeod, J. D., & Kessler, R. C. (1990). Socioeconomic status differences in vulnerability to undesirable life events. *Journal of Health and Social Behavior*, *37*(2), 162–172. doi:10.2307/2137170 PMID:2102495

Melis, R., Marengoni, A., Angleman, S., & Fratiglioni, L. (2014). Incidence andpredictors of multimorbidity in the elderly: A population-based longitudinal study. *Public Library of Science. One*, *9*, e103120. doi:10.1371/journal.pone.0103120 PMID:25058497

Mirowsky, J. (1995). Age and the sense of control. *Social Psychology Quarterly*, *58*(1), 31–43. doi:10.2307/2787141

Monaco, T.V., & Silveira, P.S. (2009). *Aging is not Senescence: A Short Computer Demonstration and Implications for Medical Practice Clinics*. Academic Press.

Morley, J. (2001). Decreased food intake in the elderly. Journal Gerontolology. *Biological Sciences Medical Sciences*, *56A*(Special Issue II), 81-88.

Mozaffarian, D., Benjamin, E. J., Go, A. S., Arnett, D. K., Blaha, M. J., Cushman, M., ... Howard, V. J. (2015). Article. *Heart Disease and Stroke*, *131*, e29–e322.

Mullins, L. C, Johnson, D. P., & Anderson, L. (1988). *Danish Medical Bulletin*. Special Supplement Series, 26–29.

National Institute on Aging. (2012). *Turning Discovery Into Health*. U.S. Department of Health and Human Services.

Neri, A. L. (2005). Palavras-chaveemgerontologia (2nd ed.). Campinas: Alínea.

Nyberg, L., & Backman, L. (2004). Cognitive ageing: A view from brain imaging. In R. Dixon, L. Bäckman, & L. Nilsson (Eds.), *New frontiers in cognitive ageing* (pp. 135–160). Oxford, UK: Oxford University Press. doi:10.1093/acprof:oso/9780198525691.003.0007

O'Neill, S., & O'Driscoll, L. (2015). Metabolic syndrome: A closer look at the growing epidemic and its associated pathologies. *Obesity Reviews*, *16*(1), 1–12. doi:10.1111/obr.12229 PMID:25407540

Oksenberg, A., Radwan, H., Arons, E., Hoffenbach, D., & Behroozi, B. (2002). Rapid Eye Movement (REM) sleep behavior disorder: A sleep disturbance affecting mainly older men. *The Israel Journal of Psychiatry and Related Sciences*, *39*, 28–35. PMID:12013707

Parkin, A. (1997). *Memory and amnesia*. Oxford, UK: Blackwall.

Pearlin, L., & Schooler, C. (1978). The structure of coping. *Journal of Health and Social Behavior*, *19*(1), 2–21. doi:10.2307/2136319 PMID:649936

Pedersen, B. K. (2009). The diseasome of physical inactivity and the role of myokines in muscle-- fat cross talk. *The Journal of Physiology*, *587*(23), 5559–5568. doi:10.1113/jphysiol.2009.179515 PMID:19752112

Peters, R. (2006). Ageing and the brain. *Postgraduate Medical Journal*, *82*(964), 84–88. doi:10.1136/pgmj.2005.036665 PMID:16461469

Phillips, B. A., Young, T., Finn, L., Asher, K., Hening, W. A., & Purvis, C. (2000). Epidemiology of restless legs symptoms in adults. *Archives of Internal Medicine*, *160*(14), 2137–2141. doi:10.1001/archinte.160.14.2137 PMID:10904456

Poloma, M. M., & Pendleton, B. F. (1989). Exploring types of prayer and quality of life: A research note. *Review of Religious Research*, *31*(1), 46–53. doi:10.2307/3511023

Poloma, M. M., & Pendleton, B. F. (1991). The effects of prayer and prayer experiences on measures of general well-being. *Journal of Psychology and Theology*, *19*, 71–83.

Posner, R. (1995). *Aging and Old Age*. University of Chicago Press.

Pressman, S. D., & Cohen, S. (2005). Does positive affect influence health? *Psychological Bulletin*, *131*(6), 925–971. doi:10.1037/0033-2909.131.6.925 PMID:16351329

Roepke, S. K., & Ancoli-Israel, S. (2010). Sleep disorders in the elderly. *The Indian Journal of Medical Research*, *131*, 302–331. PMID:20308755

Rogers, K., Sacher, G. A., Shock, N. W., Simic, P., & Guarente, L. P. (2016). *Ageing*. Encyclopaedia Britannica.

Rolls, B. A., & Drewnowski, A. (1996) Diet and nutrition. In Encyclopedia of Gerontology (vol. 1, pp. 429-440). Academic Press.

Ross, C. E., & Mirowsky, J. (1989). Explaining the social patterns of depression: Control and problem solving or support and talking? *Journal of Health and Social Behavior*, *30*(2), 206–219. doi:10.2307/2137014 PMID:2738367

Rugulies, R. (2002). Depression as a predictor for coronary heart disease. *American Journal of Preventive Medicine*, *23*(1), 51–61. doi:10.1016/S0749-3797(02)00439-7 PMID:12093424

Scheen, A. J. (2003). Pathophysiology of type 2 diabetes. *Acta Clinica Belgica*, *58*(6), 335–341. doi:10.1179/acb.2003.58.6.001 PMID:15068125

Seeman, T. E., & Robbins, R. J. (1994). Aging and hypothalamic-pituitary-adrenal response to challenge in humans. *Endocrine Reviews*, *15*, 233–260. PMID:8026389

Spaargaren, G., & VanVliet, B. (2000). Lifestyle, Consumption and the Environment: The Ecological Modernisation of Domestic Consumption. *Environmental Politics*, *9*(1), 50–75.

Steunenberg, B., Beekman, A. T., Deeg, D. J., & Kerkhof, A. J. (2006). Personality and the onset of depression in late life. *Journal of Affective Disorders*, *92*(2-3), 243–251. doi:10.1016/j.jad.2006.02.003 PMID:16545466

Sun, Z. (2015). Aging, arterial stiffness, and hypertension. *Hypertension*, *65*(2), 252–256. doi:10.1161/HYPERTENSIONAHA.114.03617 PMID:25368028

Szewczyk-Krolikowski, K., Tomlinson, P., Nithi, K., Wade-Martins, R., Talbot, K., Ben-Shlomo, Y., & Hu, M. T. M. (2014). The influence of age and gender on motorand non-motor features of early Parkinson's disease: Initial findings from the Oxford Parkinson Disease Center (OPDC) discovery cohort. *Parkinsonism & Related Disorders*, *20*(1), 99–105. doi:10.1016/j.parkreldis.2013.09.025 PMID:24183678

Talwar, P., Sinha, J., Grover, S., Rawat, C., Kushwaha, S., Agarwal, R., & Taneja, V. (2015). *Dissecting complex and multifactorial nature of Alzheimer's disease pathogenesis: A clinical, genomic, and systems biology perspective*. Academic Press.

Touitou, Y. (2001). Human aging and melatonin. Clinicalrelevance. *Experimental Gerontology*, *36*(7), 1083–1100. doi:10.1016/S0531-5565(01)00120-6 PMID:11404053

Tsugane, S., & Inoue, M. (2010). Insulin resistance and cancer: Epidemiological evidence. *Cancer Science*, *101*(5), 1073–1079. doi:10.1111/j.1349-7006.2010.01521.x PMID:20345478

Velden, P. G., Kleber, R. J., Fournier, M., Grievink, L., Drogendijk, A., & Gersons, B. P. (2007). The association between dispositional optimism and mental health problems among disaster victims and a comparison group: A prospective study. *Journal of Affective Disorders*, *102*(3), 35–45. doi:10.1016/j.jad.2006.12.004 PMID:17239959

Vijayshri. (2015). Optimistic and Pessimistic Attitude Influencing Depressive Symptoms in Older Age. *International Research Journal of Social Sciences*, *4*(5), 52-58.

Vitiello, M. V. (1996). Sleep disorders and aging. *Current Opinion in Psychiatry*, *9*(4), 284–289. doi:10.1097/00001504-199607000-00011

Vogeli, C., Shields, A. E., Lee, T. A., Gibson, T. B., Marder, W. D., Weiss, K. B., & Blumenthal, D. (2007). Multiple chronic conditions: Prevalence, health consequences, and implications for quality care management, and costs. *Journal of General Internal Medicine*, *22*(S3), 391–395. doi:10.1007/s11606-007-0322-1 PMID:18026807

Wild, S. H., Morling, J. R., McAllister, D. A., Kerssens, J., Fischbacher, C., Parkes, J., ... Byrne, C. D. (2016). Type 2 diabetes and risk of hospital admission or death for chronic liver diseases. *Journal of Hepatology*, *64*(6), 1358–1364. doi:10.1016/j.jhep.2016.01.014 PMID:26812073

Williams, R. B., & Schneiderman, N. (2002). Resolved: Psychosocial interventions can improve clinical outcomes in organic disease (pro). *Psychosomatic Medicine*, *64*, 552–557. PMID:12140342

Wilson, R. S., Krueger, K. R., Gu, L., Bienias, J. L., Mendes de Leon, C. F., & Evans, D. A. (2005). Neuroticism, extraversion, and mortality in a defined population of older persons. *Psychosomatic Medicine*, *67*(6), 841–845. doi:10.1097/01.psy.0000190615.20656.83 PMID:16314587

Woolf, A.D., & Pfleger, B., (2003). Burden of major musculoskeletal conditions. *Bulletin of the World Health Organization*, *81*, 646–656.

World Health Organization. (2002). *Active ageing: A policy framework*. Report No: WHO/NMH/NPH/02.8. Geneva: World Health Organisation. Retrieved from http://whqlibdoc.who.int/hq/2002/WHO_NMH_NPH_02.8.pdf

World Health Organization. (2017). *Ageing and Health*. WHO.

Young, T., Shahar, E., Nieto, F. J., Redline, S., Newman, A. B., & Gottlieb, D. J. (2002). Predictors of sleep-disordered breathing in community-dwelling adults: The Sleep Heart Health Study. *Archives of Internal Medicine*, *162*, 893–900. doi:10.1001/archinte.162.8.893 PMID:11966340

Zinnbauer, B. J., Pargament, K. I., Cole, B., Rye, M. S., Butter, E. M., Belavich, T. G., ... Kadar, J. L. (1997). Religion and spirituality: Unfuzzying the fuzzy. *Journal for the Scientific Study of Religion*, *36*(4), 549–564. doi:10.2307/1387689

KEY TERMS AND DEFINITIONS

Ageing: Ageing is the process of transition due to getting older, leading to decline in physical and mental capacities so that the individual is not able to function that competently.

Biological Factors: The biological factors are those factors that are occurring biologically in the individual and difficult to alter like genetic, metabolism, and wear and tear in the body.

Lifestyle Factors: Lifestyle factors are those factors that are affected by the lifestyle of a person like addiction of substances, eating behaviors, and so on.

Psychological Factors and Diseases: Psychological factors are those factors where you try to have your own psychological view of life that may constitute individual's personality including the factors like optimism, subjective wellbeing, spirituality, etc.

Sleep Disturbances: Sleep disturbances are the irregularities in sleep pattern due to certain factors that are causing disturbances in sleep.

Social Factors: Social factors are those causes where the individual is affected by social support, social networking, etc.

Chapter 23
Aging and Suicide

Hitesh Khurana
Pandit Bhagwat Dayal Sharma Post Graduate Institute of Medical Sciences, India

Aishwarya Raj
GNCT of Delhi, India

ABSTRACT

Suicide is a global phenomenon and a potential cause of preventable death. After the young (below the age of 40 years), the elderly compose the second most prominent peak in the graph of suicide attempts and suicide victims. The cause and dynamics of suicidal behavior among elderly are quite different from the younger suicides. There have been different multidisciplinary theories proposed for it. Among all mental disorders, depressive disorders are particularly associated with suicidal behavior. Alcohol use, social isolation, financial difficulties are few unique factors that identify a suicidal elder. Physical illnesses, particularly those marked with pain, increase the chances of suicide. Prevention requires a multidisciplinary approach involving community, adequate and appropriate health services near to the place of victim, legal restrictions on the methods used for suicide such as availability of firearm and insecticides, public policies to take care of the elderly are recommended.

INTRODUCTION

It may be that Gods are merciful when they make our lives more unpleasant as we grow old. In the end, death seems less intolerable than the many burdens we have to bear. - Sigmund Freud about his death due to cancer palate (Cunningham, Connell, Chin, & Lawlor, 2004)

Suicide is one of the most discussed causes of death at any stage of life. Suicidal behavior is a common cause of unnatural death and disability across the world. It accounts for 1.4% of all deaths making it 15th leading cause of mortality among all age groups. The annual global age-standardized death rate for 2012 is estimated to be 11.4 per 100,000, this is projected to remain unchanged through 2030.Besides death due to suicide, suicidal thoughts and nonfatal suicide attempts also warrant attention. of epidemiologist as this behavior strongly predict the suicide in future. Suicidal ideations are found prevalent in about 9.2% of general population surveys and attempted suicide in about 2.7% of population (Nock et al.,

DOI: 10.4018/978-1-5225-3480-8.ch023

2008). Suicide ideation and attempts can result in negative consequences such as injury, hospitalization, and loss of liberty; and exert a financial burden of billions of dollars on society. Taken together, suicide and suicidal behavior comprise the nineteenth leading cause of global disease burden (i.e., years lost to disability, ill-health, and early death), and the sixth and ninth leading cause of global disease burden among men and women 15 to 44 years of age, respectively (World Health Organization, 2014a). Those aged above 60 years make a group vulnerable to suicide. Various studies have found that elderly suicides are preceded by lesser number of attempted suicides in past and elderly used more lethal means than younger population for such purpose. Compromised physical health at late age further adds to the lethal effect of the methods of suicides for which the younger population might be resilient. By any measure, there is urgency to better understand and prevent suicidal behavior in elderly, which is the purpose of this chapter.

It is unnatural and suicide is one of the few preventable causes of death which is rising at alarming rate throughout the world. In relation to elderly, suicidal feelings and hopelessness have been considered part of ageing and understandable in the context of being elderly and having physical disabilities. The Ancient Greeks accepted these attitudes in the extreme and gave elderly people the option of assisted suicide. Such practices were based on the assumption that once an individual had reached a certain age then they no longer had any meaningful purpose in life and would be better off dead. (Cunningham et al., 2004) Although not as extreme, ageist beliefs in modern, especially industrialized, societies are based on similar assumptions. In current time too life is often valued in economic terms and, specifically, loss of productivity. And elderly age is such that is characterized by increased expenditure, increased disability, decrease productivity and hence economically not worth sustain. Thus elderly stage is often considered burden and stigmatized. Thus suicide in general and due to such myths is often incompletely not well understood in case of elder lies. Insurance companies and various other social agencies often debar the family of suicide victim from the usual benefits a deceased family gets from them. Despite all odds, the WHO estimates about 800,000 deaths every year due to suicide. The number of attempted suicide for each completed suicide is even much more. (World Health Organization, 2014b) however in comparison with younger population the ratio of completed vs attempted suicides is much smaller. (Dombrovskil1, Szanto, & Reynolds III, 2005; Gramaglia et al., 2016) Compared to younger ones, the older suicidal persons are more likely to complete suicide (Yeates Conwell, Duberstein, & Caine, 2002). Despite such trends what is rarely debated and commonly ignored is the suicide among the elderly population (Cattell, 2010). This may be partially due to the myth that death is imminent as the age advances and what makes the problem critically serious the inability of the caregivers to recognize the prodromal symptoms of suicide among elderly coupled with inability to deal with such situations (Stanley, Hom, Rogers, Hagan, & Joiner, 2016). The notion that suicide among elderly are mostly rational lack scientific support is a myth (Cattell, 2010). Such confusion can arise from the fact that the old age marked with challenges for intergenerational as well as intra-generational socialization. Despite frail health and multiple disabilities the elderly often express a zeal of living, activities, and regular contact with family members. However, the data from various studies seem to contradict this stand. Most of the elderly who attempt or commit suicide consult physician in the past one month. Physical morbidities like cardiovascular diseases, cancer and psychiatric morbidities particularly depression are commonly seen in those patients (Wearn, 2003) Henslin (1996) recorded that elderly suicides showed an upward trend between 1995 to 2010 with rates increasing from 7% to 15% of all completed suicides in US. This report extrapolated that nearly 10% of all suicides in US between 2020 – 50 are likely to be due to elderly(Henslin, 1996)The predicted global pattern is also similar across different countries, cultures and races(Crepet et al., 1991; Kumar, Anish,

& George, 2015; O'Connor & Nock, 2014) Data from other countries also show similar trends, in fact elderly make the largest proportion of suicides in many cultures and countries(Cattell, 2010; Wasserman & Ringskog, 2001) .The suicide rate in India is comparable to that of Australia and the USA; and the increasing rates during recent decades is consistent with the global trends(Radhakrishnan & Andrade, 2012) Keeping in view the rapidly graying population the absolute number of elderly dying due to suicide can be enormous. Addition to that the factors and dynamics for suicidal behavior among elderly cannot be simply extrapolated from those seen in the younger population. Thus elderly suicide is taking an epidemic form which can't be prevented on the basis of models existing for the younger population. Hence there is an urgent need of understanding and managing suicidal behavior among elderly (Gonzalez et al., 2014; Van Orden et al., 2010). Hence there is an urgent need to understand and evolve preventive strategies for suicidal behavior among elderly.

Terms and Definitions

The term suicide is derived from Latin word *suicaedere* meaning to take one's own life intentionally. Suicide is defined as conscious act of self-induced annihilation, best understood as multidimensional malaise in a needful individual who defines an issue for which suicide is perceived as the best solution. Suicide is the most severe kind of self-destructive behavior (Schneidman, 1985). This definition is most accepted definition in literature on suicide, However, for epidemiological studies World Health Organization(WHO) defined suicide in much simplistic way as an suicidal act with fatal outcome, whereas suicidal act is defined as an self-inflicted injury with varying degree of lethal intent (World Health Organisation, 1968).

Suicide is also conceptualized as the ultimate and extreme outcome of suicidal behavior evolving through many behaviors with low intent and lethality. What is common is all suicidal behaviors are presence of lethal intent which may vary in degree and self-initiated self-injurious behavior. Various such behaviors are summarized below:

- **Death Wish:** This constitute a passive content in one's thought process describing one's longing for death without and action or thought about initiating such act. Death wish as such doesn't constitute suicidal behavior but it may mark evolution of suicidal behavior.
- **Suicidal Ideas:** It constitutes one intention of taking own life deliberately It may exist in isolation without any active attempt to achieve the intended outcome.
- **Suicidal Gestures:** These behaviors are purposeful behaviors which may be confused with non-fatal suicidal attempt. However, death is not the desired goal in such gestures as evident from the circumstantial data.
- **Non-Fatal Suicidal Attempt:** It refers to behaviors which are self-inflicted and did not succeed in ending the victim's life (Schlebusch, 2005). Non-fatal suicidal behaviors are marked by different severity but a definite intention to die. The attempt may turn out to be non-fatal due to medical help available or lesser lethality of the chosen method. Para suicide and 'celebrateself harm' are the terms often used interchangeably with non-fatal suicidal attempt.
- **Consummated Suicide:** The term is often used when the consequences of the attempt reach the point of no return because of one or multiple reasons including non-availability of medical assistance to damage becoming rapidly irreversible (Venkoba Rao, 1992).

EPIDEMIOLOGY

There are some variations reported in the trends about suicide among elderly. The difference is likely to be due to the different definitions of the terms related with suicidal behavior (Table-I) differing health policies and laws of the land governing suicidal behavior. Suicide as defined by the WHO is ''the act of killing oneself deliberately initiated and performed by the person concerned in the full knowledge or expectation of its fatal outcome''. As per this definition clearly the act person has to have an unequivocal knowledge and intention about the outcome and must carry out independently It is different from euthanasia or assisted suicide where the person conveys his intentions and seeks help to achieve intended goal (Bilsen, 2000; Stanley et al., 2016; World Health Organization WHO, 1999) .Completed to attempted suicide ratio among elderly aged 75 and above is almost three times that of young adults (Conwell, 2013) They also concluded poor physical health and isolation to be the prominent factors leading to such age differences in completed suicides. Further the older people prefer not to inform other about their plans (Cox, 1998; Vanlaere, Bouckaert, & Gastmans, 2007).

The rates reported by different studies may be due cultural variations, population or sample chosen, sample selection methods and types of studies. But the suicide rate as reviewed by ICD-6 to ICD-10 category codes has remained fairly stable. The WHO requires suicide reporting by every country in absolute numbers and midyear population. The rates are recorded in WHO registers by year, age and sex wise. Updated rates for all categories are available on official website of WHO. Except suicide rates almost no country reports the rates of attempted suicide to the WHO, rates of attempted suicide which are either not collected or not adequately reported can be best estimated from the local studies (Bertolote& Fleischmann, 2002). In India too, elderly suicides make a major proportion of all deaths due to suicide. The suicide rate among aged 60 years and above is 7 per lac population against 18 per lac for younger population. This discrepancy can be accounted for due to the lack of age specific suicide data. Hence there might be over representation of younger population in Indian scenario (Radhakrishnan& Andrade, 2012) The Indian elderly suicidal victim differ from their western counterparts in some aspects. Unlike western victims most of the elderly victims in India are married, lesser educated and come from joint families. Marriage doesn't seem to offer any protective advantage especially to females. It is probably due to the fact that after marriage females in India have to deal with more stress of life in family as compared to men (Kumar et al., 2015). Women are certainly more likely to be referred to psychiatric services. But these are the men who are likely to get admitted to the hospital following an attempt. Elderly still do not make as large proportion of suicide victims and attempts as in the west. Only the rates reported for elderly suicides from the south India match the rates as in the west. The authors feel these difference from the western pattern are due to disparities in the health care availability and accessibility (Mythri & Ebenezer, 2016).

Attempted Suicide

It is commonly observed all over the world that the ratio of attempted suicide to completed suicide is lesser among older persons in comparison with any other age group. Australian data suggest this ratio to be 3.6 for people aged 60 and above as compared to 11.6 for general population (Padoani W, 2001). Similarly in a European multicentre study the rates were 1.2:1 and 3.3:1 per lac population for males and females respectively. In contrast the same ratio for younger age may be as high as 200:1(Hoxey& Shah, 2000; Wong, 2003). In India among elderly the attempted vs completed suicide ration for elderly (7:1) is almost double that of younger population (15:1). the difference as compared to western figure might be due the fact that elderly in India are still well integrated and respected in the families. Whereas, in the west social isolation adds to small ratio of attempted vs completed suicides. Physical vulnerability seem to be the predominant reason for vulnerability of elderly to suicide (Radhakrishnan & Andrade, 2012).

The data collection and reporting methods may vary from study to study. To estimate suicide behavior related studies the following types of studies and most commonly available.

- **Time Trend Analysis Studies:** Such studies are generally ecological in design and utilize crude or standardized rates from the crime records and/or census etc. Such studies are generally nation-wide or may be in the form of review of studies from different populations within the same geographical are or country. A specific consideration to the rates at various time points are reported which may encompass certain happening of interest to the population such as draught, economic recession, political change eye.
- **Cross National Comparison:** Such studies are again ecological design based that compare national mortality data from different countries either cross sectionally or on time trend pattern. Such studies are carried out to identify the cultural or inter-population differences in the suicide behavior pattern. Intra-national studies can also be carried out on similar pattern.
- **Qualitative Studies:** These studies primarily focus on the causes of suicide instead of rates. Ethnographic studies and psychological autopsy based studies are most commonly carried out qualitative studies. Content analysis and grounded theory based approach are the common methods of qualitative studies.

Suicide Across the Ages

Elderly males have recorded highest rates in most of the developed countries except for a temporary decline between 1983-1985. Similar trends have been seen in females but male to female success rate in suicide had been about 3:1. Globally the suicide rates for those >75 years age are generally twice as compared to those aged below 25 years. Such trends are common among most of high income countries except some temporary exceptions reported from UK and Ireland. Various studies examining the age trends concluded that age specific suicide rates of 1.2 for 5-14 years rises to 55.7 per lac in the age group of 75 years and above The rates are lower for females but follow the similar trends (Bertolote & Fleischmann, 2002; Yeates Conwell et al., 2002).They elderly are more likely to succeed in attempt due to their physical illness, mental morbidity, isolation, increased burden of care on family and therefore less likely to catch attention from others about their behavior and above all a false public perception that having death wish at old age is natural(Barnow, Linden, Lucht, & Freyberger, 2004; Cox, 1998; A.Dombrovski et al., 2008; Dombrovski, Szanto, & Reynolds III, 2005; Gerber & Eiser, 2001; Kumar et al., 2015)

PSYCHOLOGICAL FACTORS IN ELDERLY SUICIDE

Mental health and psychological factors play a prominent role in determining suicidal behavior among elderly. Which can be classified on state vs trait differences? The state factors primarily include psychiatric morbidities, whereas trait factors deal with the personality factors, attitude towards life etc. (Vanlaere et al., 2007).

Psychiatric Morbidity

Psychiatric morbidity is one of the major state determinants in deciding about the outcome of suicidal behavior among elderly. Almost 90% of elderly committing suicide are reported to have one or the other axis I disorder, the depressive disorders being most common (Y. Conwell, 2013; Vanlaere et al., 2007). Depression with elderly suicides is as strongly associated with age as strongly as it is in younger age groups (Harwood, Hawton, Hope, & Jacoby, 2001; Montross et al., 2008). The depressive symptoms in elderly victims are not always easy to identify. Depressive symptoms are often diagnosed on psychological autopsy. A study carried out at Finland found 75% of elderly suicide victims having history of depressive episode. But definitely recognizable symptoms were documented only in 33% of the cases. (Podgorski, Langford, Pearson, & Conwell, 2010) Suicidal ideations and attempt particularly when low self esteem and hopelessness make them particularly vulnerable to suicide (Isometsa, 2004)are prominent and they feel trapped in no escape –no rescue situations (Conwell, 1998). Various studies report prevalence of affective disorders primarily to be nearly in 54-84% and depression is the most proximal risk factor among elderly suicides (Beskow, 1979; Yeates Conwell & Thompson, 2008; Tam & Chiu, 2011) A depressive illness and help seeking any age, has multifactorial etiology in old age too. Psychosocial situations, particularly loneliness play a major role. Thus, the neurotransmitter due to degenerative process and psychosocial changes such as feeling of worthlessness as their knowledge and skills may no longer be in demand coupled with reduced cite can frequently impact upon their emotional life and mood. Such changes may include the situation where their skills and knowledge are no longer in demand, and age related. Controlling for other factors the population attributable risk studies predict that depressive illness alone among elderly contribute towards 75% probability of suicide (Beautrais, 2002; Stanley et al., 2016). Waeren et al. (2003) concluded that risk of suicide gets further compounded by the fact that the elderly especially those aged 75 years and above are less likely to get treatment, while others felt that even referral of any elderly for treatment of late life depression might be difficult (Pitkälä, Isometsä, Henriksson, & Lonnqvist, 2000). However the combination of suicidal intent and depressive episode in elderly make a strong prediction about the fatal outcome (Van Orden & Conwell, 2011).

Montross et al. (2008) reported depressive symptoms contributing prominently towards probability of suicide by elderly adults suffering from schizophrenia. Cohen and coworkers in a sample of schizophrenia patients (n=198) and community controls (n=115) in a random block design study compared the predictability of suicide attempts. They chose 15 suicide predictor variables in a regression model, They found past suicidal attempts and current syndromal depression turned out be significant variables predicting suicidal attempts in schizophrenia patients. Past attempts and suicidal ideas were more common among the patient groups in comparison with community dwellers (Wendler, 2013). More research is clearly required to elucidate to role of psychotic symptoms in suicide. As per WHO estimates lifetime risk of suicide is estimated to be 4% in patients with mood disorders, 7% in people with alcohol dependence, 8% in people with bipolar disorder and 5% in people with schizophrenia, Importantly, the risk of suicidal behavior increases with co morbidity; individuals with more than one mental disorder have significantly higher risks. The risk assessment mentioned here is not any age specific but shows the risk in general population. (World Health Organization, 2014b)

Few studies reported about the association of suicidal ideation alone with elderly suicides. In a cross-sectional study, Scocco and De Leo (2002) found 9.5% of elderly having persisting suicidal ideas over the last one year. Callahan et al found prevalence of suicidal ideas to only about 1% among elderly. However, they also commented this ideation often associated with depressive disorders. They used a stricter definition of suicide than that used by Callahan, Hendrie, Nienaber, and Tierney, (1996); Scocco and De Leo, (2002). In a Swedish study 4% of the mentally healthy elderly, reported worthlessness, 4% had death wishes, 0.9% had expressed suicidal ideations. But none thought of making an attempt seriously (Skoog et al., 1996). In the same study feelings of worthlessness and suicidal ideas were 7 to 10 times more common among the elderly with a diagnosed mental disorder. Seriousness about suicidal attempt was also three times more common among patients with mental disorders. The finding thus suggests that duration and presence of suicidal ideation is not a strong predictor of suicidal attempts but presence of a mental disorder can be. But these studies also suggest that elderly with suicidal ideas need to be followed up as such ideas are not common among healthy persons. Thus suicidal ideations, is often used as proxy measure for prediction of suicide is only has a limited local value. Myths about suicidal ideation and hopelessness being a part of normal process of aging are also prevalent in various cultures that further increases the vulnerability of elderly with such ideas to suicide (Rahimi, Ali, Md Noor, Mahmood, & Zainun, 2015). In contrast, as concluded by Dombrovski et al. (2005) from retrospective (Chiu et al., 2004), any past suicidal attempt increases the chances of similar attempts among elderly. It particularly increases the possibility of completed suicide in males.

Executive function deficits in the depressed elderly also seem to be associated with suicidal behavior in depressed elderlies. Such association continues to be significant even after controlling for the effect of dementia, substance use, medication, head injury and past suicidal behavior. Dombrovski and colleagues in a case control study found the depressed elderly patients with (n=32) and without(n=32) suicidal ideas found the patients with suicidal idea performing poorly on Dementia rating scale and executive function test interview. The sample of the study was small limiting the generalizability of the observations. (Dombrovski et al., 2008). The decision making and focusing on reward punishment based learning which are based on ventral prefrontal circuits were particularly found more affected (Dombrovski et al., 2010). Frontal executive functions which play major role in managing stressful circumstances are specifically found to be impaired in depressive elderly patients with suicidal behavior (Keilp et al., 2001; King et al., 2000). The finding receive some support from the neuroimaging studies also (Greenstein et al., 2010).

Disability seems to augment the effect of depressive symptoms and leading elderly to the path of suicidal behavior. Disabilities and physical morbidities are common among elderly males as compared to females. The randomized trials do to some extent clarify depression suicide link and gender differences(Cunningham et al., 2004). However more research is needed for unambiguous conclusion.

Loss of social support, especially among males to determine the suicidal attempts with the depression and disability. Death of a loved one (Neufeld & O'Rourke, 2009), legal problems, financial problems and physical illness were the stressors identified contributing proximally to the suicide act (Rahimi et al., 2015). Thus it is not the single or isolated state that determines the outcome of an attempt but it is the complex interplay of multiple psychosocial states.

Dementia and Suicide

Haw, Harwood, and Hawton, (2009) provided a review of the research on the association between dementia and suicidal behavior in later life. The conclusion had been equivocal and authors concluded that more research would be required to clarify association of dementia and risk of suicide. Specifically, as per authors the degree of risk conferred may vary by dementia subtype and severity. There are few studies of suicide or self-harm in vascular, front temporal, Lewy body and HIV dementia where such behavior might be expected to be more common. Rates of self-harm may be increased in mild dementia and are higher before than after predictive testing for Huntington's disease. Overall, the risk of suicide in dementia was found to be the same or less eras compared with the age-matched general population controls. However the rates were higher soon after diagnosis, in patients with dementia or Huntington's disease in hospital. The authors believed from the review of literature that depressive symptoms such as hopelessness, mild cognitive impairment, preserved insight, younger age and failure to respond to anti-dementia drugs might be the actual risk factors for such behavior in suicide (Haw et al., 2009). In the patient with cognitive impairment it might be difficult to differentiate between self-injurious behavior and suicidal attempt. Hence prediction of risk of suicide in dementia also requires robust standard methods of assessment (Pies & Popli, 1995). Another methodological flaw in dementia suicide research is reported by Keene and colleagues (Keene, Hope, Fairburn, & Jacoby, 2001). They found that in dementia research, suicide as the cause of death is often omitted especially if it has been mild or could not be confirmed clinically. A meta-analysis for the causes of death in dementia and Huntington's disease too found paucity of suicidal deaths in dementia (Harris & Barraclough, 1997).

Axis II Disorders

Not much work seems to done on association between personality disorders or trait and suicidal behavior. The studies carried out have reported timidity, shyness, hostility and independent life styles associated with late life suicides. However, anankastic and anxious traits particularly seem to distinguish between late life natural and suicidal deaths. Among the depressive traits, hopeless alone remains a significant predictor of suicidal later, even after resolution of depressive episode (Yeates Conwell & Thompson, 2008).

Physical Illness and Suicide

Physical illness being very common in the old age, it is difficult to predict their independent impact on predicting suicidal behavior. Almost half of the elderly attempting suicide have been seen suffering from physical illness (Draper, 1994). As concluded by Wearn (2003) in his review, it is reported that most of the prospective and retrospective studies using accidental death controls found physical illness getting over represented in suicidal death among elderlies. They did feel paucity of prospective studies. The studies comparing suicide victims with matched controls did suggest a strong association between elderly suicide and serious physical illness. Wearn also concluded that the type of illness really didn't matter at all (Conwell et al., 2000; Timonen et al., 2002; Wærn, 2003). Waern (2003) also opined that power of these prospective studies may be inadequate due to small number of suicidal events. Retrospective studies here seem to offer an advantage of large sample size. Risk of suicide with physical illness can be partly explained by the mediating effect of depressive features such as hopelessness. Moreover, physical illness seems to affect men more than women. The somatic illness, precipitating physical events were found more frequently associated with male victims of suicide as observed in the Finnish and Canadian studies.

Risk of suicide is more with chronic and serious illness which have a likely terminal outcome. In a case-control study compared the proportion with physical illnesses among 822 cases who committed suicide with that among 944 controls who died due to motor vehicle accident at age 55 years or over in Alberta, Canada. Compared to the prevalence of cancer, cardiovascular disease and other physical diseases among victims of accidents and suicides. The suicide victims had more prevalence of physical diseases and depression. There was no significant difference in the proportion of cerebrovascular diseases and diabetes among the case and control groups before adjustment for sociodemographic and clinical characteristics. After adjustment of these variables, the elderly with any of the following illnesses were more likely to die by suicide than those without the illness: cancer (adjusted odds ratio [95% confidence interval]: 1.73 [1.16–2.58]), prostatic disorder (excluding prostatic cancer, 1.70 [1.16–2.49]), chronic pulmonary disease among the married (1.86 [1.22–2.83]), depression (6.70 [4.72–9.50]) or other psychiatric illness (2.16 [1.68–2.76]). There was no evidence that ischemic heart disease, cerebrovascular disease, peptic ulcer and diabetes mellitus might be associated with suicide in the elderly. The authors concluded Cancer, prostatic disorder, chronic pulmonary disease among the married and psychiatric illness appear to be associated with suicide among the elderly (Quan, Arboleda-Flórez, Fick, Stuart, & Love, 2002) In a meta analysis of 63 medical disorders by Harris and Barraclough cited by Waern (2003)concluded increased suicidal risk among people with HIV/AIDS, malignant neoplasms, head and neck cancers, Huntington's chorea, multiple sclerosis, peptic ulcer, renal disease, spinal cord injury and systemic lupus erythematosus. Relative risks for suicide associated with these conditions are in the range of 1.5 to 4 times higher (Yeates Conwell, Van Orden, & Caine, 2011). Fiske, O'Riley, and Widoe (2008) also had similar observations. It is difficult to arrive at any consensus regarding variance contributed by the physical illness towards suicidal behavior. Most of such evidence linking suicidal behavior and physical illness comes from case studies. Some studies do suggest that risk for suicide increases directly with multiplicity of physical co morbidities present. If a person has 3 co morbid illnesses, then suicidal risk too increases three times in comparison with those without physical illness. Five co morbid illnesses similarly increase the risk five times and with seven co morbid illness, the risk increase 9 times (Kiriakidis, 2015). Many authors still favor the believe that even after controlling for the risk posed by physical co morbidity, chronic pain, bipolar or unipolar depression, insomnia still remain independent and significant predictors of suicide. Evidence from case control community based studies is certainly desired (Juurlink, Herrmann, Szalai, Kopp, & Redelmeier, 2004). There is no evidence that ischemic heart disease, cerebrovascular disease, peptic ulcer and diabetes mellitus might be associated with suicide in the elderly (Quan et al., 2002).

Chronic Painful Conditions

Tang and colleagues (Crane, 2006) observed that instead of diagnosis it is the distressful painful condition than increase the elderly vulnerability to suicide. They found subjects with painful condition having 2-3 times higher suicidal ideas and other behaviors in comparison with general population. Painful condition and suicidal behavior found stronger relationship among males in comparison to females (Juurlink et al., 2004; Li, Conwell, & Li Yeates, 2010). Painful condition along with a precipitating diagnosis of medical illness further increase suicidality. With relation to the physical illness it is the perceived status of quality of life that has the ultimate bearing on determination for suicidal behavior (Kaplan, Barrel, & Lusky, 1988). The impact of pain, loss of function, personal integrity play a more important role than just the diagnosis of illness. In case control multivariate studies it was found that impairment in carrying out instrumental activities of daily life was a independent of diagnosis of physical and mental disorder and a strong determinant of suicidal behavior in elderly (Conwell et al., 2010) .The rates of depression among patients with cancer range from 16.7to 34.4%. Poor control of pain depression and hopelessness were significant predictors of suicide (Fiske et al., 2008).

SOCIAL FACTORS AND SUICIDE

As noted by (Conwell et al., 2011) in a comprehensive review stressful life events preceding suicide tend to be more numerous and severe among suicides than controls. They noticed that threats associated with ill health and functional impairment, losses through bereavement or break up of relationships with family members are more saliently related to suicide in late age. Serious relationship and financial problems distinguished older adult suicides and near fatal suicide attempters from controls (Beautrais, 2002; Rubenowitz, Waern, Wilhelmson, & Allebeck, 2001). Duberstein et al also has reported that family discord and employment change distinguished suicides from controls over the age of 50 years even after adjusting for socio-demographic characteristics and mental disorders (Duberstein, Conwell, Conner, Eberly, & Caine, 2004).

Method of Suicide

Method used for suicide itself is a risk factor due to lethality associated with it. In an autopsy based study concluded that most of the elderly choose violent for suicidal attempt. Hanging was the most common method of suicide; accounting for 56.5% of the cases in their study Majority of males in the sample (62.5%) preferred hanging. Jumping from height (13.1%), exposure to unspecified chemicals (13.1%), jumping/lying before moving object (4.3%), exposure to pesticides (4.3%) and injuring oneself using sharp object (4.3%) were also chosen by many victims successfully (Rahimi et al., 2015) In the west to the trends are similar. In UK men prefer hanging whereas use of firearms is most common (60%) in US. Females generally choose poisoning as the most preferred method for suicide (Cattell, 2010). Firearm use is among the preferred methods by men in the west. But in Indian and eastern culture this method doesn't find any preference (Mythri & Ebenezer, 2016; Rahimi et al., 2015).

PROTECTIVE FACTORS

Any particular factor is difficult to be labeled as protective factor. Any factor which is a risk factor, its absence would provide protection against the possibility of suicidal behavior. However, any psychological, social or physical condition may be considered as protective if its presence or high magnitude has inverse correlation with the incidence of suicidal behavior. Participation in formal, social networks is a protecting factor against suicide and is often a buffer to ward off depression. Moving into a nursing home can also be a protecting factor against suicide. On the other hand, anticipation of moving into a nursing home can also be a major reason why some older people may display suicidal behavior. The fear of becoming dependent on other people, and the expected loss of personal possessions (and with them, their identity), privacy and control over their own lives, all have a role.

In a 24 year follow up study on 8945 participants it was seen that three factors namely marital status, social network size and religious participation significantly reduced the probability of suicide (Manuscript & Integration, 2015). Many earlier studies also found that robust social support number of friends buffers the adverse impact of risk factors for suicide in elderly. Greater number of friends, having someone to confide in reduces the possibility of suicide in comparison with controls (Friedman & Lipsedge, 1971; Harris & Barraclough, 1997; Miller, 1978; Turvey et al., 2002). Various positive and negative studies together conclude religion and spirituality generally having a very strong protective factor against suicide. Religion help individual cope with stressful situations and thus prevents from suicide. Islam condemns suicide and doesn't allow burial of suicide. Consequently, suicide rates among Islamic countries are generally the lowest. In an review of suicide rates in 71 countries Islam was found to have a lowering effect on suicide rates (Simpson & Conklin, 1989). Even in the multicultural countries e.g.US. Singapore suicide rates are lowest among Muslims (Rivallan, 2006).

Catholic religion that believe in life after death and considers suicide as a sin also acts as deterrent to suicide in comparison with protestant beliefs. Catholic countries have lower suicide rates in comparison with those reported from protestant Christian countries. Highest rates are reported generally from secular and atheist countries. China is one such country reporting highest suicide rates among females across the countries. According to Hinduism the goal in late stage of human life is to break bondage with world. On the other hand, the Geeta preaches one should neither desire for life nor death. Hinduism had been holding ambivalent views about suicide. It allows suicide under certain circumstances of having committed sins e.g. theft, incest etc. thus making some suicides allowable and religiously rational (Vijaykumar, 2009). Thus it is not surprising that India is among those countries with highest suicide rates where Hindus make majority of population. Higher rates from southern part of India (Mythri & Ebenezer, 2016) also appear to be for the similar reason where Hindus strongly belief in religious beliefs and rituals.

WHEN ELDERLY SUICIDE IS RATIONAL

This question is gaining relevance now a days as in many Scandinavian countries has legalized practice of euthanasia, whereas others are considering it. Battin (1984) as cited by Wand et al. (2016) and Pamela et al. (2016) rational suicide has been defined as occurring when a person is able to reason, possess sufficient information, have a realistic worldview, and act (to end their own life) according to their own essential interests. Suicide can be understood to rational when it is not under the influence of any psychiatric illness or symptom. He is fully dependent on others for his daily needs. Quality of life is extremely deteriorated due to pain, disability or dependence. Circumstances are such that there are no chances of recovery. Such as person has a terminal illness with painful condition. Rational suicide is invariably carried out by the person himself and he doesn't seek any assistance. The problem arises when a person has a rational choice and approaches a physician for help in the countries where euthanasia practice is ethical and legalized. This is the time for physician to be in dilemma who has to take a decision to convert the choice of rational suicide to euthanasia by proper evaluation. However, it is difficult to assess rationality as this is a dimensional concept rather than its black and white existence Just presence of depressive illness in a person with suicidal idea cannot be assumed as the suicidal ideas coming from a morbid process and therefore irrational. Additionally, the assessment of rationality may be colored by the attitude and values of physician too. On the other hand, demand for rational suicide or euthanasia itself may be a symptom of illness. In the countries where euthanasia is legal the clinician needs to have a very open mind to take decision. Elderly suicides are often explained as rational choices, especially if the person has physical illnesses, which may not reflect ageism. A realistic therapeutic nihilism in case of terminally painful illnesses may choice of suicide rational. Ageism, that is, stereotypes and assumptions about older people made purely on the basis of their age, may affect the ability of clinicians as well client to detect the psychopathology that frequently underlies suicide in late life. In the eastern countries with paternalistic attitude of physician towards their patients may again obscure the proper decision of rational suicide by unnecessarily prolonging the pain and suffering in a terminally ill provided the law of land favors euthanasia. As cited by Wand et al. (2016), however, there is little formal literature to guide clinicians in how to help older people without major psychiatric illness who wish to die. Although this lack of guidance is problematic for all jurisdictions, it is particularly relevant in settings where euthanasia is legal. In the countries where euthanasia is not legalized, the physician needs to take appropriate preventive steps to prevent the execution of rational suicide.

PREDICTING SUICIDE IN ELDERLY

It can be guessed that above all discussion was for this purpose only i.e. prediction and prevention of suicide. Despite multifactorial causation, suicide is a preventable. But it is often difficult to predict. It requires a multidimensional assessment. The risk factors which one need to assess and overcome can be concerned with the individual, his relationship and social network, community related factors, societal issues and the most important being the health care delivery system.

As explained above mental disorders especially the depressive disorder appears making a common pathway to a completed or attempted suicide. Most of the time the elderly patients visit the primary care setup where the physicians are not well trained to diagnose depressive or any psychiatric illness. They often prefer to use quick tools like Geriatric depression scale (Yesavage et al., 1983) which don't have any suicide specific items. As claimed by von Van Orden & Conwell (2011) both long and short forms of GDS are equally effective in prediction, but detection can be made more effective by adding one or more suicide specific item to it. Brief symptom rating scale(BSRS) is of limited use in comparison with previous strategy as BSRS is effective in predicting non-lethal suicides only (Liu & Chiu, 2009).

Beck et al. (1985) in a 10 years long study on patients hospitalized with suicidal ideation found that only the hopelessness scale and pessimism items on the Beck Depressive Inventory predicted suicides. A score of 10 or more on the Hopelessness Scale correctly identified 91% of eventual suicides.(Beck, Steer, Kovacs, & Garrison, 1985)Hopelessness has been found to have a strong positive correlation with degree of suicidal intent.(Beck et al., 1985) Scales used to identify suicidal risk include SAD PERSONS scale, Beck Suicidal Intent Scale and the Suicidal Intent Questionnaire (SIQ) validated in the Indian population and in many other countries too (Gupta, Anand, & Trivedi, 1983) The SIQ is a 10-item questionnaire with each item scored as 0, 1 or 2.".The scale identified suicidal ideation in about 35% of this sample. In a recent study about communicating suicidal intent among attempters, Srivastava and Kulshretha (2000) reported that the majority of the sample (73.3%) communicated suicidal intent using the SIQ. Care is to be taken if Hamilton Depression rating scale is to be used. The scores on the SIQ showed a low positive correlation with the Hamilton Depression scale. The problem of assessment may vary from culture to culture too. In Asian countries particularly India and China psychiatric symptoms may not be detectable in about 60% cases in contrast to only 10% in the western high income countries (Cavanagh, Carson, Sharpe, & Lawrie, 2003; Radhakrishnan & Andrade, 2012; Phillips et al., 2002). Hopeless along with other depressive symptoms such as loss of motivation and previous suicidal attempts may particularly signify possibility of an imminent suicidal attempt. A family history of suicide may further act as motivational or role model factors leading the person to make an attempt.

Use of alcohol and other recreational psychoactive drugs also increases the risk of suicide. The clinician should be particularly careful to the fact that co morbid substance use with depression it further increases the risk and such patients need a careful observation. Physical illnesses particularly chronic and painful must be screened out as their presence also increases the risk. Relationship conflict should also be a focus of assessment in a potentially suicidal elderly. Separation or divorce, death of a partner or a close friend are common in old age and can cause grief and situational psychological stress, and are all associated with increased risk of suicide. Unhealthy or abusive relationships can also be a risk factor. Violence, including sexual violence, against women is a common occurrence and is often committed by an intimate partner. Intimate partner violence is associated with an increase in suicide attempts and suicide risk. Globally 35% of women have experienced physical and/or sexual violence by an intimate partner or sexual violence by a non-partner

Community beliefs and culture have an important bearing on the risk of suicide. People in a community live with a bond of interdependence, common beliefs, religious feeling and past experiences etc. Generally community therefore offers a protection against suicide. In the state of conflict, the people increase their cohesiveness and tend to work together in preventing damage to the community. Thus in the event of crisis particularly when it just strikes, person try to cope up to overcome nut as the conflict resolves after the damage has occurred, is the most vulnerable period for elderly suicide when they perceive nothing is left for them which give them a sense of isolation loneliness. Another disaster that always had happening in maritime if physical neglect or abuse to the elderly. It may be because of myths as discussed. People may be incompetent in identifying the isolated and passive elderly thinking it to be a process of normal aging. In almost all communities the weapons for committing suicide are easily available. Accessibility to fire arm in the west and insecticides in agrigarian countries is almost a norm that increases the risk of suicide.

The people might also be feeling stigmatized in approaching health care services due to stigma of mental illness and fear of getting labeled. Many times as in India and many other middle and low income countries, the health system itself is inaccessible due to the need of infrastructure and manpower. Internet and use of mobile phones of by the younger generation has increased the isolation mad feeling of loneliness among elderly. The younger ones leaving their parents in the country for job abroad has further compounded the problem of suicide among elderly. There is clearly a strong need for old age homes /clubs in India where they can find someone to confide in and companionship. Compared to the west only few NGOs are working in India in this direction the mass media too particularly broadcast news about any crime/suicide in a very sensational way which may lead to copycat suicide at times. Above all the local government also needs taking care of the welfare of the elderly. Many countries like Australia, New Zealand, UK, Us and India have a policy to take care to senior citizens. However, a motivation is yet required to enforce these policies in India.

ELDERLY SUICIDE PREVENTION

Suicide prevention in late life in uphill tasks. That the specific difficulties encountered by such preventive strategies are the immobility and poor social networking of the elderly. However, health care provider can play a major role in suicide prevention among elderly persons. Quite similar to adults, various studies have demonstrated that elderly often visit family physician or primary health care provider months before contemplating suicide. Depression has been seen as an independent risk factor for suicide account for maximum variance across different studies. In a Japanese 10-year follow-up study treatment of depression lead to more than 70% reduction in suicide rates among elderly. Reduction is suicide rates was almost equal for males and females (Heisel, 2006). But the health care providers are seen often insensitive to this risk and often miss it unless trained. They often interpret potential suicide victims as non-compliant to the treatment; Due to lack of training they often fail to refer the elderly depressed patients for treatment. Heisel(2006) also commented about reduction in suicidal behavior among elderly patients referred to mental health services in the US. The PROSPECT study also highlighted that the psychosocial treatment provided at primary care level is of great help in reducing suicidal risk. Other studies reviewed by authors predicted that hospitalization may increase the suicidal risk among elderly. But a collaborative approach for management that links the primary care providers with specialist is an effective strategy.

Nursing observation and screening for depression has also been seen as effective strategies in risk management for elderly patients. Use of scale for Suicidal Ideation and Nurses Global assessment Scale has been found particularly useful for screening vulnerable individuals. When an older adult report depressive mood asking three questions? 1. Have you been feeling so sad lately that you were thinking about death or dying? 2. Have you had thoughts that life is not worth living? 3. Have you been thinking about harming yourself? Followed by more direct questioning also helps in identifying the individuals at risk (Garand, Mitchell, Dietrick, Hijjawi, & Pan, 2010; Heisel, 2006) also commented that the courier delivery boys, meter readers can also provide useful clues about the at risk individuals that can aid suicide prevention. Outreach programs can also be effective in reducing suicide risk among elderly. In Italy Tele Help-TeleCheckhelp has been shown to significantly reduce risk of suicide among elderly. The physician prescribed an alarm directly linked to a telephone network to their elderly patients. The elderly could use the alarm (Telecheck) to seek help and the volunteers used to ask about the well being (Telecheck) randomly on twice a week basis. This service reduced risk significantly among females. (De Leo, Dello Buono, & Dwyer, 2002)

CONCLUSION

To conclude suicide is one of the leading causes of preventable deaths among elderly all over the world. After the younger ones the elderly people make second most prominent peak on any graph of suicidal victims. Suicide in elderly is not a simple process but a complex interplay of personal, social, psychological and biological causes. Certain causes such as genetics causes are permanent, but most of the causes are modifiable and reversible. Psychiatric illness particularly depressive illness is commonly associated with the suicidal behavior. However, both physicians as well as community need to be sensitized for its identification. Of all this appears to the most important factor to be controlled as this is associated with about 90% of suicidal death all over the world and it is reversible with treatment. Isolation, financial and relationship problems also contribute to the suicidal behavior among elderly. These may set up a vicious circle with depressive symptoms leading to suicidal attempt by the victim. Religious and spiritual practices increase cohesiveness and prevent against suicide. In the western countries there are proper protocol and guideline to help a senior citizen and suicidal persons, but in India and other developing countries we yet need to develop such services.

What does a man need to live...good health, wealth, family, friends, and happiness. But old age lacks all of these...please give me a hand someone. - An anonymous elderly person seen everywhere.

REFERENCES

Barnow, S., Linden, M., Lucht, M., & Freyberger, H. J. (2004). *Influence of age of patients who wish to die on treatment decisions by physicians and nurses*. Academic Press.

Beautrais, A. L. (2002). A case control study of suicide and attempted suicide in older adults. *Suicide & Life-Threatening Behavior*, *32*(1), 1–9. doi:10.1521/suli.32.1.1.22184 PMID:11931007

Beck, A. T., Steer, R. A., Kovacs, M., & Garrison, B. (1985). Hopelessness and eventual suicide: A 10-year prospective study of patients hospitalized with suicidal ideation. *The American Journal of Psychiatry*, *142*(5), 559–563. doi:10.1176/ajp.142.5.559 PMID:3985195

Bertolote, J. M., & Fleischmann, A. (2002). Suicide and psychiatric diagnosis: A worldwide perspective. *World Psychiatry; Official Journal of the World Psychiatric Association (WPA)*, *1*, 181–185. PMID:16946849

Beskow, J. (1979). Suicide in mental disorder in Swedish men. *Acta Psychiatrica Scandinavica. Supplementum*, *277*, 1–138. PMID:286500

Bilsen, J. (2000). End-of-life decisions in medical practice in Flanders, Belgium: a nationwide survey. *Lancet*, *356*(9244), 1806–11. Retrieved from http://www.ncbi.nlm.nih.gov/pubmed/11117913

Callahan, C. M., Hendrie, H. C., Nienaber, N. A., & Tierney, W. M. (1996). Suicidal ideation among older primary care patients. *Journal of the American Geriatrics Society*, *44*(10), 1205–1209. doi:10.1111/j.1532-5415.1996.tb01370.x PMID:8855999

Cattell, H. (2010). *Suicide in the elderly*. Academic Press.

Cavanagh, J., Carson, A. J., Sharpe, M., & Lawrie, S. M. (2003). Psychological autopsy studies of suicide: A systematic review. *Psychological Medicine*, *33*(3), 395–405. doi:10.1017/S0033291702006943 PMID:12701661

Chiu, H. F. K., Yip, P. S. F., Chi, I., Chan, S., Tsoh, J., Kwan, C. W., … Caine, E. (2004). Elderly suicide in Hong Kong--a case-controlled psychological autopsy study. *Acta Psychiatrica Scandinavica*, *109*(4), 299–305. Retrieved from http://www.ncbi.nlm.nih.gov/pubmed/15008804

Conwell, Y. (1998). High levels of hopelessness persist in geriatric patients with remitted depression and a history of attempted suicide. *Journal of the American Geriatrics Society*, *46*(11), 1401–1406. Retrieved from http://www.ncbi.nlm.nih.gov/sites/entrez?Db=pubmed&Cmd=Retrieve&list_uids=9809762&dopt=abstractplus

Conwell, Y. (2013). Suicide and suicide prevention in later life. *Focus*, *11*(1), 39-47.

Conwell, Y., Duberstein, P. R., & Caine, E. D. (2002). Risk factors for suicide in later life. *Biological Psychiatry*, *52*(3), 193–204. doi:10.1016/S0006-3223(02)01347-1 PMID:12182926

Conwell, Y., Duberstein, P. R., Hirsch, J. K., Conner, K. R., Eberly, S., & Caine, E. D. (2010). Health status and suicide in the second half of life. *International Journal of Geriatric Psychiatry*, *25*(4), 371–379. doi:10.1002/gps.2348 PMID:19582758

Conwell, Y., Lyness, J. M., Duberstein, P., Cox, C., Seidlitz, L., DiGiorgio, A., & Caine, E. D. (2000). Completed suicide among older patients in primary care practices: A controlled study. *Journal of the American Geriatrics Society*, *48*(1), 23–29. doi:10.1111/j.1532-5415.2000.tb03024.x PMID:10642017

Conwell, Y., & Thompson, C. (2008). Suicidal Behavior in elders. *The Psychiatric Clinics of North America*, *31*(2), 333–356. doi:10.1016/j.psc.2008.01.004 PMID:18439452

Conwell, Y., Van Orden, K., & Caine, E. D. (2011). Suicide in Older Adults. *The Psychiatric Clinics of North America*, *34*(2), 451–468. doi:10.1016/j.psc.2011.02.002 PMID:21536168

Cox, C. (1998). Age Differences in Behaviors Leading to Completed Suicide. *The American Journal of Geriatric Psychiatry*, *6*(2), 122–126. doi:10.1097/00019442-199805000-00005 PMID:9581207

Crane, C. (2006). Suicidality in chronic pain : A review of the prevalence, risk factors and psychological links. *Review - Americas Society*, *36*, 575–586. doi:10.1017/S0033291705006859 PMID:16420727

Crepet, P., Caracciolo, S., Casoli, R., Fabbri, D., Florenzano, F., & Grassi, G. M. (1991). Suicidal behavior in Italy: Data, trends and guidelines for a suicide intervention/prevention policy. *Suicide & Life-Threatening Behavior*, *21*, 263–278. PMID:1759299

Cunningham, C. (2004). Recent developments: Suicide in older people. *British Medical Journal*, *329*(7471), 895–898. doi:10.1136/bmj.329.7471.895 PMID:15485967

De Leo, D., Dello Buono, M., & Dwyer, J. (2002). Suicide among the elderly: The long-term impact of a telephone support and assessment intervention in northern Italy. *The British Journal of Psychiatry*, *181*(3), 226–229. doi:10.1192/bjp.181.3.226 PMID:12204927

Dombrovski1, A. Y., Szanto, K., & Reynolds, C. F., III. (2005). Epidemiology and risk factors for suicide in the elderly: 10-year update. *Aging Health, 1*(1), 135–145.

Dombrovski, A., Clark, L., Siegle, G. J., Butters, M. A., Ichikawa, N., Sahakian, B. J., & Szanto, K. (2010). Reward/punishment reversal learning in older suicide attempters. *The American Journal of Psychiatry*, *167*(6), 699–707. doi:10.1176/appi.ajp.2009.09030407 PMID:20231320

Dombrovski, A. Y., Butters, M. A., Reynolds, C. III, Houck, F., Clark, L., Patricia, R., ... Szanto, K. (2008). Reward/punishment reversal learning in older suicide attempters. *The American Journal of Geriatric Psychiatry*, *16*(2), 109–115. doi:10.1097/JGP.0b013e3180f6338d PMID:18239196

Dombrovski, A. Y., Szanto, K., & Reynolds, C. F. III. (2005). Epidemiology and risk factors for suicide in the elderly: 10-year update. *Aging Health*, *1*(1), 135–145. doi:10.2217/1745509X.1.1.135

Draper, B. (1994). Suicidal behaviour in the elderly. *International Journal of Geriatric Psychiatry*, *9*(8), 655–661. doi:10.1002/gps.930090810

Duberstein, P. R., Conwell, Y., Conner, K. R., Eberly, S., & Caine, E. D. (2004). Suicide at 50 years of age and older: Perceived physical illness, family discord and financial strain. *Psychological Medicine*, *34*(1), 137–146. doi:10.1017/S0033291703008584 PMID:14971634

Fiske, A., O'Riley, A. A., & Widoe, R. K. (2008). Physical Health and Suicide in Late Life: An Evaluative Review. *Clinical Gerontologist*, *31*(4), 31–50. doi:10.1080/07317110801947151

Friedman, D. E., & Lipsedge, M. S. (1971). Treatment of phobic anxiety and psychogenic impotence by systematic desensitization employing methohexitone-induced relaxation. *The British Journal of Psychiatry*, *118*(542), 87–90. doi:10.1192/bjp.118.542.87 PMID:5576272

Garand, L., Mitchell, A. N., Dietrick, A., Hijjawi, S. P., & Pan, D. (2010). Suicide in older adults. *Nursing Assessment of IDAL Risk*, *27*(4), 355–370. doi:10.1080/01612840600569633.SUICIDE PMID:16546935

Gerber, B. S., & Eiser, A. R. (2001). The patient-physician relationship in the Internet Age: Future prospects and the research agenda. *Journal of Medical Internet Research*, *3*(2), 112–123. doi:10.2196/jmir.3.2.e15 PMID:11720957

Gonzalez, M. J., Miranda-Massari, J. R., Berdiel, M. J., & Duconge, J., Rodriguez-Lopez, J. L., Hunninghake, R., & Cobas-Rosario, V. J. (2014). High dose intraveneous Vitamin C and chikungunya fever: A case report. *Journal of Orthomolecular Medicine*, *29*(4), 154–156. doi:10.1016/j.biotechadv.2011.08.021. Secreted PMID:25705076

Gramaglia, C., Feggi, A., Bergamasco, P., Bert, F., Gattoni, E., Marangon, D., ... Zeppegno, P. (2016). Clinical characteristics associated with suicide attempts in clinical settings: A comparison of suicidal and non-suicidal depressed inpatients. *Frontiers in Psychiatry*, *7*, 109. doi:10.3389/fpsyt.2016.00109 PMID:27378957

Greenstein, A. S., Paranthaman, R., Burns, A., Jackson, A., Malik, R. A., Baldwin, R. C., & Heagerty, A. M. (2010). Cerebrovascular damage in late-life depression is associated with structural and functional abnormalities of subcutaneous small arteries. *Hypertension*, *56*(4), 734–740. doi:10.1161/HYPERTENSIONAHA.110.152801 PMID:20713917

Gupta, S. C., Anand, R., & Trivedi, J. K. (1983). Development of a suicidal intent questionnaire. *Indian Journal of Psychiatry*, *25*, 57–62. PMID:21847253

Harris, E. C., & Barraclough, B. (1997). Suicide as an outcome for mental disorders: A meta-analysis. *The British Journal of Psychiatry*, *170*(3), 205–228. doi:10.1192/bjp.170.3.205 PMID:9229027

Harwood, D., Hawton, K., Hope, T., & Jacoby, R. (2001). Psychiatric disorder and personality factors associated with suicide in older people: A descriptive and case-control study. *International Journal of Geriatric Psychiatry*, *16*(2), 155–165. doi:10.1002/1099-1166(200102)16:2<155::AID-GPS289>3.0.CO;2-0 PMID:11241720

Haw, C., Harwood, D., & Hawton, K. (2009). Dementia and suicidal behavior: A review of the literature. *International Psychogeriatrics*, *21*(3), 440. doi:10.1017/S1041610209009065 PMID:19368760

Heisel, M. J. (2006). Suicide and its prevention among older adults. *Canadian Journal of Psychiatry*, *51*(3), 143–154. doi:10.1177/070674370605100304 PMID:16618005

Henslin, J. A. (1996). *Social Problems.* Prentice Hall.

Hoxey, K., & Shah, A. (2000). Recent trends in elderly suicide rates in England and Wales. *International Journal of Geriatric Psychiatry*, *15*(3), 274–279. doi:10.1002/(SICI)1099-1166(200003)15:3<274::AID-GPS106>3.0.CO;2-I PMID:10713587

Isometsa, E. (2003, September). Elderly suicide attempters with depression are often diagnosed only after the attempt. *International Journal of Geriatric Psychiatry*, *19*, 35–40. doi:10.1002/gos.1031

Juurlink, D. N., Herrmann, N., Szalai, J. P., Kopp, A., & Redelmeier, D. A. (2004). Medical Illness and the Risk of Suicide in the Elderly. *Archives of Internal Medicine*, *164*(11), 1179. doi:10.1001/archinte.164.11.1179 PMID:15197042

Kaplan, G., Barrel, V., & Lusky, A. (1988). Subjective state of health and survival in elderly adults. *The Journals of Gerontology. Series B, Psychological Sciences and Social Sciences*, *43*(4), S114–S120. PMID:3385152

Keene, J., Hope, T., Fairburn, C. G., & Jacoby, R. (2001). Death and dementia. *International Journal of Geriatric Psychiatry*, *16*(10), 969–974. doi:10.1002/gps.474 PMID:11607941

Keilp, J. G., Sackeim, H. A., Brodsky, B. S., Oquendo, M. A., Malone, K. M., & Mann, J. J. (2001). Neuropsychological dysfunction in depressed suicide attempters. *The American Journal of Psychiatry*, *158*(5), 735–741. doi:10.1176/appi.ajp.158.5.735 PMID:11329395

King, D. A., Conwell, Y., Cox, C., Henderson, R. E., Denning, D. G., & Eric Caine, M. (2000). A Neuropsychological Comparison of Depressed Suicide Attempters and Nonattempters. *iThe. The Journal of Neuropsychiatry and Clinical Neurosciences*, *12*(12), 64–70. doi:10.1176/jnp.12.1.64 PMID:10678515

Kiriakidis, S. P. (2015). Elderly Suicide: Risk Factors and Preventive Strategies. *Annals of Gerontology and Geriatric Research*, *2*, 1–6.

Kumar, S., Anish, P., & George, B. (2015). Risk factors for suicide in elderly in comparison to younger age groups. *Indian Journal of Psychiatry*, *57*(3), 249. doi:10.4103/0019-5545.166614 PMID:26600577

Li, L. W., Conwell, Y., & Li Yeates, L. W. C. (2010). Pain and Self-Injury Ideation in Elderly Men and Women Receiving Home Care. *Journal of the American Geriatrics Society*, *58*(11), 2160–2165. doi:10.1111/j.1532-5415.2010.03151.x PMID:21054298

Liu, I., & Chiu, C. H. (2009). Case-control study of suicide attempts in the elderly. *International Psychogeriatrics*, *21*(05), 896–982. doi:10.1017/S1041610209990056 PMID:19538823

Manuscript, A., & Integration, S. (2015). NIH Public Access. *Annals of Internal Medicine*, *161*(2), 85–95. doi:10.7326/M13-1291.Social

Miller, M. (1978). Geriatric Suicide: The Arizona Study. *The Gerontologist*, *18*(5 Part 1), 488–495. doi:10.1093/geront/18.5_Part_1.488 PMID:263566

Montross, L. P., Kasckow, J., Golshan, S., Solorzano, E., Lehman, D., & Zisook, S. (2008). Suicidal ideation and suicide attempts among middle-aged and older patients with schizophrenia spectrum disorders and concurrent subsyndromal depression. *The Journal of Nervous and Mental Disease*, *196*(12), 884–890. doi:10.1097/NMD.0b013e31818ec823 PMID:19077855

Mythri, S. V., & Ebenezer, J. A. (2016). Suicide in India: Distinct Epidemiological Patterns and Implications. *Indian Journal of Psychological Medicine*, *38*(6), 493–498. doi:10.4103/0253-7176.194917 PMID:28031581

Neufeld, M. A., & O'Rourke, N. (2009). Impulsivity and hopelessness as predictors of suicide related ideation among older adults. *Canadian Journal of Psychiatry, 54*(10), 684–692. doi:10.1177/070674370905401005 PMID:19835675

Nock, M., Borges, G., Bromet, E., Cha, C. B., Kessler, R. C., & Lee, S. (2008). Suicide and suicidal behavior. *Epidemiologic Reviews, 30*(1), 133–154. doi:10.1093/epirev/mxn002 PMID:18653727

O'Connor, R. C., & Nock, M. K. (2014). *The psychology of suicidal behaviour. The Lancet Psychiatry.* Elsevier Ltd.; doi:10.1016/S2215-0366(14)70222-6

Padoani, W. S. P. (2001). Attempted and completed suicide in older subjects: Results from the WHO/EURO Multicentre Study of Suicidal Behaviour. *International Journal of Geriatric Psychiatry, 16*(3), 300–310. doi:10.1002/gps.337 PMID:11288165

Phillips, M. R., Yang, G., Zhang, Y., Wang, L., Ji, H., & Zhou, M. (2002). Risk factors for suicide in China: A national case-control psychological autopsy study. *Lancet, 360*(9347), 1728–1736. doi:10.1016/S0140-6736(02)11681-3 PMID:12480425

Pies, R. W., & Popli, A. P. (1995). Self-injurious behavior: Pathophysiology and implications to treatment. *Journal of Clinical Psychology, 56*, 580–588. PMID:8530335

Pitkälä, K., Isometsä, E. T., Henriksson, M. M., & Lönnqvist, J. K. (2000). Elderly suicide in Finland. *International Psychogeriatrics, 12*(2), 209–20. <ALIGNMENT.qj></ALIGNMENT>10.1017/S1041610200006335

Podgorski, C. A., Langford, L., Pearson, J. L., & Conwell, Y. (2010). Suicide Prevention for Older Adults in Residential Communities: Implications for Policy and Practice Suicide in Residential Communities. *PLoS Medicine, 7*(5), 3–7. doi:10.1371/journal.pmed.1000254 PMID:20502523

Quan, H., Arboleda-Flórez, J., Fick, G. H., Stuart, H. L., & Love, E. J. (2002). Association between physical illness and suicide among the elderly. *Social Psychiatry and Psychiatric Epidemiology, 37*(4), 190–197. doi:10.1007/s001270200014 PMID:12027246

Radhakrishnan, R., & Andrade, C. (2012). Suicide: An Indian perspective. *Indian Journal of Psychiatry, 54*(4), 304–319. doi:10.4103/0019-5545.104793 PMID:23372232

Rahimi, R., Ali, N., Md Noor, S., Mahmood, M. S., & Zainun, K. A. (2015). Suicide in the elderly in Malaysia. *The Malaysian Journal of Pathology, 37*(3), 259–263. doi:10.1097/00001504-200107000-00027 PMID:26712672

Rivallan, A. (2006). Suicide and attempted suicide in France. *Soins. Psychiatrie, 19*(246), 18–9.

Rubenowitz, E., Waern, M., Wilhelmson, K., & Allebeck, P. (2001). Life events and psychosocial factors in elderly suicides--a case-control study. *Psychological Medicine, 31*(7), 1193–1202. doi:10.1017/S0033291701004457 PMID:11681545

Schlebusch, L. (2005). *Suicidal behaviour in South Africa*. Pietermaritzburg: University of KwaZulu-Natal Press.

Schneidman, E. (1985). *Definition of Suicide*. New York: John Wiley & Sons Inc.

Scocco, P., & De Leo, D. (2002). One-year prevalence of death thoughts, suicide ideation and behaviours in an elderly population. *International Journal of Geriatric Psychiatry*, *17*(9), 842–846. doi:10.1002/gps.691 PMID:12221658

Simpson, M. E., & Conklin, G. H. (1989). Socioeconomic Development, Suicide and Religion: A Test of Durkheim's Theory of Religion and Suicide. *Social Forces*, *67*(4), 945–964. doi:10.1093/sf/67.4.945

Skoog, I., Aevarsson, Ó., Beskow, J., Larsson, L., Palsson, S., Waern, M., ... Östling, S. (1996). Suicidal feelings in a population sample of nondemented 85-year-olds. *The American Journal of Psychiatry*, *153*(8), 1015–1020. doi:10.1176/ajp.153.8.1015 PMID:8678169

Srivastava, S., & Kulshreshtha, N. (2000). Expression of suicidal intent in depressives. *Indian Journal of Psychiatry*, *42*, 184–187. PMID:21407933

Stanley, I. H., Hom, M. A., Rogers, M. L., Hagan, C. R., & Joiner, T. E. Jr. (2016). Understanding suicide among older adults: A review of psychological and sociological theories of suicide. *Aging & Mental Health*, *20*(2), 113–122. doi:10.1080/13607863.2015.1012045 PMID:25693646

Tam, C. W. C., & Chiu, H. F. K. (2011). Depression and suicide in the elderly. *Zeitschrift für Gerontologie*, *16*(9), 13–16.

Timonen, M., Viilo, K., Väisänen, E., Räsänen, P., Hakko, H., & Särkioja, T. (2002). Burden of illness and suicide in elderly people. *BMJ: British Medical Journal*, *325*(7361), 441. doi:10.1136/bmj.325.7361.441/a PMID:12193366

Turvey, C. L., Conwell, Y., Jones, M. P., Phillips, C., Simonsick, E., Pearson, J. L., & Wallace, R. (2002). Risk factors for late-life suicide: A prospective, community-based study. *The American Journal of Geriatric Psychiatry : Official Journal of the American Association for Geriatric Psychiatry*, *10*(4), 398–406. doi:10.1097/00019442-200207000-00006 PMID:12095899

Van Orden, K., & Conwell, Y. (2011). Suicides in late life. *Current Psychiatry Reports*, *13*(3), 234–241. doi:10.1007/s11920-011-0193-3 PMID:21369952

Van Orden, K., Witte, A., Tracy, K., Cukrowicz, K. C., Braithwaite, S. R., Selby, E. A., & Joiner, T. E. (2010). The interpersonal theory of suicide. *Psychological Review*, *117*(2), 575–600. doi:10.1037/a0018697 PMID:20438238

Vanlaere, L., Bouckaert, F., & Gastmans, C. (2007). Care for suicidal older people: Current clinical-ethical considerations. *Journal of Medical Ethics*, *33*(7), 376–381. doi:10.1136/jme.2006.017897 PMID:17601861

Venkoba Rao, A. (1992). Suicide. In *Postgraduae Psychiatry*. New Delhi: BI Churchil Livingstone.

Vijaykumar, L. (2009). Religion-A protective factor in suicide. In A. Sharma (Ed.), Spirituality and mental health (pp. 357–367). Mount Abu: Indian Psychiatric Society.

Wærn, M. (2003). Physical illness and depression in the elderly. *Geriatrics & Aging*, *6*, 56–59.

Waern, M., Rubenowitz, E., & Wilhelmson, K. (2003). Predictors of suicide in the old elderly. *Gerontology*, *49*(5), 328–334. doi:10.1159/000071715 PMID:12920354

Wand, A.P.F., Peisah, C., Draper, B., Jones, C., & Brodaty, H. (2016). *Case Report Rational Suicide, Euthanasia, and the Very Old: Two Case Reports*. Academic Press.

Wasserman, D., & Ringskog, S. (2001). Suicide among elderly in Sweden. Stockholm: Academic Press.

Wendler, D. S. (2013). Problems with the consensus definition of the therapeutic misconception. *The Journal of Clinical Ethics*, *24*(4), 387–394. doi:10.1038/jid.2014.371 PMID:24597427

Wong, N. (2003). Reducing Suicide: A National Imperative. American Journal of Psychiatry, 160. doi:10.1176/appi.ajp.160.8.1534

World Health Organisation. (1968). *Prevention of suicide*. Geneva: WHO.

World Health Organization. (1999). *Facts and figures about suicide*. Geneva: World Health Organisation Press Office. Retrieved from http://scholar.google.com/scholar?hl=en&btnG=Search&q=intitle:Facts+and+Figures+About+Suicide#2

World Health Organization. (2014a). *Preventing suicide: a global imperative*. Geneva: WHO.

World Health Organization. (2014b). Preventing suicide. A global imperative. *Journal de l'Association Medicale Canadienne, 143*(7), 609–610.

Yesavage, J. A., Brink, T. L., Rose, T. L., Lum, O., Huang, V., Adey, M. B., & Leirer, V. O. (1983). Development and validation of a geriatric depression screening scale: A preliminary report. *Journal of Psychiatric Research*, *17*(1), 37–49. doi:10.1016/0022-3956(82)90033-4 PMID:7183759

KEY TERMS AND DEFINITIONS

Epidemiology: Epidemiology is the study of the distribution and determinants of health-related states or events (including disease), and the application of this study to the control of diseases and other health problems.

Mental Disorders: Mental disorders are usually associated with significant distress in social, occupational, or other important activities.

Old Age: Old age is the quality or state of being old and near the end of one's life.

Physical Disorders: A physical disorder is any type of physical condition that significantly impacts one or more major life activities.

Suicide: The intent of suicidal behavior, whether consciously or unconsciously motivated, is to permanently end one's life.

Chapter 24
Aging and Sexuality

Bheemsain Tekkalaki
Jawaharlal Nehru Medical College, India

ABSTRACT

Sexual health in general and issues of old age sexuality in particular are neglected by laymen and healthcare professionals alike. Contrary to popular beliefs, elderly individuals continue to have sexual desire and sexual activities, and they believe that healthy sexual expression is an important aspect of healthy aging. Sexual problems are more frequently found in the elderly. This chapter describes the various causes of sexual dysfunction, assessment, and management of sexual problems in the elderly.

INTRODUCTION

Sexuality is defined as the dynamic outcome of physical capacity, motivation, attitudes, opportunity for partnership and sexual conduct (Gilinsky, McClintock & Waite, 2014). Sexuality is an integral part of human life and healthy sexuality is associated with better quality of life. Human sexuality is influenced by various factors like culture, ethnicity, religion, peer group, education and personal experiences. The proportion of elderly individuals is increasing worldwide, due to improved life expectancy, which is in turn due to better healthcare (Agronin, 2010). World health organization (WHO) estimates show that the proportion of people aged 60 years or more will increase from 11% in 2000 to 22% in 2050 (WHO, 2012). Hence the health issues of elderly are expected to come to forefront including the sexual heath. Researches have shown that contrary to the popular beliefs, middle aged and older individuals continue to be interested in sexual activities, and are sexually active (Gott, 2006). However, the area of sexual health in general and old age sexuality in particular are highly neglected by the lay persons and the health care professional alike (Tailor & Gosney, 2011).

In this chapter, the authors has discussed the factors affecting old age sexuality, common sexual problems of elderly and their management.

DOI: 10.4018/978-1-5225-3480-8.ch024

NORMAL SEXUAL RESPONSE CYCLE

It is important to understand the normal sexual response cycle in order to better understand the age associated changes, impact of diseases and drugs on sexuality of elderly. Willian Masters and Virginia Johnson described the model of normal sexual response consisting of four phases namely Excitement or arousal, Plateau, orgasm and resolution (Masters & Johnson, 1996). Kaplan and others added another phase called desire. In this model, sexual cycle is not a linear process but rather a waxing and waning pattern of sexual arousal which may culminate in orgasm depending on the host factors (Agronin, 2010).

Desire, the first stage is characterized by psychological urge to seek out and respond to sexual interaction. Limbic system of the brain, particularly the hypothalamus is responsible for desire. Testosterone is essential for the adequate desire to be maintained in both the sexes. Desire is closely associated with, and is often inseparable from arousal, the second stage of sexual response. Arousal is the physiological process of sexual excitement. In both the sexes, arousal is triggered by sexual fantasies, thoughts or direct sexual stimulation and is mediated by parasympathetic nervous system. In men arousal leads to penile erection, where as in women it is characterized by clitoral enlargement, swelling of other genital tissues and breast and vaginal lubrication. Plateau, the third stage relatively short lasting and is characterized by sense of impending orgasm. Orgasm is characterized by euphoria in both the sexes. There are multiple contractions of seminal vesicles, vas deference in men leading to ejaculation of seminal fluid and multiple contractions of vaginal and pelvic muscles in females. In men, orgasm is brief, lasting for few seconds and usually happening only once before the refractory period, whereas, in women orgasm may last for many seconds to minutes and multiple orgasms are possible. Resolution is a state of relaxation which follows orgasm and it is a refractory period. Refractory period is longer in males than females (Meston, 1997; Agronin, 2010; Tekkalaki, 2015).

Effect of Aging on Normal Sexual Response Cycle

Aging brings in many important physiological changes, which together affect the sexual functioning in elderly. In men, sex hormone status is relatively stable from puberty until the 5th decade of life, later on, testosterone levels decline with age. The rate of decline is 1-2% per year. Free testosterone levels fall from a 3% reduction in 5th decade to up to 30% in the 7th decade. Apart from this, the levels of sex hormone binding globulin increases with age, leading to decrease in free testosterone levels (Camecho & Reyes-Ortiz, 2005). As a result, sexual desire in elderly men is reduced.

Physiological potency, (ability to attain erection sufficient for intercourse most of the times) also decreases with age. In a cross sectional study, potency decreased from 97% in men aged 50-59 to 76% in men aged 60-69 and 51% in men aged 70-79 (Taylor & Gonsey, 2011). The time required for erection is also prolonged in elderly men. Where a young man may attain a full erection in seconds, an elderly man may require several minutes to get a similar response. Also, due to decreased penile sensitivity, maintaining erection becomes more dependent on direct physical stimulation rather than visual, psychological or non-genital stimulation. Age related changes in adrenergic and cholinergic neuronal functioning may be one of the reasons behind it. Another reason may be increased deposition of connective tissue, lowering the elasticity of penile corporeal tissue and subsequently leading to increased venous leakage (Meston, 1997).

Due to decreased penile sensitivity, the plateau stage is prolonged as the age progresses and the earlier problems of pre-mature ejaculation may improve with age. However, the duration of orgasm decreases with age. Prostatic and urethral contractions are reduced in number and strength leading to decreased expulsive ejaculatory force. The volume of ejaculate also decreases with age and occasionally, orgasm may occur without ejaculation. The resolution after orgasm is rapid in older men marked by more rapid loss of vasocongestion. Refractory period is much longer in elderly men. Compared to young men who have a refractory period of few minutes, in an 80-year-old man refractory period may extend to several days, probably secondary to delayed restoration of neurotransmitter concentrations (Meston, 1997).

Other age related changes in men are: decrease in the testicular mass, reduced elasticity of seminal vescice and vas deference, slow rate of sperm production, enlargement of prostate gland (Swain, 2015). Aging also is associated with reduced muscle mass and strength, osteopenia, increased abdominal fat (Correa, Cozzensa de Silva & Rombaldi, 2103).

Sexual response cycle in women also undergoes significant changes with age. Due to decreased production of testosterone, desire in women decreases significantly with age, leading to hypoactive sexual desire disorder. Estrogen production also decreases after menopause, leading to reduced arousal. During the excitement phase, vaginal blood flow and genital engorgement are less intense. Uterine elevation is reduced, labia majora elevate to a lesser degree, breast congestion and nipple erection is reduced. Similar to the elder men, the plateau phase is prolonged in elderly women also. In contrast to men, orgasmic experience is relatively unaffected in women with age. Women may retain multi-orgasmic capacity, although vaginal contractions are weaker than before (Meston, 1997; Yee, 2010).

Decreased estrogen in postmenopausal women is accompanied with many changes in sexual functioning. Age related genital changes like reduction in pubic hair, loss of subcutaneous fat from mons pubis, atrophy of labia majora, and lack of vaginal elasticity ensue. Vaginal secretions decrease due to atrophy of Bartholin glands and decreased number of vaginal cells. Vaginal epithelium, which is dependent on estrogen, gets atrophied and loses glycogen, which results in loss of lactobacillus, lactic acid and increase in vaginal pH. These changes affect the vaginal microbial population and predispose for vaginal infections. Decreased vaginal lubrication and thin vaginal epithelium leads to pain, bleeding and burning sensations during coitus (Meston, 1997; Yee, 2010). A brief summary of age related changes in sexual physiology and the sexual dysfunctions following these changes are mentioned in table 1.

Chronic Diseases and Sexual Functioning

Elderly population is vulnerable for many chronic diseases which also affect the sexual health through various mechanisms. Diabetes mellitus is one of the common chronic illnesses affecting middle and elderly population. Diabetes affects both microvascular and nervous systems, affecting the sexual functioning. As early as within 5 years of onset of diabetes, 60% of men experience one or the other SD. Erectile dysfunction (ED) is reported in as many as 75% of the diabetic men older than 60 years. SD are common also in diabetic women. High levels of total cholesterol and low density lipids (LDL) in men above 40 years are associated with frequent SDs (Schiavi & Rehman, 1995; Camecho & Reyes-Ortiz, 2005).Other endocrine disorders associated with SD are hypothyroidism, hyperthyroidism, hypogonadism, hyperprolactinemia, and Cushing's disease (Meston, 1997). Hypertension, another common chronic illness in elderly, results in endothelial dysfunction and hence SDs. Adequate control of blood pressure may improve sexual functioning, provided that antihypertensive medications do not worsen the same (Camecho & Reyes-Ortiz, 2005).

Erectile dysfunction is a common co-morbidity with ischemic heart disease. Moreover, ED may be a risk factor for development of IHD, given the fact that men with ED have a twofold increased risk of

Table 1. Age-related changes in sexual physiology and associated sexual dysfunctions

Sl. No	Stage of Sexual Response	Normal Physiological/Psychological Changes	Age Associated Pathology	Sexual Dysfunctions
1	Desire	Seeking sexual pleasure, sexual fantasies	Decreased levels of testosterone leading to lack of desire	Hypoactive sexual desire
2	Arousal	Penile erection, vaginal lubrication, breast and clitoris engorgement etc.	Inadequate erections due to vascular, neurological changes, and lack of testosterone in men. Lack of vaginal lubrication in females due to low estrogen levels. Reduced blood supply to vagina	1. ED in males 2. Female sexual arousal disorder 3. Sexual pain disorder in women
3	Orgasm	Ejaculation in men, contraction of genital smooth muscles and euphoric feelings in both the partners.	Reduced volume of ejaculate due to reduced testosterone levels, abnormal sperm motility and morbidity	1. PME in men 2. Anorgasmia
4	Resolution	Relaxation phase- genital revert back to normal condition	Prolonged refractory period	

developing myocardial infarction (MI). Some researchers recommend that the diabetic men with ED should be subjected for stress test (Kloner, 2004; Blumentals, Gomez-Caminero, Joo & Vannappagari, 2004). Diseases affecting liver affect sexual functioning by either directly inhibiting testosterone secretion or by modulating the gonadotrophin release. Hypogonadism, gynecomastia, and decreased libido are common complications of cirrhosis of liver. Renal failure also affects serum testosterone levels, which may be reversed by erythropoietin or by renal transplant. Long standing pulmonary diseases also lead to low testosterone levels. Arthritis is causes pain and disability in elderly population, affecting the sexual performance (Camecho & Reyes-Ortiz, 2005).

Lower urinary tract symptoms (LUTS) are associated with increased risk of SD, independent of age. Benign prostatic hypertrophy (BPH) is the commonest cause of LUTS in elderly men. Sexual dysfunctions can be improved with treatment of urinary obstructive symptoms with alpha blockers. Prostate cancer is the second most prevalent cancer, present in 90% of men older than 80. Sexual dysfunctions are common complications of prostatic cancer or its treatment. Cerebrovascular accidents lead to not only physical disability but also impair the sexual functioning. Patients with left hemisphere strokes have marked decreases in sexual desire. Frequency of sexual intercourse is reduced markedly in these patients. Patients after stroke often develop hemi neglect and, which may impair sexual functioning and partners need to be educated about this. Parkinson's disease in both men and women is also associated with higher prevalence of sexual dysfunctions (Morley, 2006) Spinal cord injuries, temporal lobe epilepsy, multiple sclerosis and sensory neuropathies are also associated with sexual dysfunctions (Morley, 2006).

Breast cancer and its surgical intervention, both are known to affect the body image of women and hence the sexual functioning. A study found that between 21% and 39% of patients with breast cancer report SD, and the incidence of SD correlated with the degree of surgical intervention (Holzapfel, 1994). Hysterectomy, one of the commonest surgeries performed on women, affects the body image of women. Women may view this procedure as loss of femininity. This surgical procedure has not been found to have direct effect on sexual functioning, but some women report decreased orgasmic pleasure due to absence of uterine contractions. Interestingly, those who were operated for pain, excessive bleeding or cramping may feel relieved and may have a better sexual functioning after surgery (Meston, 1997).

Various other medical or surgical therapies can affect sexual functioning by interfering with neurological innervation of genitals. Pelvic irradiations, lower abdominal surgeries, prostate surgeries, are some examples. Abdominal surgeries can also affect the body image of the patients for e.g. having a colostomy bag. Some researchers have suggested measures like using a "sexy scarf" to conceal the bag and dietary alterations before planned sexual intercourse to enhance sexual functioning of such patients (Holzapfel, 1994).

Dementia, which is again a common problem of elderly can affect sexual functioning in many ways ranging from difficulty in cognitive sequencing during love making to erectile dysfunction. Spouses may have difficulty in reciprocating to the sexual advances from a person who no more remembers their names or to control the frequent overtures from a spouse who forgets that he had an episode intercourse few hours before. Male caregivers express their concern over the inability of their spouses to consent for the sexual acts, fearing that, in a sense, "raping" their wives (DeLamater, & Amelia Karraker, 2009). In a survey involving 38 spousal caregivers, all participants reported alterations in sexual functioning in their partners, and also reported that no healthcare professionals have inquired about the sexuality or educated them regarding this issue. Research suggesting that sexual dysfunction in males with AD are more frequent than the similar aged healthy men (Davis, Zeiss, Shea, & Tinklenberg, 1998).

Medications and Sexual Functioning

Apart from aging process and the diseases affecting elderly, many commonly used medications may also affect sexual functioning. On an average, people older than 65 years consume three times as many medications as their younger counterparts. The homeostatic reserve in all systems is poor in the elderly, leading to the frequent undesired side effects. Patients may believe these symptoms to be part of normal aging and may not report them to their physician.

Antihypertensive drugs are the most common offenders. Among the antihypertensive drugs, thiazide diuretics are the leading group of drugs to cause SD. Compared to other group of antihypertensives angiotensin-converting enzyme inhibitors and calcium channel blockers have relatively safer profile. The frequency of SD is found to be associated with the dosage of the antihypertensive medication. The SD due to antihypertensives may be because of either the reduced blood pressure or because of interference with normal cholinergic and adrenergic system functions which are essential for erection and ejaculation (Camecho & Reyes-Ortiz, 2005; DeLamater & Sill, 2005; Morley, 2006) Apart from antihypertensives, various other groups of medications like antiandrogens (used in prostate cancer), cardiovascular drugs (such as disopyramide), and anticancer agents can also cause SD. Many psychotropics can also cause SD. Antipsychotics, antidepressants, benzodiazepines and mood stabilizers are known to cause varieties of SD.

RESEARCH ON SEXUALITY AND AGING

It is a well-known fact that research in the field of old age sexuality is poor in both qualitative and quantitative terms. Worth mentioning here is the observation made by Calasanti and King (2015) in their review. Their literature review of two leading journals of men's studies, The Journal of Men's Studies (JMS) and Men and Masculinities (MM), from the inception of these journals through the spring of

2003, reflected the lack of research. The older of these, JMS, had published approximately 233 articles; MM, approximately 89. They inferred that, no articles purported to examine old men, old age, or age relations per se and only very recently has any mention of older age or ageism even occurred. Author's PubMed search with different combination of key words – old age, elderly, aging, sexuality and sexual dysfunction revealed only 1,413 articles, which included not only original research articles but reviews, met analysis and case reports as well.

Epidemiology of Sexual Practices and Sexual Dysfunction in Elderly

Older adults continue to be sexually active, albeit with a lesser frequency than their counterparts. Most of them also believe that sexual activity is an integral part of healthy life. However, sexual dysfunctions increase in frequency and severity with age.

The Massachusetts Male Aging Study (MMAS), interviewed men between 40 and 70 years of age, and found that, the probability of complete ED triples from 5% in 40 y old men to 15% in 70 y old men. (Camecho & Reyes-Ortiz, 2005).

According to the global study of sexual attitude and behavior (GSSAB), which included 27000 men and women aged 40- 80 years across 29 countries, nearly half of the men and 21% of the women reported having sexual intercourse in past one year. Only 17% of men and 23% of women reported that 'older people no longer want sex', and around two thirds of them were in favor of elderly persons seeking medical helps to improve sexual activity (Camecho & Reyes-Ortiz, 2005). American Association of Retired Persons (AARP) study included 1,384 men and women over 45 years. The study reported that, three out of four of them were sexually active. Around half of the individuals between 45-49 years of age had sex once a week, whereas, 30% of men and 24% of women aged 60-74 years had sex once a week. Majority of men without partner masturbate but 77% of women not (American Association for Retired Persons, 2004). A study also reported that men and women, who rated their health as being poor were more likely to be either sexually inactive or having sexual problems.

In women, hypoactive sexual desire, inhibited orgasm and dyspareunia are common SDs reported. Lindau et al. (2007) have observed that among the women aged between 57-85 years, 43% reported low desire, 39% had lubrication problems and 34% had anorgasmia. A Japanese study involving 2095 females with a median age of 48 years, reported that, prevalence of the symptom of orgasmic disorder, sexual desire disorder, arousal disorder, and lubrication disorder had increased significantly from 15.2% to 32.2%, 27.7% to 57.9%, 29.7% to 57.9%, and 12.5% to 51.2%, respectively from 30 to 60 years' of age. (Hisause et al., 2005). In a latin American study, authors have used Female Sexual Function Index Scale to assess sexual dysfunction in middle aged women and have found that, 56.8% of women had sexual dysfunction. Further, bad lubrication, use of alternative menopausal therapies, partner having SD, older age, bladder problems, negative perception of female health status, were reported to be significant risk factors of sexual dysfunction. (Blumel et al., 2009)

A comparison of important epidemiological studies pertaining to old age sexuality is given in table number 2.

Table 2. Some important epidemiological studies on old age sexual problems

S.No	Authors	Study Design	Important Findings
1.	Johannes et al. 2000	Population based longitudinal study involving 847 men between 40and 69 years of age (Massachusetts Male Aging Study)	The crude incidence rate for ED was 25.9 cases per 1,000 man-years (95% CI 22.5 to 29.9). The annual incidence rate increased with each decade of age and was 12.4 cases per 1,000 man-years (95% CI 9.0 to 16.9), 29.8 (24.0 to 37.0) and 46.4 (36.9 to 58.4) for men 40 to 49, 50 to 59 and 60 to 69 years old, respectively
2.	Nicolosi et al. 2004	Cross sectional survey of 27,500 men and women aged 40 to 80 year. (The global study of sexual attitudes and behaviors.)	More than 80% of the men and 65% of the women had had sexual intercourse during the preceding year. The most common dysfunctions were early ejaculation (14%) and erectile difficulties (10%) among the men and a lack of sexual interest (21%), inability to reach orgasm (16%), and lubrication difficulties (16%) among the women. Overall, 28% of the men and 39% of the women said that they were affected by at least one sexual dysfunction.
3.	Moniz et al. 2005	Population survey involving 1,199 Brazilians of 40-80 years age.	About 92.6% of men and 58.3% of women had had sexual intercourse during the preceding year. More than half of the men and women had done so more than once a week. Premature ejaculation (30.3%) was the commonest male sexual problem, followed by anorgasmia (14.0%), erectile difficulties (13.1%) and lack of sexual interest (11.2%). For women, the commonest sexual problems were lubrication difficulties (23.4%) and lack of sexual interest (22.7%).
4.	Addis et al. 2006	Population based cross sectional study of 2,109 women of 40-69 years. The Reproductive Risk Factors for Incontinence Study at Kaiser (RRISK)	Nearly three fourths of the women were sexually active. Of the sexually active women, 60% had sexual activity at least monthly, approximately two thirds were at least some- what satisfied, and 33% reported a problem in one or more domains.
5.	Lindau et al. 2007	A cross sectional survey of a national probability sample of 3005 U.S adults of 57 to 85 years of age.	The prevalence of sexual activity decreased with age (73% among respondents who were 57 to 64 years of age, 53% among respondents who were 65 to 74 years of age, and 26% among respondents who were 75 to 85 years of age); women were significantly less likely than men at all ages to report sexual activity.
6.	Laumann et al. 2009	Telephonic survey of 1491 individuals aged 40-80 years .	Overall, 79.4% of men and 69.3% of women had engaged in sexual intercourse in preceding 12 months . Early ejaculation (26.2%) and erectile difficulties (22.5%) were the most common male sexual problems. A lack of sexual interest (33.2%) and lubrication difficulties (21.5%) were the most common female sexual problems.
7.	Hyde et al. 2010	Cohort study; Community sample of 3274 men between 75 to 95 years (Australia)	Sex was considered at least somewhat important by 48.8% (95% CI, 47.0% to 50.6%), and 30.8% (CI, 29.1% to 32.5%) had had at least 1 sexual encounter in the past 12 months. Of the latter, 56.5% were satisfied with the frequency of activity, whereas 43.0% had sex less often than preferred.
8.	Corona et al. 2010	Cross sectional multi-centric study involving 3,369 community dwelling men aged 40-79 years. European Male Ageing Study (EMAS).	Around 30% of men reported erectile dysfunction (ED) and 6% reported severe orgasmic impairment, Only 38% of men reporting ED were concerned about it. Furthermore, concern about ED increased with age, peaking in the 50-59 years age band, but decreased thereafter.
9.	Wang et al. 2014	Mail-in survey of 606 community dwelling adults of San Diego county, aged 50-99 years.	Over 80% of respondents had engaged in sexual activity in the past year, over 70% engaged in sexual activity weekly or more than once a week, and over 60% were somewhat or very satisfied with their sex lives.
10.	Rao et al. 2015	A cross sectional survey of 259 participants aged above 60. (India)	Only 27.4% of the individuals above 60 years were sexually active, and it progressively dropped as age advanced and none were sexually active after 75 years of age. Among the sexually active males, erectile dysfunction (ED) was prevalent in 43.5%, premature ejaculation in 10.9%, hypoactive sexual desire disorder (HSSD) in 0.77% and anorgasmia in 0.38% of the subjects. Among females, arousal disorder was prevalent in 28%, HSSD in 16%, anorgasmia in 20% and dyspareunia in 8% of the subjects.
11.	Lee et al. 2016	Onetime assessment (cross sectional) of a cohort of 6201 participants of 50-90 years age. (English Longitudinal study of aging)	Difficulties most frequently reported by sexually active women related to becoming sexually aroused (32%) and achieving Orgasm (27%), while for men it was erectile function (39%). Sexual health concerns most commonly reported by women related to their level of sexual desire (11%) and frequency of sexual activities (8%). Among men it was level of sexual Desire (15%) and erectile difficulties (14%)

Socio-Cultural Issues Related to Sexual Functioning in Elderly

Sexuality in general and old age sexuality in particular have significant socio-cultural implications. Callan (2006) asserted that sexuality encompasses personal, cultural and social identity rather than just sexual behaviours or orientation (Elias & Ryan, 2011). in this section, the author discusses various socio-cultural issues that affect the old age sexuality. Misconceptions about old age sexuality are prevalent in lay people and health care workers alike. Many older people believe that sexual expression is not natural and healthy for their age. They look to their younger counterparts as a reference group, leading to dissatisfaction abut one's physical appearance and hence sexual functioning (DeLamater& Moorman, 2007). Doctors also are no different. Inquiring about sexual health remains a low priority for many general practitioners, especially if the client is elderly (Andrews, 2007).

On other hand, as discussed above, researches started revealing that the older adults continue to be sexually active and consider sexuality to be important, a new norm of sexuality in older age has been established: which Hinchliff and Gott (2008) refer to as the "sexy oldie". A representation of "successful" ageing being able to maintain a "youthful" sexual performance. Within this new norm, sexual performance still adheres to a heteronormative framework of sex, with penetration considered as the "ultimate", desirable sexual act. Biomedical models of sexuality which focus on sexual "dysfunction" and age often reinforce this with a fixation on restoring penetrative capability through the facilitation of erections and remedies for vaginal dryness (Fileborn et al., 2015).

Whether this binary model of old age sexuality as asexual or "sexy oldie" accurately reflects practices, experiences or desires of older people is unknown. Indeed, a more notable finding emerging from qualitative studies is the heterogeneity of older women's sexual lives. It is argued that, the definitions of sex based around penetration and "youthful" models of sex obscure the broader range of practices, and the greater focus on intimate touch and affection that older people actually want to engage in (Fileborn et al., 2015).

Availability of sexual partner is an important issue of old age. In United States, women have about 5 years longer life expectancy than men. Gender asymmetries in physical health complicates the matter further with women having poorer health and more disability then men across all ages (Aversa et al. 2014) Those, who are devoid of partners for prolonged period of time drift into a state of sexual disinterest. Women "turn off" their sexual interest as a coping mechanism, which prevents frustration and depression (DeLamater & Moorman, 2007). For those who have sexual partner, health condition of the partner is a limiting factor. Monotony in sexual relationship and overfamiliarity with the partner may also lead to loss of sexual desire (DeLamater & Sill, 2005). "Honeymoon effect", as it has been called, is characterized by a sharp fall in the frequency of sexual activities over the first year of marriage. Kaas coined the term "Geriatric Sexuality Breakdown Syndrome" to describe the process of internalizing social attitudes towards sexuality in older age (Karraker, DeLamater& Schwartz, 2011).

Very little is understood about the sexual problems of sexual minorities. Existing literature, however, suggests that homosexual individuals continue to be sexually active and satisfied in their older ages. (Agronin, 2010). However, Fannin (2006) reported that there was a significant and invisible older gay population in care homes for whom personal identity and acceptance were important, but isolation and exclusion were the norm (Fannin, 2006). In their review, Garnets and Peplau (2006) observed that, only two studies, both by Kehoe (1986, 1988), have assessed sexual issues of lesbians over age 60. A total of 150 women aged 60 to 86 were recruited. Nearly half of the women in each study had previously been in heterosexual relationships. Most lesbians who had had sex with both men and women viewed lesbian relationships as less sexually demanding and more sexually gratifying, emotional, affectionate, and sharing than heterosexual ones (Kehoe, 1986). In both samples, a majority of women characterized sex as an important aspect of a lesbian relationship.

A majority of the women (68% in 1986 and 53% in 1988) were celibate and had had no sexual experience with a woman in the preceding year. Most celibacy was caused by lack of opportunity and was not by choice. Perhaps because of the high rates of celibacy, only 33% of lesbians in the 1988 sample reported that they were somewhat to very satisfied with their sex life during the preceding year (Kehoe, 1986).

Sexuality among the inmates of long term care centers is much more neglected and stigmatized. Staffs of the long term care facilities though acknowledge the sexual needs of the residents, most of them do not think it is necessary for the residents to be sexually active. They also are pessimistic about the possibility of active sexual life in such centers, leading to low rate of sexual life in such centers. In contrary, literature suggests that, interest in sex does not necessarily diminish with admission to care home but engagement in sexual activity diminishes (Agronin, 2010; Elias & Ryan 2011).

Unlocked door policy, shared rooms, regular room checks, and staff access to medical information are found to be hindrance to residents' perception of privacy. Furthermore, the high prevalence of chronic illnesses in residential homes and medications used to treat them also add to the problems (Frankowski & Clark, 2009).

Mental health professionals have an important role to play in eliminating these barriers. Educating both staff and residents about the residents' right to sexual expression. Policies to promote healthy sexual practices in residential care centers, wherever possible should be formed. To carry out such policies, clinical staff in residential care settings should include a detailed sexual history during the admission process, assessing the residents' concerns and capabilities with respect to normal sexual functioning. Providing private rooms for married couples or those who wish to stay together, ensuring privacy by using "Do not disturb" signs on doors are few suggested measures. A brief overview of bio-psycho-social factors affecting old age sexuality is depicted in table 3.

ASSESSMENT AND MANAGEMENT OF SEXUAL PROBLEMS OF OLDER ADULTS

Sexual history taking should include individuals earlier sexual experiences, present level of sexual functioning, attitudes towards the partner and sexuality, meanwhile caution should be taken to deal with these issues sensitively, as these are some of the most personal information patient will ever disclose to anyone. Developing a good rapport is very much essential, so is active involvement of the patient's partner in the therapeutic process (Agronin, 2010).

Wherever appropriate, post-menopausal women should be inquired directly about symptoms of urogenital atrophy as the environment of care may not feel appropriate for patients to initiate conversation even if it is causing significant distress (DeLamater & Karraker, 2007). It may be helpful to open the conversation by first asking permission to ask more personal questions. Elderly patients often attend with their adult children, and might not be comfortable discussing sexual issues in presence of them. Health care providers (HCPs) should understand that many elderly people would prefer discussing sexual issues with somebody of the same gender and as close to their age range as possible, and hence appointments with colleagues should be offered as appropriate (Taylor & Gosney, 2011) Although it is important to be aware of older people's sexuality, care must be taken not to over-sexualize the ageing

Table 3. Bio-psycho-social factors affecting old age sexuality

Sl. No	Domains	Relevant Factors Affecting Sexuality
1.	**Biological**	Decline in testosterone levels in both males and females Decline in estrogen levels in post-menopausal women Neuronal and vascular factors Chronic medical illness Multiple medications
2.	**Psychological**	Motivation Psychological health Self-perception/ Body image Cognitive functioning Sexual information Attitude towards sex
3.	**Social**	Availability of partner Sexual satisfaction Relationship satisfaction Health issues in partner Cultural beliefs

(DeLamer & Still, 2005, DeLamer & Karraker, 2007)

process, nor to over-medicalize declining sexual function and interest. The heavy involvement of drug companies in the definition of female sexual dysfunction as a medical diagnosis is potentially worrying (Taylor & Gosney, 2011). HCPs also need to be aware of and deal with their own emotional reactions and attitudes towards the clients (the countertransference) without letting any of their prejudices affect patient's management. This can be managed by appropriate supervision and a multidisciplinary approach when possible (Taylor & Gosney, 2011).

A thorough physical examination, followed by a routine blood chemistry analysis may be supplemented by tests like serum testosterone and prolactin levels, thyroid functioning test, prostate-specific antigens in men, wherever necessary. Some specialized tests for ED are nocturnal penile tumescence test and penile duplex ultrasonography (Agronin, 2010).

The PLISSIT model (Annon, 1976) is useful for management of common sexual dysfunctions by general practitioners and primary healthcare workers, which can be used in geriatric population as well with appropriate modifications. The acronym PLISSIT stands for Permission (P), Limited Information (LI) Specific Suggestions (SS), and Intensive Therapy (IT), which is briefly explained in below:

- **Permission:** It involves "permitting" the individuals to be sexual ("there is nothing wrong with masturbation, you can practice it regularly), to desire sexual activity and to discuss sexuality (Many mature adults continue to have sexual activity, and sometimes face sexual problems, you can discuss such issues with me", Permitting helps in resolving myths, misconceptions and hence promote sexual health.
- **Limited Information**: Another important step in treatment process in education of both the partners about the normal sexual functioning and the dysfunctions. Meanwhile, they can be helped to recognize sexuality as a form of physical and psychological intimacy, and not just as sexual intercourse. Educating about 'lifestyle factors' (e.g. smoking, obesity, blood sugar levels) which can affect sexual functioning may assist patients in making healthier choices (Taylor & Gosney, 2011).

- **Specific Suggestions:** Couples with one or both partners having chronic disease or disability face many practical problems. They can be educated to shift their focus from intercourse to foreplay and to find ways to perform sexual activity within their limitations such as fatigue or weakness. Palliative treatments like analgesics for pain, inhalers for shortness of breath, physiotherapy for joint pains etc. should be used judiciously. Appropriate treatment of associated psychiatric co-morbidities is also essential.
- **Intensive Therapy:** When problems are more challenging, it is advised to refer clients to specialists for intensive therapy. One such therapy is cognitive therapy, which involve training the patient to shift the focus on the pleasurable sensations of the encounter rather than the anticipation of failure. Correcting the distorted cognitions is another essential cognitive technique. Rosen, Leiblum, and Spector (1994) list eight types of cognitive distortions that may affect sexual function. These include: (1) all or nothing thinking, e.g., ''I am a complete failure because I ejaculate quickly'', (2) overgeneralization, e.g., ''If I had trouble controlling my ejaculation last night, I won't be able to today as well'', (3) disqualifying the positive, e.g. ''My wife says our lovemaking is satisfying because she doesn't want to hurt my feelings'', (4) mind reading, e.g. ''I don't need to ask, I know how she felt about last night'', (5) fortune telling, e.g., ''I am sure I will fail tonight'', (6) emotional reasoning, e.g. ''Because a man feels something is true, it must be'', (7) categorical imperatives, i.e., should, ought to and musts dominate the man's cognitive processes, and (8) catastrophizing, e.g., ''If I fail tonight my partner will leave me". Cognitive correction, an essential skill used in cognitive therapies needs to be employed to correct distorted thoughts.

Behavioral technique like sensate focus therapy is also useful. Sensate focus helps to reduce performance anxiety. In sensate focus therapy, couple practices physical relaxation techniques during non-pressured sensual touching. Once the partners feel relaxed and physically intimate together without sexual stimulation, they are asked to gradually progress to genital stimulation and then to intercourse. Squeeze technique is advised for premature ejaculation (PME), in which the partner gently squeezes the base of man's penis before penetration to reduce sensation and postpone ejaculation. However, it demands adequate co-operation from the female partner (Agronin, 2010).Many modifications in the usual sexual practices are needed in older individuals like switching to postures with minimal exertion, such as lying side by side or one partner kneeling on a soft pillow and supporting himself or herself with a soft pillow.

When sexual dysfunctions are secondary to medications, possible management options are: waiting for the side effects to come down, if no change is observed then dose reduction can be tried. Simplifying the regimen by stopping the medicines which are not absolutely essential is another useful method. Drug holidays wherever possible or replacing current drugs with the one with least possible sexual side effects can be considered. In some cases SDs due to psychotropics can be alleviated with specific antidotes. Yohimbine, amantadine, cyproheptadine, for SSRI induced SD, bethanecol, methylphenidate, bromocriptine for SD caused by antipsychotics are some examples. Phosphodiesterase 5 (PDE-5) inhibitors like sildenafil, tadalafil are also useful in reversing antidepressant induced SDs. In some unfortunate cases, when none of the above mentioned measures are helpful, the patient must be helped to choose between discontinuing the needed drug and coping with the sexual dysfunctions (Clayton, Alkis, & Votta, J.G., 2017).

ERECTILE DYSFUNCTION

Erectile dysfunction is the commonest sexual dysfunction in men. Which, according to ICD 10 is, the difficulty in developing or maintaining an erection suitable for satisfactory intercourse (WHO, 1992) Erection happening in other situations like early morning erections, erections during masturbation and during intercourse with another partner are psychogenic in nature, other cases should be thoroughly evaluated for organic causes, which are more common in elderly men (Agronin, 2010). Men often equate sexual functioning with masculinity, and hence old men with ED may perceive it as an indicator of loss of masculinity. Anxiety, stress, and depression can lead to ED in elderly men. ED in turn may lead to negative emotional states like anxiety and depression.

Pharmacological treatment of erectile dysfunction in elderly patients is similar to that of younger clients. PDE5 inhibitors are the first line treatment for ED. Sildenafil, tadalafil and vardenafil, the three PDE5 inhibitors available in market are equally efficacious in improving erectile functions in both organic and psychogenic ED. They act by inhibiting the endothelial enzyme phosphodiesterase 5. PDE 5 is responsible for breakdown of cyclic GMP to GMP. Inhibition of PDE 5 leads to increased cyclic GMP in endothelium, resulting in relaxation of endothelial smooth muscles, allowing more blood to drain in to the penile cavernous tissue and hence penile erection. These medications should be taken half an hour to 4 hour before the sexual activity. Adequate physical and psychological stimulation is essential after taking medicines, without which erection does not happen. Headache, flushing, gastric discomfort, dizziness, are potential adverse effects. PDE5 inhibitors should be avoided in patients taking nitrates (e.g. nitroglycerine) and should be used in caution in patients with abnormal penile shape, severe hepatic and renal impairments and in diseases which increases the risk of priapism, like sickle cell anemia, leukemia and multiple myeloma. Nonarthritic anterior ischemic optic neuropathy (NOIAN) is an extremely rare but potentially severe adverse effect of PDE5 inhibitors, which manifests as sudden loss of vision. (Lewis, Yaun, & Wang, 2008).

Testosterone replacement therapy may be helpful in patients with hypogonadism as a cause for ED. However, presence of prostate or bladder cancer is a contraindication for the same. Patients who have vascular causes of ED may be helped by microsurgical re-vascularization ((Lewis, Yaun, & Wang, 2008).

Penile intracavernosal self-injection of alprostadil, a synthetic prostaglandin E1 works by increasing smooth muscle relaxation and dilations of arteries of cavernous tissue. Injection of this agent into the base of penis 10-20 minutes before sex results in adequate erections in 70-80% of men. Local pain, scar formation, and rarely priapism are some adverse effects. Alprostadil is also available as urethra suppository. Vacuum suction devices and penile implants are other options available. Vacuum device consist of a plastic tube with an attached pump which fits over the penis. On creating the vacuum, blood flow increases into the penis leading to erection. A ring is placed around the base of the penis to maintain the erection. Vacuum devices are effective but require some dexterity and may cause numbness, bruises, and delayed ejaculation. Penile implants, though effective, are less frequently used. Different kinds of implants are available ranging from inflatable devises to semi rigid devices. Mechanical failures, risk associated with surgery, infections are some important problems associated with these devices. As surgical procedure to place these devices destroys the cavernous tissue, patient may need a prosthetic device permanently to achieve erections (Agronin, 2010).

PREMATURE EJACULATION

Premature ejaculation is defined in ICD 10 as the inability to control ejaculation sufficiently for both partners to enjoy sexual interaction (WHO, 1992). In severe cases ejaculation may occur even before the penetration. Unlike ED, PME is more likely to be non-organic, like secondary to erectile dysfunction. Selective serotonin reuptake inhibitors (SSRIs) have changed the way premature ejaculation was treated before. SSRIs cause delayed ejaculation, the property used to treat PME. Dapoxetine is an ultra-short acting SSRI, FDA approved for premature ejaculation. The drug can be taken on need basis, half an hour before sex. PDE5 inhibitors are also effective in treating PME, both alone and in combination with SSRIs (Rowland, & McMohan, 2008).

HYPOACTIVE SEXUAL DESIRE IN WOMEN

Hypoactive sexual desire in elderly women sometimes may be because of poor self-image due to age associated changes. Negative societal attitude towards old age sexuality may add to the problem. Treatment of low sexual desire should start with proper sex education to overcome psychological and social barriers. Estrogen replacement therapy may be helpful in improving the sexual desire. However, in post-menopausal women lack of desire may predominantly because of low testosterone levels, which may be benefitted by testosterone replacement therapy. Weight gain, virilization, liver dysfunction and Clotting factor dysfunction are some adverse effects of testosterone replacement therapy. Studies on sildenafil in female sexual dysfunction are largely inconclusive (Lankveld, 2008).

FEMALE ORGASMIC DISORDER

Orgasmic disorder is characterized by persistent or recurrent delay in or absence of orgasm after a normal sexual excitement phase. Often a comorbidity of hypoactive sexual desire and shares common socio-cultural etiologies explained above. Individual sex therapy involving relaxation exercise, sensual self-stimulation and masturbation with aid of a vibrator to enhance clitoral stimulation are suggested. Sensate focus therapy may also be helpful Dyspareunia, is recurrent pain associated with sexual intercourse. The disorder is common in old age, especially in post-menopausal women. Many medical/ gynecological conditions may cause dyspareunia like vulvitis, vulvo vestibulitis, and many surgical or gynecological procedures involving pelvis. Gynecological examination and wherever needed, treatment of underlying condition is an essential first step in treatment of dyspareunia. Sex therapies encouraging foreplay, massages, and sensate focus therapy are advised in chronic and difficult to treat cases. Estrogen replacement therapy can be helpful in post-menopausal women, in whom pain symptoms may be because of lack of lubrication. There is no data as to how common the condition of vaginismus in elderly women. It can be treated with conjoint sex therapy, use of vaginal dilators of graduated sizes to overcome involuntary vaginal contraction (Agronin, 2010).

FUTURE RESEARCH DIRECTIONS

The importance of old age sexuality will only increase in coming days. Health care providers play an important role in promoting the sexual health in elderly. The Internet is likely to play a role in knowledge dissemination and should be judiciously used by all stake holders to disseminate the proper scientific knowledge among elderly with dedicated websites and forums. If better patient care is to be provided, significantly more clinical research is needed regarding understudied and neglected populations, including older gay men and lesbians, as well as the overarching economic, cultural, and racial issues related to the sexuality of mature adults (Hillman, 2008). Currently available oral pharmacotherapy has limited efficacy in older adults due to the lack of endogenous NO supply. Some of the newer compounds such as guanylyl cyclase activators, Rho-kinaminhibitors and maxi-K channel openers bypass the NO pathway, and are therefore expected to have good efficacy in difficult to treat older patients suffering from ED (Albersen,Orabai, & Lue, 2012).

CONCLUSION

Healthy sexuality is important for elderly, and contrary to popular beliefs, elderly people continue to be sexually active, albeit with reducing frequency. Negative attitude towards old age sexuality are prevalent in laymen and in healthcare professionals alike, and negatively affect the help seeking behavior. Sexual dysfunctions are common in old age and may affect the quality of life of the subjects. Active screening for the sexual dysfunctions should be the integral part of medical evaluation. Patients with sexual dysfunctions like ED should be screened for cardiovascular risks, and modifying these risks may in turn improve sexual functioning. Appropriate use of non-pharmacological and pharmacological treatment processes may help in restoration of normal sexual functioning in elderly.

REFERENCES

Addis, I. B., Van Den Eeden, S. K., Wassel-fyr, C. L., Vittinghoff, E., Brown, J. S., & Thom, D. H. (2006). Sexual Activity and Function in Middle-Aged and Older women. *Obstetrics and Gynecology, 107*(4), 755–764. doi:10.1097/01.AOG.0000202398.27428.e2 PMID:16582109

Agronin, M. E. (2010). Sexual disorders. In D. G. Blazer & D. C. Steffens (Eds.), *The American Psychiatric Publishing Textbook of Geriatric Psychiatry* (4th ed.; pp. 357–373). Washington, DC: The American Psychiatric Publishing.

Albersen, M., & Lue, F. (2012). *Evaluation and Treatment of Erectile Dysfunction in the Aging Male: A Mini-Review*. Academic Press. 10.1159/000329598

American Association for Retired Persons. (2004). *Sexuality at Midlife and Beyond: 2004 Update of Attitude and Behaviors*. Available at http://assets.aarp.org/rgcenter/general/2004_sexuality.pdf

Andrews, C. N. (2007). Sex and the older man GP perceptions and management. *Australian Family Physician, 36*(10), 867–869. PMID:17925912

Annon, J. (1976). The PLISSIT Model: A proposed conceptual scheme for the behavioural treatment of sexual problems. *Journal of Sex Education and Therapy*, *2*(1), 1–15. doi:10.1080/01614576.1976.11074483

Aversa, A., Donini, L. M., Bruzziches, R., LaCava, R., Raso, F. M., & Sinclair, A. (2014). Coordinating Care Aspects Related to Sexual Health in the Aging Male. *International Journal of Endocrinology*, *1-3*. doi:10.1155/2014/653587 PMID:24829576

Beutel, J. E., Chedraui, P., Baron, G., Belzares, E., Bencosme, A., & Calle, A. (2009). Sexual dysfunction in middle-aged women: A multicenter Latin American study using the Female Sexual Function Index. *Menopause (New York, N.Y.)*, *16*(6), 1139–1148. doi:10.1097/gme.0b013e3181a4e317 PMID:19458559

Blumentals, W. A., Gomez-Caminero, A., Joo, S., & Vannappagari, V. (2004). Should erectile dysfunction be considered as a marker for acute myocardial infarction? Results from a retrospective cohort study. *International Journal of Impotence Research*, *16*(4), 350–353. doi:10.1038/sj.ijir.3901174 PMID:14985780

Calasanti, T., & King, N. (2005). Firming the Floppy Penis Age, Class, and Gender Relations in the Lives of Old Men. *Men and Masculinities*, *8*(1), 3–23. doi:10.1177/1097184X04268799

Camecho, M. E., & Reyes-Ortiz, C. A. (2005). Sexual dysfunction in the elderly: Age or disease? *International Journal of Impotence Research*, *17*(S1), S52–S56. doi:10.1038/sj.ijir.3901429 PMID:16391544

Clayton, A. H., Alkis, A. R., & Votta, J. G. (2017). Sexual dysfunctions due to psychotropic medications. *PsychiatrClin NA*, *39*(3), 427–463.

Corona, G., Lee, D.M., Forti, G., O'Connor, D.B., Maggi, M., O'Neill, T.W., & …, Wu, F.C. (2009). Age-related changes in general and sexual health in middle-aged and older men: Results from the European Male Ageing Study (EMAS). *Journal of Sexual Medicine*, *7*(4), 1362–1380. PMID:19929914

Correa, L.Q., Cozzensa, da Silva, M., & Rombaldi, A.J. (2013). Sexual dysfunction symptoms in men age 40 or older: Prevalence and associated factors. *Revista Brasileira de Epidemiologia*, *16*(2), 444–453. PMID:24142015

Davis, H. D., Zeiss, A. M., Shea, E. A., & Tinklenberg, J. R. (1998). Sexuality and Intimacy in Alzheimer's Patients and their partners. *Sexuality and Disability*, *16*(3), 193–283. doi:10.1023/A:1023047125906

DeLamater, J., & Amelia Karraker, A. B. (2009). Sexual Functioning in Older Adults. *Current Psychiatry Reports*, *11*(1), 6–11. doi:10.1007/s11920-009-0002-4 PMID:19187702

DeLamater, J., & Moorman, S. M. (2007). Sexual Behavior in Later Life. *Journal of Aging and Health*, *19*(6), 921–946. doi:10.1177/0898264307308342 PMID:18165289

DeLamater, J. D., & Sill, M. (2005). Sexual Desire in Later Life. *Journal of Sex Research*, *42*(2), 138–149. doi:10.1080/00224490509552267 PMID:16123844

Elias, J., & Ryan, A. (2011). A review and commentary on the factors that influence expressions of sexuality by older people in care homes. *Journal of Clinical Nursing*, *20*(11-12), 1668–1676. doi:10.1111/j.1365-2702.2010.03409.x PMID:21323776

Elias, J., Ryan, A., Elias, J., & Ryan, A. (2014). A review and commentary on the factors that influence expressions of sexuality by older people in care homes sexuality by older people in care homes. *Journal of Clinical Nursing*, *20*(11-12), 1668–1676. doi:10.1111/j.1365-2702.2010.03409.x PMID:21323776

Fannin, A. (2006). Gay and grey: Lifting the lid on sexuality and ageing. *Working With Older People*, *10*(4), 31–34. doi:10.1108/13663666200600069

Fileborn, B., Thorpe, R., Hawkes, G., Minichiello, V., Pitts, M., Dune, T., & Pitts, M. (2015). Sex, desire and pleasure: Considering the experiences of older Australian women. *Sexual and Relationship Therapy*, *30*(1), 117–130. doi:10.1080/14681994.2014.936722 PMID:25544829

Frankowski, A. C., & Clark, L. J. (2009). Sexuality and Intimacy in Assisted Living: *Residents'. Perspectives and Experiences Sexuality Research & Social Policy*, *6*(4), 25–37. doi:10.1525/srsp.2009.6.4.25 PMID:25568640

Galinsky, A., McClintock, M. K., & Waite, L. J. (2014). Sexuality and physical contact in national social life, health, and aging project wave 2. *The Journals of Gerontology. Series B, Psychological Sciences and Social Sciences*, *69*(8Suppl 2), S83–S98. doi:10.1093/geronb/gbu072 PMID:25360027

Garnets, L., & Peplau, L. A. (2006). Sexuality in the Lives of Aging Lesbian and Bisexual Women. In D. Kimmel, T. Rose, & S. David (Eds.), *Lesbian, Gay, Bisexual, and Transgender Aging* (pp. 70–90). New York: Columbia University Press. doi:10.7312/kimm13618-005

Gott, M. (2014). Sexual health and the new aging. *Age and Ageing*, *35*(2), 106–107. doi:10.1093/ageing/afj050 PMID:16431853

Hillman, J. (2008). *Sexual Issues and Aging Within the Context of Work With Older Adult Patients*. Academic Press. doi:10.1037/0735-7028.39.3.290

Hisause, S., Kumamoto, Y., Sato, Y., Masumori, N., Horita, H., Kato, R., ... Itoh, N. (2005). Prevalence of female sexual dysfunction symptoms and its relationship to quality of life: A Japanese female cohort study. *Urology*, *65*(1), 143–148. doi:10.1016/j.urology.2004.08.003 PMID:15667880

Holzapfel, S. (1994). Aging and Sexuality. *Canadian Family Physician Medecin de Famille Canadien*, *40*, 748–766. PMID:8199527

Hyde, Z., Flicker, L., Hankey, G. J., Almeda, O. P., McCaul, K. A., Paul, C., ... Yeap, B. B. (2010). Prevalence of Sexual Activity and Associated Factors in MenAged 75 to 95 Years. *Annal International Medicine*, *153*(11), 693–702. doi:10.7326/0003-4819-153-11-201012070-00002 PMID:21135292

Johannes, B. C., Araujo, A. B., Feldman, H. A., Derby, C. A., Kleinman, K. P., & McKinlay, J. B. (2000). Incidence of erectile dysfunction in men 40 to 69 years old: Longitudinal results from the Massachusetts Male Aging Study. *The Journal of Urology*, *163*(2), 460–463. doi:10.1016/S0022-5347(05)67900-1 PMID:10647654

Karraker, A., DeLamater, J., & Schwartz, C. R. (2011). Sexual frequency decline from midlife to later life. *The Journals of Gerontology. Series B, Psychological Sciences and Social Sciences*, *66*(4). PMID:21666143

Kehoe, M. (1986). Lesbians over 65: A triply invisible minority. *Journal of Homosexuality*, *12*(3-4), 139–152. doi:10.1300/J082v12n03_12 PMID:3760557

Kloner, R. A. (2004). Assessment of cardiovascular risk in patients with erectile dysfunction: Focus on the diabetic patient. *Endocrine*, *23*(2-3), 125–129. doi:10.1385/ENDO:23:2-3:125 PMID:15146090

Lankveld, J. V. (2008). Problems with Sexual Interest and Desire in Women. In D. L. Rowland & L. A. Incrocci (Eds.), *Sexual and Gender Identity Disorders* (pp. 154–187). John Wiley & Sons. doi:10.1002/9781118269978.ch6

Laumann, E. O., Glasser, D. B., Neves, R. C., & Moreira, E. D. Jr. (2009). A population-based survey of sexual activity, sexual problems and associated help-seeking behavior patterns in mature adults in the United States of America. *International Journal of Impotence Research*, *21*(3), 171–178. doi:10.1038/ijir.2009.7 PMID:19242482

Laumann, E. O., Palik, A., & Rosen, R. C. (1999). Sexual dysfunction in the United States: Prevalence and predicters. *Journal of the American Medical Association*, *281*(6), 537–544. doi:10.1001/jama.281.6.537 PMID:10022110

Lee, D. M., Nazroo, J., O'Connor, D. B., Blake, M., & Pendleton, N. (2016). Sexual Health and Well-being among Older Men and Women in England: Findings from the English Longitudinal Study of Ageing. *Archives of Sexual Behavior*, *45*(1), 133–144. doi:10.1007/s10508-014-0465-1 PMID:25624001

Lewis, R. W., Yaun, J., & Wang, R. (2008). Male sexual arousal disorder. In D. L. Rowland & L. A. Incrocci (Eds.), *Sexual and Gender Identity Disorders* (pp. 30–67). John Wiley & Sons.

Lindau, S. T., Schumm, P. L., Laumann, E. O., Levinson, W., O'Muircheartaigh, C. A., & Waite, L. J. (2007). A Study of Sexuality and Health among Older Adults in the United States. *The New England Journal of Medicine*, *357*(8), 762–774. doi:10.1056/NEJMoa067423 PMID:17715410

Masters, W. H., & Johnson, V. E. (1970). *Human sexual response*. Boston, MA: Little, Brown.

Meston, C. M. (1997). Aging and sexuality. Western Journal of Medicine, 167, 285-290.

Morley, J. E. (2005). Sexuality and Aging. In Principles and Practice of Geriatric Medicine (4th ed.). John Wiley & Sons Ltd.

Nicolosi, A., Laumann, E. O., Glasser, D. B., Brock, G., King, R., & Gingell, C. (2006). Sexual activity, sexual disorders and associated help-seeking behavior among mature adults in five Anglophone countries from the Global Survey of Sexual Attitudes and Behaviors (GSSAB). *Journal of Sex & Marital Therapy*, *32*(4), 331–342. doi:10.1080/00926230600666469 PMID:16709554

Rosen, R., Leiblum, S., & Spector, I. (1994). Psychologically based treatment for male erectile disorder: A cognitive-interpersonal model. *Journal of Sex & Marital Therapy*, *20*(2), 67–85. doi:10.1080/00926239408403419 PMID:8035472

Rowland, D. L., & McMohan, C. (2008). Premature Ejaculation. In D. L. Rowland & L. A. Incrocci (Eds.), *Sexual and Gender Identity Disorders* (pp. 68–99). John Wiley & Sons. doi:10.1002/9781118269978

Sathyanarayana, Rao, T.S., Ismail, S., Darshan, M.S., & Tandon, A. (2015). Sexual disorders among elderly: Anepidemiological study in south Indian rural population. *Indian Journal of Psychiatry*, *57*, 236–241. doi:10.4103/0019-5545.158143 PMID:26600575

Schiavi, R.C., & Rehman. (1995). Sexuality and aging. *The Urologic Clinics of North America*, *22*, 711–726. PMID:7483124

Swain, L. (2015). Human reproductive biology: Changes through life. In Developmental perspectives on human sexuality (pp. 29-34) Bhubaneshwar: Indian Institute of Sexology.

Tailor, A., & Gosney, M. A. (2011). Sexuality in older age: Essential considerations for health care professionals. *Age and Ageing*, *40*(5), 538–543. doi:10.1093/ageing/afr049 PMID:21778176

Tekkalaki, B. (2015). Issues of sexuality in geriatric population. In Developmental perspectives on human sexuality (pp. 36-43) Bhubaneshwar: Indian Institute of Sexology.

Wang, V., Depp, C. A., Ceglowski, J., Thompson, W. K., Rock, D., & Jeste, D. V. (2015). Sexual health and function in later life: A population-based study of 606 olderadults with a partner. *The American Journal of Geriatric Psychiatry*, *23*(3), 227–233. doi:10.1016/j.jagp.2014.03.006 PMID:24840610

WHO. (1992). *International Classification of Diseases, Clinical descriptions and diagnostic guidelines 1992*. Geneve: World Health Organization.

World Health Organization. (2012). *Good health adds life to years: global brief for World Health day 2012*. Geneve: World Health Organization. Retrieved on January 6, 2012 from http:// www.who.int/ world_ health_day/2012

Yee, L., & Yee, L. (2010). Aging and sexuality. *American Family Physician*, *39*(10), 8–11.

KEY TERMS AND DEFINITIONS

Aging: The term "aging" refers to the physical and psychological changes that occur with maturation.

Old Age: It is the last stage in the life processes of an individual.

Sexual Dysfunctions: Sexual dysfunction is broadly defined as the inability to fully enjoy sexual intercourse.

Chapter 25
Comorbidity of Medical and Psychiatric Disorders in Geriatric Population:
Treatment and Care

Pratima Kaushik
Amity University Uttar Pradesh, India

ABSTRACT

Ageing is a universal phenomenon that has not only social but also economic, political, and health-related implications. With the advancement in healthcare facilities and better availability of health services, the geriatric population is gradually increasing. But, this group is at an increased risk of developing both physical and psychological co-morbidities due to age-related factors and changes in the social circumstances. The present chapter proposes the concept and issues related to co-morbidity in the geriatric population. After discussing the issues and consequences of medical and psychiatric co-morbidities, their effective treatment regime and care/management in relation to the geriatric population are addressed.

INTRODUCTION

As worldwide mortality declines, people are living longer with disability and multiple comorbidities, with important implications for global healthcare needs. In developed nations, about one in four adults have at least two chronic conditions, and more than half of older adults have three or more chronic conditions. Elderly individuals (defined here as persons aged ≥65 years) are burdened by multiple concomitant medical as well as psychiatric disorders. The medical comorbid conditions, such as metabolic syndrome, respiratory and cardiovascular conditions, and endocrine abnormalities are common, while with the most common concurrent psychiatric illnesses being anxiety, depression, bipolar disorder, delirium, dementia and substance use disorders (Karlamangla et al., 2007). In older adult (persons aged ≥65 years) popu-

DOI: 10.4018/978-1-5225-3480-8.ch025

lations with depression, the presence of comorbid-anxiety is associated with more severe depressive symptoms, more chronic medical illness, greater functional impairment and lower quality of life (Hegel et al., 2005). There is also evidence to suggest that substance abuse outcomes may be particularly poor among the elderly (Patterson & Jeste, 1999; Langa et al., 2004).

CONCEPT OF CO-MORBIDITY

Feinstein described the term comorbidity as "any distinct additional entity that has existed or may occur during the clinical course of a patient who has the index disease under study." (Feinstein, 1970). In psychiatry, co-morbidity refers to the co-occurrence of two or more medical or psychiatric conditions, which may or may not directly interact with each other within the same individual. The difficulty to define comorbidity emerges from several reasons. One of them is the very nature of health problems involved. Differentiating the nature of conditions is critical to the conceptualization of comorbidity, because simultaneous occurrence of loosely defined medical entities may signal a problem with the classification system itself (Kaplan & Ong, 2007). Another reason for the problems emerged in the conceptualization of comorbidity is difficult to determine the index disease (primary disease) (Schellevis et al., 1993) considering the definition of Felstein, 1970. Depending on the research, different diseases can be considered a disease index. The conceptualization of comorbidity becomes more problematic when considering diseases that might be viewed just as possible complications of other diseases (Valderas, 2007).

Comorbidities are frequently considered in the context of an index disease (e.g., a newly diagnosed cancer); yet, the index disease focus is not sufficiently comprehensive for a general nosology, and may not be suitable for use in primary care settings. Comorbidity is the total burden of biological dysfunction. Traditionally, comorbidity assessments primarily include overt diseases; because subclinical dysfunction and impairments are highly prevalent in older adults and contribute to health outcomes, particularly when they occur in multiple systems. Lifestyle issues, socioeconomic factors, and health care access and quality, genetic factors affect health outcomes and mitigate or accentuate the effects of comorbidity on outcomes. The effect of these factors on health may be captured, at least partially, by measurements of biological processes included in this nosology. Disabilities in activities of daily living representing interaction of an individual with her/his environment are also not included in this nosology.

Older adults generally have multiple medical problems, and no single medical issue can be evaluated and treated in isolation (Van den Akker et al., 1996). In population studies, the prevalence of comorbidities and number of comorbid conditions increase with age (Wolff et al., 2002). In 1999, 24% of Medicare beneficiaries, aged 65 years or older, had four or more chronic conditions. The proportion was 31.4% among those persons 85 years or older (Wolff et al., 2002). Even healthy older adults and those with a single clinically manifest disease are likely to have subclinical pathology in multiple organ systems (Harris, 2003). Moreover, many older men and women experience a gradual decline in physical strength, gait speed, manual dexterity, memory, and cognitive skills, in the absence of a clinically manifest disease process (Fried et al., 2004). Coexistence of multiple such impairments complicates the diagnosis, treatment, and natural course of individual health conditions in older adults. Research has shown that cognitive decline, reaching the threshold for dementia, affects a large proportion of elderly in-patients and is associated with certain alterations, the treatment of which is complicated by the mental state of this segment of the population (Lopponen et al., 2004).

Patients with multiple chronic conditions have on average a higher level of morbidity, poorer physical functioning and quality of life, a greater likelihood of persistent depression, and lower levels of social well-being. Such patients incur increased risks of adverse drug events and mortality (Department of Health and Human Services Agency for Healthcare Research and Quality, 2009).

Even healthy older adults and those with a single clinically manifest disease are likely to have subclinical pathology in multiple organ systems. Moreover, many older men and women experience a gradual decline in physical strength, gait speed, manual dexterity, memory, and cognitive skills, in the absence of a clinically manifest disease process. Coexistence of multiple such impairments complicates the diagnosis, treatment, and natural course of individual health conditions in older adults (Payne, Laportte, Deber & Coyte, 2007). According to the most recent studies, the number of comorbid conditions seems to be similar in demented and non-demented subjects, but certain chronic medical conditions have been shown to be differentially associated with the cognitively impaired as compared to the unimpaired (Zekry et al., 2008). For example, heart disease, stroke and diabetes have been reported to be associated with cognitive impairment (Ferrucci et al., 1996). Not only the presence of medical conditions but also declines in the ability to perform certain activities considered important in independent functioning (e.g. activities of daily living (ADL) and instrumental activities of daily living (IADL)) were shown to be associated with cognitive impairment (Bassett & Folstein, 1991; Artero et al.2001). Gildengers and colleagues (2004) reported that a significant proportion of older bipolar patient exhibit neuropsychological deficits, and Kessing (2004) noted that the risk of dementia seems to increase with the number of episodes in individuals with BPD. The clinical implications of these findings are especially important for geriatric bipolar patients with additional comorbidity if comorbidity is untreated or under treated, e.g. comorbid substance abuse and anxiety, this is likely to lead to bipolar relapse and potentially increased rates of dementia over time.

THE 3 D'S: COGNITIVE ISSUES IN THE AGING PATIENT

Delirium or *acute* confusion is fairly common in older adult patients and may be frightening for both chiropractor and patient. Delirium is common and is a transient state, and nearly always resolves once the cause is determined and underlying issue is addressed (Robnett & Chop, 2010). Acute confusion may make it difficult to diagnose and care for the delirious chiropractic patient. Dementia is a collection of symptoms including slow, gradual onset memory loss, intellectual impairment, loss of emotional control and problem-solving ability. One type, Alzheimer's Dementia [AD] leads to a progressive loss of mental functions, and often includes disruption of speech or difficulty finding words. In recent years, research has shown that heart health and brain health are related, and patients may slow the progression of AD by making heart healthy lifestyle choices (Hybels & Blazer, 2003). Chiropractors should consider assessing confused patients with the Mini-Mental Status Exam [MMSE] and discussing the patient's score with his or her medical provider (National Institute of Health's National Institute of Neurological Disorders and Stroke the Dementias, 2004).

Depression is a common mental health concern in older adults. One in 5–10 elderly adults suffer from depression and 80% of all depression is completely treatable, once detected. Detection is of utmost importance since suicide is one of the top 10 causes of death in older patients (World Health Organization, 2008). Suicide among white males aged 85 and older was nearly six times the national U.S. rate, making this a serious concern for all health professionals. Older adults often have significant risk factors for depression such as chronic illness and/or chronic pain. Poor diet and poor absorption of B vitamins in the aging body, may also contribute to depression (Dillon, 2007). Older adults are often faced with the death of a spouse, friends or peers. Significant life events such as these, combined with all the factors above, create fertile ground for depression to take hold in the elderly patient. Chiropractors may see depressed older patients since depression often magnifies symptoms of musculoskeletal pain (Dillon, 2007).

According to World Health Organization statistics, heart disease is the number one cause of death worldwide, accounting for 7.2 million deaths annually (WHO.GBD, 2008). Cerebrovascular disease [a related disorder] is the second leading cause of death with another 3 million deaths annually. In Australia, heart disease is also the leading cause of death with nearly 50,000 deaths annually. Using America as another example, heart disease is the top killer of both men and women, with most deaths in patients over age 60 About 18 million Americans currently have heart disease, and about half of those are over age 60 (American Heart Association. Statistical Update Heart Disease and Stroke Statistics, 2011).

EPIDEMIOLOGICAL DETAILS OF CO-MORBIDITY DATA: MISDIAGNOSIS AND MISMANAGEMENT OF PRIMARY ILLNESS

As more people live to advanced old age, these demographic changes imply much more than just an increase in chronic morbidity. The same age-related susceptibility that leads to the occurrence of multiple chronic conditions in the same individual causes decrements in functional abilities as well as social and psychological problems that may have an impact on many facets of their wellbeing and quality of life. Among people aged 65 years and older in the United States, the most commonly reported condition is hypertension, followed by coronary heart disease and stroke. Arthritis and chronic joint symptoms are reported by a large proportion of older persons, and these conditions, like many on the list, have a large impact on overall health and quality of life but do not appear on the list of the most common conditions causing death (Table 1). Moreover, some differences occur in the prevalence rates of chronic conditions according to race and ethnicity (Centers for Disease Control and Prevention, National Center for Health Statistics National Health Interview Survey, sample adult questionnaire: trends in health and aging, 2008).

In purview of below mentioned rates of co-morbidity (Table 1), many older patients become more susceptible to misdiagnosis (Alemayehu & Warner, 2004). Misdiagnosis not only endangers the health of older patients but also incurs opportunity costs for health care systems due to misused clinical interventions and care of iatrogenic illness (Moynihan, Doust & Henry, 2012). Older populations may be more vulnerable to diagnostic error for reasons that relate to both patient and clinician (Mitchell, Rao & Vaze, 2010). Older persons may attribute symptoms to normal aging, and not report them, and doctors may focus unduly on clinical clues suggesting particular diseases while discounting opposing clues (Brazzale, Upward & Pretto, 2010). Commonly used diagnostic criteria for specific diseases derived and validated in younger populations may not apply to older individuals. (Skinner, Scott, & Martin, 2016). Patients with multiple chronic conditions have on average a higher level of morbidity, poorer physical functioning and quality of life, a greater likelihood of persistent depression, and lower levels of social well-being (Bayliss, Ellis & Steiner, 2007; Fortin et al., 2004, 2006, 2007). Such patients incur increased risks of adverse drug events and mortality (Gijsen et al., 2001).

One goal of a health professional in geriatric care should be to identify the diagnosis or to have a high index of suspicion of an important health concern. It is with these changes in mind that examination

Table 1. Most commonly reported chronic conditions per 100 persons aged >65 years in 2005

Condition	Men	Women
Hypertension	44.6	51.1
Arthritis diagnosis	40.4	51.4
Chronic joint symptoms	39.7	47.7
Coronary heart disease	24.3	16.5
Cancer (any type)	23.2	17.5
Vision impairment	14.9	14.9
Diabetes	16.9	14.7
Sinusitis	11.5	16.0
Ulcers	13.1	10.4
Hearing impairment	14.8	8.4
Stroke	8.9	8.2
Emphysema	6.3	4.1
Chronic bronchitis	4.5	6.3
Kidney disorders	4.1	3.9
Liver disease	1.4	1.4

Source: Ferrucci, Giallauria and Guralnik (2009)

of older patients should occur with a heightened vigilance for co-morbid conditions that may require medical care or concomitant care.

Such changes include (Kane et al., 2008):

- A decline in all five senses [vision, hearing, touch, taste and smell].
- Lower muscle mass, bone density, and ligament elasticity.
- Some amount of atherosclerosis.
- Increased risk of co-morbid conditions [higher incidences of cancers, etc.].
- Greater likelihood of chronic disease, like heart disease and arthritis.
- Potential cognitive changes.

CAUSES AND OUTCOMES OF CO-MORBIDITY

Older adults become more susceptible to infections due to several factors. As people get older, it is more frequent that they have comorbid conditions, such as diabetes, renal insufficiency and arthritis. Many comorbid conditions, both the number and type of comorbid conditions, predispose people to infections. Often, when people age, there is immunosenescence, which means that the immune system doesn't function as well or as vigorously. The combination of increased comorbid conditions and the decrease in activity of the immune system can make people more prone to infections. The other syndrome that occurs when people become old is frailty. When people become frail, their body mass index drops and they have a harder time functioning independently, in terms of their daily living activities. They become more prone to falls and injuries. All of these things predispose older people to infections. There is an increased association with being older and an increased risk of infection, but it probably has more to do with how successfully some people age. Some people age and they remain active and healthy, and individuals such as that probably do not have an increased risk of infections. But individuals who become frailer and more dependent on others for maintaining their health status and their daily activities, their risk for infections increase greatly. Treating infections in older adults is a special niche. One thing that needs to be considered is the side effects and tolerability of the medications. Sometimes, in older adults, their metabolism and their clearance of medications changes as they get older. Also, they are often on other medications. Sometimes, they can be susceptible to side effects of medications, so the side effect profile of medications must be taken into account when treating infections in the elderly. You want to take into account the other medications they are taking and also their renal function and how well you dose the medication. Other side effects of antibiotics include *Clostridium difficile*, which ironically, is caused by antibiotic use. We used to think that antibiotics were harmless. If there is any concern about whether or not people might have an infection, particularly those adults who are in institutions such as nursing homes, we need to be more thoughtful about who really needs antibiotics. It used to be that if a patient had a positive culture in their urine, you treated it regardless. But now, we have to think about whether someone truly has an infection or is just colonized, as antibiotics use can lead to super infections (Kaye et al., 2006).

PATHOPHYSIOLOGICAL PATHWAYS TO COMORBIDITY

A number of different factors determine the overall health of populations and individuals, ranging from genetic and biologic characteristics of the individual to the political and policy context (Starfield, 2007). They all play a role in the etiology of any particular disease; hence, they are also expected to play a role in co-occurring diseases. Intuitively, diseases would be expected to cluster in an individual if they shared a common pattern of influences or if the resilience or vulnerability of the individual was altered. But other reasons may explain this clustering.

There are 3 main ways in which different diseases may be found in the same individual: chance, selection bias, or by 1 or more types of causal association. Comorbidity that occurs by chance or selection bias is without causal linkage but is still important because it may lead to erroneous assumptions about causality. Two diseases can co-occur simply by chance. Consider a population with type 2 diabetes, which affects about 4% of individuals, and eczema which independently affects about 5%. By chance alone, 0.2% ($0.04*0.05 = 0.002$) of the population would have both eczema and diabetes. An association of importance would therefore need to show a significant departure from this estimate. Selection bias is an alternative explanation. In his original description of the selection bias affecting patients attending health services, Berkson observed decades ago that disease clusters appeared more frequently in patients seeking care than in the general population (Berkson, 1946), almost certainly because patients seeking care were more likely to acquire a diagnosis irrespective of what it was. This type of bias can be avoided using community samples rather than patients attending health services. Four models of genuine etiological association between conditions have been described (Figure 1): direct causation, associated risk factors, heterogeneity, and independence (Valderas et al., 2009).

In the direct causation model, the presence of 1 disease is directly responsible for another. From a clinical perspective, this model would also include the situation in which treatment for 1 disease caused another condition (eg, a anticoagulant given for a trial fibrillation causing a gastrointestinal hemorrhage). In the associated risk factors model, the risk factors for 1 disease are correlated with the risk factor for another disease, making the simultaneous occurrence of the diseases more likely. For example, smoking and alcohol consumption are correlated; the former is a risk factor for chronic obstructive pulmonary disease and the later a risk factor for liver disease, making it more likely the 2 diseases will occur together. By contrast, in the heterogeneity model, disease risk factors are not correlated, but each is capable of causing diseases associated with the other risk factor (eg, tobacco and age are independent risk factors for a number of malignancies and cardiovascular diseases). In the independence (distinct disease) model, the simultaneous presence of the diagnostic features of the co-occurring diseases actually corresponds to a third distinct disease. For example, the co-occurrence of hypertension and chronic tension headache might both be due to pheochromocytoma. These 4 models are not necessarily mutually exclusive and have yet to be applied extensively to the study of comorbidity. All models have, however, been successfully tested by means of simulation and proved empirically valid in the assessment of selected comorbidities (Johnson et al., 2004).

COMORBIDITY AND ITS IMPACT ON DISEASE MANAGEMENT

The need to classify comorbid health problems in terms of their relevance to clinical management was recognized early (Feinstein, 1970) and a number of classification systems have been suggested. These systems are useful and widely reflected in clinical care practice. For example, ischemic heart disease, cardiovascular risk factors (hypertension, hypercholesterolemia), and diabetes are commonly managed within the same cardiovascular clinics in primary care because they share important aspects of disease management. Drawing together patients who have similar clinical management needs may be efficient, but doing so runs the risk of concealing the wider range of ways in which specific diseases may interact in relation to diagnosis, prognosis, treatment, and management (including self-management) or outcomes. Even for the same pair of comorbid conditions (e.g., diabetes and chronic pulmonary disease), some interventions can be antagonistic (e.g., consider the effect of hypoglycemic drugs and corticosteroids on blood glucose), others may be agonistic (physical activity), and others may be neutral. Interactions among chronic diseases have been a particular focus of interest because they may have far-reaching effects on both health and health care (Van Weel & Schellevis, 2006). But it is no less true that any acute or subacute condition may appreciably affect the management of any other disease (Valderas et al., 2007). A minor acute injury to the right leg, for example, may impair the mobility of a person, thus affecting the management and control of her diabetes; it may also make apparent the presence of osteoarthritis of the left knee that so far had been compensated.

MEDICAL COMORBIDITY

By age 50, patients are more likely to have both hypertension and hyperlipidemia than either condition alone. The dramatic increase in prevalence of both hypertension and hyperlipidemia among patients with diabetes further emphasizes this point. Patients with diabetes and cardiovascular disease often have other health problems that complicate their management (Payne et al. 2007). Aging populations challenge existing health care systems and will increasingly do so in the future. In Western countries the proportions of the population 65 years and older were 11 to 18% in 1990 and are expected to increase to 1926% by 2025.The most rapid rate of increase will occur between 2000 and 2035 when the Baby Boomers enter retirement (Martiniet al., 2007). In the United States, one study projected health care costs due to aging will increase 20% from 2000 to 2030.17 With aging, more patients present with multiple chronic medical conditions that require appropriate management (Vitry et al., 2008).

Ageing-related physiological changes can enhance one's sensitivity to adverse effects of substance use. Substances of abuse act by altering neurotransmission in the brain; ageing related changes to the brain, drug metabolism and pharmacokinetics may interact and intensify older substance users' risk for developing neurotoxicity and severe medical consequences (Dowling et al. 2008; Simoni-Wastila & Yang,

Figure 1. Pathophysiological pathways to comorbidity
Source: Valderas et al. (2009)

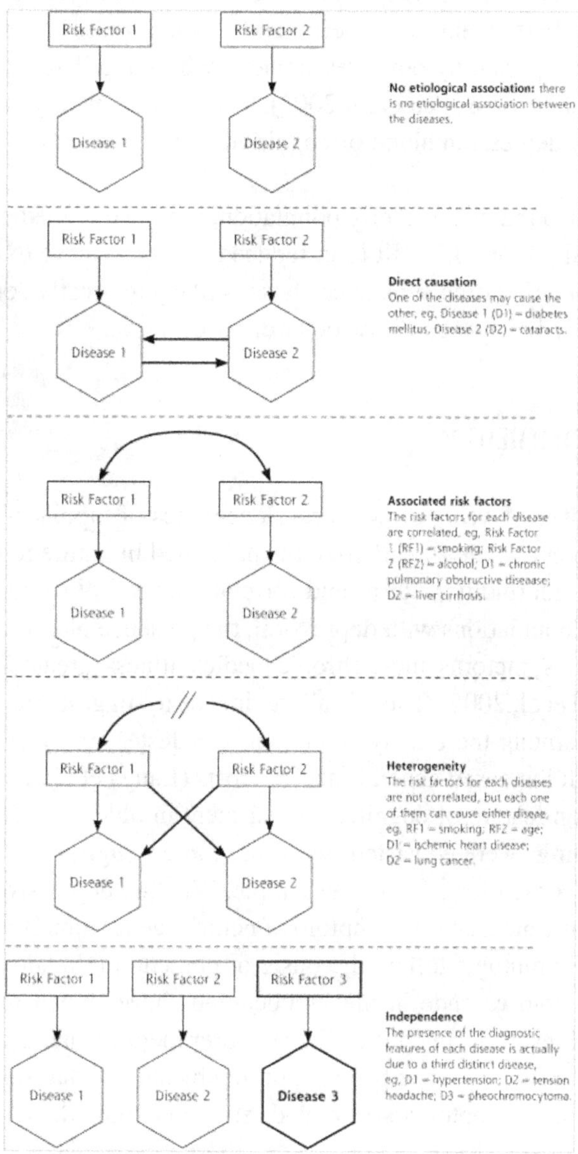

2006). Ageing-related decline in health status also increases older adults' likelihood of taking medications for either medical or psychological conditions and they may also self-medicate with non-prescription substances. For instance, approximately one in four older adults used psychoactive medications with abuse potential (Simoni-Wastila & Yang, 2006). Medication use could interact with substance use and cause adverse effects. Substance use may trigger or intensify medical conditions, such as diabetes and cardiovascular disease (Ghitza UE, Wu LT, &Tai, 2013). Use of psychoactive medications also can lead to nonmedical use or even dependence (Simoni-Wastila & Yang, 2006; Voyer et al., 2009).

Cognitive dysfunction is also a common occurrence among patients with small cell lung cancer, although prophylactic cranial irradiation has been described as one explanation for these cognitive deficits (Meyers et al., 1995). Poor cognitive performance was also highly prevalent in patients with heart disease, stroke and diabetes (Breteler et al., 1994).

Patients with arthritis, visual limitation or gastrointestinal diseases often score highly on measures of depression (Papadopoulos et al., 2005). The limited available data suggest that depression may precede the development of ulcers. Participants with peripheral vascular diseases seemed to experience more depressive symptoms than reported by other researchers, who rather stressed the importance of heart conditions and diabetes (Charlson & Peterson, 2002). The chronic medical conditions cited above are commonly associated with depression alone or cognitive impairment alone rather than co-occurrence of both.

Verduinet al. (2005) noted that in an elderly population, presence of medical disease may both make access to outpatient specialty more difficult (e.g. reduced ability to drive to appointments), and yet at the same time more essential (ongoing substance abuse is likely to greatly complicate the management of medical illness such as diabetes or cardiovascular disease).

PSYCHIATRIC COMORBIDITY

Currently, in individuals over 65 years of age, prevalence rates of bipolar disorder (BPD) range from 0.1% to 0.4% (Van Gerpen et al., 1999). Although the published literature in the area of geriatric mood disorders is growing, but comorbidity patterns and correlates among older adults with BPD are not well understood. In older adult populations with depression, the presence of comorbid anxiety is associated with more severe depressive symptoms, more chronic medical illness, greater functional impairment and lower quality of life (Hegel et al.,2005). There is also evidence to suggest that substance abuse outcomes may be particularly poor among the elderly (Patterson and Jeste, 1999). Among elderly individuals, dementia is associated with increased general medical costs (Langa et al., 2004).

Depression is a common feature of cognitive impairment in older age (Forsell et al., 2003; Gabryelewicz et al., 2004). Findings were consistent with the studies, suggesting that cognitive impairment and depressive symptoms coexist for 7.9% of the sample. Whether depressive symptoms are a reaction to cognitive deficits or constitute an early symptom of neurodegeneration is unclear. Some studies have suggested that depressive symptoms follow the onset of dementia (Vinkers et al., 2004). Conversely, research on the glucocorticoid cascade in the hippocampus have shown that older depressed adults with high or rising cortisol levels during 5 years have poorer memory and greater hippocampal atrophy (Lupien et al., 1998). These findings have been supported by studies that show that cognitive function can improve when depressive symptoms are treated, although some degree of cognitive impairment may remain even after recovery (Kessing, 1998). An alternative explanation was that the symptoms of cognitive deterioration may partially overlap with the symptoms of depression, and the underlying neuropathological condition that causes cognitive impairment also causes depressive symptoms (Panza et al., 2010). Due to the high prevalence of depression in cognitive decline and their common adverse consequences such as apathy, agitation and social withdrawal, screening for depression and cognitive impairment remains an important challenge for psychogeriatric medicine (Lyketsos et al., 2000).

In another study conducted by Sajatovic et al. (2006) demonstrated that among geriatric patients with Bipolar disorder, comorbid PTSD, substance abuse, other anxiety or dementia occur in nearly 29% of individuals, and that clinical characteristics, health resource use patterns and health care costs differ depending on the type of comorbidity. They further suggested that the reported rates are an underestimate of true prevalence of comorbidity for the following reasons: (1) underreporting of comorbid diagnoses in patients with a serious mental disorder diagnosis; (2) limited diagnostic precision in the sample by the case registry methodology; and (3) the fact that many providers might not code sub-syndromal symptoms thought to be secondary to a primary mood disorder. Simon and colleagues (2004) reported that comorbid anxiety disorders are common in mixed age bipolar samples, with over one and half of patients experiencing lifetime comorbid anxiety and 30.5% experiencing current anxiety disorder. Individuals with substance abuse in this elderly bipolar population are more likely to be younger, minority, unmarried and homeless compared to elderly bipolar populations with anxiety disorders or dementia. Other investigators have documented that comorbid substance abuse is associated with fewer psychosocial resources among mixed age populations of individuals with serious mental illness (Nolen et al., 2004; Folsom et al., 2005).

Conservative estimates from national surveys of non-institutionalized adults show that the number of Americans aged 50þ years with a substance use disorder (SUD; alcohol or drug use disorders) will double from 2.8 million (annual average) in 2002–06 to 5.7 million in 2020 (Han et al., 2009). The increase in the number of people with a SUD will occur in all sex and racial/ethnic groups because of combined effects of the growing number of older adults and of persons with a SUD (Han et al., 2009). Substance abuse can affect almost all major organs (Brick, 2004), and SUD is a relapsing condition (Wu et al., 2011). Adults aged 18–64 years (63% of the US population) who comprise the vast majority of problematic substance users continue to age and are expected to place an increasing burden on health care systems over time (Han et al., 2009; Substance Abuse and Mental Health Services Administration, 2012; Wu & Blazer, 2011). Data from the Treatment Episode Data Set (TEDS), which collects national-level admissions to substance abuse treatment facilities that receive public funds, demonstrate an escalating demand for health services for SUDs among middle-aged and older adults (Substance Abuse and Mental Health Services Administration, 2011).

INTERACTION AND SYNERGY OF MEDICAL AND PSYCHOLOGICAL SYMPTOMS

Recent studies have investigated the mechanisms through which the products of the immune system, cytokines, influence the functions of the nervous system within the brain (Figure 2). Reports on neuronal innervation of the organs of the immune system especially, sympathetic noradrenergic and peptidergic neuronal fibers that innervate the lymphoid organs, bone marrow, thymus, spleen, and lymph nodes demonstrate the network between nervous system and immune system. In these organs, neurotransmitters and neuropeptides released from the nerve endings of these neurons alter the functions of the immune

Figure 2. Bidirectional communication between the Neuroendocrine system and Immune system
Source: Srinivasan and Hannah, 2012

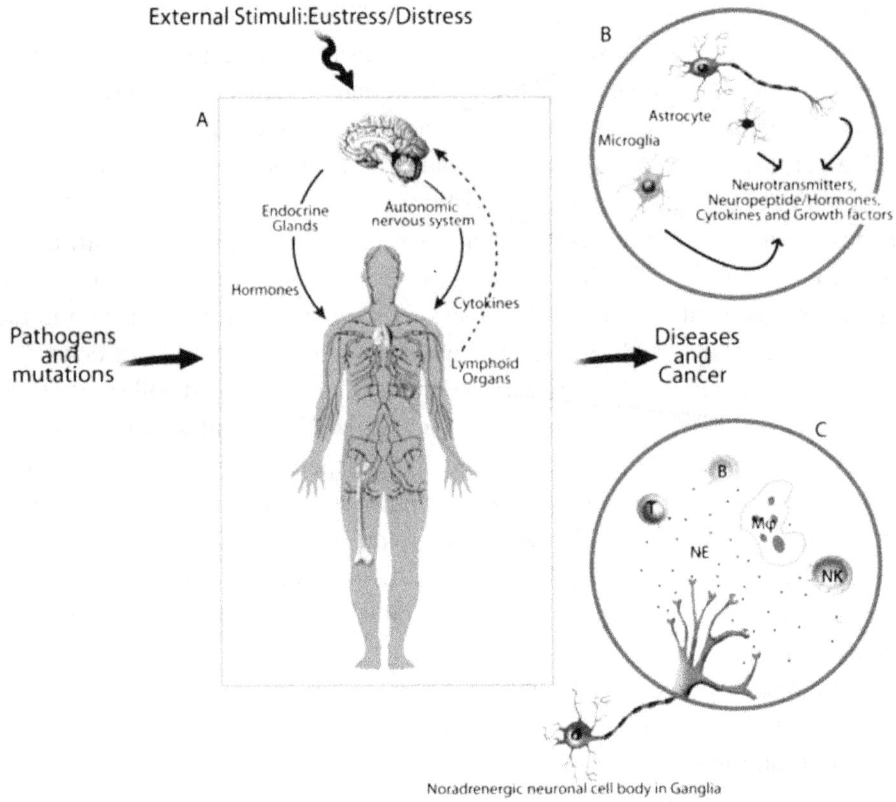

system as the lymphoid cells have receptors for hormones and neurochemicals. Behavioral and pharmacological manipulation of the neuroendocrine-immune signaling has been known to alter immunity, autoimmunity, and immunosenescence. This altered neural-immune signaling may determine the course of infectious diseases and also, response of the individuals to therapeutic strategies (Black, 1994; Srinivasan & Hannah, 2012; Srinivasan & Hannah, 2012) explained bidirectional communication between the neuroendocrine system and immune system.

1. The bidirectional interaction is mainly through neurotransmitter-, hormonal-, and cytokine-specific pathways. The CNS influences the immune system via neuroendocrine outflow, and autonomic and sensory nerves that innervate lymphoid tissue. Peripherally, cytokines produced by the immune cells under the influence of neuronal activity cross the blood-brain barrier to influence CNS functions. There is a great complexity in neural-immune interactions.
2. Neurotransmitter-specific and neuropeptidergic nerves are distributed in the rostral sections of the brain arising from the cell bodies located in the caudal portions of the brain. The neuroglial cells, astrocytes and microglia, regulate the neuronal survival through the release of cytokines and growth factors while the oligodendrocytes are critical to myelin formation. The neuroendocrine systems in the hypothalamus control metabolism and growth by influencing the release of hormones from the pituitary.

3. Noradrenergic nerves originate from ganglia and are distributed to specific lymphoid compartments in lymphoid organs and the effects are mediated through the receptors for neurotransmitters on the cells of the immune system. The presence of β2-adrenergic receptors (AR) on the subpopulations of lymphoid cells facilitates the binding of norepinephrine (NE) to alter the release of cytokines, growth factors, and immune molecules that cross the blood-brain barrier to alter brain functions.

Models are used to create comorbidity indices include interactions between various domains. Certain interactions are currently recognized. For example, hypertension confers different risk for adverse outcomes in the presence or absence of diabetes, and the same value of low-density lipoprotein cholesterol is associated with different levels of risk for cardiovascular events in those with and without coronary artery disease or diabetes (Grundy et al., 2004). Similarly, there is known synergy between depression and coronary heart disease, visual impairment and arthritis, hypertension and hyperlipidemia, and between elevated C-reactive protein levels and diabetes mellitus (Schulze et al., 2004) in the risk for adverse health outcomes. There is also likely to be synergy between domains in protective high-functioning zones, such as between positive affect and high exercise tolerance, as well as interactions between protective zones in one domain and harmful zones in another.

Some studies have found that patients with depression have more functional impairment and poorer quality of life than patients with other chronic illnesses (Wells et al. 1989; Wells & Sherbourne, 1999). Furthermore, severity of depressive symptoms is inversely related to patients' health-related quality of life, even after controlling for age, sex, and medical comorbidities (Unutzer et al., 2000; Pyne et al., 1997). Many older persons, however, have more than one chronic illness that may differentially impair health status. Elders with multiple comorbidities may be particularly vulnerable to the debilitating impact of depression. Much of the previous research examining the interconnections between depression, medical comorbidities, and health status has been conducted in restricted settings.

Noel et al. (2004) in their study found that depression severity was significantly associated with all 4 indicators of general health status in this diverse sample of depressed elders. As depression severity increased, quality of life and physical and mental functioning declined, while disability increased. Furthermore, depression severity was significantly associated with all 4 indicators of health status after controlling for sociodemographic differences, other psychological conditions, and 11 medical comorbidities. Although study participants had an average of 3.8 chronic medical illnesses, depression severity made larger independent contributions to 3 of the 4 general health indicators (mental functional status, disability, and quality of life) than the medical comorbidities. Cognitive impairment was significantly associated with physical functioning and disability. Participants with chronic lung disease, diabetes, neurological disease, heart disease, and chronic pain had significantly worse physical functioning and greater disability. Arthritis was significantly associated with both physical and mental functioning, while hypertension and gastrointestinal disease were significantly associated with decreased physical functioning only.

IMPLICATIONS FOR MANAGEMENT OF COMORBIDITIES

Multimorbidity, or multiple comorbidity, or multiple chronic conditions, is common and greatly increases the complexity of managing disease in patients. In developed nations, about one in four adults have at least two chronic conditions (Chronic Conditions: Making the case for ongoing care, 2004; Mercer et al., 2009; Barnett et al., 2012), and more than half of older adults have three or more chronic conditions (Guiding principles for the care of older adults with multimorbidity: an approach for clinicians, 2012). As worldwide mortality declines, people are living longer with disability and multiple comorbidities, with important implications for global health care needs (Global Burden of Disease Study, 2013).

Although there are guidelines for management of single chronic illnesses, the evidence base for management of multiple comorbidities is lacking. The American Geriatrics Society described a clinical approach to managing patients with multiple comorbidities in 2012 (Guiding principles for the care of older adults with multimorbidity: an approach for clinicians, 2012). The challenge of managing multiple comorbidities can be compounded by limited health literacy, which is more common in older persons, poor persons, and certain minorities, (Weiss, 2007). For a typical older patient, medical care has become more complex, comprising multiple steps with crucial exchanges of information (Nielsen-Bohlman., 2004). Most physicians have between 15 and 30 minutes for a follow-up visit, which is often insufficient to address many or all comorbidities effectively.

Ramaswamy, (2014) addressed following management strategy attempts to address clinical and system based challenges:

Prioritize

Prioritizing involves identifying concerns that need attention during this visit and those that can wait until the next visit. Focus on problems that may lead to the greatest morbidity, and possibly mortality, in the next days or weeks. A discussion of the patient's agenda, as well as your own, at the beginning of the visit will help to create a realistic framework of the items that will be addressed in the time available. The patient in this case scenario is mainly concerned about the toe amputation, the pain in the leg, and getting a motorized wheelchair for ambulation. At the beginning of the visit, create a pain management plan, discuss wound care, and follow up on his kidney function and cell counts. At the end of the visit, it would be beneficial to alert a social worker to assist the patient with procuring durable medical equipment.

Communicate Effectively

Good communication is key when interacting with older patients who have comorbidities. There are several components to facilitating effective communication with this population.

Active Listening

Start by asking the patient for his or her most pressing concerns. It is appropriate to probe for general and specific goals and values, as well as any preference for a particular plan of action. The ask-tell-ask and teach-back methods can elicit the patient's understanding of key medical concepts or recommendations.4 Avoid medical jargon, and use concrete and direct words rather than abstract terminology.

Interpreter Services

Nonverbal communication is best gauged by someone who is well versed in the patient's culture. Check whether your institution provides language interpreters, and schedule them for visits as needed. Another option is a phone interpreter service. Family members should not be used as proxy history providers or interpreters.

Reinforcement

Visual aids can clarify and reinforce comprehension of key medical issues. For example, decision aids for diabetes management are available for teaching patients about their medications' benefits, adverse effects, and dosages (Mayo Clinic, 2013). Electronic medical records can create individualized visit summaries that include instructions and educational materials.

Apply Evidence-Based Medicine

Employing a patient-specific, evidence-based approach helps balance the benefits and harms of diagnostic or therapeutic interventions. Reviewing current practice recommendations and calculating the absolute risk reduction and the number needed to treat will guide management decisions. Prognostication in patients with many chronic conditions, although imperfect, may help prioritize decisions based on the patient's life expectancy. This patient has a five-year mortality risk of roughly 69% and a 10-year mortality risk of roughly 93% based on Schonberg and Lee indices, respectively (University of California at San Francisco, 2013).

Collaborate

An interdisciplinary care team can help manage a complicated case. A social worker, nurse practitioner, or registered nurse, if available, is often able to meet with the patient or family at more frequent intervals to assist with health education, chronic care management, and psychosocial counseling. In my practice, the social worker assists with determining insurance coverage and payment sources, and the medical assistant orders supplies from our durable medical equipment vendor. In the absence of a social worker, another member of your practice can visit the Medicare website (http://www.medicare.gov) to find a list of covered medical equipment vendors in your area.

Involve the Caregiver or Family

With the patient's permission, reach out to a caregiver or responsible family member and give him or her a few tasks to complete and report back to you at a specified date. This person could be asked to obtain immunization or procedure records from other physicians or clinics or to report on the patient's response to a new medication in a week's time.

Manage Pre- and Post-Visit Factors

Alert your front-desk staff and administrative assistant to any special needs of particularly worrisome patients. Such patients may benefit from a personal phone call the day before the appointment (rather than an automated call) reminding them to bring their medication bottles to the visit and clarifying the date, time, and location. At the end of the visit, the patient should have an easy-to-understand follow-up schedule to take home. Some physicians may feel comfortable sharing their cell phone number so the patient can bypass the delay and frustration that may be associated with an answering service. The improvement in life expectancy and in survival of patients with ischemic heart disease (Jugdutt, 2010), eighty percent of patients with Heart Failure (HF) are elderly (65 years and older) whose disease differs significantly from that seen in middle aged adults (Roger, 2011). Novel therapies and other interventions have failed to show significant benefit in improving outcomes of elderly patients with HF. For instance, several medications that are proven effective in younger patients with HFREF (heart failure with reduced ejection fraction) have been tried in older patients with HFPEF and failed to show any benefit (Massie et al., 2008; Yusuf et al., 2003; Kitzman et al., 2010). Other strategies in the management of HF have also been tried in this patient population, including tele-monitoring and post-discharge care management, and showed no significant impact on mortality or re-hospitalization rates (Chaudhry et al., 2010). Relative lack of progress in improving outcomes in older persons with HF may be due to the fact that most studies have not taken into account two common and key characteristics of elderly patients with HF, frailty, and multiple comorbidities. Several diagnostic and staging criteria of frailty have been proposed, but the criteria proposed by Fried et al have been most widely used and proven clinically useful. According to Fried et al.(2001), a person is considered frail if three or more of the following criteria are present: weight loss of more than 10 lbs in one year; physical exhaustion by self-report: weakness as measured by grip strength; decline in walking speed; and low physical activity. Based on Fried criteria, it is estimated that 6.9% of older community dwelling adults are frail. This prevalence increases sharply with age, from 3.2% among persons 65-70 years old to 23.1% among persons 90 years and older (Friedet al., 2001). Once frailty is developed, both HF and its associated comorbidities can give rise to acute stressors which can lead to rapid functional decline resulting in disability, hospitalization, institutionalization, and eventually death.

Due to underrepresentation of elderly patients with HF in RCTs, especially those with frailty and multiple comorbidities, has resulted in a paucity of evidence in this patient population and rendered many aspects of their care largely empirical. It is uncertain whether trial results obtained in younger patients pertain directly to the management elderly persons with HF, as growing evidence has shown that older patients respond differently to current therapies than do younger patients with HF.

Non-adherence to medical care is common among the elderly, and is associated with poor outcomes (Hoet al., 2009). Mocker et al found that non-persistence with medication was an independent predictor of HF re-hospitalization (Mockler et al., 2009). Non-adherence to medical therapy was independently associated with higher mortality among participants in the Candesartan in Heart Failure Assessment of Reduction in Mortality and Morbidity (CHARM) trial (Granger et al., 2005). Frailty and multiple comorbidities possibly contribute to non-compliance in elderly patients with HF leading to higher rate of hospitalization, re-hospitalization, and ultimately institutionalization and death. Frail patients may have more limited access to healthy food, and medical follow-up. Patients with cognitive and sensory impairment are less likely to adhere to dietary restrictions, prescribed medications, weight monitoring, and timely reporting of symptoms. Patients with physical impairment and with disability are less likely to participate in physical exercises and cardiac rehabilitation programs. Patients with multiple comorbidities are often on complex medication regimes which may increase the risk of non-adherence, drug-to-drug interaction, and serious adverse effects (Murad, and Kitzman, 2012).

While prescribing in older patients with comorbidities, it comes as a great challenge for the medical/psychiatric practitioners. Taking medication is a choice and for the older patient with comorbidities there are few clear cut right or wrong decisions, but there are many options to consider (Gallagher et al., 2012; Melzer et al., 2015; Day, 2017):

Continue Therapy if Well Tolerated

Prescribed medication can significantly benefit many patients and the default position should be to continue therapy if it is well tolerated and supported. However, some drugs are given to manage side effects caused by other drugs. For example, diuretics are given for ankle swelling caused by amlodipine. Consider whether you could discontinue both drugs. The Screening Tool of Older People's potentially inappropriate Prescriptions (STOPP) criterion is useful.

Review Medication When Appropriate

If the intended target of treatment is not being met, discuss this again with the patient. Check that they are taking the medicine correctly. Some 50% of older patients are not taking the desired dose of statin two years after a heart attack. Dementia or increased frailty or dependency should prompt a review of medication.

Treat Distressing Symptoms

Treating distressing symptoms is always the right thing to do. This is more important than treating things that haven't happened yet, if a choice has to be made.

Use Sub-Maximal Doses

Feel free to use sub-maximal doses of medicine. It is unlikely the full dose of any drug prescribed has been tested on a patient with the combination of diseases being treated and adverse effects are more common in older patients.

Prioritize Secondary Prevention

Drugs are more effective, in absolute terms, for secondary rather than primary prevention of disease. If the patient has already had a stroke, their risk of another is as much as ten times higher than if they had not. Very few primary preventive drugs benefit more than one person in fifty each year.

Respect Your Patient's Decisions

Discuss likely risk with the patient, and ask if they want treatment. Some older people want treatment to be given to younger people who they believe have more to gain. Patient's relatives may have a different view. It is important to understand the reasoning behind the patient's informed decision. Remember that people are allowed to make different decisions to that which we would make ourselves. But usually older patients want to do what their clinician thinks is best.

Aim to 'Add Life to Years'

Remember this when managing the older patients with comorbidities. If your treatment causes more discomfort and trouble than the disease, then it is probably the wrong approach.

Lifestyle Change

It is never too late for patients to make lifestyle changes, so do discuss this with older patients. Stopping smoking, walking more and eating more vegetables are all good ways for patients to take responsibility for their health. While all patients are individuals (particularly those with multiple morbidities, who may all have different combinations of problems) it is important to remember that the final concerns and limitations for older people are often the same. Their horizons may be reduced by immobility so they become confined to the house or a room. They may feel frustration and disappointment at their loss of personal independence.

Prevention of Comorbidity

Primary prevention is a control of risk factor before it causes a disease - often requires you to treat many people to prevent one event. A decision should be made by balancing benefit with risk, and this is particularly important in older patients with comorbidities. For instance, a 75-year-old man with atrial fibrillation has a 97% chance of not having a stroke in every year that he is not taking an anticoagulant. He can improve his chances of not having a stroke to 99% by taking an anticoagulant, although this might cause him to have a gastric bleed. If the patient has advanced dementia and swallowing problems you may consider that the 2% gain in stroke prevention is not enough to outweigh the risk of death from aspiration pneumonia, for example. On the other hand, a stroke can be devastating (Gallagher et al., 2008).

It becomes important to prevent infections in elderly. There are a few different ways to prevent them, one is vaccination. Yearly influenza vaccinations are necessary. Influenza not only causes the flu, but in older adults particularly, it causes super infections with bacterial pneumonia. Getting the flu vaccine and making sure that older adults are up-to-date on their pneumococcal vaccination are important. In institutional settings, such as in hospitals and nursing homes, good hand hygiene by staff and avoiding the spread of pathogens from one patient to another is important. The final thing is for older adults to stay active. The longer they can remain independent and function without needing hands-on assistance or needing feeding tubes or urinary catheters will decrease the risk of infections, as well (Kaye et al., 2006).

CONCLUSION

Proper assessment and screening which enhances effective diagnosis is the need of the hour to manage several co-morbidities associated with old age. Also, health plans use their administrative data for planning prevention and disease management programs, programs that often range in intensity from reminder letters for health screening to case management are required. Understanding the prevalence of members with differing conditions, their management, and risks of adverse outcomes could help in planning appropriate strategies. For populations identified, as in this chapter, medical needs might be assessed and variations in health practices could be explored such as adherence with medications and health screening rates. Economic factors, ethnic variations, and geographical differences, as examples, may differentially affect patients who vary in the combinations of chronic conditions they have to manage. Future studies, in addition, might examine acute outcomes and rates of progression comparing well managed versus poorly managed patients.

REFERENCES

Alemayehu, B., & Warner, K. E. (2004). The lifetime distribution of health care costs. *Health Services Research*, *39*(3), 627–642. doi:10.1111/j.1475-6773.2004.00248.x PMID:15149482

Artero, S., Touchon, J., & Ritchie, K. (2001). Disability and mild cognitive impairment: A longitudinal population-based study. *International Journal of Geriatric Psychiatry*, *16*(11), 1092–1097. doi:10.1002/gps.477 PMID:11746656

Barnett, K., Mercer, S. W., Norbury, M., Watt, G., Wyke, S., & Guthrie, B. (2012). Epidemiology of multimorbidity and implications for health care, research, and medical education: A cross-sectional study. *Lancet*, *380*(9836), 37–43. doi:10.1016/S0140-6736(12)60240-2 PMID:22579043

Bassett, S. S., & Folstein, M. F. (1991). Cognitive impairment and functional disability in the absence of psychiatric diagnosis. *Psychological Medicine*, *21*(01), 77–84. doi:10.1017/S0033291700014677 PMID:2047508

Bayliss, E. A., Ellis, J. L., & Steiner, J. F. (2007). Barriers to self-management and quality-of-life outcomes in seniors with multimorbidities. *Annals of Family Medicine*, *5*(5), 395–402. doi:10.1370/afm.722 PMID:17893380

Berkson, J. (1946). Limitations of the application of fourfold table analysis to hospital data. *Biomet Bull*, *2*(3), 47–53. doi:10.2307/3002000 PMID:21001024

Black, P. H. (1994). Central nervous system-immune system interactions: Psychoneuroendocrinology of stress and its immune consequences. *Antimicrobial Agents and Chemotherapy*, *38*(1), 1–6. doi:10.1128/AAC.38.1.1 PMID:8141561

Boxer, H., & Snyder, S. (2009). Five communication strategies to promote self-management of chronic illness. *Family Practice Management*, *16*(5), 12–16. PMID:19751037

Brazzale, D. J., Upward, A. L., & Pretto, J. J. (2010). Effects of changing reference values and definition of the normal range on interpretation of spirometry. *Respirology (Carlton, Vic.)*, *15*(7), 1098–1103. doi:10.1111/j.1440-1843.2010.01830.x PMID:20874746

Breteler, M. M., Claus, J. J., Grobbee, D. E., & Hofman, A. (1994). Cardiovascular disease and distribution of cognitive function in elderly people: The Rotterdam study. *British Medical Journal*, *308*(6944), 1604–1608. doi:10.1136/bmj.308.6944.1604 PMID:8025427

J. Brick (Ed.). (2004). *Handbook of the Medical Consequences of Alcohol and Drug Abuse*. New York: Haworth Press.

Charlson, M., & Peterson, J. C. (2002). Medical comorbidity and late life depression: What is known and what are unmet needs? *Biological Psychiatry*, *52*(3), 226–235. doi:10.1016/S0006-3223(02)01422-1 PMID:12182928

Chaudhry, S. I., Mattera, J. A., Curtis, J. P., Spertus, J. A., Herrin, J., Lin, Z., ... Krumholz, H. M. (2010). Tele monitoring in patients with heart failure. *The New England Journal of Medicine*, *363*(24), 2301–2309. doi:10.1056/NEJMoa1010029 PMID:21080835

Chronic Conditions. Making the case for ongoing care. (2004). Johns Hopkins and the Robert Wood Johnson Foundation's Partnership for Solutions. Available at: http://www.partnershipforsolutions.org/DMS/files/chronicbook2004.pdf

Day, R. (2017, August 2). Advice on primary prevention and prescribing in older patients with comorbidities, including the impact of medication side effects [Weblog post]. Retrieved from https://www.gponline.com/comorbidities-older-people/elderly-care/article/1440520

Department of Health and Human Services Agency for Healthcare Research and Quality. (n.d.). *Optimizing prevention and healthcare management for the complex patient*. Available at: http://grants.nih.gov/grants/guide/rfafiles/RFA-HS-08-003.html

Dillon, P. (2007). *Nursing Health Assessment: A Critical Thinking Case Studies Approach*. Philadelphia: F.A. Davis Publishers.

Dowling, G. J., Weiss, S. R., & Condon, T. P. (2008). Drugs of abuse and the ageing brain. *Neuropsychopharmacology*, *33*(2), 209–218. doi:10.1038/sj.npp.1301412 PMID:17406645

Feinstein, A. R. (1970). The pre-therapeutic classification of co-morbidity in chronic disease. *Journal of Chronic Diseases*, *23*(7), 455–468. doi:10.1016/0021-9681(70)90054-8 PMID:26309916

Ferrucci, L., Giallauria, F., & Guralnik, J. M. (2009). Epidemiology of Aging. *Radiologic Clinics of North America*, *46*(4), 643–v. doi:10.1016/j.rcl.2008.07.005 PMID:18922285

Ferrucci, L., Guralnik, J. M., & Salive, M. E. (1996). Cognitive impairment and risk of stroke in the older population. *Journal of the American Geriatrics Society*, *44*(3), 237–241. doi:10.1111/j.1532-5415.1996.tb00908.x PMID:8600190

Flostein, M. F. (1983). Assessment in geriatric psychopharmacology. The Mini Mental Status Exam, 50–51.

Folsom, D. P., Hawthorne, W., Lindamer, L., Gilmer, T., Bailey, A., Golshan, S., ... Jeste, D. V. (2005). Prevalence and risk factors for homelessness and utilization of mental health services among 10.340 patients with serious mental illness in a large public mental health system. *The American Journal of Psychiatry*, *162*(2), 370–376. doi:10.1176/appi.ajp.162.2.370 PMID:15677603

Forsell, Y., Palmer, K., & Fratiglioni, L. (2003). Psychiatric symptoms/syndromes in elderly persons with mild cognitive impairment. Data from a cross-sectional study. *Acta Neurologica Scandinavica*, *107*(s179), 25–28. doi:10.1034/j.1600-0404.107.s179.4.x PMID:12603247

Fortin, M., Bravo, G., Hudon, C., Lapointe, L., Almirall, J., Dubois, M. F., & Vanasse, A. (2006). Relationship between multimorbidity and health-related quality of life of patients in primary care. *Quality of Life Research: An International Journal of Quality of Life Aspects of Treatment, Care and Rehabilitation*, *15*(1), 83–91. doi:10.1007/s11136-005-8661-z PMID:16411033

Fortin, M., Dubois, M. F., Hudon, C., Soubhi, H., & Almirall, J. (2007). Multimorbidity and quality of life: A closer look. *Health and Quality of Life Outcomes*, *5*(1), 52. doi:10.1186/1477-7525-5-52 PMID:17683600

Fortin, M., Lapooointe, L., Hudon, C., Vanasse, A., Ntetu, A. L., & Maltais, D. (2004). Multimorbidity and quality of life in primary care: A systematic review. *Health and Quality of Life Outcomes*, *2*(1), 51. doi:10.1186/1477-7525-2-51 PMID:15380021

Fox, C. S., Sullivan, L., D'Agostino, R. B., & Sr. Wilson, P. W. (2004). Framingham Heart Study. The significant effect of diabetes duration on coronary heart disease mortality: The Framingham Heart Study. *Diabetes Care*, *27*(3), 704–708. doi:10.2337/diacare.27.3.704 PMID:14988289

Fried, L. P., Ferrucci, L., Darer, J., Williamson, J. D., & Anderson, G. (2004). Untangling the concepts of disability, frailty, and comorbidity: Implications for improved targeting and care. *The Journals of Gerontology. Series A, Biological Sciences and Medical Sciences*, *59A*(3), 255–263. doi:10.1093/gerona/59.3.M255 PMID:15031310

Fried, L. P., Tangen, C. M., Walston, J., Newman, A. B., Hirsch, C., Gottdiener, J., ... McBurnie, M. A. (2001). Frailty. in older adults: Evidence for a phenotype. *The Journals of Gerontology. Series A, Biological Sciences and Medical Sciences*, *56*(3), M146–M156. doi:10.1093/gerona/56.3.M146 PMID:11253156

Gabryelewicz, T., Styczynska, M., Pfeffer, A., Wasiak, B., Barczak, A., Luczywek, E., ... Barcikowska, M. (2004). Prevalence of major and minor depression in elderly persons with mild cognitive impairment-MADRS factor analysis. *International Journal of Geriatric Psychiatry*, *19*(12), 1168–1172. doi:10.1002/gps.1235 PMID:15526303

Gallagher, P., Ryan, C., & Byrne, S. (2008). STOPP (Screening Tool of Older Person's Prescriptions) and START (Screening Tool to Alert doctors to Right Treatment). Consensus validation. *International Journal of Clinical Pharmacology and Therapeutics*, *46*(2), 72–83. doi:10.5414/CPP46072 PMID:18218287

Ghitza, U. E., Wu, L. T., & Tai, B. (2013). Integrating substance abuse care with community diabetes care: Implications for research and clinical practice. *Substance Abuse and Rehabilitation*, *4*, 3–10. doi:10.2147/SAR.S39982 PMID:23378792

Gijsen, R., Hoeymans, N., Schellevis, F. G., Ruwaard, D., Satariano, W. A., & van den Bos, G. A. (2001). Causes and consequences of comorbidity: A review. *Journal of Clinical Epidemiology*, *54*(7), 661–674. doi:10.1016/S0895-4356(00)00363-2 PMID:11438406

Gildengers, A. G., Butters, M. A., Seligman, K., McShea, M., Miller, M. D., Mulsant, B. H., ... Reynolds, C. F. III. (2004). Cognitive functioning in late-life bipolar disorder. *The American Journal of Psychiatry*, *161*(4), 736–738. doi:10.1176/appi.ajp.161.4.736 PMID:15056521

Global Burden of Disease Study 2013 Collaborators. (2015). Global, regional, and national incidence, prevalence, and years lived with disability for 301 acute and chronic diseases and injuries in 188 countries, 1990-2013: a systematic analysis for the Global Burden of Disease Study 2013. *Lancet, 386*, 743.

Granger, B., Swedberg, B., Ekman, K., Granger, I., Olofsson, C. B., Mc, B., ... Pfeffer, M. A. (2005). Adherence to candesartan and placebo and outcomes in chronic heart failure in the CHARM programme: Double-blind, randomised, controlled clinical trial. *Lancet*, *366*(9502), 2005–2011. doi:10.1016/S0140-6736(05)67760-4 PMID:16338449

Grundy, S. M., Cleeman, J. I., & Merz, C. M. B. (2004). For the Coordinating Committee of the National Cholesterol Education Program. Implications of recent clinical trials for the National Cholesterol Education Program Adult Treatment Panel III Guidelines. *Circulation, 110*(2), 227–239. doi:10.1161/01.CIR.0000133317.49796.0E PMID:15249516

Guiding principles for the care of older adults with multimorbidity: an approach for clinicians (2012). *Journal of American Geriatric Society, 60*(10), E1-E25.

Guralnik, J. M. (1996). Assessing the impact of comorbidity in the older population. *Annals of Epidemiology, 6*(5), 376–380. doi:10.1016/S1047-2797(96)00060-9 PMID:8915467

Gurwitz, J. H., Field, T. S., Harrold, L. R., Harrold, L. R., Rothschild, J., Debellis, K., ... Bates, D. W. (2003). Inciden.ce and preventability of adverse drug events among older persons in the ambulatory setting. *Journal of the American Medical Association, 289*(9), 1107–1116. doi:10.1001/jama.289.9.1107 PMID:12622580

Han, B., Gfroerer, J. C., Olliver, J. D., & Penne, M. A. (2009). Substance use disorder among older adults in the United States in 2020. *Addiction (Abingdon, England), 104*(1), 88–96. doi:10.1111/j.1360-0443.2008.02411.x PMID:19133892

Harris, T. B. (2003). Epidemiology and aging. In C. K. Cassel, R. M. Leipzig, H. J. Cohen, & ... (Eds.), *Geriatric Medicine: An Evidence-Based Approach* (4th ed.). New York: Springer Verlag. doi:10.1007/0-387-22621-4_5

Hays, R. D., Wells, K. B., Sherbourne, C. D., Rogers, W., & Spritzer, K. (1995). Functioning and well-being outcomes of patients with depression compared with chronic general medical illnesses. *Archives of General Psychiatry, 52*(1), 11–19. doi:10.1001/archpsyc.1995.03950130011002 PMID:7811158

Hegel, M. T., Unutzer, J., Tang, L., Areán, P. A., Katon, W., Noël, P. H., ... Lin, E. H. B. (2005). Impact of comorbid panic and posttraumatic stress disorder on outcomes of collaborative care for late-life depression in primary care. *The American Journal of Geriatric Psychiatry, 13*(1), 48–58. doi:10.1097/00019442-200501000-00008 PMID:15653940

Ho, P.M., Bryson, C.L., & Rumsfeld, J.S. (2009). Medication adherence: Its importance in cardiovascular outcomes. *Circulation, 119*(23), 3028–3035.

Hybels, C. F., & Blazer, D. G. (2003). Epidemiology of late-life mental disorders. *Clinics in Geriatric Medicine, 19*(4), 663–696. doi:10.1016/S0749-0690(03)00042-9 PMID:15024807

Johnson, E. O., Rhee, S. H., Chase, G. A., & Breslau, N. (2004). Comorbidity of depression with levels of smoking: An exploration of the shared familial risk hypothesis. *Nicotine & Tobacco Research Journal, 6*(6), 1029–1038. doi:10.1080/14622200412331324901 PMID:15801576

Jugdutt, B. I. (2010). Aging and heart failure: Changing demographics and implications for therapy in the elderly. *Heart Failure Reviews, 15*(5), 401–405. doi:10.1007/s10741-010-9164-8 PMID:20364319

Kane, R., Ouslander, J., Abrass, I., & Resenter, B. (2008). *Essentials of clinical geriatrics* (6th ed.). New York, NY: McGraw Hill Publishers.

Kaplan, R. M., & Ong, M. (2007). Rationale and public health implications of changing CHD risk factor definitions. *Annual Review of Public Health, 28*(1), 321–344. doi:10.1146/annurev.publhealth.28.021406.144141 PMID:17222077

Karlamangla, A., Tinetti, M., Guralnik, J., Studenski, S., Wetle, T., & Reuben, D. (2007). Comorbidity in Older Adults: Nosology of Impairment, Diseases, and Conditions. *The Journals of Gerontology. Series A, Biological Sciences and Medical Sciences, 62A*(3), 296–300. doi:10.1093/gerona/62.3.296 PMID:17389727

Kaye, K. S., Sloane, R., Sexton, D. J., & Schmader, K. A. (2006). Risk factors for surgical site infections in older people. *Journal of the American Geriatrics Society, 54*(3), 391–396. doi:10.1111/j.1532-5415.2005.00651.x PMID:16551304

Kessing, L. V., & Anderson, P. K. (2004). Does the risk of developing dementia increase with the number of episodes in patients with depressive disorder and inpatients with bipolar disorder? *Journal of Neurology, Neurosurgery, and Psychiatry, 75*(12), 1662–1666. doi:10.1136/jnnp.2003.031773 PMID:15548477

Kitzman, D. W., Hundley, W. G., Brubaker, P. H., Morgan, T. M., Moore, J. B., Stewart, K. P., & Little, W. C. (2010). A randomized double-blind trial of enalapril in older patients with heart failure and preserved ejection fraction: Effects on exercise tolerance and arterial dispensability. *Circulation: Heart Failure, 3*(4), 477–485. doi:10.1161/CIRCHEARTFAILURE.109.898916 PMID:20516425

Langa, K. M., Larson, E. B., Wallace, R. B., Fendrick, A. M., Foster, N. L., Kabeto, M. U., ... Herzog, A. R. (2004). Out-of-pocket health care expenditures among older American with dementia. *Alzheimer Disease and Associated Disorders, 18*(2), 90–98. doi:10.1097/01.wad.0000126620.73791.3e PMID:15249853

Lo¨ppo¨nen, M. K., Isoaho, R. E., Ra¨iha, I. J., Vahlberg, T. J., Loikas, S. M., Takala, T. I., ... Kivelä, S.-L. (2004). Undiagnosed diseases in patients with dementia-a potential target group for intervention. *Dementia and Geriatric Cognitive Disorders, 18*(3-4), 321–329. doi:10.1159/000080126 PMID:15305110

Lupien, S. J., de Leon, M., de Santi, S., Convit, A., Tarshish, C., Nair, N. P. V., ... Meaney, M. J. (1998). Cortisol levels during human aging predict hippocampal atrophy and memory deficits. *Nature Neuroscience, 1*(1), 69–73. doi:10.1038/271 PMID:10195112

Lyketsos, C. G., Steinberg, M., & Tschanz, J. T. (2000). Mental and behavioral disturbances in dementia: FIndings from the Cache County Study on Memory in Aging. *The American Journal of Psychiatry, 157*(5), 708–714. doi:10.1176/appi.ajp.157.5.708 PMID:10784462

Martini, E. M., Garrett, N., Lindquist, T., & Isham, G. J. (2007). The Boomers are coming: A total cost of care model of the impact of population aging on health care costs in the United States by major practice category. *Health Services Research, 42*(1 Pt 1), 201–218. doi:10.1111/j.1475-6773.2006.00607.x PMID:17355589

Massie, B. M., Carson, P. E., McMurray, J. J., Komajda, M., McKelvie, R., Zile, M. R., ... Ptaszynska, A. (2008). Irbesar.tan in patients with heart failure and preserved ejection fraction. *The New England Journal of Medicine, 359*(23), 2456–2467. doi:10.1056/NEJMoa0805450 PMID:19001508

Mayo Clinic. (2013, November 14). *Shared decisions: Diabetes medication decision aid.* Retrieved from http:// shareddecisions.mayoclinic.org/decision-aids-for-diabetes/diabetesmedication-management

Melzer, D., Delgado, J. C., & Winder, R. (2015). *The Age UK Almanac of Disease Profiles in later Life*. NIHR.

Mercer, S. W., Smith, S. M., Wyke, S., O'Dowd, T., & Watt, G. C. (2009). Multimorbidity in primary care: Developing the research agenda. *Family Practice*, *26*(2), 79–80. doi:10.1093/fampra/cmp020 PMID:19287000

Meyers, C. A., Byrne, K. S., & Komaki, R. (1995). Cognitive deficits in patients with small cell lung cancer before and after chemotherapy. *Lung Cancer (Amsterdam, Netherlands)*, *12*(3), 231–235. doi:10.1016/0169-5002(95)00446-8 PMID:7655832

Mitchell, A. J., Rao, S., & Vaze, A. (2010). Do primary care physicians have particular difficulty identifying late-life depression? A meta-analysis stratified by age. *Psychotherapy and Psychosomatics*, *79*(5), 285–294. doi:10.1159/000318295 PMID:20616623

Mockler, M., O'Loughlin, C., Murphy, N., Ryder, M., Conlon, C., McDonald, K. M., ... Ledwidge, M. T. (2009). Causes. and consequences of nonpersistence with heart failure medication Am*erica.n. Journal of Cardiology*, *103*(6), 834–838. PMID:19268741

Moynihan, R., Doust, J., & Henry, D. (2012). Preventing overdiagnosis: How to stop harming the healthy. *British Medical Journal*, *344*(may28 4), e3502. doi:10.1136/bmj.e3502 PMID:22645185

Murad, M., & Kitzman, D. W. (2012). Frailty and Multiple Comorbidities in the Elderly Patient with Heart Failure: Implications for Management. *Heart Failure Reviews*, *17*(0), 581–588. doi:10.1007/s10741-011-9258-y PMID:21626426

National Institute of Health's National Institute of Neurological Disorders and Stroke. (2004) The Dementias. Publication No. 04–2252. Bethesda, MD: Author.

Nielsen-Bohlman, L., Panzer, A. M., & Kindig, D. A. (Eds.). (2004). Health Literacy: A Prescription to End Confusion. Washington, DC: The National Academies Press.

Noël, P. H., Williams, J. W., Unützer, J., Worchel, J., Lee, S., Cornell, J., ... Hunkeler, E. (2004). Depress. ion and Comorbid Illness in Elderly Primary Care Patients. *Impact on Multiple Domains of Health Status and Well-being Annals. of Family Medicine*, *2*(6), 555–562. doi:10.1370/afm.143 PMID:15576541

Nolen, W. A., Luckenbaugh, D. A., Altshuler, L. L., Suppes, T., McElroy, S. L., Frye, M. A., ... Post, R. M. (2004). Correlates of 1-year prospective outcome in BPD: Results from the Stanley Foundation Bipolar Network. *The American Journal of Psychiatry*, *61*(8), 1447–1454. doi:10.1176/appi.ajp.161.8.1447 PMID:15285972

Panza, F., Frisardi, V., Capurso, C., D'Introno, A., Colacicco, A. M., Imbimbo, B. P., ... Solfrizzi, V. (2010). Late-life depression, mild cognitive impairment and dementia: Possible continuum? *The American Journal of Geriatric Psychiatry*, *18*(2), 98–116. doi:10.1097/JGP.0b013e3181b0fa13 PMID:20104067

Papadopoulos, F. C., Petridou, E., Argyropoulou, S., Kontaxakis, V., Dessypris, N., Anastasiou, A., ... Lyketsos, C. (2005). Prevalence and correlates of depression in late life: A population based study from a rural Greek town. *International Journal of Geriatric Psychiatry*, *20*(4), 350–357. doi:10.1002/gps.1288 PMID:15799076

Patterson, R. L., & Jeste, D. V. (1999). The potential impact of the babyboom generation on substance abuse among elderly persons. *Psychiatric Services (Washington, D.C.)*, *50*(9), 1184–1188. doi:10.1176/ps.50.9.1184 PMID:10478905

Payne, G., Laporte, A., Deberm, R., & Coyte, P. (2007). Counting backward to health care's future: Using time-todeath modeling to identify changes in end-of-life morbidity and the impact of aging on health care expenditures. *The Milbank Quarterly*, *85*(2), 213–257. doi:10.1111/j.1468-0009.2007.00485.x PMID:17517114

Piette, J. D., & Kerr, E. A. (2006). The impact of comorbid chronic conditions on diabetes care. *Diabetes Care*, *29*(3), 725–731. doi:10.2337/diacare.29.03.06.dc05-2078 PMID:16505540

Pyne, J. M., Patterson, T. L., & Kaplan, R. M. (1997). Assessment of quality of life of patients with major depression. *Psychiatric Services (Washington, D.C.)*, *48*(2), 224–230. doi:10.1176/ps.48.2.224 PMID:9021855

Reuben, D. B., Mui, S., Damesyn, M., Moore, A. A., & Greendale, G. A. (1999). The prognostic value of sensory impairment in older persons. *Journal of the American Geriatrics Society*, *47*(8), 930–935. doi:10.1111/j.1532-5415.1999.tb01286.x PMID:10443852

Robnett, R. H., & Chop, W. C. (2010). Medications. In *Gerontology for the Health Care Professional* (p. 119). Boston: Jones and Bartlett publishers.

Roger, V.L., Go, A.S., Lloyd-Jones, D.M., Adams, R.J., Berry, J.D., Brown, T.M. ,… Wylie-Rosett, J. (2011). Heart Disease and Stroke Statistics--2011 Update: A Report From the American Heart Association. *Circulation*. CIR.0b013e3182009701.

Roger, V. L., Go, A. S., Lloyd-Jones, D. M., Adams, R. J., Berry, J. D., Brown, T. M., ... Turner, M. B. (2011). Statistical Update Heart Disease and Stroke Statistics—2011 Update: A Report from the American Heart Association. *Circulation*, *123*(4), e18–e209. doi:10.1161/CIR.0b013e3182009701 PMID:21160056

Sajatovic, M., Blow, F. C., & Ignacio, R. V. (2006). Psychiatric comorbidity in older adults with bipolar disorder. *International Journal of Geriatric Psychiatry*, *21*(6), 582–587. doi:10.1002/gps.1527 PMID:16783798

Schellevis, F. G., van der Velden, J., van de Lisdonk, E., van Eijk, J. T., & van Weel, C. (1993). Comorbidity of chronic diseases in general practice. *Journal of Clinical Epidemiology*, *46*(5), 469–473. doi:10.1016/0895-4356(93)90024-U PMID:8501473

Schulze, M. B., Rimm, E. B., Li, T., Rifai, N., Stampfer, M. J., & Hu, F. B. (2004). C-reactive protein and incident cardiovascular events among men with diabetes. *Diabetes Care*, *27*(4), 889–894. doi:10.2337/diacare.27.4.889 PMID:15047644

Simon, N. M., Otto, M. W., & Wisniewsk, S. R. (2004). Anxiety disorder comorbidity in bipolar patients: Data from the first 500 participants in the Systematic Treatment Enhancement Program for Bipolar Disorder (STEP-BO). *The American Journal of Psychiatry*, *161*(12), 2222–2229. doi:10.1176/appi.ajp.161.12.2222 PMID:15569893

Simoni-Wastila, L., & Yang, H. K. (2006). Psychoactive drug abuse in older adults. *The American Journal of Geriatric Pharmacotherapy*, *4*(4), 380–394. doi:10.1016/j.amjopharm.2006.10.002 PMID:17296542

Skinner, T. R., Scott, I. A., & Martin, J. H. (2016). Diagnostic errors in older patients: A systematic review of incidence and potential causes in seven prevalent diseases. *International Journal of General Medicine*, *9*, 137–146. doi:10.2147/IJGM.S96741 PMID:27284262

Spijkerman, A. M., Dekker, J. M., Nijpels, G., Jager, A., Kostense, P. J., van Hinsbergh, V. W. M., ... Stehouwer, C. D. A. (2002). Impact of diabetes duration and cardiovascular risk factors on mortality in type 2 diabetes: The Hoorn Study. *European Journal of Clinical Investigation*, *32*(12), 924–930. doi:10.1046/j.1365-2362.2002.01090.x PMID:12534452

Srinivasan, T., & Hannah, P. P. (2012). Bidirectional communication between the neuroendocrine system and the immune system: Relevance to health and diseases. *Annals of Neurosciences*, *19*(1), 40–46. PMID:25205962

Starfield, B. (2007). Pathways of influence on equity in health. *Social Science & Medicine*, *64*(7), 1355–1362. doi:10.1016/j.socscimed.2006.11.027 PMID:17208343

Substance Abuse and Mental Health Services Administration. (2012). *Results From the 2011 National Survey on Drug Use and Health: Summary of National Findings*. NSDUH Series H-44, HHS Publication No. (SMA) 12-4713. Rockville, MD: Substance Abuse and Mental Health Services Administration, The Center for Disease Control and Prevention. Medication Safety. Retrieved from http://www.cdc.gov/medicationsafety/

Substance Abuse and Mental Health Services Administration, Office of Applied Studies. (2011). *Treatment Episode Data Set (TEDS), 1999-2009. DASIS Series: S-56, HHS Publication No. SMA 11-4646.* Rockville, MD: Substance Abuse and Mental Health Services Administration.

University of California at San Francisco. (2013, November 14). *Estimating prognosis for elders*. Retrieved from http://eprognosis.ucsf.edu/calculators

Unützer, J., Patrick, D. L., Diehr, P., Simon, G., Grembowski, D., & Katon, W. (2000). Quality adjusted life years in older adults with depressive symptoms and chronic medical disorders. *International Psychogeriatrics*, *12*(1), 15–33. doi:10.1017/S1041610200006177 PMID:10798451

Valderas, J.M., Starfield, B.&Roland, M. (2007). Multimorbidity's many challenges: A research priority in the UK. *British Medical Journal, 334*(7604), 1128.

Valderas, J. M., Starfield, B., Sibbald, B., Salisbury, C., & Roland, M. (2009). Defining Comorbidity: Implications for Understanding Health and Health Services. *Annals of Family Medicine*, *7*(4), 357–363. doi:10.1370/afm.983 PMID:19597174

Van den Akker, M., Buntinx, F., Metsemakers, J. F. M., Roos, S., & Knottnerus, J. A. (1996). Multimorbidity in general practice: Prevalence, incidence, and determinants of co-occurring chronic and recurrent diseases. *Journal of Clinical Epidemiology*, *51*(5), 367–375. doi:10.1016/S0895-4356(97)00306-5 PMID:9619963

van Weel, C., & Schellevis, F. G. (2006). Comorbidity and guidelines: Conflicting interests. *Lancet*, *367*(9510), 550–551. doi:10.1016/S0140-6736(06)68198-1 PMID:16488782

Verduin, M. L., Carter, R. E., Brady, K. T., Myrick, H., & Timmerman, M. A. (2005). Health service use among persons with comorbid bipolar and substance use disorders. *Psychiatric Services (Washington, D.C.)*, *56*(4), 475–480. doi:10.1176/appi.ps.56.4.475 PMID:15812100

Vinkers, D. J., Gussekloo, J., Stek, M. L., Westendorp, R. G., & van der Mast, R. C. (2004). Temporal relation between depression and cognitive impairment in old age: Prospective population based study. *British Medical Journal*, *329*(7471), e881. doi:10.1136/bmj.38216.604664.DE PMID:15345599

Vitry, A., & Zhang, Y. (2008). Quality of Australian clinical guidelines and relevance to the care of older people with multiple comorbid conditions. *The Medical Journal of Australia*, *189*(7), 360–365. PMID:18837677

Voyer, P., Preville, M., Roussel, M. E., Berbiche, D., & Beland, S. G. (2009). Factors associated with benzodiazepine dependence among community-dwelling seniors. *Journal of Community Health Nursing*, *26*(3), 101–113. doi:10.1080/07370010903034375 PMID:19662558

Weiss, B. D. (2007). *Health Literacy and Patient Safety: Help Patients Understand. Manual for Clinicians* (2nd ed.). AMA Foundation.

Wells, K. B., & Sherbourne, C. D. (1999). Functioning and utility for current health of patients with depression or chronic medical conditions in managed primary care practices. *Archives of General Psychiatry*, *56*(10), 897–904. doi:10.1001/archpsyc.56.10.897 PMID:10530631

Wells, K. B., Stewart, A., & Hays, R. D. (1989). The functioning and well-being of depressed patients: Results from the Medical Outcomes Study. *Journal of the American Medical Association*, *262*(7), 914–919. doi:10.1001/jama.1989.03430070062031 PMID:2754791

Wolff, J. L., Starfiled, B., & Anderson, G. F. (2002). Prevalence, expenditures, and complications of multiple chronic conditions in the elderly. *Archives of Internal Medicine*, *162*(20), 2269–2276. doi:10.1001/archinte.162.20.2269 PMID:12418941

World Health Organization (2004). *Global Burden of Disease*. WHO.

Wu, L. T., & Blazer, D. G. (2011). Illicit and nonmedical drug use among older adults: A review. *Journal of Aging and Health*, *23*(3), 481–504. doi:10.1177/0898264310386224 PMID:21084724

Wu, L. T., Woody, G. E., Yang, C., Mannelli, P., & Blazer, D. G. (2011). Differences in onset and abuse/dependence episodes between prescription opioids and heroin: Results from the National Epidemiologic Survey on Alcohol and Related Conditions. *Substance Abuse and Rehabilitation*, *2*, 77–88. doi:10.2147/SAR.S18969 PMID:21686045

Yusuf, S., Pfeffer, M. A., Swedberg, K., Granger, C. B., Held, P., McMurray, J. J., ... Östergren, J. (2003). Effects of candesartan in patients with chronic heart failure and preserved leftventricular ejection fraction: The CHARM-Preserved Trial. *Lancet*, *362*(9386), 777–781. doi:10.1016/S0140-6736(03)14285-7 PMID:13678871

Zekry, D., Herrmann, F. R., Grandjean, R., Meynet, M.-P., Michel, J.-P., Gold, G., & Krause, K.-H. (2008). Demented versus non-demented very old inpatients: The same comorbidities but poorer functional and nutritional status. *Age and Ageing*, *37*(1), 83–89. doi:10.1093/ageing/afm132 PMID:17971391

KEY TERMS AND DEFINITIONS

Comorbidity: It is the presence of one or more additional diseases or disorders co-occurring with (i.e., concomitant or concurrent with) a primary disease or disorder; in the countable sense of the term, a comorbidity (plural comorbidities) is each additional disorder or disease.

Geriatric Population: Population of elderly people (65 years and beyond).

Medical Comorbidity: A condition existing simultaneously but independently with another condition or a related medical condition.

Pathophysiological Pathways: The pathway showing the physiology of abnormal states, specifically the functional changes that accompany a particular syndrome or disease.

Psychiatric Comorbidity: Co-occurrence of two or more psychiatric diagnoses.

Chapter 26
Disability Issues, Aging, and Preventive Measures

Ashok Kori
Dharwad Institute of Mental Health and Neurosciences (DIMHANS), India

Manjunath R. Bajantri
Dharwad Institute of Mental Health and Neurosciences (DIMHANS), India

ABSTRACT

As we know, aging is an ongoing biological process from which no human being can escape. Although everyone is familiar with ageing, defining it is not so easy. There is no United Nations standard numerical criterion of old age, but, it is agreed cut off is 60 plus years. Currently, due to the availability and accessibility of effective medication and treatment at specialty hospitals that increase life expectancy of old age people, over the past century, the population, although aged with disabilities, has aged around the world. Recent advances in the field of medicine, public health, technology, and rehabilitation in different streams have reduced the discrepancy in life expectancy for persons with disabilities.

INTRODUCTION

It is very essential to understand disability, ageing and preventive measures of elder population. The population percentage of old age people varies from country to country. India's elderly population is estimated at 10 crores in 2011, and is projected to reach 20 crores by 2030. The number of elderly in India is rising rapidly. The proportion of elderly persons in the total population is expected to increase from 8.3 percent in 2011 to 12.4 percent in 2026 (Bharati & Singh 2013). According to the Census of Government of India, the elderly population accounted for 8.2% of the total population in 2011, and the number is likely to increase dramatically over the next four decades in India to 19% in 2050. The global demographic trend, however, tells us that, with the passage of time, the countries have experienced ageing of population. The proportion of older persons in the population of a country has increased. Due to economic well-being, better health care system, good medicines, etc. there is substantial reduction in mortality in the society. Reduced mortality has led to reduction in fertility too. These factors together have

DOI: 10.4018/978-1-5225-3480-8.ch026

resulted in increasing number of elderly persons in the population. This phenomenon, called population ageing, is a dynamic demographic trend all over the world.

The report on Elderly in India from Ministry of statistics and program implementation indicates that on population ageing. As per this, the population ageing, started in the last century with developed countries, is now encompassing developing countries too India, by no means, is an exception to this phenomenon. Over the years, the structure of population has changed and will further change in the time to come. Population ageing has profound social, economic and political implications for a country. The increasing number of older persons put a strain on health care and social care systems in the country. Old age comes with lot of ailment and diseases. In case of large number of elderly persons in the population, the country needs more and more health and medical services, facilities and resources. More and more number of hospitals, doctors, nurses are required. Government spending on health care is increased with the increase of average age of population (Elderly in India, 2016). Very old people, due to their reduced mobility and debilitating disabilities, need other people to do things for them. With the increasing trend of nuclear families in the society and with fewer children in the family, the care of older persons in the families gets increasingly difficult. To fulfil caring needs of aged persons more and more health care staff with appropriate skills are required.

UNDERSTANDING DISABILITY

Definition of Disability have been mentioned by various authors and defined in Acts of Government of India. It is difficult to define 'Disability' since it varies in types, form and intensity. Understanding disability will require understanding these differences. According to the World Health Organization "Disability is any restriction or lack (resulting from an impairment) of ability to perform in a manner or within the range considered normal for a human being".As per the Persons with Disability Act 1995, it has been defined as "a person suffering from not less than forty per cent of any disability as certified by a medical authority" (PWD Act, 1995).

One of the Author identified different types of disabilities like blindness, low vision, cerebral palsy, leprosy cured, hearing impairment, locomotor disability, mental illness and mental retardation as well as multiple disabilities (Baquer, 1994).

Rights of the Person with Disabilities act 2016 has been published in Gazette of India, According to this new act "person with disability" means a person with long term physical, mental, intellectual or sensory impairment which, in interaction with barriers, hinders his full and effective participation in society equally with others (RPD Act, 2016).

The International Classification of Functioning, Disability and Health (ICF) define disability as an umbrella term for impairments, activity limitations, and participation restrictions (ICF).

The NSSO considered disability as "Any restriction or lack of abilities to perform an activity in the manner or within the range considered normal for human being". It excludes illness /injury of recent origin (morbidity) resulting into temporary loss of ability to see, hear, speak or move.

Disability is a "restriction or lack (resulting from an impairment) of ability to perform an activity in the manner or within the range considered normal for a human being". It describes a functional limitation or activity restriction caused by impairment. Disabilities are descriptions of disturbances in function at the level of the person. Examples of disabilities include difficulty seeing, speaking or hearing; difficulty moving or climbing stairs; difficulty grasping, reaching, bathing, eating, toileting (The United Nations and Disabled Persons -The First Fifty Years)

As per the International Classification of Functioning (2001), Disability refers to difficulties encountered in any or all three areas of functioning given below:

- Impairments are problems in body function or alterations in body structure – for example, paralysis or blindness;
- Activity limitations are difficulties in executing activities – for example, walking or eating;
- Participation restrictions are problems with involvement in any area of life – for example, facing discrimination in employment or transportation.

Different types of Disabilities mentioned in the Persons with Disability Act 1995 like blindness, low vision, leprosy-cured, hearing impairment, loco motor disability, mental retardation and mental illness.

Country-Reported Disability Prevalence

More countries have been collecting prevalence data on disability through censuses and surveys, with many having moved from an "impairment" approach to a "difficulties in functioning" approach. Estimated prevalence rates vary widely across and within countries. (Mont, 2007, Barbotte, Guillemin., & Chau, 2011; United Nations demographic yearbook,1993)

National Policy on Older Persons

The year of 1999 is very important in the history of India, because, the Government of India adopted the National Policy on Older Persons in this year. In order to increase the need for intervention in area of old age welfare, Ministry of Social Justice and Empowerment, Government of India adopted 'National Policy on Older Persons' in January, 1999. This policy provides broad guidelines to State Governments for taking action for welfare of older persons in a proactive manner by devising their own policies and plans of action. It attempts to ensure well-being of senior citizens and improve quality of their lives through providing specific facilities, concessions, relief, services etc. and helping them cope with problems associated with old age. It also intends affirmative action on the part of Government Departments for ensuring that the existing public services for senior citizens are user friendly and sensitive to their needs. It offers a broad picture of innumerable amenities and covers many areas like financial security, health care, shelter education, welfare, protection of life and property etc. (Situation Analysis of the Elderly in India, 2011).

Trends in the Numbers of Older Persons

The number of older persons in the world has increased markedly in recent years and that growth is projected to accelerate in the coming decades. It is estimated that worldwide, there were 901 million people aged 60 years or over in 2015, an increase of 48 per cent over the 607 million older persons globally in 2000. By 2030, the number of people in the world aged 60 years or over is projected to grow by 56 per cent, to 1.4 billion, and by 2050, the global population of older persons is projected to more than double its size in 2015, reaching nearly 2.1 billion. Globally, the number of people aged 80 years or over, the "oldest-old" persons, is growing even faster than the number of older persons overall. In 2000, there were 71 million people aged 80 or over worldwide. Since then, the number of oldest-old grew by 77 per cent to 125 million in 2015, and it is projected to increase by 61 per cent over the next 15 years, reaching nearly 202 million in 2030. Projections indicate that in 2050 the oldest-old will number 434 million globally, having more than tripled in number since 2015 (World Population Ageing, 2015).

INCREASING ELDER POPULATION

According to data from World Population Prospects: the 2015 Revision (United Nations, 2015), the number of older persons those aged 60 years or over has increased substantially in recent years in most countries and regions, and that growth is projected to accelerate in the coming decades. Globally, the number of people aged 80 years or over, the "oldest-old" persons, is growing even faster than the number of older persons overall. Projections indicate that in 2050 the oldest-old will number 434 million, having more than tripled in number since 2015, when there were 125 million people over age 80. The older population is growing faster in urban areas than in rural areas. At the global level between 2000 and 2015, the number of people aged 60 years or over increased by 68 per cent in urban areas, compared to a 25 per cent increase in rural areas. As a result, older persons are increasingly concentrated in urban areas. In 2015, 58 per cent of the world's people aged 60 years or over resided in urban areas, up from 51 per cent in 2000. The oldest-old are even more likely to reside in urban areas: the proportion of people aged 80 years or over residing in urban areas increased from 56 percent in 2000 to 63 percent in 2015. Between 2015 and 2030, the number of people in the world aged 60 years or over is projected to grow by 56 per cent, from 901 million to 1.4 billion, and by 2050, the global population of older persons is projected to more than double its size in 2015, reaching nearly 2.1 billion (World population Ageing, 2015).

MAGNITUDE OF DISABILITY IN INDIA

It is estimated that approximately 30 percent of the population is affected by one or the other disability. Data on the disability on a nation-wide basis can be acquired from two sources, namely the Population Census and National Sample Surveys. After a massive public campaign, the Government of India finally yielded and has included disability as a category in Census 2001. More than one billion people in the world live with some form of disability, of whom nearly 200 million experience considerable difficulties in functioning. The following Table 1 depicts about elderly population; 60 years and above in India.

Elderly Population is at Risk

Currently, elder people are suffering from different physical, psychiatric, neurological and neurosurgical disorder due to many factors. This group constitute one of the most vulnerable groups. Due to age factors, elder persons have more chances of developing chronic disease, infections, and subsequent disabilities. Hence, this population group at greater risk of being less healthy than the nonelderly population. It has been suggested that the ageing population in India will lead to increases in the prevalence of chronic

Table 1. Elderly population (aged 60 years & above) in India (in millions)

Source	Total			Rural	Urban
	Person	Female	Male		
Census 1961	24.7	12.4	12.4	21.0	3.7
Census 1971	32.7	15.8	16.9	27.3	5.4
Census 1981*	43.2	21.1	22.0	34.7	8.5
Census 1991**	56.7	27.3	29.4	44.3	12.4
Census 2001***	76.6	38.9	37.8	57.4	19.2
Census 2011***	103.8	52.8	51.1	73.3	30.6

Source: Elderly in India (2016)
Source: Population Census Data
* The 1981 Census could not be held in Assam owing to disturbed conditions.
The population figures for 1981 of Assam were worked out by 'interpolation'.
** The 1991 Census was not held in Jammu & Kashmir.
The population figures for 1991 of Jammu & Kashmir were worked out by 'interpolation'.
*** The figures include the estimated population of Mao Maram, Paomata and Purul sub-divisions of Senapati district of Manipur.

conditions, including diabetes and hypertension, and nearly one-half (45%) of India's disease burden is projected to be borne by older adults in 2030. And Early results from a pilot phase of the Longitudinal Ageing Study in India showed that 13% of "older Indians sampled have some type of disability that affects at least one activity of daily living (Pal, 2010). Based on the survey "Report on the Status of Elderly in Select States of India, 2011" collected information on locomotor disability, and questions were asked about the about difficulty regarding vision, hearing, walking, chewing, speaking, and memory. It was found that the prevalence of locomotor disability was highest for vision (about 60%) and lowest for the speech (about 7%) (UNFPA, 2014).

Health Conditions of Older Persons

The need for health care increases with age as people above 65 years spend on average 1.5 times on health care compared to those in the 60-64 age category (Mahal & Berman, 2002). Largest proportion of expenditure is spent on out-patient treatment as well as purchase of medicines. The expenditure on health care is expected to be high for the elderly because of chronic diseases. The elderly have little recourse to insurance as insurance generally covers in-patient hospital expenditure (Shahrawat & Rao, 2011). The elderly in India suffer from cardio-vascular illnesses, circulatory diseases, cancer, arthritis, hyper tension, osteoporosis, communicable diseases, high blood pressure, kidney problems, vision problems, diabetes, rheumatism and digestive disorders (Kumari, 2001, Gajalakshmi, 2005). Other health problems can be observed if disability becomes severe in elder population. The study from western show that higher disability rates among older people reflect an accumulation of health risks across a lifespan of disease, injury, and chronic illness (Australian Institute of Health and Welfare, 2016). We can understand different types of chronic diseases in the elderly in India as the National Sample survey in 2004. The Table 2 depicts following figures which pertain different chronic diseases among the elderly in India.

Table 2. Chronic diseases among the elderly in India (Number per 1,000 persons)

	Rural			Urban		
Type of chronic Disease	**Males**	**Females**	**Persons**	**Males**	**Females**	**Persons**
Whooping cough	8	6	7	4	2	3
Ulcer	37	54	44	30	24	27
Problem of Joints	30	40	34	26	45	35
Hypertension	23	53	36	50	59	54
Heart disease	95	59	80	165	162	164
Urinary problem	78	28	57	89	33	63
Diabetes	30	52	40	68	36	53
Cancer	18	36	26	25	25	56

Source: National Sample Survey, 60th Round (2004)

PSYCHOLOGICAL WELL-BEING: DISABILITY AND COMORBIDITY

Wellbeing of elderly population is essential to know their quality of status in India. In one of the study where the investigator assessed the psychological well-being and disability status among elderly people, it was found that minimal disability was seen in 22%, moderate disability in 48.5%, and severe disability in 17%, respectively. It was also noted that as the number of morbidities increases, the psychological well-being deteriorates and disability increases(Joshi & Kumar, 2003).A number of morbidity patterns have been identified in elderly populations, which include "hypertension, diabetes, arthritis, constipation, cataracts and hearing loss" (Chandwani, Jivarajani, & Jivarajani, 2009). Many morbid conditions can be found by reviewing from another study, the authors of the study recognized many morbid conditions "pain/swelling of joints, limitation of movement, indigestion/heart bum, backache, breathlessness, giddiness/fainting, frequency/ urgency, change in bowel habits and blurring of vision" in the elderly population from a mix of rural and urban communities (Swami, Bhatia, Dutt, & Bhatia, 2002). In continuation, common presenting symptoms of the elderly were found like Headache, cough, giddiness/ fainting, backache, Itching or infection, Pain or Difficulty in urination, Chest pain, Blurring of vision, Pedal edema, wheezing and Nasal congestion in skin Change in Bowel habits,In India, Joshi reported in 2003 that 83% of the elderly people had more than three morbidities (Joshi, kumar., & Avasthi, 2003). Few research studies from India reveals that morbidity impacts the physical functioning and psychological well-being of elderly populations; (Swami et al., 2002; Joshi et al., 2003; Shankar, Tondon et al. 2006; Gupta, & Mani, 2014).

Morbidity among urban subjects was higher (90.7%) than rural (77.6%). Table 2 reveals the five common presenting symptoms of the elderly were: pain / swelling of joints (36.5%), limitation of movements (20.2%), indigestion/heartburn (17.7%), backache (17.4%), excessive tiredness/weakness (17.1%). Most common diseases in order of their magnitude were hypertension (58%) joint pains/arthritis (50.5%) cataract (19.1%), gastritis (17.7), deafness (13.5%) followed by diabetes mellitus (12.2%).

Table 3. Number of disabled per 100,000 elderly persons for different types of disability

Place of Residence	Seeing	Speech	Hearing	Movement	Mental Retardation	Mental Illness	Any Other	Multiple Disability
Rural	1467	182	1043	1425	86	86	595	708
Urban	931	230	844	1029	89	93	580	386

Sources: Elderly in India-2016, page:83

Table 4. Total Number of Disabled Elderly Persons in Different Age-Groups and their Percentage Distribution by Type of Disability

Age Group	No of PWD's in Thousands	% Distribution of Disabled Persons by Type of Disability in Each Age-Group							
		Seeing	Speech	Hearing	Movement	MR	Mental Illness	Any Other	Multiple Disability
Total									
60-69	2658	25	19	5	26	2	2	14	8
70-79	1769	26	19	3	26	1	1	10	13
80-89	724	24	20	2	24	1	1	8	19
90+	226	21	19	3	22	1	1	9	25
Rural									
60-69	1990	26	18	4	26	2	2	13	9
70-79	1374	27	19	3	26	1	1	10	14
80-89	560	25	19	2	25	1	1	7	20
90+	175	22	18	2	22	1	1	8	26
Urban									
60-69	668	22	19	7	25	3	3	16	7
70-79	396	23	21	5	25	2	2	12	10
80-89	164	21	23	4	24	1	2	10	15
90+	51	19	22	4	20	2	1	12	19

Source: Population Census (2011)

TRENDS IN HEALTH CONDITIONS ASSOCIATED WITH DISABILITY

Infectious Diseases

Infectious diseases occur due to disability reasons. Infectious diseases, may create, or be defined in terms of impairments. It was estimated to account for 9% of the years lived with disability in low-income and middle-income countries (The Global burden of disease, 2004). Lymphaticfilariasis, tuberculosis, HIV/AIDS, and other sexually transmitted diseases were prominent. Less prominent are diseases with neurological consequences, such as encephalitis (Kaiser, 1994-98; Lewis, & Glaser, 2005), meningitis (Hodgson A et al. 2001; van de Beek, D. 2006) and childhood cluster diseases – such as measles, mumps, and poliomyelitis (Galazka, Robertson, & Kraigher, 1999). Some of the trends in significant infectious diseases associated with disability can be found by reviewing some studies. In 2008 it was estimated that 33.4 million people worldwide – about 0.5% of the world population – were living with HIV. Between 2000 and 2008 the number of people living with HIV rose by 20%, but the annual global incidence of HIV infection is estimated to have declined by 17%. Sub-Saharan Africa remains the region most affected (AIDS epidemic update, 2009; WHO, 2009). Polio cases fell more than 99% in 18 years, from an estimated 350 000 cases in 1988, to 1604 in 2009 (WHO, 2008).

Morbidity Among Elderly Disability in India

The study conducted by Audinarayana et al. (2016) collected data from 750 old persons (aged 60+ years) selected from nine rural (450) and six urban (300) clusters of Tamil Nadu State, India. Data regarding physical disability from a mix of rural and urban populations among the elderly in Tamil Nadu and the disability was measured in terms of physical limitations. The information was collected about permanent loss of any of the following and resulting inability to do the normal day-to-day functions from the elderly, for "visual (loss of sight), hearing (loss of hearing), walking (loss feet or legs), dental (falling of teeth) and complete loss of arms or fingers (including fractures) and many other problems like apoplexy, speech difficulties, paralytic condition and trembling." It was found that 47% of the elderly persons were suffering from one or the other physical disability condition; the extent of physical disability was lower among the elderly belonging to higher socioeconomic background (educated, engaged in own cultivation, higher-salaried occupation, and belonging to higher family monthly income bracket). However, in this study the details of underlying morbid conditions or any other factors responsible for physical disability have not been addressed (Audinarayana & Sheela, 2016).

As quoted by Professor Stephen W Hawking in world report on disability in 2011, "Disability need not be an obstacle to success, I have had motor neurone disease for practically all my adult life. Yet it has not prevented me from having a prominent career in astrophysics and a happy family life" (World Report on Disability, 2011).

PREVENTION OF DISABILITY

- It is understood that prevention is better than cure. Hence, efforts are required to prevent disability scientifically and honestly. There is huge responsibility on health care professionals to prevent disability of elderly in India and other countries. Evidence shows that large number of cases of disability is preventable. As we know that disability caused due to poor nutrition, contaminated soil and water, accidents, wars etc are highly preventable. Data shows that 70 per cent of the visual impairment is caused either due to poor nutrition or clinical problems like cataract surgery. Concrete programs should be made so that disability caused by these can be prevented.
- Another thing, which causes disability, is old age. The incidence of disability can be significantly reduced through well-designed social and medical disability rather than only providing clinical corrections.

- Poverty is the most important cause of disability. Every year millions of people go below the poverty line. This makes them more vulnerable to disability. Many people suffering from poverty are facing lack of nutritious food.
- The WHO estimates that worldwide there are 1.5 million blind children, mainly in Asia and Africa. In developing countries up to 70 percent of blindness is either preventable or treatable. The WHO also estimates that around 50 per cent of disabling hearing impairment is also preventable. In 1995 this affected a total of 120 million people worldwide (Chaudhuri, 2006).

CONCLUSION

Recent advancement in modern medicine led elderly population to live longer period. But, bearing expenses of medicines for old age people belong to lower socio-economic status is not easy to pay it. Hence, there is a need to create awareness of disabilities in elder population. And these types of disabilities may be prevented by understanding different psychosocial issues faced by elder population in the world. Different stake holders in Government level and Non- Government level need to put efforts to create awareness to prevent diseases and disabilities could yield better results and help elderly population.

REFERENCES

AIDS Epidemic Update. (2009). Geneva: Joint United Nations Programme on HIV/AIDS and World Health Organization.

Audinarayana, N., & Sheela, J. (2016). Physical disability among the elderly in Tamil Nadu: Patterns differentials and determinants. *Health and Population; Perspectives and Issues*, *25*(1), 26–37.

Australian Institute of Health and Welfare. (2017). *Disability and its relationship to health conditions and other factors*. Retrieved from: https://www.aihw.gov.au/reports-statistics

Baquer, A. (1994). *Disabled, disablement, disablism*. New Delhi: Voluntary Health Association of India.

Barbotte, E., Guillemin, F., & Chau, N. (2001). Lorhandicap Group Prevalence of impairments, disabilities, handicaps and quality of life in the general population: A review of recent literature. *Bulletin of the World Health Organization*, *79*, 1047–1055. PMID:11731812

Bharati & Singh. (2013). *Ageing in India: Need for a Comprehensive Policy*. Academic Press.

Chandwani, H., Jivarajani, P., & Jivarajani, H. (2009). Health and social problems of geriatric population in an urban setting of Gujarat, India. *International Journal of Health, 9.*

Chaudhuri, L. (2006). *Disability in India: Issues and concerns*. Academic Press.

Elderly in India. (2016). Ministry of Statistics and Program Implementation, Central Statistics Office (Social Statistics Division).

Galazka, A. M., Robertson, S. E., & Kraigher, A. (1999). Mumps and mumps vaccine: A global review. *Bulletin of the World Health Organization*, *77*, 3–14. PMID:10063655

Global burden of disease: 2004 update. (2008). Geneva: World Health Organization.

Gupta, P., & Mani, K. (2014). Functional disability among elderly persons in a rural area of Haryana. *Indian Journal of Public Health*, *58*(1), 11. doi:10.4103/0019-557X.128155 PMID:24748351

International Classification of Functioning. (2001). *Disability and Health*. Geneva: World Health Organization.

Gajalakshmi, & Jha, P. V. (2005). Prospective study of one million deaths in India: Rationale, design, and validation results. *PLOS Medicine, 3*(2), e18.

Joshi, K., Kumar, R., & Avasthi, A. (2003). Morbidity profile and its relationship with disability and psychological distress among elderly people in Northern India. *International Journal of Epidemiology*, *32*(6), 978–987. doi:10.1093/ije/dyg204 PMID:14681260

Kaiser, R. (1999). The clinical and epidemiological profile of tick-borne encephalitis in southern Germany 1994–98: A prospective study of 656 patients. *Brain*, *122*(11), 2067–2078. doi:10.1093/brain/122.11.2067 PMID:10545392

Kumari, R. S. (2001). *Socio-economic conditions, morbidity pattern and social support among the elderly women in a rural area*. Sreekarym-Panchayat.

Hodgson, A. (2001). Survival and sequelae of meningococcal meningitis in Ghana. *International Journal of Epidemiology*, *30*, 1440–1446. PubMed. doi:10.1093/ije/30.6.1440

Lewis, P., & Glaser, C. A. (2005). Encephalitis. *Pediatrics in Review/American Academic Pediatrics*, *26*, 353–363.

Mahal, A., & Berman, P. (2002). Estimating baseline health expenditures on the elderly in India. In *Draft*. Boston, MA: Harvard School of Public Health, Department of Population and International Health.

Mont, D. (2007). *Measuring disability prevalence*. Washington, DC: World Bank (SP Discussion Paper No. 0706). Retrieved from (http://siteresources.worldbank.org/DISABILITY/Resources/Data/MontPrevalence.pdf

Pal, R. (2010). *Analysing catastrophic OOP health expenditure in India: Concepts, determinants and policy implications*. Mumbai, India: Indira Gandhi Institute of Development Research.

RPD Act. (2016). The Rights of Person with Disabilities Act, Ministry of Law and Justice. *The Gazette of India*, p. 3.

Shahrawat, R., & Rao, K. D. (2011). Insured yet vulnerable: Out-of-pocket payments and India's poor. *Health Policy and Planning*, czr029. PMID:21486910

Shankar, R., & Tondon, J. (2006). Health status of elderly population in rural area of Varanasi district. *Indian Journal of Public Health*, *51*(1), 56–58. PMID:18232146

Swami, H. M., Bhatia, V., Dutt, R., & Bhatia, S. P. (2002). A community based study of the morbidity profile among the elderly in Chandigarh, India. *Bahrain Medical Bulletin*, *24*, 13–16.

van de Beek, D., de Gans, J., Tunkel, A. R., & Wijdicks, E. F. M. (2006). Community-acquired bacterial meningitis in adults. *The New England Journal of Medicine*, *354*(1), 44–53. doi:10.1056/NEJMra052116 PMID:16394301

United Nations demographic yearbook, special issue: Population ageing and the situation of elderly persons. (1993). New York: United Nations.

World Population Ageing. (2015). *United Nations*. Department of Economic and Social Affairs, Population Division.

World Report on Disability. (2011). World Health Organization.

World Health Organization. (2015). *World Report on Ageing and Health*. Geneva: WHO.

KEY TERMS AND DEFINITIONS

Ageing: The process of growing old or developing the appearance and characteristics of old age.

Morbidity: Morbidity is an incidence of ill health. It is measured in various ways, often by the probability that a randomly selected individual in a population at some date and location would become seriously ill in some period of time.

Prevention: The goals of medicine are to promote and to preserve health, to restore health when it is impaired, and to minimize suffering and distress.

Compilation of References

551-565

A National Clinical guideline. (2006). *Management of Patients with Dementia SIGN*. Scottish Intercollegiate Guidelines Network.

Achermann, P., & Borbely, A. A. (2003). Mathematical models of sleep regulation. *Frontiers in Bioscience*, *8*(6), S683–S693. doi:10.2741/1064 PMID:12700054

Action on Elder Abuse. (1995). *Action on elder abuse's definition of elder abuse*. London: Bulletin, May/June.

Action on elder abuse. (n. d.) Retrieved October 12, 2007 from elderabuse.org.uk

Addis, I. B., Van Den Eeden, S. K., Wassel-fyr, C. L., Vittinghoff, E., Brown, J. S., & Thom, D. H. (2006). Sexual Activity and Function in Middle-Aged and Older women. *Obstetrics and Gynecology*, *107*(4), 755–764. doi:10.1097/01.AOG.0000202398.27428.e2 PMID:16582109

Adler, A. I., Stevens, R. J., Manley, S. E., Bilous, R. W., Cull, C. A., Holman, R. R., & Ukpds, G. (2003). Development and progression of nephropathy in type 2 diabetes: theUnited Kingdom prospective diabetes study (UKPDS 64). *Kidney International*, *63*(1), 225–232. doi:10.1046/j.1523-1755.2003.00712.x PMID:12472787

Advocare Incorporated. (2017). Signs and symptoms of elder abuse and neglect in care. Advocare Incorporated. Retrieved 16 December 2012 from http://www.advocare.org.au/help-with-aged-care-complaints/signs-and-symptoms-of-eld/

Agrawal, Y., Platz, E. A., & Niparko, J. K. (2008). Prevalence of hearing loss and differences by demographic characteristics among US adults: Data from the National Health and Nutrition Examination Survey, 1999-2004. *Archives of Internal Medicine*, *168*(14), 1522–1530. doi:10.1001/archinte.168.14.1522 PMID:18663164

Agronin, M. E. (2010). Sexual disorders. In D. G. Blazer & D. C. Steffens (Eds.), *The American Psychiatric Publishing Textbook of Geriatric Psychiatry* (4th ed.; pp. 357–373). Washington, DC: The American Psychiatric Publishing.

AIDS Epidemic Update. (2009). Geneva: Joint United Nations Programme on HIV/AIDS and World Health Organization.

Aitken, L., & Griffin, G. (1996). *Gender issues in elder abuse*. London: Sage Publication.

Albersen, M., & Lue, F. (2012). *Evaluation and Treatment of Erectile Dysfunction in the Aging Male: A Mini-Review*. Academic Press. 10.1159/000329598

Albert, S. G. (1960). *Introduction to a Submolecular Biology*. New York: AP.

Albert, M. S., DeKosy, S. T., Dickson, D., Dubois, B., Feldman, H. H., Fox, N. C., ... Phelps, C. H. (2011). The diagnosis of mild cognitive impairment due to Alzheimer's disease: Recommendations from the National Institute on Aging-Alzheimer's Association workgroups on diagnostic guidelines for Alzheimer's disease. *Alzheimer's & Dementia: The Journal of the Alzheimer's Association, 7*(3), 270–279. doi:10.1016/j.jalz.2011.03.008 PMID:21514249

Aldwin, C. M. (2007). *Stress, coping and development: An integrative perspective* (2nd ed.). New York: Guilford.

Alemayehu, B., & Warner, K. E. (2004). The lifetime distribution of health care costs. *Health Services Research, 39*(3), 627–642. doi:10.1111/j.1475-6773.2004.00248.x PMID:15149482

Alexander, C. N., Langer, E. J., Newman, R. I., Chandler, H. M., & Davies, J. L. (1989). Transcendental meditation, mindfulness, and longevity: An experimental study with the elderly. *Journal of Personality and Social Psychology, 57*(6), 950–964. doi:10.1037/0022-3514.57.6.950 PMID:2693686

Alex, J. A., & George, P. O. (2004). Ageing: A Christian perspective. *Global Ageing: Issues and Action, 2*, 36–43.

Alexopoulos, G. S., Meyers, B. S., Young, R. C., Mattis, S., & Kakuma, T. (1993). The course of geriatric depression with "reversible dementia": A controlled study. *The American Journal of Psychiatry, 150*(11), 1693–1699. doi:10.1176/ajp.150.11.1693 PMID:8105707

Algarabel González, S., Fuentes, M., Escudero, J., Pitarque, A., Peset, V., Mazón, J. F., & Meléndez Moral, J. C. (2012). Recognition memory deficits in mild cognitive impairment. *Neuropsychology, Development, and Cognition. Section B, Aging, Neuropsychology and Cognition, 19*(5), 608–619. doi:10.1080/13825585.2011.640657 PMID:22247955

Allen, S. M., & Mor, V. (1997). The prevalence and consequences of unmet need. Contrasts between older and younger adults with disability. *Medical Care, 35*(11), 1132–1148. doi:10.1097/00005650-199711000-00005 PMID:9366892

Altgeld, T., Cohen, S., & Brussels, J. (2012). Healthy and active ageing. (A report commissioned by Bundeszentrale-fürgesundheitlicheAufklärung (BZgA).). Euro Health Net.

Alzheimer's Association. (2010). Retrieved November 25, 2012 from http://www.alz.org/alzheimers_disease_trajectory

Alzheimer's disease facts and figures. (2015). *Alzheimer's & Dementia, The Journal of Alzheimer Association, 11*(3), 332-84.

Alzheimer's disease facts and figures. (2016). *Alzheimer's & Dementia, The Journal of Alzheimer Association, 12*(4), 459-509.

Amarya, S., Singh, K., & Sabharwal, M. (2014). Health consequences of obesity in the elderly. *Journal of Clinical Gerontology and Geriatrics, 5*(3), 63–67. doi:10.1016/j.jcgg.2014.01.004

Ambrose, A. F., Paul, G., & Hausdorff, J. M. (2013). Risk factors for falls among older adults: A review of the literature. *Maturitas, 75*(1), 51–61. doi:10.1016/j.maturitas.2013.02.009 PMID:23523272

American Academy of Sleep Medicine. (2005). *International Classification of Sleep Disorders. Diagnostic and Coding Manual* (2nd ed.). Westchester, IL: American Academy of Sleep Medicine.

American Academy of Sleep Medicine. (2014). *International classification of Sleep Disorders* (3rd ed.). Darien, IL: American Academy of Sleep Medicine.

American Association for Retired Persons. (2004). *Sexuality at Midlife and Beyond: 2004 Update of Attitude and Behaviors*. Available at http://assets.aarp.org/rgcenter/general/2004_sexuality.pdf

American Diabetes Association. (2014). Diagnosis and classification of diabetes mellitus. *Diabetes Care, 37*(1), 81-90.

American Medical Association White Paper on Elderly Health. (1990). Report on the Council on Scientific Affairs. *Archives of Internal Medicine*, *150*, 2459–2472. doi:10.1001/archinte.1990.00390230019004 PMID:2288622

American Psychiatric Association. (2000). *Diagnostic and Statistical Manual of Mental Disorders, Text Revision* (4th ed.). Washington, DC: American Psychiatric Association.

American Psychiatric association. (2012). *Diagnostic and statistical mannual of mental disorder* (5th edn, revised). Washington, DC: American Psychiatric Association.

American Psychiatric Association. (2013). *Diagnostic and Statistical Manual of Mental Disorders: DSM 5* (5th ed.). Washington, DC: American Psychiatric Association.

Ananthakrishnan, R., Kumar, K., Ganesh, M., Kumar, A. M., Krishnan, N., Swaminathan, S., ... Gupta, D. (2013). The profile and treatment outcomes of the older (aged 60 years and above) tuberculosis patients in Tamilnadu, South India. *PLoS One*, *8*(7), e67288. doi:10.1371/journal.pone.0067288 PMID:23861755

Ancoli-I, S., Kripke, D. F., Klauber, M. R., Mason, W. J., Fell, R., & Kaplan, O. (1991). Periodic limb movements in sleep in community-dwelling elderly. *Sleep*, *14*(6), 496–500. doi:10.1093/sleep/14.6.496 PMID:1798881

Ancoli-Israel, S. (2000). Insomnia in the elderly: A review for the primary care practitioner. *Sleep*, *23*, S23–S30. PMID:10755805

Ancoli-Israel, S., & Ayalon, L. (2006). Diagnosis and treatment of sleep disorders in older adults. *The American Journal of Geriatric Psychiatry*, *14*(2), 95–103.

Anderson, R. J., Freedland, K. E., Clouse, R. E., & Lustman, P. J. (2001). The prevalence of comorbid depression in adults with diabetes: A meta-analysis. *Diabetes Care*, *24*(6), 1069–1078. doi:10.2337/diacare.24.6.1069 PMID:11375373

Andrews, H. K. (2002) National Strategy for an Ageing Australia: an older Australia, challenges and opportunities for all.

Andrews, A. O., Bartels, S. J., Sie, H., & Peacock, W. J. (2009). Increased risk of nursing home admission among middle aged and older adults with schizophrenia. *The American Journal of Geriatric Psychiatry*, *17*(8), 697–705. doi:10.1097/JGP.0b013e3181aad59d PMID:19625787

Andrews, C. N. (2007). Sex and the older man GP perceptions and management. *Australian Family Physician*, *36*(10), 867–869. PMID:17925912

Angevaren, M., Aufdemkampe, G., Verhaar, H. J. J., Aleman, A., & Vanhees, L. (2008). Physical activity and enhanced fitness to improve cognitive function in older people without known cognitive impairment. *Cochrane Database of Systematic Reviews*, *2*. doi:10.1002/14651858.CD005381

Annon, J. (1976). The PLISSIT Model: A proposed conceptual scheme for the behavioural treatment of sexual problems. *Journal of Sex Education and Therapy*, *2*(1), 1–15. doi:10.1080/01614576.1976.11074483

Antonovsky, A. (1979). *Health, Stress and Coping*. San Francisco: Jossey-Bass Publishers.

Antonucci, T. C., & Akiyama, H. (1987). An examination of sex differences in social support among older men and women. *Sex Roles*, *17*(11–12), 737–749. doi:10.1007/BF00287685

Apfelbaum, E. P., Krendl, A. C., & Ambady, N. (2010). Age-related decline in executive function predicts better advice-giving in uncomfortable social contexts. *Journal of Experimental Social Psychology*, *46*(6), 1074–1077. doi:10.1016/j.jesp.2010.07.017

Apostolova, L. G., & Cummings, J. L. (2008). Neuropsychiatric manifestations in mild cognitive impairment: A systematic review of the literature. *Dementia and Geriatric Cognitive Disorders*, *25*(2), 115–126. doi:10.1159/000112509 PMID:18087152

Appelbaum, F. R., Gundacker, H., Head, D. R., Slovak, M. L., Willman, C. L., & Godwin, J. E. (2006). Age and acute myeloid leukemia. *Blood*, *107*(9), 3481–3485. doi:10.1182/blood-2005-09-3724 PMID:16455952

Arden Close, E., Gidron, Y., & Moss Morris, R. (2008). Psychological distress and its correlates in ovarian cancer: A systematic review. *Psycho-Oncology*, *17*(11), 1061–1072. doi:10.1002/pon.1363 PMID:18561287

Arean, P. A., Alviderz, J., Barrera, A., Robinson, G. S., & Hicks, S. (2002). Would older medical patients use psychological services? *The Gerontologist*, *42*(3), 392–398. doi:10.1093/geront/42.3.392 PMID:12040142

Arndt, J., Goldenberg, J. L., Greenberg, J., Pyszczynsky, T., & Solomon, S. (2000). In P. R. Duberstein & J. M. Masling (Eds.), (pp. 201–257). Washington, D.C., US: Psychodynamic Perspectives on Sickness and Health. Empirical Studies of Psychoanalytic Theories.

Arnett, J. J. (2000). Emerging adulthood: A theory of development from the late teens through the twenties. *The American Psychologist*, *55*(5), 469–480. doi:10.1037/0003-066X.55.5.469 PMID:10842426

Artero, S., Touchon, J., & Ritchie, K. (2001). Disability and mild cognitive impairment: A longitudinal population-based study. *International Journal of Geriatric Psychiatry*, *16*(11), 1092–1097. doi:10.1002/gps.477 PMID:11746656

Arthur, H. M. (2006). Depression, isolation, social support, and cardiovascular disease in older adults. *The Journal of Cardiovascular Nursing*, *21*(Suppl. 5), 2–7. doi:10.1097/00005082-200609001-00002 PMID:16966925

Arve, S., Tilvis, R. S., Lehtonen, A., Valvanne, J., & Sairanen, S. (1999). Coexistence of lowered mood and cognitive impairment of elderly people in five birth cohorts. *Aging (Milan, Italy)*, *11*(2), 90–95. PMID:10386168

Aspinwall, L. G., & Tedeschi, R. G. (2010). The Value of Positive Psychology for Health Psychology: Progress and Pitfalls in Examining the Relation of Positive Phenomena to Health. *Annals of Behavioral Medicine*, *39*(1), 4–15. doi:10.1007/s12160-009-9153-0 PMID:20091429

Atzmon, G., Barzilai, N., Hollowell, J. G., Surks, M. I., & Gabriely, I. (2009). Extreme longevity is associated with increased serum thyrotropin. *The Journal of Clinical Endocrinology and Metabolism*, *94*(4), 1251–1254. doi:10.1210/jc.2008-2325 PMID:19158193

Atzmon, G., Barzilai, N., Surks, M. I., & Gabriely, I. (2009). Genetic predisposition to elevated serum thyrotropin is associated with exceptional longevity. *The Journal of Clinical Endocrinology and Metabolism*, *94*(12), 4768–4775. doi:10.1210/jc.2009-0808 PMID:19837933

Audiffren, M., Tomporowski, P., & Zagrodnik, J. (2008). Acute aerobic exercise and information processing: Energizing motor processes during a choice reaction time task. *Acta Psychologica*, *129*(3), 410–419. doi:10.1016/j.actpsy.2008.09.006 PMID:18930445

Audinarayana, N., & Sheela, J. (2016). Physical disability among the elderly in Tamil Nadu: Patterns differentials and determinants. *Health and Population; Perspectives and Issues*, *25*(1), 26–37.

Australian Institute of Health and Welfare. (2017). *Disability and its relationship to health conditions and other factors*. Retrieved from: https://www.aihw.gov.au/reports-statistics

Ausubel, K. (2000). *When Healing Becomes a Crime: The amazing Story of Hoxsey Cancer Clinics and the Return of Alternative Therapies*. Healing Arts Press.

Aversa, A., Donini, L. M., Bruzziches, R., LaCava, R., Raso, F. M., & Sinclair, A. (2014). Coordinating Care Aspects Related to Sexual Health in the Aging Male. *International Journal of Endocrinology, 1-3.* doi:10.1155/2014/653587 PMID:24829576

Azuamah, Y. C., Imaseun, A. F., Onoseta, O. H., & Onuoha, P. C. (2013). A review of sociological factors associated with diabetes mellitus. *The International Journal of Social Sciences (Islamabad), 11*(1), 131–137.

Bablas, V., Yap, K., Cunnington, D., Swieca, J., & Greenwood, K. M. (2015). Mindfulness-based stress reduction for restless legs syndrome: A proof of concept trial. *Mindfulness, 7*(2), 396–408. doi:10.1007/s12671-015-0457-9

Baddeley, A. (2000). The episodic buffer: A new component of working memory? *Trends in Cognitive Sciences, 4*(11), 417–423. doi:10.1016/S1364-6613(00)01538-2 PMID:11058819

Bailer, J. C., & Gornik, H. L. (1997). Cancer Undefeated. *The New England Journal of Medicine, 336*(22), 1569–1574. doi:10.1056/NEJM199705293362206 PMID:9164814

Baird, A., & Samson, S. (2015). Music and dementia. *Programme Brain Research, 217*, 207–235. doi:10.1016/bs.pbr.2014.11.028 PMID:25725917

Baird, B. M., Lucas, R. E., & Donnellan, M. B. (2010). Life satisfaction across the lifespan: Findings from two nationally representative panel studies. *Social Indicators Research, 99*(2), 183–203. doi:10.1007/s11205-010-9584-9 PMID:21113322

Bajpai, S., Tripathi, M., Dey, A. B., & Nehra, A. (in press). Enhancing Memory & Activities of Daily Living (ADLs) In Patients with Early Alzheimer's disease using Memory Stimulation Intervention: A Randomized Controlled Trial. *International Journal of Advanced Medical and Health Research.*

Bajpai, S., Tripathi, M., & Nehra, A. (2015). Cognitive Rehabilitation: A State Of The Art For Long Term Management Of Alzheimer Disease For Indian Population. In *Proceedings of 12th International Conference on Alzheimer's and Parkinson's Disease*. Nice, France.

Baker, F. (2002). The effects of live, taped and no music on people experiencing posttraumatic amnesia. *Journal of Music Therapy, 38*, 82–104. PMID:11570931

Balhara, Y. P., & Sagar, R. (2011). Correlates of anxiety and depression among patients with type 2 diabetes mellitus. *Indian Journal of Endocrinology and Metabolism, 15*(5 Suppl. 1), S50–S54. doi:10.4103/2230-8210.83057 PMID:21847456

Baltes, P. B. (1987). Theoretical propositions of life-span developmental psychology: On the dynamic between growth and decline. *Developmental Psychology, 23*(5), 611–626. doi:10.1037/0012-1649.23.5.611

Baltes, P. B., & Baltes, M. M. (1990). Psychological perspectives on successful aging: The model of selective optimization with compensation. In P. B. Baltes & M. M. Baltes (Eds.), *Successful aging: Perspectives from the behavioral sciences* (pp. 1–34). New York, NY: Cambridge University Press. doi:10.1017/CBO9780511665684.003

P. B. Baltes, & M. M. Baltes (Eds.). (1990b). *Successful aging: Perspectives from the behavioural sciences*. Cambridge, UK: Cambridge University Press. doi:10.1017/CBO9780511665684

Bandura, A. (1986). *Social foundation of thoughts and actions*. Englewood Cliffs, CA: Prentice Hall.

Bandura, A. (1997). *Self-efficacy: The exercise of control*. New York: Freeman and Co.

Banks, M., Klein, S., Sinacore, D. R., Siener, C., & Villareal, D. (2005). Effects of weight loss and exercise on frailty in obese elderly subjects. *Journal of the American Geriatrics Society, 53*, S16.

Baquer, A. (1994). *Disabled, disablement, disablism*. New Delhi: Voluntary Health Association of India.

Baranoski, S. (2001). Skin tears. *Nursing Management*, *32*(8), 25–31. doi:10.1097/00006247-200108000-00010 PMID:15129526

Barbagallo, M., & Dominguez, L. J. (2014). Type 2 diabetes mellitus and Alzheimer'sdisease. *World Journal of Diabetes*, *5*(6), 889–893. doi:10.4239/wjd.v5.i6.889 PMID:25512792

Barbara, A. (1988). Hands of Light: A Guide to Healing Through the Human Energy Field. Bantam publishers.

Barbaresko, J., Koch, M., Schulze, M. B., & Nothlings, U. (2013). Dietary pattern analysis and biomarkers of low-grade inflammation: A systematic literature review. *Nutrition Reviews*, *71*(8), 511–527. doi:10.1111/nure.12035 PMID:23865797

Barbotte, E., Guillemin, F., & Chau, N. (2001). Lorhandicap Group Prevalence of impairments, disabilities, handicaps and quality of life in the general population: A review of recent literature. *Bulletin of the World Health Organization*, *79*, 1047–1055. PMID:11731812

Barker, P. J., & Buchanan-Barker, P. (2005). *The Tidal Model: A guide for mental health professionals*. Psychology Press. doi:10.4324/9780203340172

Barnes, H., & Parry, J. (2004). Renegotiating identity and relationships: Men and women's adjustment to retirement. *Ageing and Society*, *24*(2), 213–233. doi:10.1017/S0144686X0300148X

Barnett, J. H., Salmond, C. H., Jones, P. B., & Sahakian, B. J. (2006). Cognitive reserve in neuropsychiatry. *Psychological Medicine*, *36*(08), 1053–1064. doi:10.1017/S0033291706007501 PMID:16854246

Barnett, K., Mercer, S. W., Norbury, M., Watt, G., Wyke, S., & Guthrie, B. (2012). Epidemiology of multimorbidity and implications for health care, research, and medical education: A cross-sectional study. *Lancet*, *380*(9836), 37–43. doi:10.1016/S0140-6736(12)60240-2 PMID:22579043

Barnow, S., Linden, M., Lucht, M., & Freyberger, H. J. (2004). *Influence of age of patients who wish to die on treatment decisions by physicians and nurses*. Academic Press.

Baron, R. A. (2001) States of consciousness: Psychology, 5th eds, Pearson education, New work.

Bartels, S. J. (2004). Caring for the whole person: Integrated health care for older adults with severe mental illness and medical comorbidity. *Journal of the American Geriatrics Society*, *52*, 249–257. doi:10.1111/j.1532-5415.2004.52601.x PMID:15541165

Bartlett, Z. (2014). The Hayflick Limit. In *The Embryo Project Encyclopaedia*. Arizona State University.

Bassett, S. S., & Folstein, M. F. (1991). Cognitive impairment and functional disability in the absence of psychiatric diagnosis. *Psychological Medicine*, *21*(01), 77–84. doi:10.1017/S0033291700014677 PMID:2047508

Bastid, E., & Pagan, J. A. (2002). Impact of Diabetes on adult employment and earning of Mexican American finding from a community based study. *Health Economics*, *11*(5), 403–413. doi:10.1002/hec.676 PMID:12112490

Bayliss, E. A., Ellis, J. L., & Steiner, J. F. (2007). Barriers to self-management and quality-of-life outcomes in seniors with multimorbidities. *Annals of Family Medicine*, *5*(5), 395–402. doi:10.1370/afm.722 PMID:17893380

Bazin, N., Perruchet, P., De Bonis, M., & Feline, A. (1994). The dissociation of explicit and implicit memory in depressed patients. *Psychological Medicine*, *24*(01), 239–245. doi:10.1017/S0033291700027008 PMID:8208889

Beautrais, A. L. (2002). A case control study of suicide and attempted suicide in older adults. *Suicide & Life-Threatening Behavior*, *32*(1), 1–9. doi:10.1521/suli.32.1.1.22184 PMID:11931007

Beck, A. T., Steer, R. A., Kovacs, M., & Garrison, B. (1985). Hopelessness and eventual suicide: A 10-year prospective study of patients hospitalized with suicidal ideation. *The American Journal of Psychiatry*, *142*(5), 559–563. doi:10.1176/ajp.142.5.559 PMID:3985195

Becker, E. (1973). *The denial of death*. New York: The Free Press.

Beekman, A. T. F., De Beurs, E., van Balkom, A. J. L. M., Deeg, D. J. H., Van Dyck, R., & Van Tilburg, W. (2000). Anxiety and depression in later life: Co-occurrence and communality of risk factors. *The American Journal of Psychiatry*, *157*(1), 89–95. doi:10.1176/ajp.157.1.89 PMID:10618018

Begin, M. E., Langlois, M. F., Lorrain, D., & Cunnanem, S. C. (2008). Thyroid function and cognition during aging. *Current Gerontology and Geriatrics Research*, *2008*, 1–11. doi:10.1155/2008/474868 PMID:19415145

Bell-McGinty, S., Lopez, O. L., Meltzer, C. C., Scanlon, J. M., Whyte, E. M., Dekosky, S. T., & Becker, J. T. (2005). Differential cortical atrophy in subgroups of mild cognitive impairment. *Archives of Neurology*, *62*(9), 1393–1397. doi:10.1001/archneur.62.9.1393 PMID:16157746

Benington, J. H., & Heller, H. C. (1995). Brain energy metabolism as the function of sleep. *Progress in Neurobiology*, *45*(4), 347–360. doi:10.1016/0301-0082(94)00057-O PMID:7624482

Benner, D. G. (1989). Toward a psychology of spirituality: Implications for personality and psychotherapy. *Journal of Psychology and Christianity*.

Bennet, J. A., Winters-Stone, K., Nail, L. M., & Scherer, J. (2006). Definitions of Sedentary in physical-activity-intervention trials: A summary of the literature. *Journal of Aging and Physical Activity*, *14*(4), 456–477. doi:10.1123/japa.14.4.456 PMID:17215562

Bennett, R., & Eckman, J. (1973). Attitudes toward aging: A critical examination of recent literature and implications for future research. In C. Eisdorfer, & M.P. Lawton (Eds.), The psychology of adult development and aging. (pp. 575–597). Washington, DC: American Psychological Association doi:10.1037/10044-018

Bennett, D. A., Wilson, R. S., Schneider, J. A., Evans, D. A., Beckett, L. A., Aggarwal, N. T., ... Bach, J. (2002). Natural history of mild cognitive impairment in older persons. *Neurology*, *59*(2), 198–205. doi:10.1212/WNL.59.2.198 PMID:12136057

Benson, P. (1997). Spirituality and the Adolescent Journey. *Reclaiming Children and Youth*, *5*(4), 206.

Benz, S., Sellaro, R., Hommel, B., & Colzato, L. S. (2016). Music makes the world go round: The impact of musical training on non-musical cognitive functions—a review. *Frontiers in Psychology*, *6*, 2023. doi:10.3389/fpsyg.2015.02023 PMID:26779111

Berard, D. M., VanDenKerkhof, E. G., Harrison, M., & Tranmer, J. E. (2012). Gender differences in the influence of social support on one-year changes in functional status in older patients with heart failure. *Cardiology Research and Practice*, *2012*, 1–10. doi:10.1155/2012/616372 PMID:22957296

Berenson, G. S., Srinivasan, S. R., Hunter, S. M., Nicklas, T. A., Freedman, D. S., Shear, C. L., & Webber, L. S. (1989). Risk factors in early life as predictors of adult heart disease: The Bogalusa Heart Study. *The American Journal of the Medical Sciences*, *298*(3), 141–151. doi:10.1097/00000441-198909000-00001 PMID:2679086

Bergin, A.E. (1983). *Religiosity and mental health: A critical reevaluation and meta-analysis*. Academic Press.

Bergin, A. E., Masters, K. S., & Richards, P. S. (1987). Religiousness and mental health reconsidered: A study of an intrinsically religious sample. *Journal of Counseling Psychology*, *34*(2), 197–204. doi:10.1037/0022-0167.34.2.197

Bergström, A., Pisani, P., Tenet, V., Wolk, A., & Adami, H. O. (2001). Overweight as an avoidable cause of cancer in Europe. *International Journal of Cancer, 91*(3), 421–430. doi:10.1002/1097-0215(200002)9999:9999<::AID-IJC1053>3.0.CO;2-T PMID:11169969

Berkson, J. (1946). Limitations of the application of fourfold table analysis to hospital data. *Biomet Bull, 2*(3), 47–53. doi:10.2307/3002000 PMID:21001024

Berntsson, L., Lundberg, U., & Krantz, G. (2006). Gender differences in work-home interplay and symptom perception among Swedish white-collar employees. *Journal of Epidemiology and Community Health, 60*(12), 1070–1076. doi:10.1136/jech.2005.042192 PMID:17108304

Bertolote, J. M., & Fleischmann, A. (2002). Suicide and psychiatric diagnosis: A worldwide perspective. *World Psychiatry; Official Journal of the World Psychiatric Association (WPA), 1*, 181–185. PMID:16946849

Berwick, D. M., Nolan, T. W., & Whittington, J. (2008). The triple aim: Care, health, and cost. *Health Affairs, 27*(3), 759–769. doi:10.1377/hlthaff.27.3.759 PMID:18474969

Beskow, J. (1979). Suicide in mental disorder in Swedish men. *Acta Psychiatrica Scandinavica. Supplementum, 277*, 1–138. PMID:286500

Besset, A., Villemin, E., Tafti, M., & Billiard, M. (1998). Homeostatic process and sleep spindles in patients with sleep-maintenance insomnia:Effect of partial sleep deprivation. *Electroencephalography and Clinical Neurophysiology, 107*(2), 122–132. doi:10.1016/S0013-4694(98)00048-0 PMID:9751283

Beutel, M. E., Glaesmer, H., Wiltink, J., Marian, H., & Brahler, E. (2010). Life satisfaction, anxiety, depression and resilience across the life span of men. *The aging male: The official journal of the International Society for the Study of the Aging Male, 13*(1), 32-39.

Beutel, J. E., Chedraui, P., Baron, G., Belzares, E., Bencosme, A., & Calle, A. (2009). Sexual dysfunction in middle-aged women: A multicenter Latin American study using the Female Sexual Function Index. *Menopause (New York, N.Y.), 16*(6), 1139–1148. doi:10.1097/gme.0b013e3181a4e317 PMID:19458559

Bewernick, B., & Schlaepfer, T. (2013). Chronic depression as a model disease for cerebral aging. *Dialogues in Clinical Neuroscience, 15*(1), 77–85. PMID:23576891

Bharati & Singh. (2013). *Ageing in India: Need for a Comprehensive Policy*. Academic Press.

Bhasin, B. B., &Kumari, R. (2015).Essence of 'preventive medicine and holistic health'.

Bhatia, H. S. (1983). *Aging and society: A society: A sociological study of retired public servant*. Udaipur: Arya's Book Centre Publication.

Bhatia, M. S., Srivastava, S., & Bansal, S. (2008). Elder abuse. *Delhi Psychiatry Journal, 11*(2), 150–154.

Bhattacharjee, D., Rai, A. K., Singh, N. K., Kumar, P., Munda, S. K., & Das, B. (2011). Psychoeducation: A measure to strengthen psychiatric treatment. *Delhi Psychiatric Journal, 14*(1), 33–39.

Bhawuk, D. P. (1999). Who attains peace? An Indian model of personal harmony. *Indian Psychological Review, 52*(3/4), 40–48.

Bhushan, B., Kajal, N. C., Maske, A., & Singh, S. P. (2012). Manifestations of tuberculosis in elderly versus young hospitalised patients in Amritsar, India. *The International Journal of Tuberculosis and Lung Disease, 16*(9), 1210–1213. doi:10.5588/ijtld.11.0778 PMID:22794086

Bianchi, E. (1997). *Aging as a spiritual journey*. New York: Crossroads.

Bianchi, G. S., Meunier, P., Courpron, P., Edouard, E., Bernard, J., & Vignon, G. (1972). Osseous effects of hyperthyroidism. *Revue du Rhumatisme et des Maladies Osteo-Articulaires*, *39*(1), 19–32. PMID:4342875

Bianchini, F., Kaaks, R., & Vainio, H. (2002). Overweight, obesity, and cancer risk. *The Lancet Oncology*, *3*(9), 565–574. doi:10.1016/S1470-2045(02)00849-5 PMID:12217794

Bieliauskas, L. A., Boczar, J., & Lamberty, G. (1991). Lack of depression effects on cognitive functions in the elderly. Journal of Clinical and Experimental Neuropsychology, 13(3), 433-433).

Bieliauskas, L. A., Costello, S., & Terpenning, M. (1991). Depression and screening for cognitive deficit in elderly patients. Journal of Clinical and Experimental Neuropsychology, 13(1), 101-101).

Biessels, G. J., Koffeman, A., & Scheltens, P. (2006). Diabetes and cognitive impairment. Clinical diagnosis and brain imaging in patients attending a memory clinic. *Journal of Neurology*, *253*(4), 477–482. doi:10.1007/s00415-005-0036-4 PMID:16283097

Bilsen, J. (2000). End-of-life decisions in medical practice in Flanders, Belgium: a nationwide survey. *Lancet, 356*(9244), 1806–11. Retrieved from http://www.ncbi.nlm.nih.gov/pubmed/11117913

Binder, E. F., Schechtman, K. B., Ehsani, A. A., Steger-May, K., Brown, M., Sinacore, D. R., ... Holloszy, J. O. (2002). Effects of exercise training on frailty in community-dwelling older adults: Results of a randomized, controlled trial. *Journal of the American Geriatrics Society*, *50*(12), 1921–1928. doi:10.1046/j.1532-5415.2002.50601.x PMID:12473001

Biondi, B., Palmieri, E. A., & Fazio, S. (2004). Endogenous subclinical hyperthyroidism affects quality of life and cardiac morphology and function in young and middle-aged patients. *The Journal of Clinical Endocrinology and Metabolism*, *85*(12), 4701–4705. PMID:11134131

Birditt, K. S., Antonucci, T. C., & Tighe, L. (2012). Enacted support during stressful life events in middle and older adulthood: An examination of the interpersonal context. *Psychology and Aging*, *27*(3), 728–741. doi:10.1037/a0026967 PMID:22308999

Birns, J., & Kalra, L. (2009). Cognitive function and hypertension. *Journal of Human Hypertension*, *23*(2), 86–96. doi:10.1038/jhh.2008.80 PMID:18650838

Bjoro, T., Holmen, J., Kruger, O., Midthjell, K., Hunstad, K., Schreiner, T., ... Brochmann, H. (2000). Prevalence of thyroid disease, thyroid dysfunction and thyroid peroxidase antibodies in a large, unselected population. The Health Study of Nord-Trondelag (HUNT). *European Journal of Endocrinology*, *143*(5), 639–647. doi:10.1530/eje.0.1430639 PMID:11078988

Black, P. H. (1994). Central nervous system-immune system interactions: Psychoneuroendocrinology of stress and its immune consequences. *Antimicrobial Agents and Chemotherapy*, *38*(1), 1–6. doi:10.1128/AAC.38.1.1 PMID:8141561

Blaum, C., Cigolle, C. T., Boyd, C., Wolff, J. L., Tian, Z., Langa, K. M., & Weir, D. R. (2010). Clinical complexity in middle-aged and older adults with diabetes: The Health and Retirement Study. *Medical Care*, *48*(4), 327–334. doi:10.1097/MLR.0b013e3181ca4035 PMID:20355264

Blazer, D. G., Sachs-Ericsson, N., & Hybels, C. F. (2005). Perception of unmet basic needs as a predictor of mortality among community-dwelling older adults. *American Journal of Public Health*, *95*(2), 299–304. doi:10.2105/AJPH.2003.035576 PMID:15671468

Blazer, D. G., & Wu, L. T. (2009). The epidemiology of substance use and disorders among middle aged and elderly community adults: National Survey on drug use and health. *The American Journal of Geriatric Psychiatry*, *17*(3), 237–245. doi:10.1097/JGP.0b013e318190b8ef PMID:19454850

Blumberg, J. (1997). Nutritional needs of seniors. *Journal of the American College of Nutrition*, *16*, 517–523. PMID:9430078

Blumentals, W. A., Gomez-Caminero, A., Joo, S., & Vannappagari, V. (2004). Should erectile dysfunction be considered as a marker for acute myocardial infarction? Results from a retrospective cohort study. *International Journal of Impotence Research*, *16*(4), 350–353. doi:10.1038/sj.ijir.3901174 PMID:14985780

Boehnlein, J. K. (2008). *Psychiatry and religion: The convergence of mind and spirit*. Washington, DC: American Psychiatric Publishing.

Boericke, W. (1901). *Pocket Manual of Homeopathic Materia Medica* (1st Ed.), San Francisco: Retrieved from www.materiamedica.info/en/materia-medica/william-boericke/index

Boericke, W. (1927). Pocket manual of homoeopathic materia medica: comprising the characteristic and guiding symptoms of all remedies (clinical and pathogenetic).

Bombois, S., Derambure, P., Pasquier, F., & Monaca, C. (2010). Sleep disorders in aging and dementia. *The Journal of Nutrition, Health & Aging*, *14*(3), 212–217. doi:10.1007/s12603-010-0052-7 PMID:20191256

Bonham, L. W., Geier, E. G., Fan, C. C., Leong, J. K., Besser, L., Kukull, W. A., ... Yokoyama, J. S. (2016). Age-dependent effects of APOE ε4 in preclinical Alzheimer's disease. *Annals of Clinical and Translational Neurology*, *3*(9), 668–677. doi:10.1002/acn3.333 PMID:27648456

Bonsang, E., & Klein, T. (2012). Retirement and subjective wellbeing. *Journal of Economic Behavior & Organization*, *45*, 251–278.

Booth, B. K., Bruno, A. A., & Marin, R. (1996). Psychological therapy with abused and neglected patients. In Abuse, neglect and exploitation of older patients: Strategies for assessment and intervention (pp. 185-206). Baltimore, MD: Health Professions Press.

Booth, F. W., Roberts, C. K., & Laye, J. (2012). Lack of exercise is a major cause of chronic diseases. *Comprehensive Physiology*, *2*(2), 1143–1211. doi:10.1002/cphy.c110025 PMID:23798298

Bootzin, R., & Epstein, D. (2011). Understanding and Treating Insomnia. *Annual Review of Clinical Psychology*, *7*, 435–458.

Borbely, A. A., & Tobler, I. (1985). Brain Mechanisms of Sleep. Academic Press.

Bowen, R. L., & Atwood, C. S. (2004). Living and Dying for Sex. *Gerontology*, *50*(5), 265–290. doi:10.1159/000079125 PMID:15331856

Bowling, A., Gabriel, Z., Dykes, J., Dowding, L. M., Evans, O., Fleissig, A., ... Sutton, S. (2003). Let's ask them: Definitions of quality of life and its enhancement among people aged 65 and over. *International Journal of Aging & Human Development*, *56*(4), 269–306. doi:10.2190/BF8G-5J8L-YTRF-6404 PMID:14738211

Boxer, H., & Snyder, S. (2009). Five communication strategies to promote self-management of chronic illness. *Family Practice Management*, *16*(5), 12–16. PMID:19751037

Boyd, C. M., Darer, J., Boult, C., Fried, L. P., Boult, L., & Wu, A. W. (2005). Clinical practice guidelines and quality of care for older patients with multiple comorbid diseases: Implications for pay for performance. *Journal of the American Medical Association*, *294*(6), 716–724. doi:10.1001/jama.294.6.716 PMID:16091574

Bradley, L., Siddique, C. M., & Dufron, B. (1995). Reducing the use of physical restraints in long-term care facilities. *Journal of Gerontological Nursing*, *21*(9), 21–34. doi:10.3928/0098-9134-19950901-07 PMID:7560818

Bratic, I., & Trifunovic, A. (2010). Mitochondrial energy metabolism and ageing. *Biochimicaet Biophysica Acta (BBA) – Bioenergetics, 1797*(6-7), 961–967. doi:10.1016/j.bbabio.2010.01.004

Braverman, A. (1991). Medical Oncology in the 90s. *Lancet, 337*(8746), 901–902. doi:10.1016/0140-6736(91)90218-E PMID:1672980

Brazzale, D. J., Upward, A. L., & Pretto, J. J. (2010). Effects of changing reference values and definition of the normal range on interpretation of spirometry. *Respirology (Carlton, Vic.), 15*(7), 1098–1103. doi:10.1111/j.1440-1843.2010.01830.x PMID:20874746

Bremner, A. P., Feddema, P., Leedman, P. J., Brown, S. J., Beilby, J. P., Lim, E. M., ... Walsh, J. P. (2012). Age-related changes in thyroid function: A longitudinal study of a community-based cohort. *The Journal of Clinical Endocrinology and Metabolism, 97*(5), 1554–1562. doi:10.1210/jc.2011-3020 PMID:22344200

Breteler, M. M., Claus, J. J., Grobbee, D. E., & Hofman, A. (1994). Cardiovascular disease and distribution of cognitive function in elderly people: The Rotterdam study. *British Medical Journal, 308*(6944), 1604–1608. doi:10.1136/bmj.308.6944.1604 PMID:8025427

Brewer, L. D., Thibault, V., Chen, K. C., Langub, M. C., Landfield, P. W., & Porter, N. M. (2001). Vitamin D hormone confers neuroprotection in parallel with downregulation of L-type calcium channel expression in hippocampal neurons. *The Journal of Neuroscience, 21*(1), 98–108. PMID:11150325

J. Brick (Ed.). (2004). *Handbook of the Medical Consequences of Alcohol and Drug Abuse*. New York: Haworth Press.

Bridget, B. K. (2010). Promoting Cardiovascular Health in the Developing World: A Critical Challenge to Achieve Global Health (V. Fuster Ed.). Washington, D.C: National Academies Press.

Bristowe, E., & Collins, J. B. (1989). Family mediated abuse of non-institutionalized elder men and women living in British Columbia. *Journal of Elder Abuse & Neglect, 1*(1), 45–54. doi:10.1300/J084v01n01_05

Brockman, G., Tsaih, S., Neuschi, C., Churchill, G., & Li, R. (2008). Genetic factors contributing to obesity and body weight can act through mechanisms affecting muscle weight, fat weight or both. *Physiological Genomics, 10*, 1152. PMID:18984673

Bronfenbrenner, U., & Ceci, S. J. (1994). Nature-nutureреconceptualized in developmental perspective: A bioecological model. *Psychological Review, 101*(4), 568–586. doi:10.1037/0033-295X.101.4.568 PMID:7984707

Brosius, F. C. III, Waller, B. F., & Roberts, W. C. (1981). Radiation heart disease. Analysis of 16 young (aged 15 to 33 years) necropsy patients who received over 3,500 rads to the heart. *The American Journal of Medicine, 70*(3), 519–530. doi:10.1016/0002-9343(81)90574-X PMID:6782873

Browne, J. L., Ventura, A., Mosely, K., & Speight, J. (2013). I call it the blame and the shame disease: A qualitative study about perceptions of social stigma surrounding type 2 diabetes. *BMJ Open, 3*(11), 1–10. doi:10.1136/bmjopen-2013-003384 PMID:24247325

Brown, J. S., Seeley, D. G., Fong, J., Black, D. M., Ensrud, K. E., & Grady, D.Study of Osteoporotic Fractures Research Group. (1996). Urinary incontinence in older women: Who is at risk? *Obstetrics and Gynecology, 87*(5), 715–721. doi:10.1016/0029-7844(96)00013-0 PMID:8677073

Brown, J. S., Vittinghoff, E., Lin, F., Nyberg, L. M., Kusek, J. W., & Kanaya, A. M. (2006). Prevalence and risk factors for urinary incontinence in women with type 2 diabetes and impaired fasting glucose: Findings from the National Health and Nutrition Examination Survey (NHANES) 2001-2002. *Diabetes Care, 29*(6), 1307–1312. doi:10.2337/dc05-2463 PMID:16732013

Brown, J., Wimpenny, P., & Maughan, H. (2004). Skin problems in people with obesity. *Nursing Standard, 18*(35), 38–42. doi:10.7748/ns2004.05.18.35.38.c3609 PMID:15160455

Brown, L. A. (2016). Spatial-Sequential Working Memory in Younger and Older Adults: Age Predicts Backward Recall Performance within Both Age Groups. *Frontiers in Psychology, 7*, 1514. doi:10.3389/fpsyg.2016.01514 PMID:27757096

Brownlee, M. (2001). Biochemistry and molecular cell biology of diabetic complications. *Nature, 414*(6865), 813–820. doi:10.1038/414813a PMID:11742414

Brown, P. J., Liu, X., Sneed, J. R., Pimontel, M. A., Devanand, D. P., & Roose, S. P. (2013). Speed of processing and depression affect function in older adults with mild cognitive impairment. *The American Journal of Geriatric Psychiatry, 21*(7), 675–684. doi:10.1016/j.jagp.2013.01.005 PMID:23567401

Brown, S. A., Upchurch, S., Anding, R., Winter, M., & Ramirez, G. (1996). Promoting weight loss in Type II diabetes. *Diabetes Care, 19*(3), 613–624. doi:10.2337/diacare.19.6.613 PMID:8725861

Brummett, B. H., Helms, M. J., Dahlstrom, W. G., & Siegler, I. C. (2006). Prediction of all-cause mortality by the Minnesota Multiphasic Personality Inventory Optimism-Pessimism Scale scores: Study of a college sample during a 40-year follow-up period. *Mayo Clinic Proceedings, 81*(12), 1541–1544. doi:10.4065/81.12.1541 PMID:17165632

Bruscoli, M., & Lovestone, S. (2004). Is MCI really just early dementia? A systematic review of conversion studies. *International Psychogeriatrics, 16*(02), 129–140. doi:10.1017/S1041610204000092 PMID:15318760

Bryant, T., Daiski, I., & Lines, E. (2010). Type 2 diabetes: poverty, priorities and policy: the social determinants of the incidence and management of Type 2 diabetes [monograph on the Internet] Toronto, Ontario, Canada: York University School of Health Policy and Management; Retrieved March 16, 2017 from www.hpclearinghouse.ca/pdf/Diabetes%20 Fact%20Sheet%202010%20-%20March%2016%20-%20final%20.pdf

Bryden, K. S., Dunger, D. B., Mayou, R. A., Peveler, R. C., & Neil, H. A. (2003). Poor prognosis of young adults with type 1 diabetes: A longitudinal study. *Diabetes Care, 26*(4), 1052–1057. doi:10.2337/diacare.26.4.1052 PMID:12663572

Buchman, A. S., Tanne, D., Boyle, P. A., Shah, R. C., Leurgans, S. E., & Bennett, D. A. (2009). Kidney function is associated with the rate of cognitive decline in the elderly. *Neurology, 73*(12), 920–927. doi:10.1212/WNL.0b013e3181b72629 PMID:19657107

Buddy, T. (2006). Drinking alcohol and diabetes. Retrieved from http://alcoholism.about.com

Budge, M., Johnston, C., Hogervorst, E., De Jager, C., Milwain, E., Iversen, S. D., ... Smith, A. D. (2000). Plasma total homocysteine and cognitive performance in a volunteer elderly population. *Annals of the New York Academy of Sciences, 903*(1), 407–410. doi:10.1111/j.1749-6632.2000.tb06392.x PMID:10818531

Bunker, P., Gomby, D. S., & Kehrer, B. H. (1989). *Pathways to health: the role of social factors.* Menlo Park, CA: Kaiser Family Foundation.

Burkhardt, M. A. (1989). Spirituality: An analysis of the concept. *Holistic Nursing Practice, 3*(3), 69–77. doi:10.1097/00004650-198905000-00011 PMID:2670980

Burkhardt, M. A., & Nagai-Jacobson, M. G. (1985). Dealing with spiritual concerns of clients in the community. *Journal of Community Health Nursing, 2*(4), 191–198. doi:10.1207/s15327655jchn0204_3 PMID:3852858

Burkhardt, M. A., & Nagai-Jacobson, M. G. (2002). *Spirituality: Living our connectedness.* Cengage Learning.

Burnett, A. K., & Eden, O. B. (1997). The treatment of leukemia. *Lancet, 349*(9047), 270–275. doi:10.1016/S0140-6736(96)08086-5 PMID:9014927

Buschert, V., Bokde, A. L. W., & Hampel, H. (2010). Cognitive intervention in Alzheimer disease. *Nature Reviews. Neurology*, *6*(9), 508–517. PMID:20717104

Buschkuehl, M., Jaeggi, S. M., Hutchison, S., Perrig-Chiello, P., Däpp, C., Müller, M., ... Perrig, W. J. (2008). Impact of working memory training on memory performance in old-old adults. *Psychology and Aging*, *23*(4), 743–753. doi:10.1037/a0014342 PMID:19140646

Buskin, S. E., Gale, J. L., Weiss, N. S., & Nolan, C. M. (1994). Tuberculosis risk factors in adults in King County, Washington, 1988 through 1990. *American Journal of Public Health*, *84*(11), 1750–1756. doi:10.2105/AJPH.84.11.1750 PMID:7977912

Busse, A., Hensel, A., Gühne, U., Angermeyer, M. C., & Riedel-Heller, S. G. (2006). Mild cognitive impairment: Long-term course of four clinical subtypes. *Neurology*, *67*(12), 2176–2185. doi:10.1212/01.wnl.0000249117.23318.e1 PMID:17190940

Bussema, K. E., & Bussema, E. F. (2000). Is there a balm in Gilead? The implications of faith in coping with a psychiatric disability. *Psychiatric Rehabilitation Journal*, *24*(2), 117–124. doi:10.1037/h0095109

Butters, M. A., Becker, J. T., Nebes, R. D., Zmuda, M. D., Mulsant, B. H., Pollock, B. G., & Reynolds, C. F. III. (2000). Changes in cognitive functioning following treatment of late-life depression. *The American Journal of Psychiatry*, *157*(12), 1949–1954. doi:10.1176/appi.ajp.157.12.1949 PMID:11097959

Butters, M. A., Whyte, E. M., Nebes, R. D., Begley, A. E., Dew, M. A., Mulsant, B. H., ... Reynolds, C. F. (2004). The nature and determinants of neuropsychological functioning in late-life depression. *Archives of General Psychiatry*, *61*(6), 587–595. doi:10.1001/archpsyc.61.6.587 PMID:15184238

Byng-Maddick, R., & Noursadeghi, M. (2016). Does tuberculosis threaten our ageing populations? *BMC Infectious Diseases*, *16*(1), 119. doi:10.1186/s12879-016-1451-0 PMID:26968654

Byrne, R. (2006). *The Secret*. New York, NY: Atria Books.

Cabeza, R. (2004). Commentary: neuroscience frontiers of cognitive ageing: approaches to cognitive neuroscience of ageing. In R. Dixon, L. Bäckman, & L. Nilsson (Eds.), *New frontiers in cognitive ageing* (pp. 179–198). Oxford, UK: Oxford University Press. doi:10.1093/acprof:oso/9780198525691.003.0009

Cabeza, R., Daselaar, S., Dolcos, F., Prince, S. E., Budde, M., & Nyberg, L. (2004). Task-independent and task-specific age effects on brain activity during working memory, visual attention and episodic retrieval. *Cerebral Cortex*, 14364–14375. PMID:15028641

Cade, W. T. (2008). Diabetes-related microvascular and macrovascular diseases inthe physical therapy setting. *Physical Therapy*, *88*(11), 1322–1335. doi:10.2522/ptj.20080008 PMID:18801863

Cairney, J., McCabe, L., Veldhuizen, S., Corna, L. M., Streiner, D., & Herrmann, N. (2007). Epidemiology of social phobia in later life. *The American Journal of Geriatric Psychiatry*, *15*(3), 224–233. doi:10.1097/01.JGP.0000235702.77245.46 PMID:17213375

Calasanti, T., & King, N. (2005). Firming the Floppy Penis Age, Class, and Gender Relations in the Lives of Old Men. *Men and Masculinities*, *8*(1), 3–23. doi:10.1177/1097184X04268799

Callahan, C. M., Hendrie, H. C., Nienaber, N. A., & Tierney, W. M. (1996). Suicidal ideation among older primary care patients. *Journal of the American Geriatrics Society*, *44*(10), 1205–1209. doi:10.1111/j.1532-5415.1996.tb01370.x PMID:8855999

Camecho, M. E., & Reyes-Ortiz, C. A. (2005). Sexual dysfunction in the elderly: Age or disease? *International Journal of Impotence Research*, *17*(S1), S52–S56. doi:10.1038/sj.ijir.3901429 PMID:16391544

Campanelli, A., Rendace, L., Parisi, F., D'Antonio, F., Imbriano, L., de Lena, C., & Trebbastoni, A. (2016). Musical cognition in Alzheimer's disease: Application of the Montreal Battery of Evaluation of Amusia. *Annals of the New York Academy of Sciences*, *1375*(1), 28–37. doi:10.1111/nyas.13155 PMID:27447536

Campbell, V.A., Crews, J.E., Moriarty, D.G., Zack, M.M., & Blackman, D.K. (1999). Surveillance for sensory impairment, activity limitation, and health-related quality of life among older adults – United States.

Campbell, A., Converse, P. E., & Rodgers, W. L. (1976). *The quality of American Life: Perceptions, evaluations and satisfactions*. New York: Russell Sage Foundation.

Canaris, G. J., Manowitz, N. R., Mayor, G., & Ridgway, E. C. (2000). The Colorado thyroid disease prevalence study. *Archives of Internal Medicine*, *160*(4), 526–534. doi:10.1001/archinte.160.4.526 PMID:10695693

Cancer Tutor. (2017). Death by doctoring, Fraught with risks and side effects. Retrieved from https://www.cancertutor.com/deathbydoctoring4/

Candy, B., Jackson, K. C., Jones, L., Leurent, B., Tookman, A., & King, M. (2012). Drug therapy for delirium in terminally ill adult patients. *Cochrane Database of Systematic Reviews*, *9*(4), 285–288. PMID:23152226

Caracciolo, B., Gatz, M., Xu, W., Pedersen, N. L., & Fratiglioni, L. (2012). Differential distribution of subjective and objective cognitive impairment in the population: A nation-wide twin-study. *Journal of Alzheimer's Disease*, *29*(2), 393–403. PMID:22233768

Carey, G. W. (1894). *Biochemic System of Medicine*. The Theory, Pathological Action, Therapeutical Application, MateriaMedica, and Repertory of Schuessler's Twelve Tissue Remedies.

Carey, J. R. (2003). Life span: A conceptual overview. In J. R. Carey & S. Tuljapurkar (Eds.), *Life span evolutionary: Ecological and demographical perspectives, supplement to population and development review* (Vol. 29). New York: Population Council.

Carlson, M. C., Hasher, L., Connelly, S. L., & Zacks, R. T. (1995). Aging, distraction, and the benefits of predictable location. *Psychology and Aging*, *10*(3), 427–436. doi:10.1037/0882-7974.10.3.427 PMID:8527063

Carpenter, I., & Hirdes, J. P. (2013). Using interRAI assessment systems to measure and maintain quality of long-term care. In A Good Life in Old Age. Monitoring and Improving Quality in Long-term Care (pp. 93–139). OECD Health Policy Studies. doi:10.1787/9789264194564-7-en

Cassel, C. K., Leipzig, R. M., Cohen, H. J., & Larson, E. B. (2003). Geriatric Medicine: An Evidence-Based Approach (4th ed.). Springer-Verlag.

Cassels, A., & Moyninan, R. (2005). *Selling Sickness: How Drug Companies Are Turning Us All into Patients*. Greystone Books.

Casson, A. G., Evans, S. C., Gillis, A., Porter, G. A., Veugelers, P., Darnton, S. J., ... Hainaut, P. (2003). Clinical implications of p53 tumor suppressor gene mutation and protein expression in esophageal adenocarcinomas: Results of a ten-year prospective study. *The Journal of Thoracic and Cardiovascular Surgery*, *125*(5), 1121–1131. doi:10.1067/mtc.2003.176 PMID:12771886

Cattell, H. (2010). *Suicide in the elderly*. Academic Press.

Cavaliere, R., Antonangeil, L., & Vitti, P. (2002). The aging thyroid in a mild to moderate iodine deficient area of Italy. *Journal of Endocrinological Investigation*, *25*(10l), 66–68. Retrieved from https://www.ncbi.nlm.nih.gov/pubmed/12508922 PMID:12508922

Cavanagh, J., Carson, A. J., Sharpe, M., & Lawrie, S. M. (2003). Psychological autopsy studies of suicide: A systematic review. *Psychological Medicine*, *33*(3), 395–405. doi:10.1017/S0033291702006943 PMID:12701661

CDC Manual. (2013). *Introduction to the core curriculum on tuberculosis: what the clinician should know*. Retrieved from www.cdc.gov/tb

Center on an Aging Society (2003). *Obesity among older Americans.* Retrieved July 23, 2008, from http://ihcrp.georgetown.edu/agingsociety/pdfs/obesity2.pdf

Centers for Disease Control and Prevention and the Merck Company Foundation. (2007). *The state of ageing and health in America 2007*. Whitehouse Station, NJ: The Merck Company Foundation. Retrieved from http://www.cdc.gov/ageing/pdf/saha_2007.pdf

Centorrino, F., Mark, T. L., Talamo, A., Oh, K., & Chang, J. (2009). Health and economic burden of metabolic comorbidity among individuals with bipolar disorder. *Journal of Clinical Psychopharmacology*, *29*(6), 595–600. doi:10.1097/JCP.0b013e3181bef8a6 PMID:19910727

Central Tuberculosis Division. (2012). *Tuberculosis India. Annual Report of the Revised National Tuberculosis Control Programme*. Directorate General of Health Services, Ministry of Health and Family Welfare, Government of India.

Ceresini, G., Lauretani, F., Maggio, M., Ceda, G. P., Morganti, S., Usberti, E., ... Ferrucci, L. (2009). Thyroid function abnormalities and cognitive impairment in elderly people: Results of the Invecchiare in Chianti study. *Journal of the American Geriatrics Society*, *57*(1), 89–93. doi:10.1111/j.1532-5415.2008.02080.x PMID:19054181

Chambers, R. (1989). Vulnerability, Coping and Policy. *Institute of Development Studies-Bulletin*, *20*(2), 1–7. doi:10.1111/j.1759-5436.1989.mp20002001.x

Chandler, E. (1999). Spirituality. *The Hospice Journal*, *14*(3/4), 63–74. doi:10.1300/J011v14n03_05 PMID:10839002

Chandwani, H., Jivarajani, P., & Jivarajani, H. (2009). Health and social problems of geriatric population in an urban setting of Gujarat, India. *International Journal of Health, 9.*

Chapman, I. M. (2006). Nutritional disorders in the elderly. *The Medical Clinics of North America*, *90*(5), 887–907. doi:10.1016/j.mcna.2006.05.010 PMID:16962848

Chapman, L. S. (1987). Developing a useful perspective on spiritual health: Love, joy, peace and fulfillment. *American Journal of Health Promotion*, *2*(2), 12–17. doi:10.4278/0890-1171-2.2.12 PMID:22208509

Charlson, M., & Peterson, J. C. (2002). Medical comorbidity and late life depression: What is known and what are unmet needs? *Biological Psychiatry*, *52*(3), 226–235. doi:10.1016/S0006-3223(02)01422-1 PMID:12182928

Chasteen, A. L., Park, D. C., & Schwarz, N. (2001). Implementation intentions and facilitation of prospective memory. *Psychological Science*, *12*(6), 457–461. doi:10.1111/1467-9280.00385 PMID:11760131

Chaturvedi, S. K. (1991). What's important for quality of life to Indians—in relation to cancer. *Social Science & Medicine*, *33*(1), 91–94. doi:10.1016/0277-9536(91)90460-T PMID:1882246

Chaudhry, S. I., Mattera, J. A., Curtis, J. P., Spertus, J. A., Herrin, J., Lin, Z., ... Krumholz, H. M. (2010). Tele monitoring in patients with heart failure. *The New England Journal of Medicine*, *363*(24), 2301–2309. doi:10.1056/NEJMoa1010029 PMID:21080835

Chaudhuri, L. (2006). *Disability in India: Issues and concerns*. Academic Press.

Chen, C. H., Chen, J. F., & Yang, B. Y. (2004). Bone mineral density in women receiving thyroxine suppressive therapy for differentiated thyroid carcinoma. *Journal of the Formosan Medical Association, 103*(6), 442–447. PMID:15278189

Chengxuan, Q., & Miia, K., & Eva von S. (2009). Epidemiology of Alzheimer's disease: Occurrence, determinants, and strategies toward intervention Dialogues. *Clinical Neuroscience (New York, N.Y.), 11*(2), 111–128.

Chen, L., Magliano, D. J., & Zimmet, P. Z. (2011). The worldwide epidemiology of type 2 diabetes mellitus--present and future perspectives. *Nature Reviews. Endocrinology, 8*(4), 228–236. doi:10.1038/nrendo.2011.183 PMID:22064493

Chen, P., Ganguli, M., Mulsant, B. H., & DeKosky, S. T. (1999). The temporal relationship between depressive symptoms and dementia: A community-based prospective study. *Archives of General Psychiatry, 56*(3), 261–266. doi:10.1001/archpsyc.56.3.261 PMID:10078504

Chen, P., Ratcliff, G., Belle, S. H., Cauley, J. A., DeKosky, S. T., & Ganguli, M. (2001). Patterns of cognitive decline in presymptomatic Alzheimer disease: A prospective community study. *Archives of General Psychiatry, 58*(9), 853–858. doi:10.1001/archpsyc.58.9.853 PMID:11545668

Chertkow, H., Massoud, F., Nasreddine, Z., Belleville, S., Joanette, Y., Bocti, C., ... Bergman, H. (2008). Diagnosis and treatment of dementia: 3. Mild cognitive impairment and cognitive impairment without dementia. *Canadian Medical Association Journal, 178*(10), 1273–1285. doi:10.1503/cmaj.070797 PMID:18458258

Chesnokova, V., Pechnick, R. N., & Wawrowsky, K. (2016). Chronic peripheral inflammation, hippocampal neurogenesis, and behavior. *Brain Behavior and Immunity, 22*. doi:1016/j.bbi.2016.01.017

Cheung, C. K., & Kam, P. K. (2012). Resiliency in older Hong Kong Chinese: Using the grounded theory approach to reveal social and spiritual conditions. *Journal of Aging Studies, 26*(3), 355–367. doi:10.1016/j.jaging.2012.03.004

Chida, Y., & Steptoe, A. (2008). Positive psychological well-being and mortality: A quantitative review of prospective observational studies. *Psychosomatic Medicine, 70*(7), 741–756. doi:10.1097/PSY.0b013e31818105ba PMID:18725425

Chiesa, A., & Serretti, A. (2009). Mindfulness-based stress reduction for stress management in healthy people: A review and meta-analysis. *Journal of Alternative and Complementary Medicine (New York, N.Y.), 15*(5), 593–600. doi:10.1089/acm.2008.0495 PMID:19432513

Chintala, K. K., Krishna, B. H., & Reddy, M. (2015). Heart rate variability in overweight health care students: Correlation with visceral fat. *Journal of Clinical and Diagnostic Research: JCDR, 9*(1), CC06. PMID:25737980

Chiovato, L., Mariotti, S., & Pinchera, A. (1997). Thyroid diseases in the elderly. *Baillieres Clinical Endocrinology Metabolism, 11*(2), 251–70. Retrieved from https://www.ncbi.nlm.nih.gov/pubmed/9403122

Chiu, H. F. K., Yip, P. S. F., Chi, I., Chan, S., Tsoh, J., Kwan, C. W., … Caine, E. (2004). Elderly suicide in Hong Kong--a case-controlled psychological autopsy study. *Acta Psychiatrica Scandinavica, 109*(4), 299–305. Retrieved from http://www.ncbi.nlm.nih.gov/pubmed/15008804

Choi, N. G., & Dinitto, D. M. (2011). Heavy/binge drinking and depressive symptoms in older adults: Gender differences. *International Journal of Geriatric Psychiatry, 26*(8), 860–868. doi:10.1002/gps.2616 PMID:20886659

Chollet, F. (2013). Pharmacologic approaches to cerebral aging and neuroplasticity: Insights from the stroke model. *Dialogues in Clinical Neuroscience, 15*(1), 69–78. PMID:23576890

Chou, C. Y., Lin, C. H., Lin, C. C., Huang, C. C., Liu, C. S., & Lai, S. W. (2008). Association between waist-to-hip ratio and chronic kidney disease in the elderly. *Internal Medicine Journal*, *38*(6a), 402–406. doi:10.1111/j.1445-5994.2007.01587.x PMID:18336543

Chou, K. L., & Chi, I. (2001). Stressful life events and depressive symptoms: Social support and sense as mediator or moderators. *International Journal of Aging & Human Development*, *52*(2), 155–171. doi:10.2190/9C97-LCA5-EWB7-XK2W PMID:11352200

Chrisoulidou, A., Boudina, M., Tzemailas, A., Doumala, E., Iliadou, P. K., Patakiouta, F., & Pazaitou-Panayiotou, K. (2011). Histological subtype is the most important determinant of survival in metastatic papillary thyroid cancer. *Thyroid Research*, *4*(1), 12. doi:10.1186/1756-6614-4-12 PMID:21771294

Chronic Conditions. Making the case for ongoing care. (2004). Johns Hopkins and the Robert Wood Johnson Foundation's Partnership for Solutions. Available at: http://www.partnershipforsolutions.org/DMS/files/chronicbook2004.pdf

Chu, J. W., & Crapo, L. M. (2001). The treatment of subclinical hypothyroidism is seldom necessary. *The Journal of Clinical Endocrinology and Metabolism*, *86*(10), 4591–4599. doi:10.1210/jcem.86.10.7961 PMID:11600508

Chyun, D. A., Melkus, G. D., Katten, D. M., Price, W. J., Davey, J. A., & Grey, N. (2006). The association of psychological factors, physical activity, neuropathy, and quality of life in type 2 diabetes. *Biological Research for Nursing*, *7*(4), 279–288. doi:10.1177/1099800405285748 PMID:16581898

Ciarrochi, J., Atkins, P. W. B., Hayes, L. L., Sahdra, B. K., & Parker, P. (2016). Contextual Positive Psychology: Policy Recommendations for Implementing Positive Psychology into Schools. *Frontiers in Psychology*, *7*, 1561. doi:10.3389/fpsyg.2016.01561 PMID:27777564

Ciarrochi, J., & Kashdan, T. (2013). The foundations of flourishing. In J. Ciarrochi (Ed.), *Mindfulness, Acceptance, and Positive Psychology*. Oakland, CA: Context Press.

Cincotta, A. L., Gehrman, P., Gooneratne, N. S., & Baime, M. J. (2011). The effects of amindfulness-based stress reduction programme on pre-sleep cognitive arousal and insomnia symptoms: A pilot study. *Stress and Health*, *27*(3), E299–E305. doi:10.1002/smi.1370

Circadian Rhythm. (2007). *American Heritage Science Dictnarary*. Houghton Mifflin.

Clare, L., & Woods, R. T. (2004). Cognitive training and cognitive rehabilitation for people with early-stage Alzheimer's disease: A review. *Neuropsychological Rehabilitation*, *14*(4), 385–401. doi:10.1080/09602010443000074

Clare, L., Woods, R. T., Cook, E. D. M., Orrell, M., & Spector, A. (2003). Cognitive rehabilitation and cognitive training for early-stage Alzheimer's disease and vascular dementia. *Cochrane Database of Systematic Reviews*, *4*. PMID:14583963

Clark, F. (1987). Traditional Indian medicine/western medical measure hope. *Paper presented at Traditional Indian Medical conference*, Tucson, Arizona.

Clark, A. E., Diener, E., Georgellis, Y., & Lucas, R. E. (2008). Lags and leads in life satisfaction: A test of the baseline hypothesis. *Economic Journal (London)*, *118*(529), F222–F243. doi:10.1111/j.1468-0297.2008.02150.x

Clark, C. M., Xie, S., Chittams, J., Ewbank, D., Peskind, E., Galasko, D., ... Trojanowski, J. Q. (2003). Cerebrospinal fluid tau and beta-amyloid: How well do these biomarkers reflect autopsy-confirmed dementia diagnoses? *Archives of Neurology*, *60*(12), 1696–1702. doi:10.1001/archneur.60.12.1696 PMID:14676043

Clark, C., Cross, J., Deane, D., & Lowry, L. (1991). Spirituality: Integral to quality care. *Holistic Nursing Practice*, *5*(3), 67–76. doi:10.1097/00004650-199104000-00012 PMID:2045441

Clarke, M. F., & Fuller, M. (2006). Stem cells and cancer: Two faces of eve. *Cell, 124*(6), 1111–1115. doi:10.1016/j.cell.2006.03.011 PMID:16564000

Clarke, R., Birks, J., Nexo, E., Ueland, P. M., Schneede, J., Scott, J., ... Evans, J. G. (2007). Low vitamin B-12 status and risk of cognitive decline in older adults. *The American Journal of Clinical Nutrition, 86*(5), 1384–1391. PMID:17991650

Clark, L. J., Gatz, M., Zheng, L., Chen, Y. L., McCleary, C., & Mack, W. J. (2009). Longitudinal verbal fluency in normal aging, preclinical and prevalent Alzheimer disease. *American Journal of Alzheimer's Disease and Other Dementias, 24*(6), 461–468. doi:10.1177/1533317509345154 PMID:19759254

Clayton, A. H., Alkis, A. R., & Votta, J. G. (2017). Sexual dysfunctions due to psychotropic medications. *PsychiatrClin NA, 39*(3), 427–463.

Clem, M. A., Holliday, R. P., Pandya, S., Hynan, L. S., Lacritz, L. H., & Woon, F. L. (2017). Predictors That a Diagnosis of Mild Cognitive Impairment Will Remain Stable 3 Years Later. *Cognitive and Behavioral Neurology, 30*(1), 8–15. doi:10.1097/WNN.0000000000000119 PMID:28323681

Cobb, S. (1976). Social support as moderator in life stress. *Journal of Psychosomatic Medicine, 38*(5), 300–314. doi:10.1097/00006842-197609000-00003 PMID:981490

Cochran, J. K., & Beeghley, L. (1991). The influence of religion on attitudes toward nonmarital sexuality: A preliminary assessment of reference group theory. *Journal for the Scientific Study of Religion, 30*(1), 45–62. doi:10.2307/1387148

Coffey, D. S. (2006). Hyperthermic biology and Cancer therapies. *Journal of the American Medical Association*, 296. PMID:16868303

Cohen, G. D. (1992). The future of mental health and aging. In J. E. Birren, R. B. Sloane, & G. D. Cohen (Eds.), *Handbook of mental health and aging* (2nd ed.; pp. 893–914). San Diego, CA: Academic Press. doi:10.1016/B978-0-12-101277-9.50037-1

Cohen, M. (1990). Caring for ourselves can be funny business. *Holistic Nursing Practice, 4*(4), 1–11. doi:10.1097/00004650-199007000-00004 PMID:2365748

Cohen-Mansfield, J., & Werner, P. (1997). Management of verbally disruptive behaviours in the nursing home. *Journal of Gerantology Nursing, 24*, 10–17.

Cohen, R. A. (1993). *The Neuropsychology of Attention*. New York: Plenum Press. doi:10.1007/978-1-4419-7463-1

Cohen, S. (2004). Social relationships and health. *The American Psychologist, 59*(8), 676–684. doi:10.1037/0003-066X.59.8.676 PMID:15554821

Cohen, S., Gottlieb, B. H., & Underwood, L. G. (2000). Social relationships and health. In S. Cohen, L. G. Underwood, & B. H. Gottlieb (Eds.), *Social Support measurement and intervention: A guide for health and social scientists* (pp. 3–25). Oxford: Oxford University Press. doi:10.1093/med:psych/9780195126709.003.0001

Cohen, S., Janicki-Deverts, D., & Miller, G. E. (2007). Psychological stress and disease. *Journal of the American Medical Association, 298*(14), 1685–1687. doi:10.1001/jama.298.14.1685 PMID:17925521

Cohen, S., & Syne, S. L. (1985). Issues in the study and application of social support. In S. Cohen & S. L. Syne (Eds.), *Social support and health* (pp. 3–22). New York: Academic Press.

Cohen, S., & Wills, T. A. (1985). Stress social support and buffering hypothesis. *Psychological Bulletin, 98*(2), 310–357. doi:10.1037/0033-2909.98.2.310 PMID:3901065

Cohler, B. J. (1993). Aging, morale, and meaning: The nexus of narrative. In T. R. Cole, W. A. Achenbaum, P. L. Jakobi, & R. Kastenbaum (Eds.), *Voices and visions of aging: Toward a critical gerontology* (pp. 107–133). New York: Springer.

Colantonio, A., Kasl, S. V., & Ostfeld, A. M. (1992). Depressive symptoms and other psychosocial factors as predictors of stroke in the elderly. *American Journal of Epidemiology*, *136*(7), 884–894. doi:10.1093/aje/136.7.884 PMID:1442754

Colantonio, A., Kasl, S. V., Ostfeld, A. M., & Berkman, L. F. (1993). Psychosocial predictors of stroke outcomes in an elderly population. *Journal of Gerontology*, *48*(5), S261–S268. doi:10.1093/geronj/48.5.S261 PMID:8366275

Cole, B., & Pargament, K. (1999). Re-creating your life: A spiritual/psychotherapeutic intervention for people diagnosed with cancer. *Psycho-Oncology*, *8*(5), 395–407. doi:10.1002/(SICI)1099-1611(199909/10)8:5<395::AID-PON408>3.0.CO;2-B PMID:10559799

Collet, T.H., Gussekloo, J., Bauer, D.C., den Elzen, W.P., & Cappola, A.R., Balmer, P., … Rodondi, N. (2012). Thyroid Studies Collaboration: Subclinical hyperthyroidism and the risk of coronary heart disease and mortality. *Archieves International Medcine*, *172*, 799–809. doi:10.1001/archinternmed.2012.402 PMID:22529182

Collins, A., & Koechlin, E. (2012). Reasoning, learning, and creativity: Frontal lobe function and human decision-making. *PLoS Biology*, *10*(3), e1001293. doi:10.1371/journal.pbio.1001293 PMID:22479152

Collins, M. M., Corcoran, P., & Perry, I. J. (2009). Anxiety and depression symptoms in patients with diabetes. *Diabetic Medicine*, *26*(2), 153–161. doi:10.1111/j.1464-5491.2008.02648.x PMID:19236618

Comijs, H. C., Penninx, B. W., Knipscheer, K. P., & Van Tilburg, W. (1999). Psychological distress in victims of elder mistreatment: The effects of social support and coping. *Journal of Gerontology Series B: Psycholical Science and Social Science*, *54*(4), 240–245. doi:10.1093/geronb/54B.4.P240 PMID:12382593

Constant, E. L., Adam, S., Seron, X., Bruyer, R., Seghers, A., & Daumerie, C. (2005). Anxiety and depression, attention, and executive functions in hypothyroidism. *Journal of the International Neuropsychological Society*, *11*(05), 535–544. doi:10.1017/S1355617705050642 PMID:16212680

Conti, C., Carrozzino, D., Patierno, C., Vitacolonna, E., & Fulcheri, M. (2016). The Clinical Link between Type D Personality and Diabetes. *Frontiers in Psychiatry*, *7*, 113. doi:10.3389/fpsyt.2016.00113 PMID:27445869

Conwell, Y. (1998). High levels of hopelessness persist in geriatric patients with remitted depression and a history of attempted suicide. *Journal of the American Geriatrics Society, 46*(11), 1401–1406. Retrieved from http://www.ncbi.nlm.nih.gov/sites/entrez?Db=pubmed&Cmd=Retrieve&list_uids=9809762&dopt=abstractplus

Conwell, Y. (2013). Suicide and suicide prevention in later life. *Focus, 11*(1), 39-47.

Conwell, Y., Duberstein, P. R., & Caine, E. D. (2002). Risk factors for suicide in later life. *Biological Psychiatry*, *52*(3), 193–204. doi:10.1016/S0006-3223(02)01347-1 PMID:12182926

Conwell, Y., Duberstein, P. R., Hirsch, J. K., Conner, K. R., Eberly, S., & Caine, E. D. (2010). Health status and suicide in the second half of life. *International Journal of Geriatric Psychiatry*, *25*(4), 371–379. doi:10.1002/gps.2348 PMID:19582758

Conwell, Y., Lyness, J. M., Duberstein, P., Cox, C., Seidlitz, L., DiGiorgio, A., & Caine, E. D. (2000). Completed suicide among older patients in primary care practices: A controlled study. *Journal of the American Geriatrics Society*, *48*(1), 23–29. doi:10.1111/j.1532-5415.2000.tb03024.x PMID:10642017

Conwell, Y., & Thompson, C. (2008). Suicidal Behavior in elders. *The Psychiatric Clinics of North America*, *31*(2), 333–356. doi:10.1016/j.psc.2008.01.004 PMID:18439452

Conwell, Y., Van Orden, K., & Caine, E. D. (2011). Suicide in Older Adults. *The Psychiatric Clinics of North America, 34*(2), 451–468. doi:10.1016/j.psc.2011.02.002 PMID:21536168

Cook-Daniels, L. (2003b). 2003 is the year elder abuse hits the international state. *Victimization of the Elderly and Disabled, 5*, 65-66, 76.

Coolidge, F. L., Segal, D. L., Hook, J. N., & Stewart, S. (2000). Personality disorders and coping among anxious older adults. *Journal of Anxiety Disorders, 14*(2), 157–172. doi:10.1016/S0887-6185(99)00046-8 PMID:10864383

Cooney, C., & Mortimer, A. (1995). Elder abuse and dementia: A pilot study. *The International Journal of Social Psychiatry, 41*(4), 276–283. doi:10.1177/002076409504100405 PMID:8815051

Cooper, C., Selwood, A., & Livingston, G. (2008). The prevalence of elder abuse and neglect: A systematic review. *Age and Ageing, 37*(2), 151–160. doi:10.1093/ageing/afm194 PMID:18349012

Cooper, D. S. (2004). Thyroid disease in the oldest old: The exception to the rule. *Journal of the American Medical Association, 292*(21), 2651–2654. doi:10.1001/jama.292.21.2651 PMID:15572724

Cooper, H. C., Booth, K., & Gill, G. (2003). Patients' perspectives on diabetes health care education. *Health Education Research, 18*(2), 191–206. doi:10.1093/her/18.2.191 PMID:12729178

Corman, J.C., Lynch, S. M., Goldman, N., Weinstein, M., & Lin, H. (2004). Stability and change in perceived social support of older Taiwanese adults. *Journal of Gerontology: Series B: Psychological sciences and social sciences, 59*(6), 350-3357.

Cornelis, M. C., Glymour, M., Kawachi, I., & Chivue, S. (2013). Marital status and risk of type 2 diabetes in the health professionals. *American Heart Foundation*. Retrieved from http://www.ahajournals.org

Corona, G., Lee, D.M., Forti, G., O'Connor, D.B., Maggi, M., O'Neill, T.W., & …, Wu, F.C. (2009). Age-related changes in general and sexual health in middle-aged and older men: Results from the European Male Ageing Study (EMAS). *Journal of Sexual Medicine, 7*(4), 1362–1380. PMID:19929914

Corpas, E., Harman, S., & Blackman, M. (1993). Human growth hormone and human aging. *Endocrinology Review, 14*(1), 20–39. doi:10.1210/edrv-14-1-20 PMID:8491152

Correa-de-Araujo, R., McDermott, K., & Moy, E. (2006). Gender differences across racial and ethnic groups in the quality of care for diabetes. *Women's Health Issues, 16*(2), 56–65. doi:10.1016/j.whi.2005.08.003 PMID:16638522

Correa, L.Q., Cozzensa, da Silva, M., & Rombaldi, A.J. (2013). Sexual dysfunction symptoms in men age 40 or older: Prevalence and associated factors. *Revista Brasileira de Epidemiologia, 16*(2), 444–453. PMID:24142015

Correia, N., Mullally, S., Cooke, G., Tun, T. K., Phelan, N., Feeney, J., ... Gibney, J. (2009). Evidence for a specific defect in hippocampal memory in overt and subclinical hypothyroidism. *The Journal of Clinical Endocrinology and Metabolism, 94*(10), 3789–3797. doi:10.1210/jc.2008-2702 PMID:19584178

Corriher, C. T., & Corriher, S. G. (2013). *Defy Your Doctor and Be Healed*. Health Wyze Media.

Corsentino, E. A., Collins, N., Sachs-Ericsson, N., & Blazer, D. G. (2009). Religious attendance reduces cognitive decline among older women with high levels of depressive symptoms. *The Journals of Gerontology. Series A, Biological Sciences and Medical Sciences, 64*(12), 1283–1289. doi:10.1093/gerona/glp116 PMID:19675176

Corsi, M., Di Raimo, T., Di Lorenzo, C., Rapp-Ricciardi, M., Archer, T., & Ricci, S. B. (2016). Cognitive disability in Alzheimer's disease and its management. *Research in Clinical Therapy, 167*(5), e123–e126. doi:10.7417/CT.2016.1955 PMID:27845490

Coşar, B., Kocal, N., Arikan, Z., & Işik, E. (1997). Suicide attempts among Turkish psychiatric patients. *Canadian Journal of Psychiatry*, *42*(10), 1072–1075. doi:10.1177/070674379704201009 PMID:9469240

Costa, M. M., Reus, V. I., Wolkowitz, O. M., Manfredi, F., & Lieberman, M. (1999). Estrogen replacement therapy and cognitive decline in memory-impaired post-menopausal women. *Biological Psychiatry*, *46*(2), 182–188. doi:10.1016/S0006-3223(98)00355-2 PMID:10418692

Cotran, R. S., & Robbins, S. L. (1997). Basic Pathology (6th ed.). W.B. Saunders Company.

Cottrell, L. (1942). The adjustment of an individual to his age and roles. *American Sociological Review*, *7*(5), 617–620. doi:10.2307/2085687

Cox, C. (1998). Age Differences in Behaviors Leading to Completed Suicide. *The American Journal of Geriatric Psychiatry*, *6*(2), 122–126. doi:10.1097/00019442-199805000-00005 PMID:9581207

Crane, C. (2006). Suicidality in chronic pain : A review of the prevalence, risk factors and psychological links. *Review - Americas Society*, *36*, 575–586. doi:10.1017/S0033291705006859 PMID:16420727

Crepet, P., Caracciolo, S., Casoli, R., Fabbri, D., Florenzano, F., & Grassi, G. M. (1991). Suicidal behavior in Italy: Data, trends and guidelines for a suicide intervention/prevention policy. *Suicide & Life-Threatening Behavior*, *21*, 263–278. PMID:1759299

Crimmins, E. M., Hayward, M. D., & Saito, Y. (1994). Changing mortality and morbidity rates and health status and life expectancy of the older population. *Demography*, *31*(1), 159–175. doi:10.2307/2061913 PMID:8005340

Crowther, M. R., Parker, M. W., Achenbaum, W. A., Larimore, W. L., & Koenig, H. G. (2002). Rowe and Kahn's model of successful aging revisited: Positive spirituality. The forgotten factor. *The Gerontologist*, *42*(5), 613–620. doi:10.1093/geront/42.5.613 PMID:12351796

Cugati, S., Cumming, R. G., Smith, W., Burlutsky, G., Mitchell, P., & Wang, J. J. (2007). Visual impairment, age-related macular degeneration, cataract, and long-term mortality: The Blue Mountains Eye Study. *Archives of Ophthalmology*, *125*(7), 917–924. doi:10.1001/archopht.125.7.917 PMID:17620571

Cumming, E., & Henry, W. E. (1961). *Growing old, the process of disengagement*. Basic Books.

Cumming, E., & Henry, W. E. (1961). *Growing old: The process of Disengagement*. New York: Basic Book.

Cumming, E., Newell, D. S., & McCaffery, I. (1960). Disengagement: A tentative theory of aging. *Sociometry*, *23*(1), 23–35. doi:10.2307/2786135

Cunningham, C. (2004). Recent developments: Suicide in older people. *British Medical Journal*, *329*(7471), 895–898. doi:10.1136/bmj.329.7471.895 PMID:15485967

Cure Naturali Cancro. (n.d.). 75% of the physicians refuses chemotherapy themselves. Retrieved from http://www.curenaturalicancro.com/en/75-percent-of-the-physicians-refuses-chemotherapy-themselves/

Cutolo, M., Sulli, A., Capellino, S., Villaggio, B., Montagna, P., Seriolo, B., & Straub, R. H. (2004). Sex hormones influence on the immune system: Basic and clinical aspects in autoimmunity. *Lupus*, *13*(9), 635–638. doi:10.1191/0961203304lu1094oa PMID:15485092

D'Adamo, E., Guardamagna, O., Chiarelli, F., Bartuli, A., Liccardo, D., Ferrari, F., & Nobili, V. (2015). Atherogenic dyslipidemia and cardiovascular risk factors in obese children. *International Journal of Endocrinology*, *912047*. doi:10.1155/2015/912047 PMID:25663838

Dahlin, E., Neely, A. S., Larsson, A., Backman, L., & Nyberg, L. (2008). Transfer of learning after updating training mediated by the striatum. *Science*, *320*(5882), 1510–1512. doi:10.1126/science.1155466 PMID:18556560

Daichman, L. S. (2005). Elder abuse in developing nations. In M. L. Johnson, V. L. Bengston, P. G. Coleman, & T. B. L. Kirkwood (Eds.), *The Cambridge handbook of age and ageing* (pp. 323–331). Cambridge: Cambridge University Press. doi:10.1017/CBO9780511610714.032

Dammeyer, J. (2010). Prevalence and aetiology of congenitally deafblind people in Denmark. *International Journal of Audiology*, *49*(2), 76–82. doi:10.3109/14992020903311388 PMID:20151880

Daniels, J. (2006). Obesity: America's epidemic. *The American Journal of Nursing*, *106*(1), 40–49. doi:10.1097/00000446-200601000-00028 PMID:16481779

Danion, J. M., Kauffmann-Muller, F., Grangé, D., Zimmermann, M. A., & Greth, P. (1995). Affective valence of words, explicit and implicit memory in clinical depression. *Journal of Affective Disorders*, *34*(3), 227–234. doi:10.1016/0165-0327(95)00021-E PMID:7560551

Darwin, C. (1888). *The life and letters of Charles Darwin*. New York: D. Appleton and Company.

Das-Munshi, J., Stewart, R., Ismail, K., Bebbington, P. E., Jenkins, R., & Prince, M. J. (2007). Diabetes, common mental disorders, and disability: Findings from the UK National Psychiatric Morbidity Survey. *Psychosomatic Medicine*, *69*(6), 543–550. doi:10.1097/PSY.0b013e3180cc3062 PMID:17636148

Dassa, A., & Amir, D. (2014). The role of singing familiar songs in encouraging conversation among people with middle to late stage Alzheimer's disease. *Journal of Music Therapy*, *51*(2), 131–153. doi:10.1093/jmt/thu007 PMID:25013944

Datta, H.S., Mitra, S.K., Paramesh, R., & Patwardhan, B. (2011). Theories and Management of Aging: Modern and Ayurveda Perspectives. In *Evidence-Based Complementary and Alternative Medicine*. doi:10.1093/ecam/nep005

Datta, P. P., Gangopadhyay, N., & Sengupta, B. (2013). Association of psychological morbidity with socio-demographic characteristics among elderly: A cross-sectional study from Eastern Indian. *International Journal of Medicine and Public Health*, *3*(2), 94–99. doi:10.4103/2230-8598.115172

Dauncey, M. J. (2014). Nutrition, the brain and cognitive decline: Insights from epigenetics. *European Journal of Clinical Nutrition*, *68*(11), 1179–1185. doi:10.1038/ejcn.2014.173 PMID:25182020

Davey, J., & Glasgow, K. (2006). Positive Ageing – A Critical Analysis. *Police Quarterly*, *4*(4), 21–28.

Davidson, K. W., Mostofsky, E., & Whang, W. (2010). Don't worry, be happy: Positive affect and reduced 10-year incident coronary heart disease: *The Canadian Nova Scotia Health Survey. European Heart Journal*, *31*(9), 1065–1070. doi:10.1093/eurheartj/ehp603 PMID:20164244

Davis, H. D., Zeiss, A. M., Shea, E. A., & Tinklenberg, J. R. (1998). Sexuality and Intimacy in Alzheimer's Patients and their partners. *Sexuality and Disability*, *16*(3), 193–283. doi:10.1023/A:1023047125906

Davis, P. J., & Davis, F. B. (1974). Hyperthyroidism in patients over the age of 60 years. Clinical features in 85 patients. *Medicine; Analytical Reviews of General Medicine, Neurology, Psychiatry, Dermatology, and Pediatries*, *53*(3), 161–181. doi:10.1097/00005792-197405000-00001 PMID:4133091

Davydov, D. M., Stewart, R., Ritchie, K., & Chaudieu, I. (2010). Resilience and mental health. *Clinical Psychology Review*, *30*(5), 479–495. doi:10.1016/j.cpr.2010.03.003 PMID:20395025

Day, R. (2017, August 2). Advice on primary prevention and prescribing in older patients with comorbidities, including the impact of medication side effects [Weblog post]. Retrieved from https://www.gponline.com/comorbidities-older-people/elderly-care/article/1440520

Day, J. J., & Sweatt, J. D. (2012). Epigenetic treatments for cognitive impairments. *Neuropsychopharmacology*, *37*(1), 247–260. doi:10.1038/npp.2011.85 PMID:21593731

Day, P. (2000). *Cancer: Why we're still Dying to Know the Truth*. Credence Publications.

de l'Etoile, S. (2011). Processes of music therapy: clinical and scientific rationales and models. In S. Hallam, I. Cross, & M. Thaut (Eds.), *The Oxford handbook of music psychology* (pp. 493–502). Oxford, UK: Oxford University Press.

De Leo, D., Dello Buono, M., & Dwyer, J. (2002). Suicide among the elderly: The long-term impact of a telephone support and assessment intervention in northern Italy. *The British Journal of Psychiatry*, *181*(3), 226–229. doi:10.1192/bjp.181.3.226 PMID:12204927

De Paula Couto, M. C., Koller, S. H., & Novo, R. (2011). Stressful Life Events and Psychological Well-being in a Brazilian Sample of Older Persons: The Role of Resilience. *Ageing International*, *36*(4), 492–505. doi:10.1007/s12126-011-9123-2

Deanfield, J., Donald, A., Ferri, C., Giannattasio, C., Halcox, J., Halligan, S., ... Lerman, A. (2005). Endothelial function and dysfunction. Part I: Methodological issues for assessment in the different vascular beds: a statement by the Working Group on Endothelin and Endothelial Factors of the European Society of Hypertension. *Journal of Hypertension*, *23*(1), 7–17. doi:10.1097/00004872-200501000-00004 PMID:15643116

Deary, I. J., Corley, J., Gow, A. J., Harris, S. E., Houlihan, L. M., Marioni, R. E., ... Starr, J. M. (2009). Age associated cognitive decline. *British Medical Bulletin*, *92*(1), 135–152. doi:10.1093/bmb/ldp033 PMID:19776035

Deary, I. J., & Johnson, W. (2010). Intelligence and education: Causal perceptions drive analytic processes and therefore conclusions. *International Journal of Epidemiology*, *39*(5), 1362–1369. doi:10.1093/ije/dyq072 PMID:20504860

Deary, I. J., Johnson, W., & Houlihan, L. M. (2009). Genetic foundations of human intelligence. *Human Genetics*, *126*(1), 215–232. doi:10.1007/s00439-009-0655-4 PMID:19294424

Deary, I. J., Penke, L., & Johnson, W. (2010). The neuroscience of human intelligence differences. *Nature Reviews. Neuroscience*, *11*, 201–211. PMID:20145623

deJongh, R. T., Lips, P., van Schoor, N. M., Rijs, K. J., Deeg, D. J. H., Comijs, H. C., ... Dekkers, O. M. (2011). Endogenous subclinical thyroid disorders, physical and cognitive function, depression, and mortality in older individuals. *European Journal of Endocrinology*, *165*(4), 545–554. doi:10.1530/EJE-11-0430 PMID:21768248

Delahanty, L. M., Grant, R. W., Wittenberg, E., Bosch, J. L., Wexler, D. J., Cagliero, E., & Meigs, J. B. (2007). Association of diabetes-related emotional distress with diabetes treatment in primary care patients with Type 2 diabetes. *Diabetic Medicine*, *24*(1), 48–54. doi:10.1111/j.1464-5491.2007.02028.x PMID:17227324

DeLamater, J. D., & Sill, M. (2005). Sexual Desire in Later Life. *Journal of Sex Research*, *42*(2), 138–149. doi:10.1080/00224490509552267 PMID:16123844

DeLamater, J., & Amelia Karraker, A. B. (2009). Sexual Functioning in Older Adults. *Current Psychiatry Reports*, *11*(1), 6–11. doi:10.1007/s11920-009-0002-4 PMID:19187702

DeLamater, J., & Moorman, S. M. (2007). Sexual Behavior in Later Life. *Journal of Aging and Health*, *19*(6), 921–946. doi:10.1177/0898264307308342 PMID:18165289

Delaney, C., Barrere, C., & Helming, M. (2011). The influence of a spirituality-based intervention on quality of life, depression, and anxiety in community-dwelling adults with cardiovascular disease: A pilot study. *Journal of Holistic Nursing, 29*(1), 21–32. doi:10.1177/0898010110378356 PMID:20713655

Denburg, N. L., Cole, C. A., Hernandez, M., Yamada, T. H., Tranel, D., Bechara, A., & Wallace, R. B. (2007). The orbitofrontal cortex, real-world decision-making, and normal aging. *Annals of the New York Academy of Sciences, 1121*(1), 480–498. doi:10.1196/annals.1401.031 PMID:17872394

Denollet, J. (2005). DS14: Standard assessment of negative affectivity, social inhibition, and Type D personality. *Psychosomatic Medicine, 67*(1), 89–97. doi:10.1097/01.psy.0000149256.81953.49 PMID:15673629

Department of Health and Human Services Agency for Healthcare Research and Quality. (n.d.). *Optimizing prevention and healthcare management for the complex patient.* Available at: http://grants.nih.gov/grants/guide/rfafiles/RFA-HS-08-003.html

Depp, C. A., & Jeste, D. V. (2006). Definitions and predictors of successful aging: A comprehensive review of larger quantitative studies. *The American Journal of Geriatric Psychiatry, 14*(1), 6–20. doi:10.1097/01.JGP.0000192501.03069.bc PMID:16407577

Desai, M. M., Lentzner, H. R., & Weeks, J. D. (2001). Unmet need for personal assistance with activities of daily living among older adults. *The Gerontologist, 41*(1), 82–88. doi:10.1093/geront/41.1.82 PMID:11220818

Dey, A. B. (2003). *Aging in India: Situational analysis and planning for the future. Ministry of health and family welfare.* New Delhi: Ramko Press.

Dhaval, D., Inas, R., & Spasojevic, J. (2006). The effects of retirement on physical and mental health outcomes. *National Bureau of Economic Research,* w12123.

Diamond, A. (2013). Executive functions. *Annual Review of Psychology, 64*(1), 135–168. doi:10.1146/annurev-psych-113011-143750 PMID:23020641

Dickens, A. P., Richards, S. H., Greaves, C. J., & Campbell, J. L. (2011). Interventions targeting social isolation in older people: A systematic review. *BMC Public Health, 11*(1), 647. doi:10.1186/1471-2458-11-647 PMID:21843337

Dickerson, B. C., Sperling, R. A., Hyman, B. T., Albert, M. S., & Blacker, D. (2007). Clinical prediction of Alzheimer disease dementia across the spectrum of mild cognitive impairment. *Archives of General Psychiatry, 64*(12), 1443–1450. doi:10.1001/archpsyc.64.12.1443 PMID:18056553

Dickson, D. W., Farlo, J., Davies, P., Crystal, H., Fuld, P., & Yen, S. H. (1988). Alzheimer'sdisease. A double-labeling immunohistochemical study of senile plaques. *American Journal of Pathology, 132,* 86–101. PMID:2456021

Diener, E. (2000). Subjective well-being: The science of happiness and a proposal for a national index. *The American Psychologist, 55*(1), 34–43. doi:10.1037/0003-066X.55.1.34 PMID:11392863

Diener, E. D., Sandvik, E., Seidlitz, L., & Diener, M. (1993). The relationship between income and wellbeing. Relative or absolute? *Social Indicators Research, 28*(3), 195–223. doi:10.1007/BF01079018

Diesfeldt, H. F., Vander Elst, W., & Jolles, J. (2009). Category fluency (animals, professions) in normal cognitive ageing and dementia. *Tijdschriftvoor Gerontologie en Geriatrie., 40*(2), 54-71. Retrieved from https://www.ncbi.nlm.nih.gov/pubmed/19472572

Dillin, A., Gottschling, D. E., & Nyström, T. (2014). The good and the bad of being connected: The integrons of aging. *Current Opinion in Cell Biology, 26C,* 107–112. doi:10.1016/j.ceb.2013.12.003 PMID:24529252

Dillion, C. F., Gu, Q., Hoffman, H. J., & Ko, C. (2010). Vision, hearing, balance, and sensory impairment in Americans aged 70 years and over. *United States, 1999–2006* (Data Brief No. 31). Retrieved from http://www.cdc.gov/nchs/data/databriefs/db31.pdf

Dillon, P. (2007). *Nursing Health Assessment: A Critical Thinking Case Studies Approach.* Philadelphia: F.A. Davis Publishers.

Diniz, B. S., Pinto, J. A. Jr, & Forlenza, O. V. (2008). Do CSF total tau, phosphorylated tau, and β-amyloid 42 help to predict progression of mild cognitive impairment to Alzheimer's disease? A systematic review and meta-analysis of the literature. *The World Journal of Biological Psychiatry*, *9*(3), 172–182. doi:10.1080/15622970701535502 PMID:17886169

Dirven, L., Reijneveld, J. C., Aaronson, N. K., Bottomley, A., Uitdehaag, B. M., & Taphoorn, M. J. (2013). Health-related quality of life in patients with brain tumors: Limitations and additional outcome measures. *Current Neurology and Neuroscience Reports*, *13*(7), 359. doi:10.1007/s11910-013-0359-y PMID:23666388

Dobie, D. J., Miller, M. A., Raskind, M. A., & Dorsa, D. M. (1992). Testosterone reverses a senescent decline in extra hypothalamic vasopressin MRNA. *Brain Research*, *583*(1-2), 247–252. doi:10.1016/S0006-8993(10)80030-7 PMID:1504830

Dobson, K. S., & Dozois, D. J. A. (2001). Historical and philosophical bases of the cognitive behavioural therapies. In K. S. Dobson (Ed.), *Handbook of cognitive-behavioral therapies* (2nd ed.; pp. 3–39). New York: Guilford.

Doctors Against Vivisection. (n.d.). Doctors Against animal Research Experiments. Retrieved from https://doctorsagainstvivisection.wordpress.com/

Dokal, I. (2000). Dyskeratosis congenital in all its forms. *British Journal of Haematology*, *110*(4), 768–779. doi:10.1046/j.1365-2141.2000.02109.x PMID:11054058

Dolan, P., & White, M. P. (2007). How can measures of subjective well-being be used to inform public policy? *Perspectives on Psychological Science*, *2*(1), 71–84. doi:10.1111/j.1745-6916.2007.00030.x PMID:26151920

Dombrovski1, A. Y., Szanto, K., & Reynolds, C. F., III. (2005). Epidemiology and risk factors for suicide in the elderly: 10-year update. *Aging Health, 1*(1), 135–145.

Dombrovski, A. Y., Butters, M. A., Reynolds, C. III, Houck, F., Clark, L., Patricia, R., ... Szanto, K. (2008). Reward/punishment reversal learning in older suicide attempters. *The American Journal of Geriatric Psychiatry*, *16*(2), 109–115. doi:10.1097/JGP.0b013e3180f6338d PMID:18239196

Dombrovski, A. Y., Szanto, K., & Reynolds, C. F. III. (2005). Epidemiology and risk factors for suicide in the elderly: 10-year update. *Aging Health*, *1*(1), 135–145. doi:10.2217/1745509X.1.1.135

Dombrovski, A., Clark, L., Siegle, G. J., Butters, M. A., Ichikawa, N., Sahakian, B. J., & Szanto, K. (2010). Reward/punishment reversal learning in older suicide attempters. *The American Journal of Psychiatry*, *167*(6), 699–707. doi:10.1176/appi.ajp.2009.09030407 PMID:20231320

Donaldson, I. M. (2004). Bon sante: Is wine good for your health? *International Medical Journal*, *34*(5), 221–223. doi:10.1111/j.1444-0903.2004.00583.x PMID:15151665

Dong, X. (2005). Medical implications of elder abuse and neglect. *Clinics in Geriatric Medicine*, *21*(2), 293–313. doi:10.1016/j.cger.2004.10.006 PMID:15804552

Dong, X., Tong, F., Qian, C., Zhang, R., Dong, J., Wu, G., & Hu, Y. (2015). NEMO modulatesradiation-induced endothelial senescence of human umbilical veinsthrough NF-kappaB signal pathway. *Radiation Research*, *183*(1), 82–93. doi:10.1667/RR13682.1 PMID:25536232

Donini, L., Chumlea, W., Vellas, B., delBalzo, V., & Cannalla, C. (2006). In preparation for the International Symposium on 'Obesity in the Elderly'. *Aging Health, 2*(1), 47–51. Retrieved August 12, 2008 from www.futuremedicine.com.doi/abs/ doi:10.2217/1745509X.2.1.47

Donmez, L., Gokkoca, Z., & Dedeoglu, N. (2005). Disability and its effects on quality of life among older people living in Antalya city centre. *Turkey Archives of Gerontology and Geriatrics, 40*(2), 213–223. doi:10.1016/j.archger.2004.08.006 PMID:15680503

Dorr, M., Wolff, B., Robinson, D. M., John, U., Lüdemann, J., Meng, W., ... Völzke, H. (2005). The associations of thyroid function with cardiac mass and left ventricular hypertrophy. *The Journal of Clinical Endocrinology and Metabolism, 90*(2), 673–677. doi:10.1210/jc.2004-1554 PMID:15522926

Dossey, L. (2001). *Healing beyond the body* (pp. 10–22). Boston: Shambala.

Dowling, G. J., Weiss, S. R., & Condon, T. P. (2008). Drugs of abuse and the ageing brain. *Neuropsychopharmacology, 33*(2), 209–218. doi:10.1038/sj.npp.1301412 PMID:17406645

Dozois, D. J. A., Frewen, P. A., & Covin, R. (2006). Cognitive theories. In J. C. Thomas & D. L. Segal (Eds.), Personality and everyday functioning. Hoboken, NJ: John Wiley & Sons, Inc.

Draper, B. (1994). Suicidal behaviour in the elderly. *International Journal of Geriatric Psychiatry, 9*(8), 655–661. doi:10.1002/gps.930090810

Drzezga, A., Grimmer, T., Riemenschneider, M., Lautenschlager, N., Siebner, H., Alexopoulus, P., ... Kurz, A. (2005). Prediction of individual clinical outcome in MCI by means of genetic assessment and (18)F-FDG PET. *Journal of Nuclear Medicine, 46*(10), 1625–1632. PMID:16204712

Duberstein, P. R., Conwell, Y., Conner, K. R., Eberly, S., & Caine, E. D. (2004). Suicide at 50 years of age and older: Perceived physical illness, family discord and financial strain. *Psychological Medicine, 34*(1), 137–146. doi:10.1017/S0033291703008584 PMID:14971634

Dubrow, E. L. (1976). Reactivation of tuberculosis: A problem of aging. *Journal of the American Geriatrics Society, 24*(11), 481–487. doi:10.1111/j.1532-5415.1976.tb03269.x PMID:972234

Duckworth, A. L., Steen, T. A., & Seligman, M. E. P. (2005). Positive psychology in clinical practice. *Annual Review of Clinical Psychology, 1*(1), 629–651. doi:10.1146/annurev.clinpsy.1.102803.144154 PMID:17716102

Duckworth, A., & Gross, J. J. (2014). Self-Control and Grit: Related but Separable Determinants of Success. *Current Directions in Psychological Science, 23*(5), 319–325. doi:10.1177/0963721414541462 PMID:26855479

Dunkle-Blatter, S. E., Jean, M. R. S., Whitehead, C., Strodel, W., Bennotti, P. N., Still, C., & Petrick, A. T. (2007). Outcomes among elderly bariatric patients at a high-volume center. *Surgery for Obesity and Related Diseases, 3*(2), 163–169. doi:10.1016/j.soard.2006.12.004 PMID:17331804

Dupuis, K., Pichora-Fuller, M. K., Chasteen, A. L., Marchuk, V., Singh, G., & Smith, S. L. (2015). Effects of hearing and vision impairments on the Montreal Cognitive Assessment. *Neuropsychological Development Cognition Brain Aging Neuropsychol Cognition, 22*(4), 413–437. doi:10.1080/13825585.2014.968084 PMID:25325767

Dutra, M., Uliano, E., Machado, D., Martins, T., Vinholes, D., Trevisol, F., & Trevisol, D. (2013). Obesity prevalence among elderly people using different measurement methods: A population-base study. *International Journal of Diseases and Disorders, 1*(2), 24–32.

Dy, S. M., Apostol, C., Martinez, K. A., & Aslakson, R. A. (2013). Continuity, coordination, and transitions of care for patients with serious and advanced illness: A systematic review of interventions. *Journal of Palliative Medicine*, *16*(4), 436–445. doi:10.1089/jpm.2012.0317 PMID:23488450

Eckel, R. H. (1997). Obesity and Heart Disease: A Statement for Healthcare Professionals From the Nutrition Committee. American Heart Association.

Eddy, D. M. (1989). Screening for lung cancer. *Annals of Internal Medicine*, 111. PMID:2665590

Elderly in India. (2016). Ministry of Statistics and Program Implementation, Central Statistics Office (Social Statistics Division).

Elias, J., & Ryan, A. (2011). A review and commentary on the factors that influence expressions of sexuality by older people in care homes. *Journal of Clinical Nursing*, *20*(11-12), 1668–1676. doi:10.1111/j.1365-2702.2010.03409.x PMID:21323776

Elisabeth, M. H., Vliegen, M., Basdevant, A., & Finer, N. (2012). Prevalence, Pathophysiology, Health Consequences and Treatment Options of Obesity in the Elderly: A Guideline. *Obesity Facts*, *5*(3), 460–483. doi:10.1159/000341193 PMID:22797374

Elkins, D. N., Hedstrom, L. J., Hughes, L. L., Leaf, J. A., & Saunders, C. (1988). Toward a humanistic-phenomenological spirituality: Definition, description, and measurement. *Journal of Humanistic Psychology*, *28*(4), 5–18. doi:10.1177/0022167888284002

Ellis, D. (1980). Whatever happened to the spiritual dimension? *The Canadian Nurse*, *76*(8), 42–43. PMID:6901632

Ellison, C. G., & Levin, J. S. (1998). The religion-health connection: Evidence, theory, and future directions. *Health Education & Behavior*, *25*(6), 700–720. doi:10.1177/109019819802500603 PMID:9813743

Elżbieta, G. (2015). Music therapy in neurological rehabilitation settings. *Psychiatria Polska*, *49*(4), 835–846. PMID:26488358

Emma, P., Phillip, F., & Christine, R. (2017). Management of Acute Stroke in the Older Person. *Geriatrics*, *2*(3), 27. doi:10.3390/geriatrics2030027

Erickson's, S. H. (1963). Childhood and society (2nd ed.). New York: W.W. Norton.

Erickson's, S. H. (1968). *Identity: Youth and crisis*. New York: W.W. Norton.

Erickson, K. I., Gildengers, A., & Butters, M. (2013). Physical activity and brain plasticity in late adulthood. *Dialogues in Clinical Neuroscience*, *15*(1), 99–108. PMID:23576893

Erickson, K. I., Leckie, R. L., & Weinstein, A. M. (2014). Physical activity, fitness, and gray matter volume. *Neurobiology of Aging*, *35*, 20–28. doi:10.1016/j.neurobiolaging.2014.03.034 PMID:24952993

Erikson, E. H. (1959). *Childhood and society*. New York: Norton.

Erikson, E. H. (1982). *The life cycle completed*. New York, London: W. W. Norton & Company.

Erikson, E. H. (1984). Reflections on the last stage-and the first. *The Psychoanalytic Study of the Child*, *39*(1), 155–165. doi:10.1080/00797308.1984.11823424 PMID:6514889

Erikson, E. H., & Erikson, J. M. (1998). *The life cycle completed (extended version)*. New York: WW Norton & Company.

Erikson, E. H., Erikson, J. M., & Kivnic, J. (1989). *Vital involvement in old age*. New York, London: W.W. Norton & Company.

Erikson, J. M. (1995). *On old age 1: A conversation with Joan Erikson at 90*. California: Davidson Films.

Erikson, J. M. (1997). *The life cycle completed: Extended version with new chapters on the ninth stage of development*. New York, London: W.W. Norton & Company.

Ershler, W. B., Stewart, J. A., Hacker, M. P., Moore, A. L., & Tindle, B. A. (1984). B16 melanoma and aging: Slower growth and longer survival in old mice. *Journal of the National Cancer Institute*, *72*(1), 161–164. doi:10.1093/jnci/72.1.161 PMID:6582296

Erwin, C. W., Somerville, E. R., & Radtke, R. A. (1984). A review of electroencephalographic features of normal sleep. *Journal of Clinical Neurophysiology*, *1*(3), 253–274. doi:10.1097/00004691-198407000-00001 PMID:6399909

Espie, C. A. (2002). Insomnia: Conceptual issues in the development, persistence, and treatment of sleep disorder in adults. *Annual Review of Psychology*, *53*(1), 215–243. doi:10.1146/annurev.psych.53.100901.135243 PMID:11752485

Essays, U. K. (2013). Cardiovascular Disease. Retrieved from https://www.ukessays.com/essays/health/cardiovascular-disease.php?cref=1

Etgen, T., Bickel, H., & Förstl, H. (2010). Metabolic and endocrine factors in mild cognitive impairment. *Ageing Research Reviews*, *9*(3), 280–288. doi:10.1016/j.arr.2010.01.003 PMID:20109582

Etgen, T., Sander, D., Chonchol, M., Briesenick, C., Poppert, H., Förstl, H., & Bickel, H. (2009). Chronic kidney disease is associated with incident cognitive impairment in the elderly: The INVADE study. *Nephrology, Dialysis, Transplantation*, *24*(10), 3144–3150. doi:10.1093/ndt/gfp230 PMID:19461010

Everard, K. M., Lach, H. W., Fisher, E. B., & Baum, M. C. (2000). Relationship of activity and social support to the functional health of older *adults. The Journals of Gerontology. Series B, Psychological Sciences and Social Sciences*, *55*(4), 208–212. doi:10.1093/geronb/55.4.S208 PMID:11584883

Exline, J. J. (2002). Stumbling blocks on the religious road: Fractured relationships, nagging vices, and the inner struggle to believe. *Psychological Inquiry*, *13*(3), 182–189. doi:10.1207/S15327965PLI1303_03

Exline, J. J., Yali, A. M., & Lobel, M. (1999). When God disappoints: Difficulty forgiving God and its role in negative emotion. *Journal of Health Psychology*, *4*(3), 365–379. doi:10.1177/135910539900400306 PMID:22021604

Exline, J. J., Yali, A. M., & Sanderson, W. C. (2000). Guilt, discord, and alienation: The role of religious strain in depression and suicidality. *Journal of Clinical Psychology*, *56*(12), 1481–1496. doi:10.1002/1097-4679(200012)56:12<1481::AID-1>3.0.CO;2-A PMID:11132565

Fabbri, E., An, Y., Zoli, M., Simonsick, E. M., Guralnik, J. M., Bandinelli, S., ... Ferrucci, L. (2015). Aging and the burden of multimorbidity: Associations within flammatory and anabolic hormonal biomarkers. *The Journals of Gerontology. Series A, Biological Sciences and Medical Sciences*, *70*(1), 63–70. doi:10.1093/gerona/glu127 PMID:25104822

Faigin, C. A., & Pargament, K. I. (2011). Strengthened by the Spirit: Religion, Spirituality, and Resilience Through Adulthood and Aging. In B. Resnick, L. P. P. Gwyther, & K. A. A. Roberto (Eds.), *Resilience in Aging: Concepts*. Research, and Outcomes. doi:10.1007/978-1-4419-0232-0_11

Fannin, A. (2006). Gay and grey: Lifting the lid on sexuality and ageing. *Working With Older People*, *10*(4), 31–34. doi:10.1108/13663666200600069

Farooqi, S., Bochukova, E., Huang, N., Keogh, J., Henning, E., Purmann, C., & Blaszczyk, K. (2010). Large, rare chromosomal deletions associated with severe early-onset obesity. *Nature Journal*, *463*(7281), 666–670. doi:10.1038/nature08689 PMID:19966786

Farzian, P. F., Arab, M., Hosseini, S. M., Pirozi, B., & Shadi, H. (2012). Quality of life of the elderly residents in Marivan Evaluation of quality of life of the elderly population covered by healthcare centers of Marivan and the influencing demographic and background factors in 2010. *Iranian Red Crescent Medical Journal*, *14*(11), 695–696. PMID:23397047

Fässberg, M. M., Van Orden, K. A., Duberstein, P., Erlangsen, A., Lapierre, S., & Bodner, E. (2012). A systematic review of social factors and suicidal behavior in older adulthood. *International Journal of Environmental Research and Public Health*, *9*(3), 722–745. doi:10.3390/ijerph9030722 PMID:22690159

Fazio, S., Palmieri, E. A., Lombardi, G., & Biondi, B. (2004). Effects of Thyroid Hormone on the Cardiovascular System. *Recent Progress in Hormone Research*, *59*(1), 31–50. doi:10.1210/rp.59.1.31 PMID:14749496

Féart, C., Samieri, C., & Barberger-Gateau, P. (2010). Mediterranean diet and cognitive function in older adults. *Current Opinion in Clinical Nutrition and Metabolic Care*, *13*(1), 14–18. doi:10.1097/MCO.0b013e3283331fe4 PMID:19834324

Feinstein, A. R. (1970). The pre-therapeutic classification of co-morbidity in chronic disease. *Journal of Chronic Diseases*, *23*(7), 455–468. doi:10.1016/0021-9681(70)90054-8 PMID:26309916

Ferlay, J., Shin, H. R., & Bray, F. (2010). GLOBOCAN 2008 v2.0, Cancer incidence and mortality worldwide. Lyon: *International agency for Research on Cancer*. Retrieved from http://globocan.iarc.fr

Ferrucci, L., Giallauria, F., & Guralnik, J. M. (2009). Epidemiology of Aging. *Radiologic Clinics of North America*, *46*(4), 643–v. doi:10.1016/j.rcl.2008.07.005 PMID:18922285

Ferrucci, L., Guralnik, J. M., & Salive, M. E. (1996). Cognitive impairment and risk of stroke in the older population. *Journal of the American Geriatrics Society*, *44*(3), 237–241. doi:10.1111/j.1532-5415.1996.tb00908.x PMID:8600190

Fetzer Institute. (1999). Multidimensional measurement of religiousness/ spirituality for use in health research.

Fiatarone, M. A., O'Neill, E. F., Ryan, N. D., Clements, K. M., Solares, G. R., Nelson, M. E., ... Evans, W. J. (1994). Exercise training and nutritional supplementation for physical frailty in very elderly people. *The New England Journal of Medicine*, *330*(25), 1769–1775. doi:10.1056/NEJM199406233302501 PMID:8190152

Figueira, H. A., Figueira, O. A., & Figueira, A. A. (2010). Elderly quality of life impacted by traditional Chinese medicine techniques. *Clinical Interventions in Aging*, *5*, 301–305. doi:10.2147/CIA.S10615 PMID:21103400

Figueira, H., Figueira, J., Mello, D., & Dantas, E. (2008). Quality of life throughout aging. *ActaMedicaLituanica*, *15*, 169–172.

Fileborn, B., Thorpe, R., Hawkes, G., Minichiello, V., Pitts, M., Dune, T., & Pitts, M. (2015). Sex, desire and pleasure: Considering the experiences of older Australian women. *Sexual and Relationship Therapy*, *30*(1), 117–130. doi:10.1080/14681994.2014.936722 PMID:25544829

Finegold, J. A., Asaria, P., & Francis, D. P. (2012). Mortality from ischaemic heart disease by country, region, and age: Statistics from World Health Organisation and United Nations. *International Journal of Cardiology*, *168*(2), 934–945. doi:10.1016/j.ijcard.2012.10.046 PMID:23218570

Fingerman, K. L., Miller, L. M., & Seidel, A. J. (2009). Functions families serve in old age. In S. H. Qualls & S. H. Zarit (Eds.), *Aging families and caregiving* (pp. 19–44). Hoboken, NJ: John Wiley & Sons, Inc.

Fisher, J. E., & Noll, J. P. (1996). Anxiety disorders. In L. L. Carstensen, B. A. Edelstein, & L. Dornobrand (Eds.), The practical handbook of clinical gerontology (pp. 304-323). Thousand Oaks, CA: Sage.

Fisher, D., Li, C.-M., Chiu, M. A., Themann, C. L., Petersen, H., & Jonasson, F. (2014). Impairments in hearing and vision impact on mortality in older people. *International Journal of Audiology*, *54*(9), 634–641. doi:10.3109/14992027.2015.1024889 PMID:25816699

Fiske, A., O'Riley, A. A., & Widoe, R. K. (2008). Physical Health and Suicide in Late Life: An Evaluative Review. *Clinical Gerontologist*, *31*(4), 31–50. doi:10.1080/07317110801947151

Fiske, A., Wetherell, J. L., & Gatz, M. (2009). Depression in older adults. *Annual Review of Clinical Psychology*, *5*(1), 363–389. doi:10.1146/annurev.clinpsy.032408.153621 PMID:19327033

Fleck, M. P. A., Chachamovisch, E., & Trentini, C. M. (2003). Projeto WHOQOL-OLD: Método e resultados de grupos-focais no Brasil. *Revista de Saude Publica*, *37*(6), 793–799. doi:10.1590/S0034-89102003000600016 PMID:14666311

Flessner, M. F., Wyatt, S. B., Akylbekova, E. L., Coady, S., Fulop, T., Lee, F., ... Crook, E. (2009). Prevalence and awareness of CKD among African Americans: The Jackson heart study. *American Journal of Kidney Diseases*, *53*(2), 238–247. doi:10.1053/j.ajkd.2008.08.035 PMID:19166799

Flint, Alastair J. "Epidemiology and comorbidity of anxiety disorders in the elderly." *The American Journal of Psychiatry* 151.5 (1994): 640.

Flood, M., & Newman, A. (2007). Obesity in older adults: Synthesis of findings and recommendations for clinical practice. *Journal of Gerontological Nursing*, *33*, 19–35. PMID:18183745

Flostein, M. F. (1983). Assessment in geriatric psychopharmacology. The Mini Mental Status Exam, 50–51.

Foley, D. J., Monjan, A. A., Brown, S. L., Simonsick, E. M., Wallace, R. B., & Blazer, D. G. (1995). Sleep complaints among elderly persons: An epidemiologic study of three communities. *Sleep*, *18*, 425–432.

Folkman, J., & Shing, Y. (1992). Angiogenesis. *The Journal of Biological Chemistry*, *267*, 10931–10934. PMID:1375931

Folsom, D. P., Depp, C., Palmer, B. W., Mausbach, B. T., Golshan, S., Fellows, I., ... Jeste, D. V. (2009). Physical and mental health related quality of life among older people with schizophrenia. *Schizophrenia Research*, *108*(1-3), 207–213. doi:10.1016/j.schres.2008.12.008 PMID:19168328

Folsom, D. P., Hawthorne, W., Lindamer, L., Gilmer, T., Bailey, A., Golshan, S., ... Jeste, D. V. (2005). Prevalence and risk factors for homelessness and utilization of mental health services among 10.340 patients with serious mental illness in a large public mental health system. *The American Journal of Psychiatry*, *162*(2), 370–376. doi:10.1176/appi.ajp.162.2.370 PMID:15677603

Folstein, M. F., Folstein, S. E., & McHugh, P. R. (1975). Mini-mental state: A practical method for grading the cognitive state of patients for the clinician. *Journal of Psychiatric Research*, *12*(3), 189–198. doi:10.1016/0022-3956(75)90026-6 PMID:1202204

Fontbonne, A., Berr, C., Ducimetiere, P., & Alperovitch, A. (2001). Changes in cognitive abilities over a 4-year period are unfavorably affected in elderly diabetic subjects: Results of the epidemiology of vascular aging study. *Diabetes Care*, *24*(2), 366–370. doi:10.2337/diacare.24.2.366 PMID:11213894

Forbes, A. (1996). Education and debate, caring for older people: Loneliness. *BMJ (Clinical Research Ed.)*, *313*(7053), 352–354. doi:10.1136/bmj.313.7053.352 PMID:8760749

Forette, F., Seux, M. L., Staessen, J. A., Thijs, L., Babarskiene, M. R., & Babeanu, S., ... Systolic Hypertension in Europe Investigators. (2002). The prevention of dementia with antihypertensive treatment: New evidence from the Systolic Hypertension in Europe (Syst-Eur) study. *Archives of Internal Medicine*, *162*(18), 2046–2052. doi:10.1001/archinte.162.18.2046 PMID:12374512

Forfar, J. C., Miller, H. C., & Toft, A. D. (1979). Occult thyrotoxicosis: A reversible cause of "idiopathic" atrial fibrillation. *The American Journal of Cardiology*, *44*(1), 9–12. doi:10.1016/0002-9149(79)90243-1 PMID:110126

Forsberg, A., Engler, H., Almkvist, O., Blomquist, G., Hagman, G., Wall, A., ... Nordberg, A. (2008). PET imaging of amyloid deposition in patients with mild cognitive impairment. *Neurobiology of Aging*, *29*(10), 1456–1465. doi:10.1016/j.neurobiolaging.2007.03.029 PMID:17499392

Forsell, Y., Palmer, K., & Fratiglioni, L. (2003). Psychiatric symptoms/syndromes in elderly persons with mild cognitive impairment. Data from a cross-sectional study. *Acta Neurologica Scandinavica*, *107*(s179), 25–28. doi:10.1034/j.1600-0404.107.s179.4.x PMID:12603247

Fortin, M., Bravo, G., Hudon, C., Lapointe, L., Almirall, J., Dubois, M. F., & Vanasse, A. (2006). Relationship between multimorbidity and health-related quality of life of patients in primary care. *Quality of Life Research: An International Journal of Quality of Life Aspects of Treatment, Care and Rehabilitation*, *15*(1), 83–91. doi:10.1007/s11136-005-8661-z PMID:16411033

Fortin, M., Dubois, M. F., Hudon, C., Soubhi, H., & Almirall, J. (2007). Multimorbidity and quality of life: A closer look. *Health and Quality of Life Outcomes*, *5*(1), 52. doi:10.1186/1477-7525-5-52 PMID:17683600

Fortin, M., Lapoointe, L., Hudon, C., Vanasse, A., Ntetu, A. L., & Maltais, D. (2004). Multimorbidity and quality of life in primary care: A systematic review. *Health and Quality of Life Outcomes*, *2*(1), 51. doi:10.1186/1477-7525-2-51 PMID:15380021

Foskett, J., Marriott, J., & Wilson-Rudd, F. (2004). Mental health, religion and spirituality: Attitudes, experience and expertise among mental health professionals and religious leaders in Somerset. *Mental Health, Religion & Culture*, *7*(1), 5–22. doi:10.1080/13674670310001602490

Fowler, J. W. (1981). *Stages of faith: The psychology of human developmet and the quest for meaning*. San Francisco: Harper & Row.

Fox, C. S., Sullivan, L., D'Agostino, R. B., & Sr. Wilson, P. W. (2004). Framingham Heart Study. The significant effect of diabetes duration on coronary heart disease mortality: The Framingham Heart Study. *Diabetes Care*, *27*(3), 704–708. doi:10.2337/diacare.27.3.704 PMID:14988289

Franchini, G., Fukumoto, R., & Fullen, J. R. (2003). T-Cell control by human T cell leukemia/lymphoma virus type 1. *International Journal of Hematology*, *78*(4), 280–296. doi:10.1007/BF02983552 PMID:14686485

Frankl, V. E. (1959). The spiritual dimension in existential analysis and logotherapy. *Journal of Individual Psychology*, *15*(2), 157.

Frankowski, A. C., & Clark, L. J. (2009). Sexuality and Intimacy in Assisted Living: *Residents'. Perspectives and Experiences Sexuality Research & Social Policy*, *6*(4), 25–37. doi:10.1525/srsp.2009.6.4.25 PMID:25568640

Frazier, P. A., Tix, A. P., Klein, C. D., & Arikian, N. J. (2000). Testing theoretical models of the relations between social support, coping, and adjustment to stressful life events. *Journal of Social and Clinical Psychology*, *19*(3), 314–335. doi:10.1521/jscp.2000.19.3.314

Fredrickson, B. L. (2001). The role of positive emotions in positive psychology -The broaden-and-build theory of positive emotions. *The American Psychologist*, *56*(3), 218–226. doi:10.1037/0003-066X.56.3.218 PMID:11315248

Fredrickson, B. L., Cohn, M. A., Coffey, K. A., Pek, J., & Finkel, S. M. (2008). Open Hearts Build Lives: Positive Emotions, Induced Through Loving-Kindness Meditation, Build Consequential Personal Resources. *Journal of Personality and Social Psychology*, *95*(5), 1045–1062. doi:10.1037/a0013262 PMID:18954193

Fried, L. P., Ferrucci, L., Darer, J., Williamson, J. D., & Anderson, G. (2004). Untangling the concepts of disability, frailty, and comorbidity: Implications for improved targeting and care. *The Journals of Gerontology. Series A, Biological Sciences and Medical Sciences*, *59A*(3), 255–263. doi:10.1093/gerona/59.3.M255 PMID:15031310

Fried, L. P., Tangen, C. M., Walston, J., Newman, A. B., Hirsch, C., Gottdiener, J., ... McBurnie, M. A. (2001). Frailty. in older adults: Evidence for a phenotype. *The Journals of Gerontology. Series A, Biological Sciences and Medical Sciences*, *56*(3), M146–M156. doi:10.1093/gerona/56.3.M146 PMID:11253156

Friedland, R. P., Fritsch, T., Smyth, K. A., Koss, E., Lerner, A. J., Chen, C. H., & Debanne, S. M. (2001). Patients with Alzheimer's disease have reduced activities in midlife compared with healthy control-group members. *Proceedings of the National Academy of Sciences of the United States of America*, *98*(6), 3440–3445. doi:10.1073/pnas.061002998 PMID:11248097

Friedman, A. S. (1964). Minimal effects of severe depression on cognitive functioning. *Journal of Abnormal and Social Psychology*, *69*(3), 237–243. doi:10.1037/h0048608 PMID:14210773

Friedman, D. E., & Lipsedge, M. S. (1971). Treatment of phobic anxiety and psychogenic impotence by systematic desensitization employing methohexitone-induced relaxation. *The British Journal of Psychiatry*, *118*(542), 87–90. doi:10.1192/bjp.118.542.87 PMID:5576272

Fulop, T., Larbi, A., Kotb, R., de Angelis, F., & Pawelec, G. (2011). Aging, immunity, and cancer. *Discovery Medicine*, *11*(61), 537–550. PMID:21712020

Gabriel, Z., & Bowling, A. (2004). Quality of life from the perspectives of older people. *Ageing and Society*, *24*(05), 675–691. doi:10.1017/S0144686X03001582

Gabryelewicz, T., Styczynska, M., Pfeffer, A., Wasiak, B., Barczak, A., Luczywek, E., ... Barcikowska, M. (2004). Prevalence of major and minor depression in elderly persons with mild cognitive impairment-MADRS factor analysis. *International Journal of Geriatric Psychiatry*, *19*(12), 1168–1172. doi:10.1002/gps.1235 PMID:15526303

Gajalakshmi, & Jha, P. V. (2005). Prospective study of one million deaths in India: Rationale, design, and validation results. *PLOS Medicine, 3*(2), e18.

Galanter, M. (2008). The concept of spirituality in relation to addiction recovery and general psychiatry. In Recent developments in alcoholism (pp. 125-140). Springer New York. doi:10.1007/978-0-387-77725-2_8

Galazka, A. M., Robertson, S. E., & Kraigher, A. (1999). Mumps and mumps vaccine: A global review. *Bulletin of the World Health Organization*, *77*, 3–14. PMID:10063655

Galinsky, A., McClintock, M. K., & Waite, L. J. (2014). Sexuality and physical contact in national social life, health, and aging project wave 2. *The Journals of Gerontology. Series B, Psychological Sciences and Social Sciences*, *69*(8Suppl 2), S83–S98. doi:10.1093/geronb/gbu072 PMID:25360027

Gallacher, J., Mitchell, C., Heslop, L., & Christopher, G. (2012). Resilience to health related adversity in older people. *Emerald Quality in Ageing and Older Adults*, *13*(3), 197–204. doi:10.1108/14717791211264188

Gallagher, D., Fischer, C. E., & Iaboni, A. (2017). Neuropsychiatric Symptoms in Mild Cognitive Impairment. *Canadian Journal of Psychiatry*, *62*(3), 161–169. doi:10.1177/0706743716648296 PMID:28212495

Gallagher, P., Ryan, C., & Byrne, S. (2008). STOPP (Screening Tool of Older Person's Prescriptions) and START (Screening Tool to Alert doctors to Right Treatment). Consensus validation. *International Journal of Clinical Pharmacology and Therapeutics*, *46*(2), 72–83. doi:10.5414/CPP46072 PMID:18218287

Galmi, R. (2010). Insomnia in the elderly: An update and future challenges. *Journal of Gerontology*, *58*, 231–247.

Gameiro, G.R., & Minguini, P. I., & FerrazAlves, T.C. (2014). The role of stress and life events in the onset of depression in the elderly. *Review of Medicine*, *93*(1), 31–40.

Ganguli, M. (2009). Depression, cognitive impairment and dementia: Why should clinicians care about the web of causation? *Indian Journal of Psychiatry*, *51*(5), 29. PMID:21416013

Ganguli, M., Dodge, H. H., Shen, C., & DeKosky, S. T. (2004). Mild cognitive impairment, amnestic type: An epidemiologic study. *Neurology*, *63*(1), 115–121. doi:10.1212/01.WNL.0000132523.27540.81 PMID:15249620

Garand, L., Mitchell, A. N., Dietrick, A., Hijjawi, S. P., & Pan, D. (2010). Suicide in older adults. *Nursing Assessment of IDAL Risk*, *27*(4), 355–370. doi:10.1080/01612840600569633.SUICIDE PMID:16546935

Garnets, L., & Peplau, L. A. (2006). Sexuality in the Lives of Aging Lesbian and Bisexual Women. In D. Kimmel, T. Rose, & S. David (Eds.), *Lesbian, Gay, Bisexual, and Transgender Aging* (pp. 70–90). New York: Columbia University Press. doi:10.7312/kimm13618-005

Gates, N. J., Sachdev, P. S., Fiatarone Singh, M. A., & Valenzuela, M. (2011). Cognitive and memory training in adults at risk of dementia: A systematic review. *BMC Geriatrics*, *11*(1), 55. doi:10.1186/1471-2318-11-55 PMID:21942932

Gatz, M., Kasl-Godley, J. E., & Karel, M. J. (1996). Aging and mental disorders. In J. E. Birren & K. W. Schaie (Eds.), *Handbook of the psychology of aging* (4th ed.; pp. 365–382). San Diego, CA: Academic Press.

Gaugler, J. E., Yu, F., Krichbaum, K., & Wyman, J. F. (2009). Predictors of nursing home admission for persons with dementia. *Medical Care*, *47*(2), 191–198. doi:10.1097/MLR.0b013e31818457ce PMID:19169120

Gaugler, J., Roth, D., Haley, W., & Mitterlman, M. (2008). Can counselling and support reduce burden and depressive symptoms in caregivers of people with Alzheimer's disease during the transition to institutionalization. Results from the New York University Caregiver Intervention Study. *Journal of the American Geriatrics Society*, *56*(3), 421–428. doi:10.1111/j.1532-5415.2007.01593.x PMID:18179495

Gazzaley, A., Clapp, W., Kelley, J., McEvoy, K., Knight, R. T., & D'Esposito, M. (2008). Age related top-down suppression deficit in the early stages of cortical visual memory processing. *Proceedings of the National Academy of Sciences of the United States of America*, *105*(35), 13122–13126. doi:10.1073/pnas.0806074105 PMID:18765818

Gazzalley, A. (2009). Normal aging. UCSF Memory and Aging Center. Retrieved August 4, 2009 from http://memory.ucsf.edu/Education/Topics/normalaging.html

GBD 2013 Mortality and Causes of Death, Collaborators. (2014). Global, regional, and national age-sex specific all-cause and cause-specific mortality for 240 causes of death, 1990-2013: a systematic analysis for the Global Burden of Disease Study 2013.". *Lancet, 385*(9963), 117–71. doi:10.1016/S0140-6736(14)61682-2

GBD 2015 Mortality and Causes of Death, Collaborators. (2016). "Global, regional, and national life expectancy, all-cause mortality, and cause-specific mortality for 249 causes of death, 1980-2015: a systematic analysis for the Global Burden of Disease Study 2015.". *Lancet, 388*(10053), 1459–1544. doi:10.1016/S0140-6736(16)31012-1

Geerlings, M. I., Bouter, L. M., Schoevers, R., Beekman, A. T. F., Jonker, C., & Deeg, D. J. H. (2000). Depression and risk of cognitive decline and Alzheimer's disease: Results of two prospective community-based studies in The Netherlands. *The British Journal of Psychiatry*, *176*(6), 56875. doi:10.1192/bjp.176.6.568 PMID:10974964

Gehrman, P. R., Martin, J. L., Shochat, T., Nolan, S., Corey-Bloom, J., & Ancoli-Israel, S. (2003). Sleep disordered breathing and agitation in institutionalized adults with Alzheimer's disease. *The American Journal of Geriatric Psychiatry*, *11*(4), 426–433. doi:10.1097/00019442-200307000-00005 PMID:12837671

George, L. (1989). Stress, social support and depression over the life course.IN K. Markides & C. Cooper (Eds.), Aging, stress, social support and health (pp. 241-267). New York: John Wiley & Sons.

Gerber, B. S., & Eiser, A. R. (2001). The patient-physician relationship in the Internet Age: Future prospects and the research agenda. *Journal of Medical Internet Research*, *3*(2), 112–123. doi:10.2196/jmir.3.2.e15 PMID:11720957

Getahun, H., Harrington, M., O'Brien, R., & Nunn, P. (2007). Diagnosis of smear-negative pulmonary tuberculosis in people with HIV infection or AIDS in resource-constrained settings: Informing urgent policy changes. *Lancet*, *369*(9578), 2042–2049. doi:10.1016/S0140-6736(07)60284-0 PMID:17574096

Gharib, H., Tuttle, R. M., Baskin, H. J., Fish, L. H., Singer, P. A., & McDermott, M. T. (2005). Subclinical thyroid dysfunction: A joint statement on management from the American Association of Clinical Endocrinologists, the American Thyroid Association, and the Endocrine Society. *The Journal of Clinical Endocrinology and Metabolism*, *90*(1), 581–585. doi:10.1210/jc.2004-1231 PMID:15643019

Ghitza, U. E., Wu, L. T., & Tai, B. (2013). Integrating substance abuse care with community diabetes care: Implications for research and clinical practice. *Substance Abuse and Rehabilitation*, *4*, 3–10. doi:10.2147/SAR.S39982 PMID:23378792

Gifford, J., & Jones, R. (2009). Assessment and treatment of cognitive deficits in dementia. *The Prescriber*, *20*(6), 45–49. doi:10.1002/psb.490

Gijsen, R., Hoeymans, N., Schellevis, F. G., Ruwaard, D., Satariano, W. A., & van den Bos, G. A. (2001). Causes and consequences of comorbidity: A review. *Journal of Clinical Epidemiology*, *54*(7), 661–674. doi:10.1016/S0895-4356(00)00363-2 PMID:11438406

Gilchrest, B. A., & Bohr, V. A. (1997). Aging processes, DNA damage, and repair. *The FASEB Journal*, *11*, 322–330. PMID:9141498

Gildengers, A. G., Butters, M. A., Seligman, K., McShea, M., Miller, M. D., Mulsant, B. H., ... Reynolds, C. F. III. (2004). Cognitive functioning in late-life bipolar disorder. *The American Journal of Psychiatry*, *161*(4), 736–738. doi:10.1176/appi.ajp.161.4.736 PMID:15056521

Gioia, G. A., Isquith, P. K., Guy, S. C., & Kenworthy, L. (2000). *BRIEF: Behavior Rating Inventory of Executive Function Professional Manual*. Lutz, FL: PAR.

Glanz, K., Rimer, B. K., & Viswanath, K. (2008). Health behavior and health education: Theory, research, and practice. In K. Glanz, B. K. Rimer, & K. Viswanath (Eds.), *Health behavior and health education: Theory, research, and practice* (4th ed.). San Francisco, CA: Jossey-Bass.

Glenn, G. C. (1996). Practice parameter on laboratory panel testing for screening and case finding in asymptomatic adults.Laboratory Testing Task Force of the College of the American Pathologists. *Archives of Pathology & Laboratory Medicine*, *120*(10), 929–943. PMID:12049072

Glick, I. D., Weiss, R. S., & Parkes, C. M. (1974). The first year of bereavement following suicide: A review of the literature. *Current Psychological Research & Reviews*, *3*(2), 53–61.

Glidden, P. (2010). *The MD Emperor has No Clothes*.

Glisky, E. L. (2007). Changes in cognitive function in human aging. In *Brain aging: Models, methods, and mechanisms* (pp. 3-20).

Glisky, E. L. (2007). Changes in cognitive function in human aging. In D.R. Riddle (Ed.), Brain aging: Models, methods, mechanisms. Boca Raton, FL: CRC Press. Retrieved July 30, 2009 from http://www.ncbi.nlm.nih.gov/bookshelf/br.fcgi?book=frbrainage&part=ch1

Global Burden of Disease (GBD). (2013). Risk Factors Collaborators. Global, regional, and national comparative risk assessment of 79 behavioral, environmental and occupational, and metabolic risks or clusters of risks in 188 countries, 1990–2013: a systematic analysis for the Global Burden of Disease Study 2013. *Lancet, 386*, 2287–323.

Global Burden of Disease Study 2013 Collaborators. (2015). Global, regional, and national incidence, prevalence, and years lived with disability for 301 acute and chronic diseases and injuries in 188 countries, 1990-2013: a systematic analysis for the Global Burden of Disease Study 2013. *Lancet, 386*, 743.

Global burden of disease: 2004 update. (2008). Geneva: World Health Organization.

Go, A. S., Mozaffarian, D., Roger, V. L., Benjamin, E. J., Berry, J. D., Borden, W. B., ... Turner, M. B. (2013). Heart disease and stroke statistics--2013 update: A report from the American Heart Association. *Circulation, 127*(1), e6–e245. doi:10.1161/CIR.0b013e31828124ad PMID:23239837

Goldbourt, U., Yaari, S., & Medalie, J. H. (1993). Factors predictive of long-term coronary heart disease mortality among 10,059 male Israeli civil servants and municipal employees. *Cardiology, 82*(2-3), 100–121. doi:10.1159/000175862 PMID:8324774

Gold, D. A. (2012). An examination of instrumental activities of daily living assessment in older adults and mild cognitive impairment. *Journal of Clinical and Experimental Neuropsychology, 34*(1), 11–34. doi:10.1080/13803395.2011.614598 PMID:22053873

Golden, H.L., Clark, C.N., Nicholas, J.M., Cohen, M.H., Slattery, C.F., Paterson, R.W., ... Warren, J.D. (2016). Music Perception in Dementia. *Journal Alzheimer's Disorder, 11.*

Goldman, N., Korenman, S., & Weinstein, R. (1995). Marital status and health among the elderly. *Social Science & Medicine, 40*(12), 1717–1730. doi:10.1016/0277-9536(94)00281-W PMID:7660185

Goldney, R. D., Phillips, P. J., Fisher, L. J., & Wilson, D. H. (2004). Diabetes, depression, and quality of life: A population study. *Diabetes Care, 27*(5), 1066–1070. doi:10.2337/diacare.27.5.1066 PMID:15111522

Goldstein, M. (1996). Elder mistreatment and PTSD. In Ageing and post-traumatic stress disorder (pp. 126-135). American Psychiatric Association.

Gomez-Pinilla, F., & Tyagi, E. (2013). Diet and cognition: Interplay between cell metabolism and neuronal plasticity. *Current Opinion in Clinical Nutrition and Metabolic Care, 16*(6), 726–733. doi:10.1097/MCO.0b013e328365aae3 PMID:24071781

Gonzalez, J. S., Safren, S. A., Cagliero, E., Wexler, D. J., Delahanty, L., Wittenberg, E., ... Grant, R. W. (2007). Depression, self-care, and medication adherence in type 2 diabetes: Relationships across the full range of symptom severity. *Diabetes Care, 30*(9), 2222–2227. doi:10.2337/dc07-0158 PMID:17536067

Gonzalez, M. J., Miranda-Massari, J. R., Berdiel, M. J., & Duconge, J., Rodriguez-Lopez, J. L., Hunninghake, R., & Cobas-Rosario, V. J. (2014). High dose intraveneous Vitamin C and chikungunya fever: A case report. *Journal of Orthomolecular Medicine, 29*(4), 154–156. doi:10.1016/j.biotechadv.2011.08.021.Secreted PMID:25705076

Gooding, P. A., Hurst, A., Johnson, J., & Tarrier, N. (2012). Psychological resilience in young and older adults. *International Journal of Geriatric Psychiatry, 27*(3), 262–270. doi:10.1002/gps.2712 PMID:21472780

Gopinath, B., Schneider, J., McMahon, C. M., Burlutsky, G., Leeder, S. R., & Mitchell, P. (2013). Dual sensory impairment in older adults increases the risk of mortality: A population-based study. *PLoS One, 8*(3), e55054. doi:10.1371/journal.pone.0055054 PMID:23469161

Goswami, S. (2017). Proteomics in Personalized Medicine: An Evolution Not a Revolution. In Applying big Data Analytics in Bioinformatics & Medicine. Hershey, PA: IGI Global.

Gott, M. (2014). Sexual health and the new aging. *Age and Ageing*, *35*(2), 106–107. doi:10.1093/ageing/afj050 PMID:16431853

Government Accountability Office. (2011). Elder justice: Stronger federal leadership could enhance national response to elder abuse. Retrieved from http://aging.senate.gov/events/hr230kb2.pdf

Government, H. M. (2005). *Opportunity Age: meeting the challenges of ageing in the 21st century*. London: HM Government.

Graf, C. (2006). Functional decline in hospitalized older adults. *The American Journal of Nursing*, *106*(1), 58–67. doi:10.1097/00000446-200601000-00032 PMID:16481783

Gramaglia, C., Feggi, A., Bergamasco, P., Bert, F., Gattoni, E., Marangon, D., ... Zeppegno, P. (2016). Clinical characteristics associated with suicide attempts in clinical settings: A comparison of suicidal and non-suicidal depressed inpatients. *Frontiers in Psychiatry*, *7*, 109. doi:10.3389/fpsyt.2016.00109 PMID:27378957

Graney, M. (1975). Happiness and social participation in aging. *Journal of Gerontology*, *30*(6), 701–706. doi:10.1093/geronj/30.6.701 PMID:1184930

Granger, B., Swedberg, B., Ekman, K., Granger, I., Olofsson, C. B., Mc, B., ... Pfeffer, M. A. (2005). Adherence to candesartan and placebo and outcomes in chronic heart failure in the CHARM programme: Double-blind, randomised, controlled clinical trial. *Lancet*, *366*(9502), 2005–2011. doi:10.1016/S0140-6736(05)67760-4 PMID:16338449

Grant, D. (2004). Spiritual interventions: How, when, and why nurses use them. *Holistic Nursing Practice*, *18*(1), 36–41. doi:10.1097/00004650-200401000-00007 PMID:14765691

Gray, J. W., Rattan, A. I., & Dean, R. S. (1986). Differential diagnosis of dementia and depression in the elderly using neuropsychological methods. *Archives of Clinical Neuropsychology*, *1*(4), 341–349. doi:10.1093/arclin/1.4.341 PMID:14591414

Gredig, D., & Bartelsen-Raemy, A. (2016). Diabetes-related stigma affects the quality of life of people living with diabetes mellitus in Switzerland: implications for healthcare providers. *Journal of Health & Social Care in the Community*. doi.10.1111/hsc.12376

Greenspan, S. L., & Greenspan, F. S. (1999). The effect of thyroid hormone on skeletal integrity. *Annals of Internal Medicine*, *130*(9), 750–758. doi:10.7326/0003-4819-130-9-199905040-00016 PMID:10357695

Greenstein, A. S., Paranthaman, R., Burns, A., Jackson, A., Malik, R. A., Baldwin, R. C., & Heagerty, A. M. (2010). Cerebrovascular damage in late-life depression is associated with structural and functional abnormalities of subcutaneous small arteries. *Hypertension*, *56*(4), 734–740. doi:10.1161/HYPERTENSIONAHA.110.152801 PMID:20713917

Gregg, E. W., Beckles, G. L., Williamson, D. F., Leveille, S. G., Langlois, J. A., Engelgau, M. M., & Narayan, K. M. (2000). Diabetes and physical disability among older U.S. adults. *Diabetes Care*, *23*(9), 1272–1277. doi:10.2337/diacare.23.9.1272 PMID:10977018

Gregg, E. W., Mangione, C. M., Cauley, J. A., Thompson, T. J., Schwartz, A. V., Ensrud, K. E., & Nevitt, M. C. (2002). Diabetes and incidence of functional disability in older women. *Diabetes Care*, *25*(1), 61–67. doi:10.2337/diacare.25.1.61 PMID:11772902

Gregg, E. W., & Narayan, K. M. V. (2000). Type 2 diabetes and cognitive function: Are cognitive impairment and dementia complications of type 2 diabetes? *Clinics in Geriatric Medicine*, *8*, 57–72.

Grenade, L., & Boldy, D. (2008). Social isolation and loneliness among older people: Issues and future challenges in community and residential settings. *Australian Health Review*, *32*(3), 468–478. doi:10.1071/AH080468 PMID:18666874

Griffith, H. R., Belue, K., Sicola, A., Krzywanski, S., Zamrini, E., Harrell, L., & Marson, D. C. (2003). Impaired financial abilities in mild cognitive impairment A direct assessment approach. *Neurology*, *60*(3), 449–457. doi:10.1212/WNL.60.3.449 PMID:12578926

Grozinsky-Glasberg, S., Fraser, A., Nahshoni, E., Weizman, A., & Leibovici, L. (2006). Thyroxine-triiodothyronine combination therapy versus thyroxinemonotherapy for clinical hypothyroidism: Meta-analysis of randomized controlled trials. *The Journal of Clinical Endocrinology and Metabolism*, *91*(7), 2592–2599. doi:10.1210/jc.2006-0448 PMID:16670166

Grubbs, E. G., Rich, T. A., Li, G., Sturgis, E. M., Younes, M. N., Myers, J. N., ... Evans, D. B. (2008). Recent advances in thyroid cancer. *Current Problems in Surgery*, *45*(3), 156–250. doi:10.1067/j.cpsurg.2007.12.010 PMID:18346477

Gruenewald, T. L., & Kemeny, M. E. (2007). Psychoneuroimmunological process in aging and health. In C. M. Aldwin, C. L. Park, & A. Spiro (Eds.), *Handbook of health psychology and aging* (pp. 97–118). New York: Guilford.

Grundy, S. M. (2004). Obesity, metabolic syndrome, and cardiovascular disease. *The Journal of Clinical Endocrinology and Metabolism*, *89*(6), 2595–2600. doi:10.1210/jc.2004-0372 PMID:15181029

Grundy, S. M., Cleeman, J. I., & Merz, C. M. B. (2004). For the Coordinating Committee of the National Cholesterol Education Program. Implications of recent clinical trials for the National Cholesterol Education Program Adult Treatment Panel III Guidelines. *Circulation*, *110*(2), 227–239. doi:10.1161/01.CIR.0000133317.49796.0E PMID:15249516

Grunnet, J. (2008). Heredity and Diabetes. *Annals of Internal Medicine*, *6*(10), 1272–1274.

Guerra-Laso, J. M., González-García, S., González-Cortés, C., Diez-Tascón, C., López-Medrano, R., & Rivero-Lezcano, O. M. (2013). Macrophages from elders are more permissive to intracellular multiplication of Mycobacterium tuberculosis. *Age*, 1–16. PMID:22791369

Guetin, S., Charras, K., Berard, A., Arbus, C., Berthelon, P., & Leger, J. M. (2013). An overview of the use of music therapy in the context of Alzheimer's disease: A report of a French expert group. *Dementia (London)*, *12*(5), 619–634. doi:10.1177/1471301212438290 PMID:24337333

Guiding principles for the care of older adults with multimorbidity: an approach for clinicians (2012). *Journal of American Geriatric Society, 60*(10), E1-E25.

Gullo, D., Latina, A., Frasca, F., Le Moli, R., Pellegriti, G., & Vigneri, R. (2011). Levothyroxine monotherapy cannot guarantee euthyroidism in all athyreotic patients. *PLoS One*, *6*(8), e22552. doi:10.1371/journal.pone.0022552 PMID:21829633

Gupta, K. L. (1995). Neoplasm of the thyroid gland. *Clinical Geriatric Medicine*, *11*, 271–90. Retrieved from https://www.ncbi.nlm.nih.gov/pubmed/16440564

Gupta, P., & Mani, K. (2014). Functional disability among elderly persons in a rural area of Haryana. *Indian Journal of Public Health*, *58*(1), 11. doi:10.4103/0019-557X.128155 PMID:24748351

Gupta, R., Sharma, S., Gupta, V. P., & Gupta, K. D. (1995). Smoking and alcohol intake in a rural Indian population and correlation with hypertension and coronary heart disease prevalence. *The Journal of the Association of Physicians of India*, *43*, 243–248. PMID:8713264

Gupta, S. C., Anand, R., & Trivedi, J. K. (1983). Development of a suicidal intent questionnaire. *Indian Journal of Psychiatry*, *25*, 57–62. PMID:21847253

Guralnik, J. M. (1996). Assessing the impact of comorbidity in the older population. *Annals of Epidemiology*, *6*(5), 376–380. doi:10.1016/S1047-2797(96)00060-9 PMID:8915467

Gureje, O., Ogunniyi, A., Kola, L., & Afolabi, E. (2006). Functional disability in elderly Nigerians: Results from the Ibadan study of aging. *Journal of the American Geriatrics Society*, *54*(11), 1784–1789. doi:10.1111/j.1532-5415.2006.00944.x PMID:17087709

Gurwitz, J. H., Field, T. S., Harrold, L. R., Harrold, L. R., Rothschild, J., Debellis, K., ... Bates, D. W. (2003). Inciden. ce and preventability of adverse drug events among older persons in the ambulatory setting. *Journal of the American Medical Association*, *289*(9), 1107–1116. doi:10.1001/jama.289.9.1107 PMID:12622580

Guskiewicz, K. M., Marshall, S. W., Bailes, J., McCrea, M., Cantu, R. C., Randolph, C., & Jordan, B. D. (2005). Association between recurrent concussion and late-life cognitive impairment in retired professional football players. *Neurosurgery*, *57*(4), 719–726. doi:10.1093/neurosurgery/57.4.719 PMID:16239884

Gussekloo, J., van Exel, E., & de Craen, A. J. (2006). Thyroid function, activities of daily living and survival in extreme old age: The 'Leiden 85-plus Study'. *Nederlands Tijdschrift voor Geneeskunde*, *150*(2), 90–96. Retrieved from https://www.ncbi.nlm.nih.gov/pubmed/16440564 PMID:16440564

Gussekloo, J., van Exel, E., de Craen, A. J. M., & Meinders, A. E. M. (2004). Thyroid status, disability and cognitive function, and survival in old age. *Journal of the American Medical Association*, *292*(21), 2591–2599. doi:10.1001/jama.292.21.2591 PMID:15572717

Gutmann, D. (1978). Personal Transformations in the Post-Parental Period: A Cross-Cultural View.

Gutmann, D. L. (1987). *Reclaimed powers: Toward a new psychology of men and women in later life*. New York: Basic Books.

Guttman, M. (2001). The aging brain. *USC Health Magazine*. Retrieved August 4, 2009 from http://www.usc.edu/hsc/info/pr/hmm/01spring/brain.html

Gyorgyi, A. S. (1960). Introduction to a Submolecular Biology (1st ed.). Academic Press.

Haag, M. D. M., Hofman, A., Koudstaal, P. J., Stricker, B. H. C., & Breteler, M. M. B. (2009). Statins are associated with a reduced risk of Alzheimer disease regardless of lipophilicity. The Rotterdam Study. *Journal of Neurology, Neurosurgery, and Psychiatry*, *80*(1), 13–17. doi:10.1136/jnnp.2008.150433 PMID:18931004

Habra, M., & Sarlis, N. J. (2005). Thyroid and aging. *Reviews in Endocrine & Metabolic Disorders*, *6*(2), 145–154. doi:10.1007/s11154-005-1494-9 PMID:15843886

Hagedoorn, M., Kuijer, R. G., Buunk, B. P., DeJong, G. M., Wobbes, T., & Sanderman, R. (2000). Marital satisfaction in patients with cancer: Does support from intimate partners benefit those who need it most? *Health Psychology*, *19*(3), 274–282. doi:10.1037/0278-6133.19.3.274 PMID:10868772

Haley, K. C., Koenig, H. G., & Bruchett, B. M. (2001). Relationship between private religious activity and physical functioning in older adults. *Journal of Religion and Health*, *40*(2), 305–312. doi:10.1023/A:1012561909054

Hallal, P. C., & Lee, I. M. (2013). Prescription of physical activity: An undervalued intervention. *Lancet*, *381*(9864), 356–357. doi:10.1016/S0140-6736(12)61804-2 PMID:23199848

Hall, C. B., Derby, C., LeValley, A., Katz, M. J., Verghese, J., & Lipton, R. B. (2007). Education delays accelerated decline on a memory test in persons who develop dementia. *Neurology*, *69*(17), 1657–1664. doi:10.1212/01.wnl.0000278163.82636.30 PMID:17954781

Hammen & Constance. (2005). Stress and depression. *Annual Review of Clinical Psychology, 1,* 293-319.

Han, B., Gfroerer, J. C., Olliver, J. D., & Penne, M. A. (2009). Substance use disorder among older adults in the United States in 2020. *Addiction (Abingdon, England)*, *104*(1), 88–96. doi:10.1111/j.1360-0443.2008.02411.x PMID:19133892

Hanley, I. G., McGuire, R. J., & Boyd, W. D. (1981). Reality orientation and dementia: A controlled trial of two approaches. *The British Journal of Psychiatry*, *138*(1), 10–14. doi:10.1192/bjp.138.1.10 PMID:7023589

Hanninen, T., Koivisto, K., Reinikainen, K. J., Helkala, E. L., Soininen, H., Mykkanen, L., & Riekkinen, P. J. (1996). Prevalence of ageing-associated cognitive decline in an elderly population. *Age and Ageing*, *25*(3), 201–205. doi:10.1093/ageing/25.3.201 PMID:8670552

Hans, G., & Dar, M. M. (2015). Psychiatric co-morbidity in patients suffering from cancer and its relationship to disease awareness. *Delhi Journal of Psychiatry*, *18*(1), 40–47.

Hansson, O., Zetterberg, H., Buchhave, P., Londos, E., Blennow, K., & Minthon, L. (2006). Association between CSF biomarkers and incipient Alzheimer's disease in patients with mild cognitive impairment: A follow-up study. *Lancet Neurology*, *5*(3), 228–234. doi:10.1016/S1474-4422(06)70355-6 PMID:16488378

Han, T. S., Tajar, A., & Lean, M. E. J. (2011). Obesity and weight management in the elderly. *British Medical Bulletin*, *97*(1), 169–196. doi:10.1093/bmb/ldr002 PMID:21325341

Han, T., & Bchir, M. (2013). Obesity and weight management in the elderly: A focus on men. *Best Practice & Research. Clinical Endocrinology & Metabolism*, *27*(4), 509–525. doi:10.1016/j.beem.2013.04.012 PMID:24054928

Harada, C. N., Love, M. C. N., & Triebel, K. L. (2013). Normal cognitive aging. *Clinics in Geriatric Medicine*, *29*(4), 737–752. doi:10.1016/j.cger.2013.07.002 PMID:24094294

Hara, E., Smith, R., Parry, D., Tahara, H., Stone, S., & Peters, G. (1996). Regulation of p16CDKN2 expression and its implications for cell immortalization and senescence. *Molecule Cell Biology*, *16*(3), 859–867. doi:10.1128/MCB.16.3.859 PMID:8622687

Hardy, S. E., Concato, J.& Gill, T. H. (2014). Resilience of community-dwelling older persons. *Journal of the American Geriatrics Society, 52*(2), 257-262.

Harley, C. B., & Villeponteau, B. (1995). Telomeres and telomerase in aging and cancer. *Current Opinion in Genetics & Development*, *5*(2), 249–255. doi:10.1016/0959-437X(95)80016-6 PMID:7613096

Harman, D. (1956). Aging: A theory based on free radical and radiation chemistry. *Journal of Gerontology*, *11*(3), 298–300. doi:10.1093/geronj/11.3.298 PMID:13332224

Harman, D. (1981). The aging process. *Proceedings of the National Academy of Sciences of the United States of America*, *78*(11), 7124–7128. doi:10.1073/pnas.78.11.7124 PMID:6947277

Harris, L. (1975). The Myth and Reality of Aging in America: Conducted for the National Council on the Aging.

Harris, E. C., & Barraclough, B. (1997). Suicide as an outcome for mental disorders: A meta-analysis. *The British Journal of Psychiatry*, *170*(3), 205–228. doi:10.1192/bjp.170.3.205 PMID:9229027

Harris, T. B. (2003). Epidemiology and aging. In C. K. Cassel, R. M. Leipzig, H. J. Cohen, & ... (Eds.), *Geriatric Medicine: An Evidence-Based Approach* (4th ed.). New York: Springer Verlag. doi:10.1007/0-387-22621-4_5

Harris, T. B., Launer, L. J., Madans, J., & Feldman, J. J. (1997). Cohort study of effect of being overweight and change in weight on risk of coronary heart disease in old age. *BMJ (Clinical Research Ed.)*, *314*(7097), 1791. doi:10.1136/bmj.314.7097.1791 PMID:9224080

Hart, R. P., & Kwentus, J. A. (1987). Psychomotor slowing and subcortical-type dysfunction in depression. *Journal of Neurology, Neurosurgery, and Psychiatry*, *50*(10), 1263–1266. doi:10.1136/jnnp.50.10.1263 PMID:3681304

Hartshorne, J. K., & Germine, L. T. (2015). When does cognitive functioning peak? The asynchronous rise and fall of different cognitive abilities across the life span. *Psychological Science*, *26*(4), 433–443. doi:10.1177/0956797614567339 PMID:25770099

Harvey, A. G. (2002). A cognitive model of insomnia. *Behaviour Research and Therapy*, *40*, 869–893.

Harvey, A., Montezano, A. C., & Touyz, R. M. (2015). Vascular biology ofageing-implications in hypertension. *Journal of Molecular and Cellular Cardiology*, *83*, 112–121. doi:10.1016/j.yjmcc.2015.04.011 PMID:25896391

Harwood, D., Hawton, K., Hope, T., & Jacoby, R. (2001). Psychiatric disorder and personality factors associated with suicide in older people: A descriptive and case-control study. *International Journal of Geriatric Psychiatry*, *16*(2), 155–165. doi:10.1002/1099-1166(200102)16:2<155::AID-GPS289>3.0.CO;2-0 PMID:11241720

Havasi, P. (2012). The Education of Cancer Healing (Vol. 2: Specialists).

Haw, C., Harwood, D., & Hawton, K. (2009). Dementia and suicidal behavior: A review of the literature. *International Psychogeriatrics*, *21*(3), 440. doi:10.1017/S1041610209009065 PMID:19368760

Hawkley, L. C., Hughes, M. E., Waite, L. J., Masi, C. M., Thisted, R. A., & Cacioppo, J. T. (2008). From social structural factors to perceptions of relationship quality and loneliness: The Chicago health, aging, and social relations study. *The Journals of Gerontology. Series B, Psychological Sciences and Social Sciences*, *63*(6), 375–384. doi:10.1093/geronb/63.6.S375 PMID:19092047

Hawley, P. J., & Klaukev, M. R. (1988). Health practices and perception of social support in person over 60. *Journal of Gerontology*, *36*(1), 112–121.

Hayden, K. M., & Welsh-Bohmer, K. A. (2011). Epidemiology of cognitive aging and Alzheimer's disease: contributions of the cache county utah study of memory, health and aging. In *Behavioral Neurobiology of Aging* (pp. 3–31). Springer Berlin Heidelberg. doi:10.1007/7854_2011_152

Hayes, S. C., Strosahl, K., & Wilson, K. (2011). *Acceptance and Commitment Therapy: The Process and Practice of Mindful Change* (2nd ed.). New York, NY: The Guilford Press.

Hay, M. W. (1989). Principles in building spiritual assessment tools. *The American Journal of Hospice Care*, *6*(5), 25–31. doi:10.1177/104990918900600514 PMID:2604991

Haynes, S. N., Adams, A., & Franzen, M. (1981). The effects of pre-sleep stress on sleep-onset insomnia. *Journal of Abnormal Psychology*, *90*, 601–606.

Hays, R. D., & Stewart, A. L. (1992). Sleep measures. In A. L. Stewart & J. E. Ware (Eds.), *Measuring functioning and wellbeing:the Medical Outcomes Study Approach*. Durham, NC: Duke University.

Hays, R. D., Wells, K. B., Sherbourne, C. D., Rogers, W., & Spritzer, K. (1995). Functioning and well-being outcomes of patients with depression compared with chronic general medical illnesses. *Archives of General Psychiatry*, *52*(1), 11–19. doi:10.1001/archpsyc.1995.03950130011002 PMID:7811158

He, W., Goodkind, D., &Kowal, P. (2016). An aging world: 2015. International population reports.

Headey, B. (2010). The set point theory of well-being has serious flaws: On the eve of a scientific revolution? *Social Indicators Research*, *97*(1), 7–21. doi:10.1007/s11205-009-9559-x

Healing Cancer Naturally. (2004). Cancer causes statistics drugs. Retrieved from http://www.healingcancernaturally.com/cancer-causes-statistics-drugs.html

Healing Cancer Naturally. (n.d.). Quotes animal models of human disease. Retrieved from http://www.healingcancernaturally.com/quotes-animal-models-of-human-disease.html

Healing Cancer Naturally. (n.d.). Quotes on cancer diagnosing. Retrieved from http://www.healingcancernaturally.com/quotes-on-cancer-diagnosing.html

Health Guides on Thyroid Disease. (2017). *Graves' Eye Disease (Ophthalmopathy)*. Retrieved from http://www.thyroid.ca/ophthalmopathy.php

Hebert, L. E., Scherr, P. A., Beckett, L. A., Albert, M. S., Pilgrim, D. M., Chown, M. J., ... Evans, D. A. (1995). Age-specific incidence of Alzheimer's disease in a community population. *Journal of the American Medical Association*, *273*(17), 1354–1359. doi:10.1001/jama.1995.03520410048025 PMID:7715060

Hegde, B. M. (2014). What Doctors Don't Get to Study. In *Medical School* (4th ed.). Paras Medical Publisher.

Hegel, M. T., Unutzer, J., Tang, L., Areán, P. A., Katon, W., Noël, P. H., ... Lin, E. H. B. (2005). Impact of comorbid panic and posttraumatic stress disorder on outcomes of collaborative care for late-life depression in primary care. *The American Journal of Geriatric Psychiatry*, *13*(1), 48–58. doi:10.1097/00019442-200501000-00008 PMID:15653940

Heidenreich, T., Strohle, G., & Michalak, J. (2006). Mindfulness: Conceptual aspects and results of the Freiburg mindfulness inventory. *Verhaltenstherapie*, *16*, 33–40. doi:10.1159/000091521

Heikkinen, R., Berg, S., & Avland, K. (1995). Depressive symptoms in late life. *Journal of Cross-Cultural Gerontology*, *10*(4), 315–330. doi:10.1007/BF00972332 PMID:24389881

Heisel, M. J. (2006). Suicide and its prevention among older adults. *Canadian Journal of Psychiatry*, *51*(3), 143–154. doi:10.1177/070674370605100304 PMID:16618005

Helzner, E. P., Scarmeas, N., Cosentino, S., Portet, F., & Stern, Y. (2007). Leisure activity and cognitive decline in incident Alzheimer disease. *Archives of Neurology*, *64*(12), 1749–1754. doi:10.1001/archneur.64.12.1749 PMID:18071038

Henderson, B. (n.d.). Cancer-Free. Retrieved from http://www.beating-cancer-gently.com/doctors-comments.html

Henderson, V. W. (1997). Estrogen replacement therapy for the prevention and treatment of Alzheimer's disease. *CNS Drugs*, *8*(5), 343–351. doi:10.2165/00023210-199708050-00001

Henoch, I., Bergman, B., Gustafsson, M., Gaston-Johansson, F., & Danielson, E. (2007). The impact of symptoms, coping capacity, and social support on quality of life experience over time in patients with lung cancer. *Journal of Pain and Symptom Management*, *34*(4), 370–379. doi:10.1016/j.jpainsymman.2006.12.005 PMID:17616335

Henslin, J. A. (1996). *Social Problems*. Prentice Hall.

Hering, C. (1836). Preface to the first American edition. In the Organon of Homeopathic Medicine. New-York: William Radde.

Hering, C. (1879). *The Guiding Symptoms of our MateriaMedica*. Philadelphia: The American Publishing Society.

Herth, K. (1990). Fostering hope in terminally-ill people. *Journal of Advanced Nursing*, *15*(11), 1250–1259. doi:10.1111/j.1365-2648.1990.tb01740.x PMID:2269747

Herth, K. A. (1989). The relationship between level of hope and level of coping response and other variables in patients with cancer. *Oncology Nursing Forum*, *16*(1), 67–72. PMID:2911529

Hertzog, C., & Hultsch, D. F. (2000). Metacognition in adulthood and old age. In F. I. M. Craik & T. A. Salthouse (Eds.), *The handbook of aging and cognition* (2nd ed., pp. 417–466). Mahwah, NJ: Erlbaum.

Herukka, S.-K., Simonsen, A. H., Andreasen, N., Baldeiras, I., Bjerke, M., Blennow, K., ... Waldemar, G. (2017). Recommendations for cerebrospinal fluid Alzheimer's disease biomarkers in the diagnostic evaluation of mild cognitive impairment. *Alzheimer's & Dementia. The Journal of the Alzheimer's Association, 13*(3), 285–295. doi:10.1016/j.jalz.2016.09.009 PMID:28341066

Hessler, R. M., Jia, S., Madsen, R., & Pazaki, H. (1995). Gender, social networks and survival time: A 20-year study of the rural elderly. *Archives of Gerontology and Geriatrics, 21*(3), 291–306. doi:10.1016/0167-4943(95)00669-C PMID:15374205

Hess, T. M. (2006). Attitudes toward aging and their effects on behavior. In J. E. Birren & K. W. Schaie (Eds.), *Handbook of the psychology of aging* (6th ed., pp. 379–406). San Diego, CA: Academic Press. doi:10.1016/B978-012101264-9/50020-3

Hickam, D. H., Weiss, J. W., Guise, J.-M., Buckley, D., Motu'apuaka, M., Graham, E., & Saha, S. (2013). Outpatient case management for older adults with medical illness and complex care needs. Rockville, MD: Agency for Healthcare Research and Quality.

Hildebrand, H. P. (1982). Psychotherapy with older patients. *The British Journal of Medical Psychology, 55*(1), 19–28. doi:10.1111/j.2044-8341.1982.tb01477.x PMID:7059528

Hildon, Z., Montgomery, S. M., Blane, D., Wiggins, R. D., & Netuveli, G. (2010). Examining Resilience of Quality of Life in the Face of Health Related and Psychosocial Adversity at Older Ages: What is "Right" About the Way We Age? *The Gerontologist, 50*(1), 36–47. doi:10.1093/geront/gnp067 PMID:19549715

Hildreth, C. J. (2011). *Elder Abuse. Jama, 306*(5), 568. doi:10.1001/jama.306.5.568

Hill, J., Nielsen, M., & Fox, M. H. (2013). Understanding the Social Factors That Contribute to Diabetes: A Means to Informing Health Care and Social Policies for the Chronically Ill. *The Permanente Journal, 17*(2), 67–72. doi:10.7812/TPP/12-099

Hillecke, T., Nickle, A., & Bolay, H.V. (2005). Scientific perspectives on music therapy *Annals of New York Academy of Science, 1060*, 271-282.

Hillman, J. (2008). *Sexual Issues and Aging Within the Context of Work With Older Adult Patients*. Academic Press. doi:10.1037/0735-7028.39.3.290

Hill, P. C., Pargament, K. I., Hood, R. W., McCullough, M. E. Jr, Swyers, J. P., Larson, D. B., & Zinnbauer, B. J. (2000). Conceptualizing religion and spirituality: Points of commonality, points of departure. *Journal for the Theory of Social Behaviour, 30*(1), 51–77. doi:10.1111/1468-5914.00119

Hill, V., & Towfighi, A. (2017). Factors for Stroke and Strategies for Stroke Prevention. *Seminars in Neurology, 37*(3), 237–258. doi:10.1055/s-0037-1603685 PMID:28759906

Hilmer, S. N., McLachlan, A. J., & Le Couteur, D. G. (2007). Clinical pharmacology in the geriatric patient. *Fundamental & Clinical Pharmacology, 21*(3), 217–230. doi:10.1111/j.1472-8206.2007.00473.x PMID:17521291

Hin, H., Clarke, R., Sherliker, P., Atoyebi, W., Emmens, K., Birks, J., ... Evans, J. G. (2006). Clinical relevance of low serum vitamin B12 concentrations in older people: The Banbury B12 study. *Age and Ageing, 35*(4), 416–422. doi:10.1093/ageing/afl033 PMID:16709605

Hirshkowitz, M. (2004). Normal human sleep: An overview. *The Medical Clinics of North America*, 88.

Hisause, S., Kumamoto, Y., Sato, Y., Masumori, N., Horita, H., Kato, R., ... Itoh, N. (2005). Prevalence of female sexual dysfunction symptoms and its relationship to quality of life: A Japanese female cohort study. *Urology*, *65*(1), 143–148. doi:10.1016/j.urology.2004.08.003 PMID:15667880

Ho, P.M., Bryson, C.L., & Rumsfeld, J.S. (2009). Medication adherence: Its importance in cardiovascular outcomes. *Circulation, 119*(23), 3028–3035.

Ho, A. J., Stein, J. L., Hua, X., Lee, S., Hibar, D. P., Leow, A. D., & Foroud, T. (2010). A commonly carried allele of the obesity-related FTO gene is associated with reduced brain volume in the healthy elderly. *Proceedings of the National Academy of Sciences of the United States of America*, *107*(18), 8404–8409. doi:10.1073/pnas.0910878107 PMID:20404173

Hodgson, A. (2001). Survival and sequelae of meningococcal meningitis in Ghana. *International Journal of Epidemiology*, *30*, 1440–1446. PubMed. doi:10.1093/ije/30.6.1440

Hogan, B. E., Linden, W., & Najarian, B. (2002). Social support interventions: Do they work? *Clinical Psychology Review*, *22*(3), 381–440. doi:10.1016/S0272-7358(01)00102-7 PMID:17201192

Hollowell, J. G., Staehling, N. W., Flanders, W. D., Hannon, W. H., & Gunter, E. W. (2001). Cohort study of thyroid cancer in a San Francisco Bay area population. *International Journal of Cancer*, *93*(5), 745–750. doi:10.1002/ijc.1377 PMID:11477590

Hollowell, J. G., Staehling, N. W., Flanders, W. D., Hannon, W. H., Gunter, E. W., Spencer, C. A., & Braverman, L. E. (2002). Serum TSH, T(4), and thyroid antibodies in the United States population (1988 to 1994): National Health and Nutrition Examination Survey (NHANES III). *The Journal of Clinical Endocrinology and Metabolism*, *87*(2), 489–499. doi:10.1210/jcem.87.2.8182 PMID:11836274

Holmes, J., Powell-Griner, E., Lethbridge-Cejku, M., & Heyman, K. (2009). *Aging differently: Physical limitations among adults aged 50 years and over: United States, 2001-2007 (NCHS Data Brief No. 20)*. Atlanta, GA: Centers for Disease Control.

Holsinger, T., Deveau, J., Boustani, M., & Williams, J. W. (2007). Does this patient have dementia? *Journal of the American Medical Association*, *297*(21), 2391–2404. doi:10.1001/jama.297.21.2391 PMID:17551132

Holt-Lunstad, J., Smith, T. B., & Layton, J. B. (2010). Social relationships and mortality risk: A meta-analytic review. *PLoS Medicine*, *7*(7). doi:10.1371/journal.pmed.1000316 PMID:20668659

Holt, R. I., & Katon, W. J. (2012). Dialogue on Diabetes and Depression: Dealing with the double burden of co-morbidity. *Journal of Affective Disorders*, *142*, S1–S3. doi:10.1016/S0165-0327(12)00632-5 PMID:23062852

Holzapfel, S. (1994). Aging and Sexuality. *Canadian Family Physician Medecin de Famille Canadien*, *40*, 748–766. PMID:8199527

Honda, K., & Goodwin, R. D. (2004). Cancer and mental disorders in a national community sample: Findings from the National Comorbidity Survey. *Psychotherapy and Psychosomatics*, *73*(4), 235–242. doi:10.1159/000077742 PMID:15184718

Hood Jr, R. W., Spilka, B., Hunsberger, B., & Gorsuch, R. (1996). Religion, coping, and adjustment. *The psychology of religion: An empirical approach*, 377-405.

Houry, D., Florence, C., Baldwin, G., Stevens, J., & McClure, R. (2016). The CDC injury center's response to the growing public health problem of falls among older adults. *American Journal of Lifestyle Medicine*, *10*(1), 74–77. doi:10.1177/1559827615600137 PMID:26688674

House, J. S., & Kahn, R. L. (1985). Measures and concepts of social support. *See Cohen & Syme*, *1985*, 83–108.

Howden, J. (1992). Development and psychometric characteristics of the Spirituality Assessment Scale [Doctoral dissertation].

Howieson, D. B., Holm, L. A., Kaye, J. A., Oken, B. S., & Howieson, J. (1993). Neurologic function in the optimally healthy oldest old Neuropsychological evaluation. *Neurology, 43*(10), 1882–1882. doi:10.1212/WNL.43.10.1882 PMID:8413942

Hoxey, K., & Shah, A. (2000). Recent trends in elderly suicide rates in England and Wales. *International Journal of Geriatric Psychiatry, 15*(3), 274–279. doi:10.1002/(SICI)1099-1166(200003)15:3<274::AID-GPS106>3.0.CO;2-I PMID:10713587

Hoyer, W. J., & Roodin, P. A. (2003). *Adult development and aging* (5th ed.). New York: McGraw-Hill.

Hozumi, S., Hori, H., Okawa, M., Hishikawa, Y., & Sato, K. (1996). Favorable effect of transcranialelectrostimulation on behavior disorders in elderly patients with dementia: A double-blind study. *The International Journal of Neuroscience, 88*(1-2), 1–10. doi:10.3109/00207459608999809 PMID:9003961

Hsu, C. Y., Iribarren, C., McCulloch, C. E., Darbinian, J., & Go, A. S. (2009). Risk factors for end-stage renal disease: 25-year follow-up. *Archives of Internal Medicine, 169*(4), 342–350. Retrieved from http://win.niddk.gov/publications/understanding.htm doi:10.1001/archinternmed.2008.605 PMID:19237717

Hu, F., Li, T., Colditz, G., Willett, W., & Manson, J. (2003). Television watching and other Sedentary

Huber, M., Knottnerus, J. A., Green, L., van der Horst, H., Jadad, A. R., Kromhout, D., & Smid, H. (2011). How should we define health? *British Medical Journal, 343*(2), d4163. doi:10.1136/bmj.d4163 PMID:21791490

Huckans, M., Hutson, L., Twamley, E., Jak, A., Kaye, J., & Storzbach, D. (2013). Efficacy of cognitive rehabilitation therapies for mild cognitive impairment (MCI) in older adults: Working toward a theoretical model and evidence-based interventions. *Neuropsychology Review, 23*(1), 63–80. doi:10.1007/s11065-013-9230-9 PMID:23471631

Hughes, V. A., Frontera, W. R., Wood, M., Evans, W. J., Dallal, G. E., Roubenoff, R., & Singh, M. A. F. (2001). Longitudinal muscle strength changes in older adults: Influence of muscle mass, physical activity, and health. *The Journals of Gerontology, Series A: Biological Sciences & Medical Sciences, 56*, B209-B217. doi:.B20910.1093/gerona/56.5

Huguelet, P., Mohr, S., Borras, L., Gillieron, C., & Brandt, P. Y. (2006). Spirituality and religious practices among outpatients with schizophrenia and their clinicians. *Psychiatric Services (Washington, D.C.), 57*(3), 366–372. doi:10.1176/appi.ps.57.3.366 PMID:16524995

Hummer, R. A., Rogers, R. G., Nam, C. B., & Ellison, C. G. (1999). Religious involvement and US adult mortality. *Demography, 36*(2), 273–285. doi:10.2307/2648114 PMID:10332617

Hummert, M. L. (2011). Age stereotypes and aging. In K. W. Schaie & S. L. Willis (Eds.), *Handbook of the psychology of aging* (7th ed., pp. 249–262). San Diego, CA: Academic Press. doi:10.1016/B978-0-12-380882-0.00016-4

Hungelmann, J., Kenkel-Rossi, E., Klassen, L., & Stollenwerk, R. M. (1985). Spiritual well-being in older adults: Harmonious interconnectedness. *Journal of Religion and Health, 24*(2), 147–153. doi:10.1007/BF01532258 PMID:24306074

Hunskaar, S. (2008). A systematic review of overweight and obesity as risk factors and targets for clinical intervention for urinary incontinence in women. *Neurourology and Urodynamics, 27*(8), 749–757. doi:10.1002/nau.20635 PMID:18951445

Hunsley, J., & Lee, C. M. (2010). *Introduction to clinical psychology: An evidence-based approach.* New York: John Wiley & Sons, Inc.

Huskamp, H. A., Kaufmann, C., & Stevenson, D. G. (2011). The intersection of long-term care and end-of-life care. *Medical Care Research and Review, 69*(1), 3–44. doi:10.1177/1077558711418518 PMID:21903662

Hutchens, R. L., Kinsella, G. J., Ong, B., Pike, K. E., Clare, L., Ames, D., ... Parsons, S. (2013). Relationship between control beliefs, strategy use, and memory performance in amnestic mild cognitive impairment and healthy aging. *The Journals of Gerontology. Series B, Psychological Sciences and Social Sciences*, *68*(6), 862–871. doi:10.1093/geronb/gbt016 PMID:23550087

Hutter, N., Schnurr, A., & Baumeister, H. (2010). Healthcare costs in patients with diabetes mellitus and comorbid mental disorders--a systematic review. *Diabetologia*, *53*(12), 2470–2479. doi:10.1007/s00125-010-1873-y PMID:20700575

Hybels, C. F., & Blazer, D. G. (2003). Epidemiology of late-life mental disorders. *Clinics in Geriatric Medicine*, *19*(4), 663–696. doi:10.1016/S0749-0690(03)00042-9 PMID:15024807

Hyde, Z., Flicker, L., Hankey, G. J., Almeda, O. P., McCaul, K. A., Paul, C., ... Yeap, B. B. (2010). Prevalence of Sexual Activity and Associated Factors in MenAged 75 to 95 Years. *Annal International Medicine*, *153*(11), 693–702. doi:10.7326/0003-4819-153-11-201012070-00002 PMID:21135292

Idler, E. L., & Kasl, S. V. (1997). Religion among disabled and nondisabled persons I: Cross-sectional patterns in health practices, social activities, and well-being. *The Journals of Gerontology. Series B, Psychological Sciences and Social Sciences*, *52*(6), S294–S305. doi:10.1093/geronb/52B.6.S294 PMID:9403523

Idler, E. L., & Kasl, S. V. (1997). Religion among disabled and nondisabled persons II: Attendance at religious services as a predictor of the course of disability. *The Journals of Gerontology. Series B, Psychological Sciences and Social Sciences*, *52*(6), S306–S316. doi:10.1093/geronb/52B.6.S306 PMID:9403524

In Holt, R. I. G., de Groot, M., & Huang, E. S. (2007). Appropriate application of evidence to the care of elderly patients with diabetes. *Current Diabetes Reviews*, *3*(4), 260–263. doi:10.2174/1573399810703040260 PMID:18220684

Indian Health Service. (2014). Indian health disparities. Retrieved from www.ihs.gov/newsroom/includes/themes/newihstheme/display_objects/documents/factsheets/Disparities.pdf

Inouye, S. K., Westendorp, R. G., & Saczynski, J. S. (2014b). Delirium in elderly people. *Lancet*, *383*(9920), 911–922. doi:10.1016/S0140-6736(13)60688-1 PMID:23992774

Institute of Medicine. (2012). *The Mental Health and Substance Use Workforce for Older Adults: In Whose Hands?* Retrieved from: http://www.iom.edu/reports/2012/The-Mental-Health-and-Substance-Use-Workforce-for-Older-Adults.aspx

International Classification of Functioning. (2001). *Disability and Health*. Geneva: World Health Organization.

International Diabetes Federation (IDF). (2013). *Diabetes* (6th ed.). Brussels: Atlas.

Irudaya Rajan, S., Mishra, U. S., & Sarma, P. S. (1999). Review: India's Elderly: Burden or Challenge? *The Journal of Asian Studies*, *60*(2).

Isometsa, E. (2003, September). Elderly suicide attempters with depression are often diagnosed only after the attempt. *International Journal of Geriatric Psychiatry*, *19*, 35–40. doi:10.1002/gos.1031

Jack, C. R., Wiste, H. J., Vemuri, P., Weigand, S. D., Senjem, M. L., Zeng, G., ... Knopman, D. S. (2010). Brain beta-amyloid measures and magnetic resonance imaging atrophy both predict time-to-progression from mild cognitive impairment to Alzheimer's disease. *Brain*, *133*(11), 3336–3348. doi:10.1093/brain/awq277 PMID:20935035

Jackson, J. H. (1984). Remarks on the evolution and dissolution of the nervous system. *The Journal of Mental Science*, *33*, 25–48.

Jackson, S., & Hafemeister, T. (2012). Pure financial exploitation vs. Hybrid financial exploitation co-occurring with physical abuse and/or neglect of elderly persons. *Psychology of Violence*, *2*(3), 285–296. doi:10.1037/a0027273

Jacobson, J. M. (1992). Alcoholism and tuberculosis. *Alcohol Research & Health, 16*(1), 39.

Jacobs, P., & Johnson, J. A. (2001). Productivity Losses Associated with Diabetes in the US. *Diabetes Care, 24*(3), 257–261. PMID:11213875

Jadad, A. R., & O'Grady, L. (2008). How should health be defined? *British Medical Journal, 337.* doi:.a290010.1136/bmj

Jaeggi, S. M., Buschkuehl, M., Jonides, J., & Perrig, W. J. (2008). Improving fluid intelligence with training on working memory. *Proceedings of the National Academy of Sciences of the United States of America, 105*(19), 6829–6833. doi:10.1073/pnas.0801268105 PMID:18443283

Jagger, C. (2006). Can we live longer, healthier lives? In Y. Zeng (Ed.), Longer life and healthy aging. Springer.

Jahangir, S. F. (1995). Third force therapy and its impact on treatment outcome. *The International Journal for the Psychology of Religion, 5*(2), 125–129. doi:10.1207/s15327582ijpr0502_7

Jani, B., & Rajkumar, C. (2006). Ageing and vascular ageing. *Postgraduate Medical Journal, 82*(968), 357–362. doi:10.1136/pgmj.2005.036053 PMID:16754702

Jantos, M., & Kiat, H. (2007). Prayer as medicine: How much have we learned? *The Medical Journal of Australia, 186*(10), S51. PMID:17516884

Jean, L., Bergeron, M.-E., Thivierge, S., & Simard, M. (2010). Cognitive intervention programs for individuals with mild cognitive impairment: Systematic review of the literature. *The American Journal of Geriatric Psychiatry, 18*(4), 281–296. doi:10.1097/JGP.0b013e3181c37ce9 PMID:20220584

Jee, J. J., Wang, J. J., Rose, K. A., Lindley, R., Landau, P., & Mitchell, P. (2005, January). Wang, K. A. Rose, R. Lindley, P. Landau, & P. Mitchell, "Vision and hearing impairment in aged care clients. *Ophthalmic Epidemiology, 12*(3), 199–205. doi:10.1080/09286580590969707 PMID:16036479

Jeon, C. Y., & Murray, M. B. (2008). Diabetes mellitus increases the risk of active tuberculosis: A systematic review of 13 observational studies. *PLoS Medicine, 5*(7), e152. doi:10.1371/journal.pmed.0050152 PMID:18630984

Jeste, D. V., Twamley, E. W., Eyler Zorrilla, L. T., Golshan, S., Patterson, T. L., & Palmer, B. W. (2003). Aging and outcome in schizophrenia. *Acta Psychiatrica Scandinavica, 107*(5), 336–343. doi:10.1034/j.1600-0447.2003.01434.x PMID:12752029

Jewell, A. (1999). *Spirituality and ageing.* Jessica Kingsley Publishers.

Jimbo, D., & Urakami, K. (2008). Aromatherapy [in Japanese]. *Japanese Journal of Geriatric Psychiatry, 19*, 1365–1372.

Jimbo, D., & Urakami, K. (2008). Effect of aromatherapy on patients with severe Alzheimer's disease [in Japanese]. *Journal of Japanese Society of Aromatherapy, 7*, 43–48.

Johannes, B. C., Araujo, A. B., Feldman, H. A., Derby, C. A., Kleinman, K. P., & McKinlay, J. B. (2000). Incidence of erectile dysfunction in men 40 to 69 years old: Longitudinal results from the Massachusetts Male Aging Study. *The Journal of Urology, 163*(2), 460–463. doi:10.1016/S0022-5347(05)67900-1 PMID:10647654

Johns, M. W. (1991). A new method for measuring daytime sleepiness: The Epworth Sleepiness Scale. *Sleep*, 50–55. PMID:1798888

Johnson, E. O., Rhee, S. H., Chase, G. A., & Breslau, N. (2004). Comorbidity of depression with levels of smoking: An exploration of the shared familial risk hypothesis. *Nicotine & Tobacco Research Journal, 6*(6), 1029–1038. doi:10.1080/14622200412331324901 PMID:15801576

Jokela, M., Batty, G. D., & Kivimäki, M. (2013). Ageing and the prevalence and treatment of mental health problems. *Psychological Medicine*, *43*(10), 2037–2045. doi:10.1017/S0033291712003042 PMID:23324208

Jones, H. (n.d.). Cancer cures more deadly than disease. Rethinking Cancer, Foundation for Advancement in Cancer Therapy. Retrieved from http://www.rethinkingcancer.org/resources/magazine-articles/2_1-2/cancer-cures-more-deadly-than-disease.php

Jonklaas, J., Bianco, A. C., Bauer, A. J., Burman, K. D., Cappola, A. R., Celi, F. S., ... Sawka, A. M. (2014). Guidelines for the treatment of hypothyroidism: Prepared by the American Thyroid Association task force on thyroid hormone replacement. *Thyroid*, *24*(12), 1670–1751. doi:10.1089/thy.2014.0028 PMID:25266247

Jordan, R. M. (1995). Myxedema coma. Pathophysiology, therapy, and factors affecting prognosis. *The Medical Clinics of North America*, *79*(1), 185–194. doi:10.1016/S0025-7125(16)30091-8 PMID:7808091

Jorm, A. F. (2001). History of depression as a risk factor for dementia: An updated review. *The Australian and New Zealand Journal of Psychiatry*, *35*(6), 776–781. doi:10.1046/j.1440-1614.2001.00967.x PMID:11990888

Jorm, A. F., Korten, A. E., & Henderson, A. S. (1987). The prevalence of dementia: A quantitative integration of the literature. *Acta Psychiatrica Scandinavica*, *76*(5), 465–479. doi:10.1111/j.1600-0447.1987.tb02906.x PMID:3324647

Jose, N., & Taylor, E. (1986). Spiritual health: A look at barriers to its inclusion in the health education curriculum. *The Eta Sigma Gamman*, *18*(2), 16–29.

Joshi, K., Kumar, R., & Avasthi, A. (2003). Morbidity profile and its relationship with disability and psychological distress among elderly people in Northern India. *International Journal of Epidemiology*, *32*(6), 978–987. doi:10.1093/ije/dyg204 PMID:14681260

Jourard, S. M. (1971). *Self-disclosure: An experimental analysis of the transparent self.* New York: Wiley-Interscience.

Jousilahti, V., & Tuomilehto, P. (1999). Sex, Age, Cardiovascular Risk Factors, and coronary heart disease. *Circulation*, *99*(9), 1165–1172. doi:10.1161/01.CIR.99.9.1165 PMID:10069784

Joyner, M., & Pedersen, B. (2011). Ten Questions about Systems Biology. *The Journal of Physiology*, *589*(5), 1017–1030. doi:10.1113/jphysiol.2010.201509 PMID:21224238

Jugdutt, B. I. (2010). Aging and heart failure: Changing demographics and implications for therapy in the elderly. *Heart Failure Reviews*, *15*(5), 401–405. doi:10.1007/s10741-010-9164-8 PMID:20364319

Jung, C. G. (1971). The stages of life. In *The portable Jung* (pp. 3-22).

Jurjanz, L., Donix, M., Amanatidis, E. C., Meyer, S., Poettrich, K., Huebner, T., ... Holthoff, V. A. (2011). Visual personal familiarity in amnestic mild cognitive impairment. *PLoS One*, *6*(5), e20030. doi:10.1371/journal.pone.0020030 PMID:21625502

Juurlink, D. N., Herrmann, N., Szalai, J. P., Kopp, A., & Redelmeier, D. A. (2004). Medical Illness and the Risk of Suicide in the Elderly. *Archives of Internal Medicine*, *164*(11), 1179. doi:10.1001/archinte.164.11.1179 PMID:15197042

Kabat-Zinn, J. (2005). Bringing mindfulness to medicine: An interview with Jon Kabat-Zinn, PhD. Interview by Karolyn Gazella. *Advances in Mind-Body Medicine*, *21*, 22–27. PMID:16170903

Kabat-Z, J., Wheeler, E., Light, T., Skillings, A., Scharf, M. J., & Cropley, T. G. (1998). Influence of a mindfulness meditation based stress reduction intervention on rates of skin clearing in patients with moderate to severe psoriasis undergoing phototherapy (UVB) and photochemotherapy (PUVA). *Psychosomatic Medicine*, *60*(5), 625–632. doi:10.1097/00006842-199809000-00020 PMID:9773769

Kaesberg, P. R., & Ershler, W. B. (1989). The importance of immune senescence in the incidence and malignant properties of cancer in hosts of advanced age. *Journal of Gerontology*, *44*(6), 63–66. doi:10.1093/geronj/44.6.63 PMID:2681365

Kahana, E., & Kahana, B. (1996). Conceptual and empirical advances in understanding aging well through proactive adaptation. In V. L. Bengtson (Ed.), *Adulthood and aging: Research on continuities and discontinuities* (pp. 18–40). New York, NY: Springer.

Kaiser, R. (1999). The clinical and epidemiological profile of tick-borne encephalitis in southern Germany 1994–98: A prospective study of 656 patients. *Brain*, *122*(11), 2067–2078. doi:10.1093/brain/122.11.2067 PMID:10545392

Kane, R., Ouslander, J., Abrass, I., & Resenter, B. (2008). *Essentials of clinical geriatrics* (6th ed.). New York, NY: McGraw Hill Publishers.

Kang, H., Zhao, F., You, L., Giorgetta, C., Venkatesh, D., Sarkhel, S., & Prakash, R. (2014). Pseudo-dementia: A neuropsychological review. *Annals of Indian Academy of Neurology*, *17*(2), 147. doi:10.4103/0972-2327.132613 PMID:25024563

Kannel, W.B., &Feinleib, M. (1972). Natural history of angina pectoris in the Framingham Institute (NHLBI), Women and Cardiovascular Diseases—Statistics.

Kaplan, G., Barrel, V., & Lusky, A. (1988). Subjective state of health and survival in elderly adults. *The Journals of Gerontology. Series B, Psychological Sciences and Social Sciences*, *43*(4), S114–S120. PMID:3385152

Kaplan, J. R., Chen, H., & Manuck, S. B. (2009). The relationship between social status and atherosclerosis in male and female monkeys as revealed by meta-analysis. *American Journal of Primatology*, *71*(9), 732–741. doi:10.1002/ajp.20707 PMID:19452517

Kaplan, R. M., & Ong, M. (2007). Rationale and public health implications of changing CHD risk factor definitions. *Annual Review of Public Health*, *28*(1), 321–344. doi:10.1146/annurev.publhealth.28.021406.144141 PMID:17222077

Karel, M. J., Gatz, M., & Smyer, M. (2012). Ageing and mental health in the decade ahead: What psychologists need to know. *The American Psychologist*, *67*(3), 184–198. doi:10.1037/a0025393 PMID:21942364

Karin, M., & Greten, F. R. (2005). NF-kappaB: Linking inflammation and immunity to cancer development and progression. *Nature Reviews. Immunology*, *5*(10), 749–759. doi:10.1038/nri1703 PMID:16175180

Karlamangla, A., Tinetti, M., Guralnik, J., Studenski, S., Wetle, T., & Reuben, D. (2007). Comorbidity in Older Adults: Nosology of Impairment, Diseases, and Conditions. *The Journals of Gerontology. Series A, Biological Sciences and Medical Sciences*, *62A*(3), 296–300. doi:10.1093/gerona/62.3.296 PMID:17389727

Karlsson, I., Widerlöv, E., Melin, E. V., Nyth, A., Brane, G. A. M., Rybo, E., ... Nemeroff, C. B. (1985). Changes of CSF neuropeptides after environmental stimulation in dementia. *Nordisk Psykiatrisk Tidsskrift [Nordic Journal of Psychiatry]*, *39*, 75–81.

Karpa, M. J., Gopinath, B., Beath, K., Rochtchina, E., Cumming, R. G., Wang, J. J., & Mitchell, P. (2010). Associations between hearing impairment and mortality risk in older persons: The Blue Mountains Hearing Study. *Annals of Epidemiology*, *20*(6), 452–459. doi:10.1016/j.annepidem.2010.03.011 PMID:20470972

Karraker, A., DeLamater, J., & Schwartz, C. R. (2011). Sexual frequency decline from midlife to later life. *The Journals of Gerontology. Series B, Psychological Sciences and Social Sciences*, *66*(4). PMID:21666143

Kashdan, T. B., & Ciarrochi, J. (2013). *Mindfulness, Acceptance, and Positive Psychology: The Seven Foundations of Well-being*. Oakland, CA: Context Press.

Kasl-Godley, J., & Gatz, M. (2000). Psychosocial interventions for individuals with dementia: An integration of theory, therapy, and a clinical understanding of dementia. *Clinical Psychology Review*, *20*(6), 755–782. doi:10.1016/S0272-7358(99)00062-8 PMID:10983267

Katona, C., Cooper, C., & Robertson, M. (2016). *Psychiatry at a glance*. New Delhi: Wiley Blackwell.

Kautzky-Willer, A., Dorner, T., Jensby, A., & Rieder, A. (2012). Women show a closer association between educational level and hypertension or diabetes mellitus than males: A secondary analysis from the Austrian HIS. *BMC Public Health*, *12*(1), 392. doi:10.1186/1471-2458-12-392 PMID:22646095

Kawabata, K., Yoshii, Y., & Tamizu, S. (2000). *Medical aromatherapy using in the clinical*. Medicus Shuppan, Osaka Publisher Co. Ltd, in Japanese.

Kawachi, I., Colditz, G. A., Stampfer, M. J., Willett, W. C., Manson, J. E., Rosner, B., & Hennekens, C. H. (1993). Smoking cessation and decreased risk of stroke in women. *Journal of the American Medical Association*, *269*(2), 232–236. doi:10.1001/jama.1993.03500020066033 PMID:8417241

Kawai, M., Negoro, K., & Kanda, T. (2007). Olfactory disorder in the Alzheimer disease. [in Japanese.]. *Neurological Medicine*, *66*, 366–369.

Kaye, K. S., Sloane, R., Sexton, D. J., & Schmader, K. A. (2006). Risk factors for surgical site infections in older people. *Journal of the American Geriatrics Society*, *54*(3), 391–396. doi:10.1111/j.1532-5415.2005.00651.x PMID:16551304

Keene, J., Hope, T., Fairburn, C. G., & Jacoby, R. (2001). Death and dementia. *International Journal of Geriatric Psychiatry*, *16*(10), 969–974. doi:10.1002/gps.474 PMID:11607941

Kehoe, M. (1986). Lesbians over 65: A triply invisible minority. *Journal of Homosexuality*, *12*(3-4), 139–152. doi:10.1300/J082v12n03_12 PMID:3760557

Keilp, J. G., Sackeim, H. A., Brodsky, B. S., Oquendo, M. A., Malone, K. M., & Mann, J. J. (2001). Neuropsychological dysfunction in depressed suicide attempters. *The American Journal of Psychiatry*, *158*(5), 735–741. doi:10.1176/appi.ajp.158.5.735 PMID:11329395

Keller, M. L., Leventhal, E. A., & Larson, B. (1989). Aging: The lived experience. *International Journal of Aging & Human Development*, *29*(1), 67–82. doi:10.2190/DEQQ-AAUV-NBU0-3RMY PMID:2628349

Kelly, M. E., Loughrey, D., Lawlor, B. A., Robertson, I. H., Walsh, C., & Brennan, S. (2014). The impact of cognitive training and mental stimulation on cognitive and everyday functioning of healthy older adults: A systematic review and meta-analysis. *Ageing Research Reviews*, *15*, 28–43. doi:10.1016/j.arr.2014.02.004 PMID:24607830

Kennedy, J. W., & Caro, J. F. (1996). The ABC of managing hyperthyroidism in the older patient. *Geriatric, 51*, 22–32. Retrieved from https://www.ncbi.nlm.nih.gov/pubmed/8621100

Kennedy, J. (2001). Unmet and undermet need for activities of daily living and instrumental activities of daily living assistance among adults with disabilities: Estimates from the 1994 and 1995 disability follow-back surveys. *Medical Care*, *39*(12), 1305–1312. doi:10.1097/00005650-200112000-00006 PMID:11717572

Kent, J. T. (1929). *Lectures on Homeopathic Philosophy* (2nd ed.). Chicago: Ehrhardt & Karl.

Kessels, P. C., Overbeek, A., & Bouman, Z. (2015). Assessment of verbal and visuospatial working memory in mild cognitive impairment and Alzheimer's dementia. *Dementia &Neuropsycholgia, 9*(3), 301-305. Retrieved http://www.scielo.br/pdf/dn/v9n3/1980-5764-dn-9-03-00301.pdf

Kessing, L. V., & Andersen, P. K. (2004). Does the risk of developing dementia increase with the number of episodes in patients with depressive disorder and in patients with bipolar disorder? *Journal of Neurology, Neurosurgery, and Psychiatry*, *75*(12), 1662–1666. doi:10.1136/jnnp.2003.031773 PMID:15548477

Kessler, R. C., Berglund, P. A., Demler, O., Jin, R., & Walters, E. E. (2005). Lifetime prevalence and age of onset distributions of DSM-IV disorders in the National Comorbidity Survey Replication (NCS-R). *Archives of General Psychiatry*, *62*(6), 593–602. doi:10.1001/archpsyc.62.6.593 PMID:15939837

Keyes, C. L. (2002). The mental health continuum: From languishing to flourishing in life. *Journal of Health and Social Behavior*, *43*(2), 207–222. doi:10.2307/3090197 PMID:12096700

Keyes, C. L. M. (1998). Social well-being. *Social Psychology Quarterly*, *61*(2), 121–140. doi:10.2307/2787065

Keyes, C. L. M., & Haidt, J. (2003). *Flourishing: positive psychology and the life well-lived*. Washington, DC: American Psychological Association. doi:10.1037/10594-000

Kilfoy, B. A., Devesa, S. S., Ward, M. H., Zhang, Y., Rosenberg, P. S., Holford, T. R., & Anderson, W. F. (2009). Gender is an age-specific effect modifier for papillary cancers of the thyroid gland. *Cancer Epidemiology, Biomarkers & Prevention*, *18*(4), 1092–1100. doi:10.1158/1055-9965.EPI-08-0976 PMID:19293311

Kimble, M. A. (1995). Pastoral care. In M. A. Kimble, S. H. McFadden, J. W. Ellor, & J. J. Seeber (Eds.), *Aging, spirituality, and religion: A handbook* (pp. 131–147). Minneapolis, MN: Fortress Press.

Kim, H. J., Kim, B. H., & Kim, O. S. (2011). The Effect of Visual and Hearing Impairment on Depression and Cognitive Function in Community-dwelling Elderly. *Journal of Aging and Health*, *19*(7), 658–665.

King, D. A., Conwell, Y., Cox, C., Henderson, R. E., Denning, D. G., & Eric Caine, M. (2000). A Neuropsychological Comparison of Depressed Suicide Attempters and Nonattempters. *iThe. The Journal of Neuropsychiatry and Clinical Neurosciences*, *12*(12), 64–70. doi:10.1176/jnp.12.1.64 PMID:10678515

King, L. A. (2001). The health benefits of writing about life goals. *Personality and Social Psychology Bulletin*, *27*(7), 798–807. doi:10.1177/0146167201277003

King, M. B., & Dein, S. (1998). The spiritual variable in psychiatric research. *Psychological Medicine*, *28*(6), 1259–1262. doi:10.1017/S003329179800703X PMID:9854267

Kiriakidis, S. P. (2015). Elderly Suicide: Risk Factors and Preventive Strategies. *Annals of Gerontology and Geriatric Research*, *2*, 1–6.

Kirkwood, T. B. (2008). Gerontology: Healthy old age. *Nature*, *455*(7214), 739–740. doi:10.1038/455739a PMID:18843351

Kitzman, D. W., Hundley, W. G., Brubaker, P. H., Morgan, T. M., Moore, J. B., Stewart, K. P., & Little, W. C. (2010). A randomized double-blind trial of enalapril in older patients with heart failure and preserved ejection fraction: Effects on exercise tolerance and arterial dispensability. *Circulation: Heart Failure*, *3*(4), 477–485. doi:10.1161/CIRCHEARTFAILURE.109.898916 PMID:20516425

Kivipelto, M., Helkala, E. L., Hänninen, T., Laakso, M. P., Hallikainen, M., Alhainen, K., ... Nissinen, A. (2001). Midlife vascular risk factors and late-life mild cognitive impairment: A population-based study. *Neurology*, *56*(12), 1683–1689. doi:10.1212/WNL.56.12.1683 PMID:11425934

Klein, J. (2011). How lifestyle habits affect diabetes. Retrieved from http://www.Life.guiam.com

Klein, I., & Ojamaa, K. (2001). Thyroid hormone and the cardiovascular system. *The New England Journal of Medicine*, *344*(7), 501–509. doi:10.1056/NEJM200102153440707 PMID:11172193

Kleinspehn-Ammerlahn, A., Kotter-Grühn, D., & Smith, J. (2008). Self-perceptions of aging: Do subjective age and satisfaction with aging change during old age? *The Journals of Gerontology. Series B, Psychological Sciences and Social Sciences*, *63B*(6), 377–385. doi:10.1093/geronb/63.6.P377 PMID:19092041

Kloner, R. A. (2004). Assessment of cardiovascular risk in patients with erectile dysfunction: Focus on the diabetic patient. *Endocrine*, *23*(2-3), 125–129. doi:10.1385/ENDO:23:2-3:125 PMID:15146090

Knight, B. G., & Satre, D. D. (1999). Cognitive behavioural psychotherapy with older adults. *Clinical Psychology: Science and Practice*, *6*(2), 188–203. doi:10.1093/clipsy.6.2.188

Koehler, E. M., Schouten, J. N., Hansen, B. E., van Rooij, F. J., Hofman, A., Stricker, B. H., & Janssen, H. L. (2012). Prevalence and risk factors of non-alcoholic fatty liver disease in the elderly: Results from the Rotterdam study. *Journal of Hepatology*, *57*(6), 1305–1311. doi:10.1016/j.jhep.2012.07.028 PMID:22871499

Koenen, K. C., Moffitt, T. E., Roberts, A. L., Martin, L. T., Kubzansky, L., Harrington, H., ... Caspi, A. (2009). Childhood IQ and adult mental disorders: A test of the cognitive reserve hypothesis. *The American Journal of Psychiatry*, *166*(1), 50–57. doi:10.1176/appi.ajp.2008.08030343 PMID:19047325

Koenig, H. G. (1994). Religion and hope. In *Religion in aging and health: Theoretical foundations and methodological frontiers* (pp. 18-51).

Koenig, H. G. (1989). Research on religion and mental health in later life: A review and commentary. *Journal of Geriatric Psychiatry*, *23*, 23–53. PMID:2212522

Koenig, H. G. (1998). *Handbook of religion and mentaldisorders*. San Diego, CA: Elsevier.

H. G. Koenig, & H. J. Cohen (Eds.). (2002). *The link between religion and health: Psychoneuroimmunology and the faith factor*. Oxford University Press. doi:10.1093/acprof:oso/9780195143607.001.0001

Koenig, H. J., Cohen, D. G., Blazer, C., Pieper, K. G., & Meador, F. S. (1992). Religious coping and depression among elderly, hospitalized medically ill men. *The American Journal of Psychiatry*, *149*(12), 1693–1700. doi:10.1176/ajp.149.12.1693 PMID:1443246

Koenig, H., King, D., & Carson, V. B. (2012). *Handbook of religion and health*. US: Oxford University Press.

Koepsell, T. D., & Monsell, S. E. (2012). Reversion from mild cognitive impairment to normal or near-normal cognition Risk factors and prognosis. *Neurology*, *79*(15), 1591–1598. doi:10.1212/WNL.0b013e31826e26b7 PMID:23019264

Koger, S. M., Chapin, K., & Brotons, M. (1999). Is Music Therapy an Effective Intervention for Dementia? A Meta-Analytic Review of Literature. *Journal of Music Therapy*, *36*(1), 2–15. doi:10.1093/jmt/36.1.2 PMID:10519841

Kohn, M. L., & Schooler, C. (1983). *Work and personality: An inquiry into the impact of social stratification*. Norwood, NJ: Ablex.

Koh, S., Blank, K., Cohen, C. I., Cohen, G., Faison, W., Kennedy, G., ... Streim, J. (2010). Public's view of mental health services for the elderly: Responses to dea Abby. *Psychiatric Services (Washington, D.C.)*, *61*(11), 1146–1149. doi:10.1176/ps.2010.61.11.1146 PMID:21041356

Koivunen, J., Pirttilä, T., Kemppainen, N., Aalto, S., Herukka, S.-K., Jauhianen, A. M., ... Soininen, H. (2008). PET amyloid ligand [11C]PIB uptake and cerebrospinal fluid beta-amyloid in mild cognitive impairment. *Dementia and Geriatric Cognitive Disorders*, *26*(4), 378–383. doi:10.1159/000163927 PMID:18931497

Kollman, C., Howe, C. W., Anasetti, C., Antin, J. H., Davies, S. M., & Filipovich, A. H. (2001). Donor characteristics as risk factors in recipients after transplantation of bone marrow from unrelated donors: The effect of donor age. *Blood*, *98*(7), 2043–2051. doi:10.1182/blood.V98.7.2043 PMID:11567988

Koseberg, J. I., & Garcia, J. L. (1995). Common and unique themes on elder abuse from a worldwide perspective. In J. I. Kosberg & J. L. Garcia (Eds.), *Elder abuse: International and cross-cultural perspectives*. Binghamton, NY: Haworth Press.

Kosowicz, J., Baszko-Błaszyh, D., Horst-Sikorska, W., & Baumann-Antczak, A. (1999). Bone mineral density in primary hyperparathyroidism. Polskie Archiwum Medycyny Wewnetrznej, 101(2), 133–138.

Kotter-Grühn, D., & Hess, T. M. (2012). The impact of age stereotypes on self-perceptions of aging across the adult lifespan. *The Journals of Gerontology. Series B, Psychological Sciences and Social Sciences*, *67*(5), 563–571. doi:10.1093/geronb/gbr153 PMID:22367710

Kotter-Grühn, D., Kleinspehn-Ammerlahn, A., Gerstorf, D., & Smith, J. (2009). Self-perceptions of aging predict mortality and change with approaching death: 16-year longitudinal results from the Berlin Aging Study. *Psychology and Aging*, *24*(3), 654–667. doi:10.1037/a0016510 PMID:19739922

Kraaij, V., Arensman,E., & Spinhoven, P. (2002). Negative Life Events and Depression in Elderly Persons: A Meta-Analysis. *Journal of Gerontology*, *57B*(1), 87–94.

Kraepelin, E. (1971). *Dementia praecox and paraphrenia* (R. M. Barclay, Trans.). Huntington, NY: Rovert E. Kreiger. (Original work published 1919)

Krag, M. O., Hasselbalch, L., Siersma, V., Nielsen, A. B., Reventlow, S., Malterud, K., & de Fine Olivarius, N. (2016). The impact of gender on the long-term morbidity and mortality of patients with type 2 diabetes receiving structured personal care: A 13 year follow-up study. *Diabetologia*, *59*(2), 275–285. doi:10.1007/s00125-015-3804-4 PMID:26607637

Kral, V. A. (1962). Senescent forgetfulness: Benign and malignant. *Canadian Medical Association Journal*, *86*(6), 257–260. PMID:14459267

Kramer, C., Von Muhlen, D., Kritz-Silverstein, D., & Barrett-Connor, E. (2009). Treated hypothyroidism, cognitive function, and depressed mood in old age: The Rancho Bernardo Study. European. *The Journal of Endocrinology*, *161*, 917–921. doi:10.1530/EJE-09-0606 PMID:19755406

Kramer, J. H., Nelson, A., Johnson, J. K., Yaffe, K., Glenn, S., Rosen, H. J., & Miller, B. L. (2006). Multiple cognitive deficits in amnestic mild cognitive impairment. *Dementia and Geriatric Cognitive Disorders*, *22*(4), 306–311. doi:10.1159/000095303 PMID:16931884

Kramer, S. E., Kapteyn, T. S., Kuik, D. J. H., & Deeg, D. J. H. (2002). The association of hearing impairment and chronic diseases with psychosocial health status in older age. *Journal of Aging and Health*, *14*(1), 122–137. doi:10.1177/089826430201400107 PMID:11892756

Krause, N. (1995a). Stress and well-being in later life: *Using research findings to inform intervention design*. In L. A. Bond, S. J. Cutler, & A. Grams (Eds.), *Promoting successful and productive aging* (pp. 203–219). Thousand Oaks, CA: Sage.

Krause, N. (1998). Neighborhood deterioration, religious coping, and changes in health during late life. *The Gerontologist*, *38*(6), 653–664. doi:10.1093/geront/38.6.653 PMID:9868846

Krishnam, S., Cozier, Y., Rosenberg, L., & Palmer, J. (2009). Socioeconomic status and incidence of type 2 diabetes: Results from the black women's health study. *American Journal of Epidemiology*, *171*(5), 564–570. doi:10.1093/aje/kwp443 PMID:20133518

Krumholz, H. M. (2013). Post-hospital syndrome--an acquired, transient condition of generalized risk. *The New England Journal of Medicine*, *68*(2), 100–102. doi:10.1056/NEJMp1212324 PMID:23301730

Kuchenbuch, A., Paraskevopoulos, E., Herholz, S. C., & Pantev, C. (2014). Audio-tactile integration and the influence of musical training. *PLoS One*, *9*(1), e85743. doi:10.1371/journal.pone.0085743 PMID:24465675

Kueider, A., & Rebok, G. (2014). Cognitive Training for Older Adults: What Is It and Does It Work? Center on Ageing, American Institutes for Research.

Kumari, R. S. (2001). *Socio-economic conditions, morbidity pattern and social support among the elderly women in a rural area*. Sreekarym-Panchayat.

Kumar, S., Anish, P., & George, B. (2015). Risk factors for suicide in elderly in comparison to younger age groups. *Indian Journal of Psychiatry*, *57*(3), 249. doi:10.4103/0019-5545.166614 PMID:26600577

Kumar, V., Fausto, N., & Abbas, A. (2008). *Pathologic Basis of Disease* (7th ed., pp. 1189–1206). Saunders Company.

Kuppers, R. B. (2003). Cells under influence: Transformation of B cells by Epstein –Barr virus. *Nature Reviews. Immunology*, *3*(10), 801–812. doi:10.1038/nri1201 PMID:14523386

Kurella, M., Chertow, G. M., Fried, L. F., Cummings, S. R., Harris, T., Simonsick, E., ... Yaffe, K. (2005). Chronic kidney disease and cognitive impairment in the elderly: The health, aging, and body composition study. *Journal of the American Society of Nephrology*, *16*(7), 2127–2133. doi:10.1681/ASN.2005010005 PMID:15888561

La Pierre, L. L. (2003). JCAHO safeguards spiritual care. *Holistic Nursing Practice*, *17*(4), 219. doi:10.1097/00004650-200307000-00009 PMID:12889550

Laidlaw, K., Davidson, K., Toner, H., Jackson, G., Clark, S., Law, J., ... Cross, S. (2008). A randomised controlled trial of cognitive behaviour therapy vs treatment as usual in the treatment of mild to moderate late life depression. *International Journal of Geriatric Psychiatry*, *23*(8), 843–850. doi:10.1002/gps.1993 PMID:18311844

Laiteerapong, N., Iveniuk, J., John, P. M., Laumann, E. O., & Huang, E. S. (2012). Classification of older adults who have diabetes by comorbid conditions, United States, 2005-2006. *Preventing Chronic Disease*, *9*, 3–8. PMID:22595321

LaMantia, M. A., Alder, C. A., Callahan, C. M., Gao, S., French, D. D., Austrom, M. G., & Boustani, M. A. (2015). The aging brain care medical home: Preliminary data. *Journal of the American Geriatrics Society*, *63*(6), 1209–1213. doi:10.1111/jgs.13447 PMID:26096394

Landau, S. M., Harvey, D., Madison, C. M., Reiman, E. M., Foster, N. L., Aisen, P. S., ... Jagust, W. J. (2010). Comparing predictors of conversion and decline in mild cognitive impairment. *Neurology*, *75*(3), 230–238. doi:10.1212/WNL.0b013e3181e8e8b8 PMID:20592257

Lane, J. A. (1987). The care of the human spirit. *Journal of Professional Nursing*, *3*(6), 332–337. doi:10.1016/S8755-7223(87)80121-7 PMID:3429744

Langa, K. M., Larson, E. B., Wallace, R. B., Fendrick, A. M., Foster, N. L., Kabeto, M. U., ... Herzog, A. R. (2004). Out-of-pocket health care expenditures among older American with dementia. *Alzheimer Disease and Associated Disorders*, *18*(2), 90–98. doi:10.1097/01.wad.0000126620.73791.3e PMID:15249853

Langa, K. M., & Levine, D. A. (2014). The diagnosis and management of mild cognitive impairment: A clinical review. *Journal of the American Medical Association*, *312*(23), 2551–2561. doi:10.1001/jama.2014.13806 PMID:25514304

Langer, E. J. (1989). Minding matters: The consequences of mindlessness mindfulness. *Advances in Experimental Social Psychology*, *22*, 137–173. doi:10.1016/S0065-2601(08)60307-X

Langford, C. P., Bowsher, J., Maloney, J. P., & Lillis, P. P. (1997). Social support: A conceptual analysis. *Journal of Advanced Nursing*, *25*(1), 95–100. doi:10.1046/j.1365-2648.1997.1997025095.x PMID:9004016

Lankveld, J. V. (2008). Problems with Sexual Interest and Desire in Women. In D. L. Rowland & L. A. Incrocci (Eds.), *Sexual and Gender Identity Disorders* (pp. 154–187). John Wiley & Sons. doi:10.1002/9781118269978.ch6

LaPlante, M. P., Kaye, H. S., Kang, T., & Harrington, C. (2004). Unmet need for personal assistance services: Estimating the shortfall in hours of help and adverse consequences. *Journal of Gerontology: Psychological Sciences and Social Sciences*, *59*(2), S98–S108. doi:10.1093/geronb/59.2.S98 PMID:15014097

Larbi, A., & Fulop, T. (2014). From "truly naïve" to "exhausted senescent" T cells: When markers predict functionality. *Cytometry. Part A*, *85*(1), 25–35. doi:10.1002/cyto.a.22351 PMID:24124072

Larrieu, S., Peres, K., Letenneur, L., Berr, C., Dartigues, J. F., Ritchie, K., & Barberger-Gateau, P. (2004). Relationship between body mass index and different domains of disability in older persons: The 3C study. *International Journal of Obesity*, *28*(12), 1555–1560. doi:10.1038/sj.ijo.0802755 PMID:15314627

D. B. Larson, J. P. Swyers, & M. E. McCullough (Eds.). (1998). *Scientific research on spirituality and health: A report based on the Scientific Progress in Spirituality Conferences*. National Institute for Healthcare Research.

Larson, E. B., & Kukull, W. A. (1996). Prevention of Alzheimer disease: A perspective based on successes in the prevention of other chronic diseases. *Alzheimer Disease and Associated Disorders*, *10*(1), 9–12. doi:10.1097/00002093-199601031-00003 PMID:8876781

Latovich, M. A. (1995). The Clergyperson and the Fifth Step, in Spirituality and Chemical Dependency.

Laumann, E. O., Glasser, D. B., Neves, R. C., & Moreira, E. D. Jr. (2009). A population-based survey of sexual activity, sexual problems and associated help-seeking behavior patterns in mature adults in the United States of America. *International Journal of Impotence Research*, *21*(3), 171–178. doi:10.1038/ijir.2009.7 PMID:19242482

Laumann, E. O., Nicolosi, A., Glasser, D. B., Paik, A., Gingell, C., Moreira, E., & Wang, T. (2005). Sexual problems among women and men aged 40-80 years: Prevalence and correlates identified in the Global Study of Sexual Attitudes and Behaviours. *International Journal of Impotence Research*, *17*(1), 39–57. doi:10.1038/sj.ijir.3901250 PMID:15215881

Laumann, E. O., Palik, A., & Rosen, R. C. (1999). Sexual dysfunction in the United States: Prevalence and predicters. *Journal of the American Medical Association*, *281*(6), 537–544. doi:10.1001/jama.281.6.537 PMID:10022110

Lavretsky, H. (2010). Spirituality and aging. *Aging Health*, *6*(6), 749–769. doi:10.2217/ahe.10.70

Lawn, S. D., Mwaba, P., Bates, M., Piatek, A., Alexander, H., Marais, B. J., & Abubakar, I. (2013). Advances in tuberculosis diagnostics: The Xpert MTB/RIF assay and future prospects for a point-of-care test. *The Lancet Infectious Diseases*, *13*(4), 349–361. doi:10.1016/S1473-3099(13)70008-2 PMID:23531388

Layous, K., Chancellor, J., Lyubomirsky, S., Wang, L. H., & Doraiswamy, P. M. (2011). Delivering Happiness: Translating Positive Psychology Intervention Research for Treating Major and Minor Depressive Disorders. *Journal of Alternative and Complementary Medicine (New York, N.Y.)*, *17*(8), 675–683. doi:10.1089/acm.2011.0139 PMID:21721928

Lazar, M. A. (1993). Thyroid hormone receptors: Multiple forms, multiple possibilities. *Endocrinology Review*, *24*, 184–193. PMID:8325251

Lazarus, R. S. (2003). Does the positive psychology movement have legs? *Psychological Inquiry*, *14*(2), 93–109. doi:10.1207/S15327965PLI1402_02

Lazarus, R. S., & Folkman, S. (1984). *Stress, appraisal and coping*. New York: Springer.

LeBlanc, E. S., Janowsky, J., Chan, B. K. S., & Nelson, H. D. (2001). Hormone replacement therapy and cognition. *Journal of the American Medical Association*, *285*(11), 1489–1499. doi:10.1001/jama.285.11.1489 PMID:11255426

Lee, D. C., Artero, E. G., Sui, X., & Blair, S. N. (2010). Mortality trends in the general population: The importance of cardiorespiratory fitness. *Journal of Psychopharmacology (Oxford, England)*, *24*(4 Suppl.), 27–35. doi:10.1177/1359786810382057 PMID:20923918

Lee, D. M., Nazroo, J., O'Connor, D. B., Blake, M., & Pendleton, N. (2016). Sexual Health and Well-being among Older Men and Women in England: Findings from the English Longitudinal Study of Ageing. *Archives of Sexual Behavior*, *45*(1), 133–144. doi:10.1007/s10508-014-0465-1 PMID:25624001

Lee, D. S., Kim, Y. J., & Han, H. R. (2013). Sex differences in the association between socio-economic status and type 2 diabetes: Data from the 2005 Korean National Health and Nutritional Examination Survey (KNHANES). *Public Health*, *127*(6), 554–560. doi:10.1016/j.puhe.2013.02.001 PMID:23706862

Leith, C. P., Kopecky, K. J., Godwin, J., McConnell, T., Slovak, M. L., & Chen, I. M. (1997). Acute myeloid leukemia in the elderly: Assessment of multidrug resistance (MDR1) and cytogenetics distinguishes biologic subgroups with remarkably distinct responses to standard chemotherapy. A Southwest Oncology Group study. *Blood*, *89*, 3323–3329. PMID:9129038

Leon, A. S., Franklin, B. A., Costa, F., Balady, G. J., & Berra, K. A. (2005). Cardiac rehabilitation and secondary prevention of coronary heart disease. *Circulation*, *111*(3), 369–376. doi:10.1161/01.CIR.0000151788.08740.5C PMID:15668354

Leonarda, G., & Gabriella, L. (2015). Short communication, gender differences in cardiovascular disease. *Journal of Interventional Cardiology*, *1*(1), 20–22. doi:10.15761/JIC.1000107

Leonard, R., & Horowitz, A. (2004). Hearing problems of and the need for hearing services by consumers of vision rehabilitation services. *Journal of Visual Impairment & Blindness*, *98*, 168–172.

Lerner, D. J., & Kannel, W. B. (1986). Patterns of coronary heart disease morbidity and mortality in the sexes: A 26-year follow-up of the Framingham population. *American Heart Journal*, *111*(2), 383–390. doi:10.1016/0002-8703(86)90155-9 PMID:3946178

Lethaby, A., Hogervorst, E., Richards, M., Yesufu, A., & Yaffe, K. (2008). Hormone replacement therapy for cognitive function in postmenopausal women. *Cochrane Database of Systematic Reviews*, (1): CD003122. PMID:18254016

Leung, N. T. Y., Tam, H. M. K., Chu, L. W., Kwok, T. C. Y., Chan, F., Lam, L. C. W., ... Lee, T. M. C. (2015). Neural Plastic Effects of Cognitive Training on Aging Brain. *Neural Plasticity*, *2015*, 1–9. doi:10.1155/2015/535618 PMID:26417460

Levine, S. A., & Sturgis, C. C. (1924). Hyperthyroidism masked as heart disease. *Boston Medical and Surgical Journal*, *190*(7), 23–237. doi:10.1056/NEJM192402141900703

Levin, J. S., & Vanderpool, H. Y. (1991). Religious factors in physical health and the prevention of illness. *Prevention in Human Services*, *9*(2), 41–64. doi:10.1300/J293v09n02_03

Levy, B. (1996). Improving memory in old age through implicit self-stereotyping. *Journal of Personality and Social Psychology*, *71*(6), 1092–1107. doi:10.1037/0022-3514.71.6.1092 PMID:8979380

Levy, B. (2009). Stereotype embodiment: A psychological approach to aging. *Current Directions in Psychological Science*, *18*(6), 332–336. doi:10.1111/j.1467-8721.2009.01662.x PMID:20802838

Levy, B. R. (2003). Mind matters: Cognitive and physical effects of aging self-stereotype. *The Journals of Gerontology. Series B, Psychological Sciences and Social Sciences*, *58B*(4), 203–211. doi:10.1093/geronb/58.4.P203 PMID:12878645

Levy, B. R., & Myers, L. M. (2004). Preventive health behaviors influenced by self-perceptions of aging. *Preventive Medicine*, *39*(3), 625–629. doi:10.1016/j.ypmed.2004.02.029 PMID:15313104

Levy, B. R., Slade, M. D., Kunkel, S. R., & Kasl, S. V. (2002). Longevity increased by positive self-perceptions of aging. *Journal of Personality and Social Psychology*, *83*(2), 261–270. doi:10.1037/0022-3514.83.2.261 PMID:12150226

Levy, B. R., Slade, M. D., Murphy, T. E., & Gill, T. M. (2012). Association between positive age stereotypes and recovery from disability in older persons. *Journal of the American Medical Association*, *308*(19), 1972–1973. doi:10.1001/jama.2012.14541 PMID:23168819

Levy, B., & Langer, E. (1994). Aging free from negative stereotypes: Successful memory in China and among the American deaf. *Journal of Personality and Social Psychology*, *66*(6), 989–997. doi:10.1037/0022-3514.66.6.989 PMID:8046582

Lew, H. L., Weihing, J., Myers, P. J., Pogoda, T. K., & Goodrich, G. L. (2010). Dual sensory impairment (DSI) in traumatic brain injury (TBI)- an emerging interdisciplinary challenge. *NeuroRehabilitation*, *26*, 213–222. doi:10.3233/nre-2010-0557 PMID:20448311

Lewis, P., & Glaser, C. A. (2005). Encephalitis. *Pediatrics in Review/American Academic Pediatrics*, *26*, 353–363.

Lewis, R. W., Yaun, J., & Wang, R. (2008). Male sexual arousal disorder. In D. L. Rowland & L. A. Incrocci (Eds.), *Sexual and Gender Identity Disorders* (pp. 30–67). John Wiley & Sons.

Ley, D. C., & Corless, I. B. (1988). Spirituality and hospice care. *Death Studies*, *12*(2), 101–110. doi:10.1080/07481188808252227 PMID:10302346

Lezak, M. D., Howieson, D. B., & Loring, D. W. (2004). *Neuropsychological assessment* (4th ed.). New York: Oxford UniversityPress.

Liang, X. H., Jackson, S., Seaman, M., Brown, K., Kempkes, B., Hibshoosh, H., & Levine, B. (1999). Induction of autophagy and inhibition of tumorigenesis by beclin1. *Nature*, *402*(6762), 672–676. doi:10.1038/45257 PMID:10604474

Liehr, P. R. (1989). The core of true presence: A loving center. *Nursing Science Quarterly*, *2*(1), 7–8. doi:10.1177/089431848900200105 PMID:2648211

Li, L. W., Conwell, Y., & Li Yeates, L. W. C. (2010). Pain and Self-Injury Ideation in Elderly Men and Women Receiving Home Care. *Journal of the American Geriatrics Society*, *58*(11), 2160–2165. doi:10.1111/j.1532-5415.2010.03151.x PMID:21054298

Lima, J. C., & Allen, S. M. (2001). Targeting risk for unmet need: Not enough help versus no help at all. *Journal of Gerontology: Psychological Sciences and Social Sciences*, *56*(5), 302–310. doi:10.1093/geronb/56.5.S302 PMID:11522812

Lindau, S. T., Schumm, L. P., Laumann, E. O., Levinson, W., O'Muircheartaigh, C. A., & Waiter, L. J. (2007). A study of sexuality and health among older adults in the United States. *The New England Journal of Medicine*, *357*(8), 762–774. doi:10.1056/NEJMoa067423 PMID:17715410

Lindholm, L., & Eriksson, K. (1993). To understand and alleviate suffering in a caring culture. *Journal of Advanced Nursing*, *18*(9), 1354–1361. doi:10.1046/j.1365-2648.1993.18091354.x PMID:8258592

Lin, J. S., O'Connor, E., Rossom, R. C., Perdue, L. A., & Eckstrom, E. (2013). Screening for cognitive impairment in older adults: A systematic review for the US Preventive Services Task Force. *Annals of Internal Medicine*, *159*(9), 601–612. PMID:24145578

Lin, M. C., Hsu, F. M., Bee, Y. S., & Ger, L.-P. (2008). Age influences the severity of Graves' ophthalmopathy. *The Kaohsiung Journal of Medical Sciences*, *24*(6), 283–288. doi:10.1016/S1607-551X(08)70154-2 PMID:18635413

Lin, M. P., Ovbiagele, B., Markovic, D., & Towfighi, A. (2016). Association of Second hand Smoke with Stroke Outcomes. *Stroke*, *47*(11), 2828–2835. doi:10.1161/STROKEAHA.116.014099 PMID:27729574

Lipscombe, C., Smith, K. J., Gariepy, G., & Schmitz, N. (2016). Gender differences in the association between lifestyle behaviors and diabetes distress in a community sample of adults with type 2 diabetes. *Journal of Diabetes*, *8*(2), 269–278. doi:10.1111/1753-0407.12298 PMID:25850582

Lipton, B. (2015). *The Biology of Belief.* Hay House Publishers Pvt. Ltd.

Lipton, B. H. (2017). *The Biology of belief: Unleashing the power of consciousness, Matter & Miracles.* New York: Hay House, Inc.

Li, S. C., Schmiedek, F., Huxhold, O., Rocke, C., Smith, J., & Lindenberger, U. (2008). Working memory plasticity in old age: Transfer and maintenance. *Psychology and Aging*, *23*(4), 731–742. doi:10.1037/a0014343 PMID:19140644

Li, T. M. (2002). Hypothyroidism in elderly people. *Geriatric Nursing*, *23*(2), 88–93. doi:10.1067/mgn.2002.124325 PMID:11956521

Liu, I., & Chiu, C. H. (2009). Case-control study of suicide attempts in the elderly. *International Psychogeriatrics*, *21*(05), 896–982. doi:10.1017/S1041610209990056 PMID:19538823

Liu, R. Y., Zhou, J. N., Hoogendijk, W. J. G., Van Heerikhuize, J. J., Kamphorst, W., Unmehopa, U. A., ... Swaab, D. F. (2000). Decreased vasopressin gene expression in the biological clock of Alzheimer's disease patients with and without depression. *Journal of Neuropathology and Experimental Neurology*, *59*(4), 314–322. doi:10.1093/jnen/59.4.314 PMID:10759187

Liu, S., Semeciw, R., Ugnat, A. M., & Mao, Y. (2001). Increasing thyroid cancer incidence in Canada, 1970–1996: Time trends and age-period-cohort effects. *British Journal of Cancer*, *86*(9), 1335–1339. doi:10.1054/bjoc.2001.2061 PMID:11720471

LiveT. T. A. C. (2017). Retrieved from https://www.cancertutor.com/ttac-live-2017-hope-cancer-free-future/

Lloyd, C. E., Dyer, P. H., & Barnett, A. H. (2000). Prevalence of symptoms of depression and anxiety in a diabetes clinic population. *Diabetic Medicine*, *17*(3), 198–202. doi:10.1046/j.1464-5491.2000.00260.x PMID:10784223

Lo¨ppo¨nen, M. K., Isoaho, R. E., Ra¨iha, I. J., Vahlberg, T. J., Loikas, S. M., Takala, T. I., ... Kivelä, S.-L. (2004). Undiagnosed diseases in patients with dementia-a potential target group for intervention. *Dementia and Geriatric Cognitive Disorders*, *18*(3-4), 321–329. doi:10.1159/000080126 PMID:15305110

Logroscino, G., Kang, J. H., & Grodstein, F. (2004). Prospective study of type 2 diabetes and cognitive decline in women aged 70-81 years. *BMJ (Clinical Research Ed.)*, *328*(7439), 548. doi:10.1136/bmj.37977.495729.EE PMID:14980984

Lopez, A. D. (1993). Assessing the burden of mortality from cardiovascular diseases. *World Health Statistics Quarterly. Rapport Trimestriel de Statistiquess Anitairesmondiales*, *46*(2), 91–96.

Lopez, O. L., Becker, J. T., Chang, Y. F., Sweet, R. A., DeKosky, S. T., Gach, M. H., ... Kuller, L. H. (2012). Incidence of mild cognitive impairment in the Pittsburgh Cardiovascular Health Study–Cognition Study. *Neurology*, *79*(15), 1599–1606. doi:10.1212/WNL.0b013e31826e25f0 PMID:23019262

Lopez, O. L., Jagust, W. J., DeKosky, S. T., Becker, J. T., Fitzpatrick, A., Dulberg, C., ... Carlson, M. (2003). Prevalence and classification of mild cognitive impairment in the Cardiovascular Health Study Cognition Study: Part 1. *Archives of Neurology*, *60*(10), 1385–1389. doi:10.1001/archneur.60.10.1385 PMID:14568808

Lorig, K., & Fries, J. (2006). *The arthritis helpbook* (6th ed.). Reading, MA: Perseus.

Lorig, K., Holman, H., Sobel, D., Laurent, D., Gonzalez, V., & Minor, M. (2006). *Living a healthy life with chronic conditions* (3rd ed.). Boulder, CO: Bull.

Lucas, R. E., & Donnellan, M. B. (2011). Personality development across the life span: Longitudinal analyses with a national sample from Germany. *Journal of Personality and Social Psychology*, *101*(4), 847–861. doi:10.1037/a0024298 PMID:21707197

Luchsinger, J. A., Reitz, C., Patel, B., Tang, M. X., Manly, J. J., & Mayeux, R. (2007). Relation of diabetes to mild cognitive impairment. *Archives of Neurology*, *64*(4), 570–575. doi:10.1001/archneur.64.4.570 PMID:17420320

Luchsinger, J. A., Tang, M., Stern, Y., Shea, S., & Mayeux, R. (2001). Diabetes mellitus and risk of Alzheimer's disease and dementia with stroke in a multiethnic cohort. *American Journal of Epidemiology*, *154*(7), 635–641. doi:10.1093/aje/154.7.635 PMID:11581097

Ludwig, E. (1943). *The Hippocratic Oath: Test, Translation and Interpretation*. Baltimore: John Hopkins Press.

Lu, H., Ouyang, W., & Huang, C. (2006). Inflammation, a key event in cancer development. *Molecular Cancer Research*, *4*(4), 221–233. doi:10.1158/1541-7786.MCR-05-0261 PMID:16603636

Luis, A. U. C., Rosalinda, D., Israel, V. P., & Juan, F. R. (2015). The Effect of Spatial Working Memory Deterioration on Strategic Visuomotor Learning across Aging. *Behavioural Neurology*. Retrieved from https://www.hindawi.com/journals/bn/2015/512617/

Lundberg, U. (2005). Stress hormones in health and illness: The roles of work and gender. *Psychoneuroendocrinology*, *30*(10), 1017–1021. doi:10.1016/j.psyneuen.2005.03.014 PMID:15963652

Lundh, L. G. (2005). The Role of Acceptance and mindfulness in the treatment of insomnia. *Journal of Cognitive Psychotherapy*, *19*(1), 29–39. doi:10.1891/jcop.19.1.29.66331

Lunn, J. S. (2004). Spiritual care in a multi-religious context. *Journal of Pain & Palliative Care Pharmacotherapy*, *17*(3-4), 153–166. doi:10.1080/J354v17n03_23 PMID:15022959

Lunt, L., Bramham, J., Morris, R. G., Bullock, P. R., Selway, R. P., Xenitidis, K., & David, A. S. (2012). Prefrontal cortex dysfunction and 'Jumping to Conclusions': Bias or deficit? *Journal of Neuropsychology*, *6*(1), 65–78. doi:10.1111/j.1748-6653.2011.02005.x PMID:22257612

Lupien, S. J., de Leon, M., de Santi, S., Convit, A., Tarshish, C., Nair, N. P. V., ... Meaney, M. J. (1998). Cortisol levels during human aging predict hippocampal atrophy and memory deficits. *Nature Neuroscience*, *1*(1), 69–73. doi:10.1038/271 PMID:10195112

Lustig, C., & Buckner, R. (2004). Preserved neural correlates of priming in old age and dementia. *Neuron*, 42865–42875. PMID:15182724

Lustman, P. J., Anderson, R. J., Freedland, K. E., de Groot, M., Carney, R. M., & Clouse, R. E. (2000). Depression and poor glycemic control: A meta-analytic review of the literature. *Diabetes Care*, *23*(7), 934–942. doi:10.2337/diacare.23.7.934 PMID:10895843

Lutz, W., Sanderson, W., & Scherbov, S. (2008). The coming acceleration of global population ageing. *Nature*, *451*(7179), 716–719. doi:10.1038/nature06516 PMID:18204438

Lyketsos, C. G., Lopez, O., Jones, B., Fitzpatrick, A. L., Breitner, J., & DeKosky, S. (2002). Prevalence of neuropsychiatric symptoms in dementia and mild cognitive impairment: Results from the cardiovascular health study. *Journal of the American Medical Association*, *288*(12), 1475–1483. doi:10.1001/jama.288.12.1475 PMID:12243634

Lyketsos, C. G., Steinberg, M., & Tschanz, J. T. (2000). Mental and behavioral disturbances in dementia: FIndings from the Cache County Study on Memory in Aging. *The American Journal of Psychiatry*, *157*(5), 708–714. doi:10.1176/appi.ajp.157.5.708 PMID:10784462

Lynes, B. (1990). *The Healing of Cancer: the Cures the cover ups and the solution now*. Marcus Books.

Lyubomirsky, S., King, L., & Diener, E. (2005). The benefits of frequent positive affect: Does happiness lead to success? *Psychological Bulletin*, *131*(6), 803–855. doi:10.1037/0033-2909.131.6.803 PMID:16351326

MacGreen, D. (1997). Spirituality as a coping resource. *Behavior Therapy*, *20*, 28.

Mackay, J., Mensah, G. A., Mendis, S., & Greenlund, K. (2004). The atlas of heart disease and stroke (tech. Rep.). World Health Organization, Geneva, Switzerland.

MacKinlay, E. B., & Trevitt, C. (2007). Spiritual care and ageing in a secular society. *The Medical Journal of Australia*, *186*(10), S74. PMID:17516891

MacRae, C.A., & Vasan, R. S. (2016). The Future of Genetics and Genomics: Closing the Phenotype Gap in Precision Medicine. *Circulation*, *133*(25), 2634–2639. doi:10.1161/CIRCULATIONAHA.116.022547

Magomedova, S., & Damadaeva, A. (2014). Application of physical education in the rehabilitation of patients with cardiovascular disease. *Biological Medicine*, 6.

Mahal, A., & Berman, P. (2002). Estimating baseline health expenditures on the elderly in India. In *Draft*. Boston, MA: Harvard School of Public Health, Department of Population and International Health.

Mahfouz, E., Sameh, E., & Areny, T. (2006). Prevalence and correlates of overweight and obesity among elderly population residing a rural community, Minia, Egypt. Faculty of medicine, Minia University.

Mahler, R. J., & Adler, M. L. (1999). Type 2 diabetes mellitus: Update on diagnosispathophysiology, and treatment. *The Journal of Clinical Endocrinology and Metabolism*, *84*(4), 1165–1171. doi:10.1210/jcem.84.4.5612 PMID:10199747

Mahrouf-Yorgov, M., De L'Hortet, A. C., Cosson, C., Slama, A., Abdoun, E., Guidotti, J. E., & Gilgenkrantz, H. (2011). Increased susceptibility to liver fibrosis with age is correlated with an altered inflammatory response. *Rejuvenation Research*, *14*(4), 353–363. doi:10.1089/rej.2010.1146 PMID:21548759

Majnemer, A., Limperopoulos, C., Shevell, M., Rosenblatt, B., Rohlicek, C., & Tchervenkov, C. (2006). Long-term neuromotor outcome at school entry of infants with congenital heart defects requiring open-heart surgery. *The Journal of Pediatrics*, *148*(1), 72–77. doi:10.1016/j.jpeds.2005.08.036 PMID:16423601

Malek, A. H., Baradaran, E. M., Hejazi, F., Khojasteh, T., Noot, R. H., & Falahat, K. (2010). The effectiveness of educational intervention in the health promotion in elderly people. *Iranian Journal of Public Health*, *39*(2), 18–23. PMID:23113002

Manly, J. J., Tang, M. X., Schupf, N., Stern, Y., Vonsattel, J.-P. G., & Mayeux, R. (2008). Frequency and course of mild cognitive impairment in a multiethnic community. *Annals of Neurology*, *63*(4), 494–506. doi:10.1002/ana.21326 PMID:18300306

Manuscript, A., & Integration, S. (2015). NIH Public Access. *Annals of Internal Medicine*, *161*(2), 85–95. doi:10.7326/M13-1291.Social

Marais, B. J., Schaaf, H. S., & Graham, S. M. (2014). Child health and tuberculosis. *The Lancet. Respiratory Medicine*, *2*(4), 254–256. doi:10.1016/S2213-2600(14)70009-8 PMID:24717618

Marcucci, F., & Mele, A. (2011). Hepatitis viruses and non-Hodgkin lymphoma: Epidemiology, mechanism of tumorigenesis and therapeutic opportunities. *Blood*, *117*(6), 1192–1198. doi:10.1182/blood-2010-06-275818

Mariotti, S., Franceschi, C., & Cossarizza, A. (1995). The aging thyroid. *Endocrinology Review, 16*, 686–715. Retrieved from https://www.ncbi.nlm.nih.gov/pubmed/8747831

Mariotti, S., Barbesino, G., & Caturegli, P. (1993). Complex alteration of thyroid function in healthy centenarians. *The Journal of Clinical Endocrinology and Metabolism, 77*, 1130–1134. Retrieved from https://www.ncbi.nlm.nih.gov/pubmed/8077303 PMID:8077303

Mariotti, S., Franceschi, C., Cossarizza, A., & Pinchera, A. (1995). The aging thyroid. *Endocrinology Review, 16*(6), 686–715. doi:10.1210/edrv-16-6-686 PMID:8747831

Markolin, C. (n.d.). Total Health Institute. Dr. Hammer's Medical Paradigm. Retrieved from http://www.totalhealthinstitute.com/german-new-medicine/

Markov, D., & Goldman, M. (2006). Normal sleep and circadian rhythms: Neurobiologic mechanisms underlying sleep and wakefulness. *The Psychiatric Clinics of North America, 29*(4), 841–853. doi:10.1016/j.psc.2006.09.008 PMID:17118271

Marković, L. (2004). Interaction involving the thymus and the hypothalamus-pituitary axis, immunomodulation by hormones. *Srpski Arhiv za Celokupno Lekarstvo, 132*(5-6), 187–193. doi:10.2298/SARH0406187M PMID:15493593

Marmot, M. G. (2001). Alcohol and coronary heart disease. *International Journal of Epidemiology, 30*(4), 724–729. doi:10.1093/ije/30.4.724 PMID:11511592

Marshall, G. N., Wortman, C. B., Kusulas, J. W., Hervig, L. K., & Vickers, R. R. Jr. (1992). Distinguishing optimism from pessimism: Relations to fundamental dimensions of mood and personality. *Journal of Personality and Social Psychology, 62*(6), 1067–1074. doi:10.1037/0022-3514.62.6.1067

Martínez-Maldonado, M. L., Vivaldo-Martínez, M., & Mendoza-Núñez, V. M. (2016). Comprehensive Gerontological Development: A Positive View on Aging. *Gerontology & Geriatric Medicin, 2*, 1–6. PMID:28913371

Martini, E. M., Garrett, N., Lindquist, T., & Isham, G. J. (2007). The Boomers are coming: A total cost of care model of the impact of population aging on health care costs in the United States by major practice category. *Health Services Research, 42*(1 Pt 1), 201–218. doi:10.1111/j.1475-6773.2006.00607.x PMID:17355589

Martin, P., Kelly, N., Kahana, B., Kahana, E., Willcox, B. J., Willcox, D. C., & Poon, L. W. (2015). Defining successful aging: A tangible or elusive concept? *The Gerontologist, 55*(1), 14–25. doi:10.1093/geront/gnu044 PMID:24840916

Marty, M. E., & Appleby, R. S. (1991). *Fundamentalisms Observed*. Chicago: Univ.

Masayuki, S. T., Ken-ichi, T., Yukari, O., Hirotaka, K., Hajime, S., & Hidekazu, T. (2015). Music Therapy Using Singing Training Improves Psychomotor Speed in Patients with Alzheimer's disease: A Neuropsychological and fMRI Study Dementia. *Geriatric Cognition Disorder Extra, 5*(3), 296–308. doi:10.1159/000436960

Massague, L., & Norton, L. (2006). Is cancer a disease of self seeding? *Nature Medicine, 12*(8), 875–878. doi:10.1038/nm0806-875 PMID:16892025

Massar, D., & Khadi, P. B. (2016). Quality of life of elderly of Northern Karnataka and Jaintia hills region. *Journal of Pharmaceutical Sciences, 29*(4), 533–535.

Massie, B. M., Carson, P. E., McMurray, J. J., Komajda, M., McKelvie, R., Zile, M. R., ... Ptaszynska, A. (2008). Irbesar.tan in patients with heart failure and preserved ejection fraction. *The New England Journal of Medicine, 359*(23), 2456–2467. doi:10.1056/NEJMoa0805450 PMID:19001508

Massoud, F., Belleville, S., Bergman, H., Kirk, J., Chertkow, H., Nasreddine, Z., ... Freedman, M. (2007). Mild cognitive impairment and cognitive impairment, no dementia: Part B, therapy. *Alzheimer's & Dementia*, *3*(4), 283–291. doi:10.1016/j.jalz.2007.07.002 PMID:19595949

Masters, C. L., & Beyreuther, K. (1994). Alzheimer's disease: A clever definition of the genetic components, Alzheimer's Association Australia. *4th Natl. Conf.* Sydney: Alzheimer's Association.

Masters, W. H., & Johnson, V. E. (1970). *Human sexual response*. Boston, MA: Little, Brown.

Mathew, R., Gucciardi, E., De Melo, M., & Barata, P. (2012). Self-management experiences among men and women with type 2 diabetes mellitus: A qualitative analysis. *BMC Family Practice*, *13*(1), 122. doi:10.1186/1471-2296-13-122 PMID:23249410

Maton, K. I., & Wells, E. A. (1995). Religion as a community resource for well-being: Prevention, healing, and empowerment pathways. *The Journal of Social Issues*, *51*(2), 177–193. doi:10.1111/j.1540-4560.1995.tb01330.x

Max, L. S., David, J. V., Jacobijn, G., & Aartjan, T. F. (2015). Is depression in old age fatal only when people feel lonely? *The American Journal of Psychiatry*, *162*, 178–180.

Mayeroff, M. (1971). *On caring*. New York: Perennial Library.

Mayo Clinic. (2013, November 14). *Shared decisions: Diabetes medication decision aid*. Retrieved from http:// shared-decisions.mayoclinic.org/decision-aids-for-diabetes/diabetesmedication-management

Mazzaferri, E. L. (1993). Management of a solitary thyroid nodule. *New England Journal of Medicnie, 25*, 553–9. Retrieved from https://www.ncbi.nlm.nih.gov/pubmed/16399019

McAdams, D. P. (2001). Generativity in midlife. In M. Lachman (Ed.), *Handbook of midlife deveopment* (pp. 395–443). New York: Wiley.

McBee, W. L., Dailey, M. E., Dugan, E., & Shumaker, S. A. (1997). Hormone replacement therapy and other potential treatments for dementias. *Menopause Hormone and Replacement Therapy*, *26*, 329–345. PMID:9193887

McCarroll, P., O'Connor, T., & Meakes, E. (2005). Assessing plurality in spirituality definitions. In *Spirituality and health: Multidisciplinary explorations* (pp. 43-61).

McCarten, J. R. (2013). Clinical evaluation of early cognitive symptoms. *Clinics in Geriatric Medicine*, *29*(4), 791–807. doi:10.1016/j.cger.2013.07.005 PMID:24094297

McClam, T. D., Marano, C. M., Rosenberg, P. B., & Lyketsos, C. G. (2015). Interventions for Neuropsychiatric Symptoms in Neurocognitive Impairment Due to Alzheimer's Disease: A Review of the Literature. *Harvard Review of Psychiatry*, *23*(5), 377–393. doi:10.1097/HRP.0000000000000097 PMID:26332220

McDonnell, M. N., Smith, A. E., & Mackintosh, S. F. (2011). Aerobic exercise to improve cognitive function in adults with neurological disorders: A systematic review. *Archives of Physical Medicine and Rehabilitation*, *92*(7), 1044–1052. doi:10.1016/j.apmr.2011.01.021 PMID:21704783

McFadden, S. H. (1995). Religion and well-being in aging persons in an aging society. *The Journal of Social Issues*, *51*(2), 161–175. doi:10.1111/j.1540-4560.1995.tb01329.x

McFadden, S. H. (1999). Religion, personality, and aging: A life span perspective. *Journal of Personality*, *67*(6), 1081–1104. doi:10.1111/1467-6494.00083 PMID:10637989

McIntyre, R. S., Cha, D. S., Soczynska, J. K., Woldeyohannes, H. O., Gallaugher, L. A., Kudlow, P., ... Baskaran, A. (2013). Cognitive deficits and functional outcomes in major depressive disorder: Determinants, substrates, and treatment interventions. *Depression and Anxiety*, *30*(6), 515–527. doi:10.1002/da.22063 PMID:23468126

McLeod, J. D., & Kessler, R. C. (1990). Socioeconomic status differences in vulnerability to undesirable life events. *Journal of Health and Social Behavior*, *37*(2), 162–172. doi:10.2307/2137170 PMID:2102495

Mehta, K. M., Simonsick, E. M., Penninx, B. W. J. H., Schulz, R., Rubin, S. M., Satterfield, S., & Yaffe, K. (2003). Prevalence and correlates of anxiety symptoms in well-functioning older adults: Findings from the Healthy Aging and Body Composition Study. *Journal of the American Geriatrics Society*, *51*(4), 499–504. doi:10.1046/j.1532-5415.2003.51158.x PMID:12657069

Mehta, S. (2015). "Age-Related Macular Degeneration.". Primary care. Clinics in office. *Practice*, *42*(3), 377–391.

Melis, R., Marengoni, A., Angleman, S., & Fratiglioni, L. (2014). Incidence andpredictors of multimorbidity in the elderly: A population-based longitudinal study. *Public Library of Science*. *One*, *9*, e103120. doi:10.1371/journal.pone.0103120 PMID:25058497

Mellor, D., Russo, S., McCabe, M. P., Davison, T. E., & George, K. (2008). Depression training program for caregivers of elderly care recipients: Implementation and qualitative evaluation. *Journal of Gerontological Nursing*, *34*(9), 8–17. doi:10.3928/00989134-20080901-09 PMID:18795560

Melzer, D., Delgado, J. C., & Winder, R. (2015). *The Age UK Almanac of Disease Profiles in later Life*. NIHR.

Mendis, S., Puska, P., & Norrving, B. (2011). Global Atlas on Cardiovascular Disease Prevention and Control (PDF). World Health Organization.

Mendis, S. (2005). For the Pathobiological Determinants of Atherosclerosis in Youth (PBDAY) Research group. Atherosclerosis in children and young adults. *Prevention and Control; the Official Journal of the World Heart Federation*, *1*, 3–15. doi:10.1016/j.precon.2005.02.010

Menke, A., Muntner, P., Batuman, V., Silbergeld, E.K., & Guallar, E. (2006). Blood lead below 0.48 micromol/L (10 microg/dL) and mortality among US adults. *Circulation, 114*(13), 1388-1394.

Mercer, S. W., Smith, S. M., Wyke, S., O'Dowd, T., & Watt, G. C. (2009). Multimorbidity in primary care: Developing the research agenda. *Family Practice*, *26*(2), 79–80. doi:10.1093/fampra/cmp020 PMID:19287000

Merica, H., & Fortune, R. D. (1997). A neuronal transition probability model for the evolution of power in the sigma and delta frequency bands of sleep EEG. *Physiology & Behavior*, *62*(3), 585–589. doi:10.1016/S0031-9384(97)00165-0 PMID:9272668

Merz, E. M., & Huxhold, O. (2010). Wellbeing depends on social relationship characteristics: Comparing different types and providers of support to older adults. *Ageing and Society*, *30*(05), 843–857. doi:10.1017/S0144686X10000061

Messikomer, C. M., & De Craemer, W. (2002). The Spirituality of Academic Physicians: An Ethnography of a Scripture-based Group in an Academic Medical Center. *Academic Medicine*, *77*(6), 562–573. doi:10.1097/00001888-200206000-00017 PMID:12063205

Meston, C. M. (1997). Aging and sexuality. Western Journal of Medicine, 167, 285-290.

Meyer, K. C. (2005). Aging. *Proceedings of the American Thoracic Society*, *2*(5), 433–439. doi:10.1513/pats.200508-081JS PMID:16322596

Meyers, C. A., Byrne, K. S., & Komaki, R. (1995). Cognitive deficits in patients with small cell lung cancer before and after chemotherapy. *Lung Cancer (Amsterdam, Netherlands)*, *12*(3), 231–235. doi:10.1016/0169-5002(95)00446-8 PMID:7655832

Mfinanga, S. G., Mørkve, O., Kazwala, R. R., Cleaveland, S., Sharp, J. M., Shirima, G., & Nilsen, R. (2003). The role of livestock keeping in tuberculosis trends in Arusha, Tanzania. *The International Journal of Tuberculosis and Lung Disease*, *7*(7), 695–704. PMID:12870693

Michael, J., McFarlane, A.R., & Feinstein, C. K., & Wells. (1987). "The epidemiologic necroscopy": Unexpected detections, demographic selections and changing rate of lung cancer. *Journal of the American Medical Association*, 258.

Mickley, J. R., Carson, V., & Soeken, K. L. (1995). Religion and adult mental health: State of the science in nursing. *Issues in Mental Health Nursing*, *16*(4), 345–360. doi:10.3109/01612849509072529 PMID:7615381

Miller, D. K., Duckro, P. N., Videen, S. D., & Chibnall, J. T. (2001). Life threatening illness supportive±affective group experience: the LTI-SAGE program. *Supportive Care of the Dying*. Retrieved from www.CareOfDying.org/default.asp

Miller, D. I., Taler, V., Davidson, P. S. R., & Messier, C. (2012). Measuring the impact of exercise on cognitive aging: Methodological issues. *Neurobiology of Aging*, *33*(3), 622.e29–622.e43. doi:10.1016/j.neurobiolaging.2011.02.020 PMID:21514694

Miller, E., & Lewis, P. (1977). Recognition memory in elderly patients with depression and dementia: A signal detection analysis. *Journal of Abnormal Psychology*, *86*(1), 84–86. doi:10.1037/0021-843X.86.1.84 PMID:838953

Miller, J. F., & Powers, M. J. (1988). Development of an instrument to measure hope. *Nursing Research*, *37*(1), 6–10. doi:10.1097/00006199-198801000-00002 PMID:3340583

Miller, M. (1978). Geriatric Suicide: The Arizona Study. *The Gerontologist*, *18*(5 Part 1), 488–495. doi:10.1093/geront/18.5_Part_1.488 PMID:263566

Miller, R. A. (1991). Aging and immune function. *International Review of Cytology*, *124*, 187–215. doi:10.1016/S0074-7696(08)61527-2 PMID:2001916

Miller, R. A. (1996). The aging immune system: Primer and prospectus. *Science*, *273*(5271), 70–74. doi:10.1126/science.273.5271.70 PMID:8658199

Miller, W. R., & Martin, J. E. (1988). *Behavior therapy and religion: Integrating spiritual and behavioral approaches to change*. Sage Publications, Inc.

Mindful. (2008). Indicators- Determinants of health-social and cultural environment-16, Social support- Metadata, Retrieved March, 16, 2009 from http://lib.stakes.fi/mindful/metadata150.htm

Mirowsky, J. (1995). Age and the sense of control. *Social Psychology Quarterly*, *58*(1), 31–43. doi:10.2307/2787141

Mitchell, A. J., Chan, M., Bhatti, H., Halton, M., Grassi, L., Johansen, C., & Meader, N. (2011). Prevalence of depression, anxiety, and adjustment disorder in oncological, haematological, and palliative-care settings: A meta-analysis of 94 interview-based studies. *Lancet*, *12*(2), 160–174. doi:10.1016/S1470-2045(11)70002-X PMID:21251875

Mitchell, A. J., Rao, S., & Vaze, A. (2010). Do primary care physicians have particular difficulty identifying late-life depression? A meta-analysis stratified by age. *Psychotherapy and Psychosomatics*, *79*(5), 285–294. doi:10.1159/000318295 PMID:20616623

Mittelman, M. S., Ferris, S. H., Shulman, E., Steinberg, G., & Lvin, B. (1996). A family intervention to delay nursing home placement of patients with Alzheimer's disease: A randomized controlled trial. *Journal of the American Medical Association*, *276*, 1725–1731. doi:10.1001/jama.1996.03540210033030 PMID:8940320

Miyake, A., Friedman, N. P., Emerson, M. J., Witzki, A. H., Howerter, A., & Wager, T. D. (2000). The unity and diversity of executive functions and their contributions to complex "frontal lobe" tasks: A latent variable analysis. *Cognitive Psychology*, *41*(1), 49–100. doi:10.1006/cogp.1999.0734 PMID:10945922

D. O. Moberg (Ed.). (1979). *Spiritual well-being: Sociological perspectives*. University Press of America.

D. O. Moberg (Ed.). (2001). *Aging and spirituality*. New York: Haworth.

Mockler, M., O'Loughlin, C., Murphy, N., Ryder, M., Conlon, C., McDonald, K. M., ... Ledwidge, M. T. (2009). Causes. and consequences of nonpersistence with heart failure medication America.n. *Journal of Cardiology*, *103*(6), 834–838. PMID:19268741

Moher, D., Shamseer, L., Clarke, M., Ghersi, D., Liberati, A., Petticrew, M., ... Stewart, L. A. (2015). Preferred reporting items for systematic review and meta-analysis protocols (PRISMA-P) 2015 statement. *Systematic Reviews*, *4*(1), 1. doi:10.1186/2046-4053-4-1 PMID:25554246

Mohr, W. K. (2006). Spiritual issues in psychiatric care. *Perspectives in Psychiatric Care*, *42*(3), 174–183. doi:10.1111/j.1744-6163.2006.00076.x PMID:16916420

Mokdad, A. H., Ford, E. S., Bowman, B. A., Dietz, W. H., Vincor, F., Bales, V. S., & Marks, J. S. (2003). Prevalence of obesity, diabetes, and obesity-related health risk factors, 2001. *Journal of the American Medical Association*, *289*(1), 76–79. doi:10.1001/jama.289.1.76 PMID:12503980

Molano, J., Boeve, B., Ferman, T., Smith, G., Parisi, J., Dickson, D., ... Petersen, R. (2010). Mild cognitive impairment associated with limbic and neocortical Lewy body disease: A clinicopathological study. *Brain*, *133*(Pt 2), 540–556. doi:10.1093/brain/awp280 PMID:19889717

V. Molinary (Ed.). (2000). *Professional psychology in long term care: A comprehensive guide*. New York: Hatherleigh Press.

Monaco, T.V., & Silveira, P.S. (2009). *Aging is not Senescence: A Short Computer Demonstration and Implications for Medical Practice Clinics*. Academic Press.

Mondesir, F. L., White, K., Liese, A. D., & McLain, A. C. (2015). Gender, illness-related diabetes social support, and glycemic control among middle-aged and older adults. *The Journals of Gerontology. Series B, Psychological Sciences and Social Sciences*, *71*(6), 1081–1088. doi:10.1093/geronb/gbv061 PMID:26307487

Monk, T. H., Reynolds, C. F. III, Kupfer, D. J., Buysse, D. J., Coble, P. A., Hayes, A. J., ... Ritenour, A. M. (1994). The Pittsburgh Sleep Diary. *Journal of Sleep Research*, *3*(2), 111–120. doi:10.1111/j.1365-2869.1994.tb00114.x

Monroe, L. J. (1967). Psychological and physiological differences between good and poor sleepers. *Journal of Abnormal Psychology*, *72*(3), 255–264. doi:10.1037/h0024563 PMID:6045597

Mont, D. (2007). *Measuring disability prevalence*. Washington, DC: World Bank (SP Discussion Paper No. 0706). Retrieved from (http://siteresources.worldbank.org/DISABILITY/Resources/Data/MontPrevalence.pdf

Montaño, D. E., & Kasprzyk, D. (2008). Theory of reasoned action, theory of planned behavior, and the integrated behavioral model. In K. Glanz, B. K. Rimer, & K. Viswanath (Eds.), *Health behavior and health education: Theory, research, and practice* (4th ed., pp. 67–96). San Francisco, CA: Jossey-Bass.

Montross, L. P., Kasckow, J., Golshan, S., Solorzano, E., Lehman, D., & Zisook, S. (2008). Suicidal ideation and suicide attempts among middle-aged and older patients with schizophrenia spectrum disorders and concurrent subsyndromal depression. *The Journal of Nervous and Mental Disease*, *196*(12), 884–890. doi:10.1097/NMD.0b013e31818ec823 PMID:19077855

Mora, F. (2013). Successful brain aging: Plasticity, environmental enrichment, and lifestyle. *Dialogues in Clinical Neuroscience*, *15*(1), 45–52. PMID:23576888

Moran, A. E., Forouzanfar, M. H., Roth, G. A., Mensah, G. A., Ezzati, M., Murray, C. J., & Naghavi, M. (2014). Temporal trends in ischemic heart disease mortality in 21 world regions, 1980 to 2010: The Global Burden of Disease 2010 study. *Circulation*, *129*(14), 1483–1492. doi:10.1161/CIRCULATIONAHA.113.004042 PMID:24573352

Morgan, P., Simpson, J., & Smith, A. (2015). Health care workers' experiences of mindfulness training: A qualitative review. *Mindfulness*, *6*(4), 744–758. doi:10.1007/s12671-014-0313-3

Morimoto, S. S., Kanellopoulos, T., & Alexopoulos, G. S. (2014). Cognitive Impairment in Depressed Older Adults: Implications for Prognosis and Treatment. *Psychiatric Annals*, *44*(3), 138–142. doi:10.3928/00485713-20140306-05 PMID:25821256

Morin, C. M., Colecchi, C. A., Stone, J., Sood, R. D., & Brink, D. (1995). Cognitive-behavior therapy and pharmacotherapy for insomnia: Update of a placebo-controlled clinical trial. *Sleep Research*, *24*, 303.

Morin, C. M., Colecchi, C., Stone, J., Sood, R., & Brink, D. (1999). Behavioral and pharmacological therapies for late life insomnia. *Journal of the American Medical Association*, *281*(11), 991–999. doi:10.1001/jama.281.11.991 PMID:10086433

Morin, C. M., Culbert, J. P., & Schwartz, S. M. (1994). Nonpharmacological interventions for insomnia: A meta-analysis of treatment efficacy. *The American Journal of Psychiatry*, *151*(8), 1172–1180. doi:10.1176/ajp.151.8.1172 PMID:8037252

Morley, J. (2001). Decreased food intake in the elderly. Journal Gerontolology. *Biological Sciences Medical Sciences*, *56A*(Special Issue II), 81-88.

Morley, J. E. (2005). Sexuality and Aging. In Principles and Practice of Geriatric Medicine (4th ed.). John Wiley & Sons Ltd.

Morrison, J. H., & Hof, P. R. (1997). Life and death of neurons in the aging brain. *Science*, *278*(5337), 412–419. doi:10.1126/science.278.5337.412 PMID:9334292

Mortimer, J. A., & Graves, A. B. (1993). Education and other socioeconomic determinants of dementia and Alzheimer's disease. *Neurology*, *43*, S39–S544. PMID:8389010

Mosca, L., Banka, C. L., Benjamin, E. J., Berra, K., Bushnell, C., Dolor, R. J., ... Wenger, N. K. (2007). Evidence-Based Guidelines for Cardiovascular Disease Prevention in Women. *Circulation*, *115*(11), 1481–1501. doi:10.1161/CIRCULATIONAHA.107.181546 PMID:17309915

Mosca, L., Manson, J. A. E., Sutherland, S. E., Langer, R. D., & Manolio, T. (1997). Cardiovascular Disease in Women. *Circulation*, *96*, 2468–2482. doi:10.1161/01.CIR.96.7.2468 PMID:9337227

Mouton, C. P. (2003). Intimate partner violence and health status among older women. Psychological Well-being Among Older Adults: Exploring the Role of Psychosocial Resources and Deficits. *The Journals of Gerontology. Series B, Psychological Sciences and Social Sciences*, *66B*(2), 217–229. doi:10.1093/geronb/gbq096

Moyer, V. A. (2012). Prevention of falls in communitydwelling older adults: US Preventive Services Task Force recommendation statement. *Annals of Internal Medicine*, *157*(3), 197–204. doi:10.7326/0003-4819-157-3-201208070-00462 PMID:22868837

Moyle, W., Clarke, C., Gracia, N., Reed, J., Cook, G., Klein, B., ... Richardson, E. (2010). Older people maintaining mental health well-being through resilience: An appreciative inquiry study in four countries. *Journal of Nursing and Healthcare of Chronic Illness*, *2*(2), 113–121. doi:10.1111/j.1752-9824.2010.01050.x

Moynihan, R., Doust, J., & Henry, D. (2012). Preventing overdiagnosis: How to stop harming the healthy. *British Medical Journal*, *344*(may28 4), e3502. doi:10.1136/bmj.e3502 PMID:22645185

Mozaffarian, D., Benjamin, E. J., Go, A. S., Arnett, D. K., Blaha, M. J., Cushman, M., ... Howard, V. J. (2015). Article. *Heart Disease and Stroke*, *131*, e29–e322.

Mukherjee, A., Saha, I., & Paul, B. (2008). Tuberculosis in Patients Below and Above 60 years and Their Treatment Outcome Under RNTCP–A study in Rural West Bengal, India. *Journal Indian Academy of Geriatric*, *4*, 60–63.

Mullins, L. C, Johnson, D. P., & Anderson, L. (1988). *Danish Medical Bulletin*. Special Supplement Series, 26–29.

Munroe, S. (2001). *Developing a National Volunteer Registry of Persons with Deafblindness in Canada. Results from the study, 1999-2001*. Port Morien, Nova Scotia: Canadian Deafblind and Rubella Association.

Munson, S., Lauterbach, D., Newman, M., & Resnick, P. (2010). Happier Together: Integrating a Wellness Application Into a Social Network Site. doi:10.1007/978-3-642-13226-1_5

Munzel, T., Sinning, C., Post, F., Warnholtz, A., & Schulz, E. (2008). Pathophysiology, diagnosis and prognostic implications of endothelial dysfunction. *Annals of Medicine*, *40*, 180–196. doi:10.1080/07853890701854702 PMID:18382884

Murad, M., & Kitzman, D. W. (2012). Frailty and Multiple Comorbidities in the Elderly Patient with Heart Failure: Implications for Management. *Heart Failure Reviews*, *17*(0), 581–588. doi:10.1007/s10741-011-9258-y PMID:21626426

Murphy, E., Gluer, C. C., Reid, D. M., Felsenberg, D., Roux, C., Eastell, R., & Williams, G. R. (2010). Thyroid function within the upper normal range is associated with reduced bone mineral density and an increased risk of non-vertebral fractures in healthy euthyroid postmenopausal women. *The Journal of Clinical Endocrinology and Metabolism*, *95*(7), 3173–3181. doi:10.1210/jc.2009-2630 PMID:20410228

Murphy, T., Dias, G. P., & Thuret, S. (2014). Effects of diet on brain plasticity in animal and human studies: Mind the gap. *Neural Plasticity*, *14*, 563–160. PMID:24900924

Murray, C. J., & Lopez, A. D. (1996). Evidence-based health policy--lessons from the Global Burden of Disease Study. *Science*, *274*(5288), 740–743. doi:10.1126/science.274.5288.740 PMID:8966556

Musaiger, A. (2011). Overweight and obesity in eastern mediterranean region: prevalence and possible causes. Retrieved 3 June 2015 from http://www.hindawi.com/journals/jobe/2011/407237/

Musalakis, K., Mintziori, G., Kaprara, A., Tarlatzis, B., & Goulis, D. (2013). The complex interaction between obesity, metabolic syndrome and reproductive axis: A narrative review. *Metabolism: Clinical and Experimental*, *62*(4), 457–478. doi:10.1016/j.metabol.2012.08.012 PMID:22999785

Mythri, S. V., & Ebenezer, J. A. (2016). Suicide in India: Distinct Epidemiological Patterns and Implications. *Indian Journal of Psychological Medicine*, *38*(6), 493–498. doi:10.4103/0253-7176.194917 PMID:28031581

Nadkarni, A., Murthy, P., Crome, I. B., & Rao, R. (2013). Alcohol use and alcohol use disorders among older adults in India: A literature review. *Aging & Mental Health*, *17*(8), 979–991. doi:10.1080/13607863.2013.793653 PMID:23659339

Naeem, A. G. (2003). The role of culture and religion in the management of diabetes: A study of Kashiri men in Leeds. *The Journal of the Royal Society for the Promotion of Health*, *123*(2), 110–116. doi:10.1177/146642400312300216 PMID:12852196

Nagaraja, D., & Jayashree, S. (2001). Randomized study of the dopamine receptor agonist piribedil in the treatment of mild cognitive impairment. *The American Journal of Psychiatry*, *158*(9), 1517–1519. doi:10.1176/appi.ajp.158.9.1517 PMID:11532743

Nancy, A. (1999). *"The Illustrated Encyclopedia of Body Mind Disciplines", the Rosen Publishing Group Inc. New York. New York Health Department. (1932). Practical Homeopathic Therapeutics*. New York: Oxford University Press.

Narme, P., Clément, S., & Ehrlé, N. (2014). Efficacy of musical interventions in dementia: Evidence from a randomized controlled trial. *Journal of Alzheimer's Disease*, *38*, 359–369. PMID:23969994

Nasreddine, Z. S., Phillips, N. A., Bedirian, V., Charbonneau, S., Whitehead, V., Collin, I., ... Chertkow, H. (2005). The Montreal Cognitive Assessment, MoCA: A brief screening tool for mild cognitive impairment. *Journal of the American Geriatrics Society*, *53*(4), 695–699. doi:10.1111/j.1532-5415.2005.53221.x PMID:15817019

National Center for Health Statistics (NCHS). (2009). The National Heart, Lung, and Blood Study: Prognosis and survival. *The American Journal of Cardiology*, *29*, 154–163.

National Center for Health Statistics. (2013). *Health, United States, 2012: With special feature on emergency care*. Hyattsville, MD: Author.

National Collaborating Centre for Mental Health (UK). (2007). *Dementia: A NICE-SCIE Guideline on Supporting People With Dementia and Their Carers in Health and Social Care*. Leicester, UK: British Psychological Society.

National Council on Aging. (2014). *Healthy aging: Fact sheet* (p. 2). Washington, DC: Author.

National Crime Record Bureau. (2014). Accidental deaths & suicide in India. Ministry of home affairs, Government of India. Retrieved from http://ncrb.nic.in/StatPublications/ADSI/ADSI2014/chapter-2%20suicides.pdf

National Diabetes Statistics. (2011). *Department of Health and Human Services*. National Institutes of Health.

National Institute of Aging. (2008). Healthy aging: Lessons from the Baltimore Longitudinal Study of Aging. Retrieved from www.nia.nih.gov/health/publication/healthy-aging-lessons-baltimore-longitudinal-study-aging/why-study-aging

National Institute of Health's National Institute of Neurological Disorders and Stroke. (2004) The Dementias. Publication No. 04–2252. Bethesda, MD: Author.

National Institute on Aging. (2012). *Turning Discovery Into Health*. U.S. Department of Health and Human Services.

National Institutes of Aging. (2005). Blood Vessels and Aging: The Rest of the Journey in Health and Aging.

National Institutes of Health (NIH). (2017). Manifestations and management of chronic insomnia in adults. *NIH Consensus and State-of-the-Science Statements*, *22*, 5–17. Retrieved from http:// consensus.nih.gov

National Institutes of Health. (1998). Clinical guidelines on the identification, evaluation, and treatment of overweight and obesity in adults: The evidence report. *Obesity Research*, *6*(2), 51S–209S. PMID:9813653

NCCN. (2014). NCCN Distress thermometer and problem list of patients. Retrieved on 25 February 2015 from https://www.nccn.org/patients/resources/life_with_cancer/pdf/nccn_distress_thermometer.pdf

NCD Risk Factor Collaboration (NCD-RisC). (2016). Worldwide trends in diabetes since 1980: a pooled analysis of 751 population-based studies with 4*4 million participants. *Lancet*. doi:.10.1016/S0140-6736(16)00618-8

Nefs, G., Pouwer, F., Denollet, J., & Pop, V. (2012). The course of depressive symptoms in primary care patients with type 2 diabetes: Results from the Diabetes, Depression, Type D Personality Zuidoost-Brabant (DiaDDZoB) Study. *Diabetologia*, *55*(3), 608–616. doi:10.1007/s00125-011-2411-2 PMID:22198261

Nefs, G., Pouwer, F., Pop, V., & Denollet, J. (2012). Type D (distressed) personality in primary care patients with type 2 diabetes: Validation and clinical correlates of the DS14 assessment. *Journal of Psychosomatic Research*, *72*(4), 251–257. doi:10.1016/j.jpsychores.2012.01.006 PMID:22405217

Negin, J., Abimbola, S., & Marais, B. J. (2015). Tuberculosis among older adults–time to take notice. *International Journal of Infectious Diseases*, *32*, 135–137. doi:10.1016/j.ijid.2014.11.018 PMID:25809769

Nehra, A., & Bajpai, S. (2013). *The Importance of Diagnosis & Assessment of Dementia: From a Neuropsychological Perspective. Alzheimer's & related Disorders Society of India (ARSDI)* (pp. 43–46). Delhi Chapter.

Nehra, A., & Bajpai, S. (2015). *Normal Aging Versus Dementia: Which signs to look for? Alzheimer's & Related Disorders Society of India (ARSDI)*. Delhi Chapter.

Neikrug, A. B., & Ancoli-Israel, S. (2010). Sleep Disorders in the Older Adults- A Mini- Review. *Gerontology*, *56*(2), 181–189. doi:10.1159/000236900 PMID:19738366

Neri, A. L. (2005). Palavras-chaveemgerontologia (2nd ed.). Campinas: Alínea.

Netuveli, G., Wiggins, R. D., Montgomery, S. M., Hildon, Z., & Blane, D. (2008). Mental health and resilience at older ages: Bouncing back after adversity in the British Household Panel Survey. *Journal of Epidemiology and Community Health*, *62*(11), 987–991. doi:10.1136/jech.2007.069138 PMID:18854503

Netz, Y., Wu, M.-J., Becker, B. J., & Tenenbaum, G. (2005). Physical activity and psychological well-being in advanced age: A meta-analysis of intervention studies. *Psychology and Aging*, *20*(2), 272–284. doi:10.1037/0882-7974.20.2.272 PMID:16029091

Neufeld, M. A., & O'Rourke, N. (2009). Impulsivity and hopelessness as predictors of suicide related ideation among older adults. *Canadian Journal of Psychiatry*, *54*(10), 684–692. doi:10.1177/070674370905401005 PMID:19835675

Neugarten, B. L. (1973). Personality change in late life: A developmental perspective. In C. Eisdorfer & M. P. Lawton (Eds.), *The psychology of adult development and aging* (pp. 311–335). Washington, DC: American Psychological Association. doi:10.1037/10044-012

Newcomer, R., Kang, T., Laplante, M., & Kaye, S. (2005). Living quarters and unmet need for personal care assistance among adults with disabilities. *Journal of Gerontology: Psychological Sciences and Social Sciences*, *60*(4), S205–S213. doi:10.1093/geronb/60.4.S205 PMID:15980296

Newman, A. (2009). Obesity in older adults. *Online Journal of Issues in Nursing*, *14*(1).

Newton, N., Brauer, D., Gutmann, D. L., & Grunes, J. (1986). Psychodynamic therapy with the aged: A review. *Clinical Gerontologist*, *5*(3-4), 205–229. doi:10.1300/J018v05n03_01

Nicolosi, A., Laumann, E. O., Glasser, D. B., Brock, G., King, R., & Gingell, C. (2006). Sexual activity, sexual disorders and associated help-seeking behavior among mature adults in five Anglophone countries from the Global Survey of Sexual Attitudes and Behaviors (GSSAB). *Journal of Sex & Marital Therapy*, *32*(4), 331–342. doi:10.1080/00926230600666469 PMID:16709554

Nielsen, J. (2012) Exploring the sleep deprivation. (online image) Retrived August8, 2017from https;//jordannielson.blogspot.in/2012/an- introduction to – sleep.html

Nielsen-Bohlman, L., Panzer, A. M., & Kindig, D. A. (Eds.). (2004). Health Literacy: A Prescription to End Confusion. Washington, DC: The National Academies Press.

Niemann, C., Godde, B., & Voelcker-Rehage, C. (2014). Not only cardiovascular, but also coordinative exercise increases hippocampal volume in older adults. *Frontiers in Aging Neuroscience*, *6*, 170. doi:10.3389/fnagi.2014.00170 PMID:25165446

Nigosian, S. A. (1994). Islam. In World Faiths (pp. 417-457). Palgrave Macmillan UK.

NIH Publication No. 01-3680 (2006). *Understanding adult obesity.*

NIH Publication No. 01-3680 (2006). *Understanding adult obesity.* Retrieved July 23, 2008 from, http://win.niddk.gov/publications/understanding.htm

Nijhout, H. F. (1990). Metaphors and the role of genes in development. *BioEssays*, *12*(9), 441–446. doi:10.1002/bies.950120908 PMID:1979486

Nilsson, H. (2014). A four-dimensional model of mindfulness and its implications for health. *Psychology of Religion and Spirituality*, *6*(2), 162–174. doi:10.1037/a0036067

Nock, M., Borges, G., Bromet, E., Cha, C. B., Kessler, R. C., & Lee, S. (2008). Suicide and suicidal behavior. *Epidemiologic Reviews*, *30*(1), 133–154. doi:10.1093/epirev/mxn002 PMID:18653727

Noël, P. H., Williams, J. W., Unützer, J., Worchel, J., Lee, S., Cornell, J., ... Hunkeler, E. (2004). Depress.ion and Comorbid Illness in Elderly Primary Care Patients. *Impact on Multiple Domains of Health Status and Well-being Annals. of Family Medicine*, *2*(6), 555–562. doi:10.1370/afm.143 PMID:15576541

Nolen, W. A., Luckenbaugh, D. A., Altshuler, L. L., Suppes, T., McElroy, S. L., Frye, M. A., ... Post, R. M. (2004). Correlates of 1-year prospective outcome in BPD: Results from the Stanley Foundation Bipolar Network. *The American Journal of Psychiatry*, *61*(8), 1447–1454. doi:10.1176/appi.ajp.161.8.1447 PMID:15285972

Noll, D. R., Degenhardt, B. F., Morley, T. F., Blais, F. X., Hortos, K. A., Hensel, K., ... Stoll, S. T. (2010). Efficacy of osteopathic manipulation as an adjunctive treatment for hospitalized patients with pneumonia: A randomized controlled trial. *Osteopathic Medicine and Primary Care, 4*(2).

Noll, D. R., Shores, J. H., Russell, G. G., Herron, K. M., & Swift, J. (2000). Benefits of osteopathic manipulative treatment for hospitalized elderly patients with pneumonia. *JAOA*, *100*(12), 776–782. PMID:11213665

Nooyens, A. C., Baan, C. A., Spijkerman, A. M., & Verschuren, W. M. (2010). Type 2 diabetes and cognitive decline in middle-aged men and women. *Diabetes Care*, *33*(9), 1964–1969. doi:10.2337/dc09-2038 PMID:20519662

Nordberg, A. (1995). Long-term treatment with tacrine: effects on progression of Alzheimer's disease as determined by functional brain studies. In K. Iqbal, J. A. Mortimer, B. Winblad, & H. M. Wisniewski (Eds.), *Research Advances in Alzheimer's Disease and Related Disorders* (pp. 293–298). New York: John Wiley and Sons.

Nouwen, A., Nefs, G., Caramlau, I., Connock, M., Winkley, K., Lloyd, C. E., ... Pouwer, F. (2011). Prevalence of depression in individuals with impaired glucose metabolism or undiagnosed diabetes: A systematic review and meta-analysis of the European Depression in Diabetes (EDID) Research Consortium. *Diabetes Care*, *34*(3), 752–762. doi:10.2337/dc10-1414 PMID:21357362

Nowotny, M. L. (1989). Assessment of hope in patients with cancer: Development of an instrument. *Oncology Nursing Forum*, *1*(1), 57–61. PMID:2911528

Null, G. (2010). Death by Medicine (DVD ed.). Axios Press.

Nursing Home Abuse Laws (NHAL). USA. (2017). Retrieved from https://www.hg.org/nursing-home-abuse.html

Nussbaum, J. F., Thompson, T. L., & Robinson, J. D. (1989). Barriers to conversation. In J. F. Nussbaum, T. Thompson, & J. D. Robinson (Eds.), *Communication and aging*. New York: Harper & Row.

Nyberg, L., & Backman, L. (2004). Cognitive ageing: A view from brain imaging. In R. Dixon, L. Bäckman, & L. Nilsson (Eds.), *New frontiers in cognitive ageing* (pp. 135–160). Oxford, UK: Oxford University Press. doi:10.1093/acprof:oso/9780198525691.003.0007

Nyberg, L., Sandblom, J., Jones, S., Neely, A. S., Petersson, K. M., Ingvar, M., & Backman, L. (2003). Neural correlates of training related memory improvement in adulthood and aging. *Proceedings of the National Academy of Sciences of the United States of America*, *100*(23), 13728–13733. doi:10.1073/pnas.1735487100 PMID:14597711

O'Bryant, S. E., Humphreys, J. D., Smith, G. E., Ivnik, R. J., Graff-Radford, N. R., ... Lucas, J. A. (2008). Detecting Dementia with the Mini-Mental State Examination (MMSE) in Highly Educated Individuals. *Archives of Neurology*, *65*(7), 963–967. PMID:18625866

O'Connor, R. C., & Nock, M. K. (2014). *The psychology of suicidal behaviour. The Lancet Psychiatry*. Elsevier Ltd.; doi:10.1016/S2215-0366(14)70222-6

O'Neill, S., & O'Driscoll, L. (2015). Metabolic syndrome: A closer look at the growing epidemic and its associated pathologies. *Obesity Reviews*, *16*(1), 1–12. doi:10.1111/obr.12229 PMID:25407540

Oberoi, K., & Dey, S. (1991). Satisfaction level of rural and urban aged persons for various need in Samastipur district (Bihar). *Indian Psychological Review*, *37*(7&8), 6–10.

Ohayon, M. M. (2002). Epidemiology of insomnia: What we know and what we still need to learn. *Sleep Medicine Reviews*, *6*(2), 97–111. doi:10.1053/smrv.2002.0186 PMID:12531146

Ohayon, M. M., Carskadon, M. A., Guilleminault, C., & Vitiello, M. V. (2004). Meta-analysis of quantitative sleep parameters from childhood to old age in healthy individuals: Developing normative sleep values across the human lifespan. *Sleep*, *27*(7), 1255–1273. doi:10.1093/sleep/27.7.1255 PMID:15586779

Ohsumi, Y. (2001). Molecular dissection of autophagy: Two ubiquitin-like systems. *Nature Reviews. Molecular Cell Biology*, *2*(3), 211–216. doi:10.1038/35056522 PMID:11265251

Okereke, O. I., Kang, J. H., Cook, N. R., Gaziano, J. M., Manson, J. E., Buring, J. E., & Grodstein, F. (2008). Type 2 diabetes mellitus and cognitive decline in two large cohorts of community-dwelling older adults. *Journal of the American Geriatrics Society*, *56*(6), 1028–1036. doi:10.1111/j.1532-5415.2008.01686.x PMID:18384580

Oksenberg, A., Radwan, H., Arons, E., Hoffenbach, D., & Behroozi, B. (2002). Rapid Eye Movement (REM) sleep behavior disorder: A sleep disturbance affecting mainly older men. *The Israel Journal of Psychiatry and Related Sciences*, *39*, 28–35. PMID:12013707

Oldnall, A. (1996). A critical analysis of nursing: Meeting the spiritual needs of patients. *Journal of Advanced Nursing*, *23*(1), 138–144. doi:10.1111/j.1365-2648.1996.tb03145.x PMID:8708209

Oliver, N. R. (1990). Nurse, are you a healer? *Nursing Forum*, *25*(2), 11–14. doi:10.1111/j.1744-6198.1990.tb00843.x PMID:2235650

Olson, E. J., Boeve, B. F., & Silber, M. H. (2000). Rapid eye movement sleep behaviour disorder: Demographic, clinical and laboratory findings in93 cases. *Brain*, *123*, 331–339.

Oman, D., & Thoresen, C. E. (2002). 'Does religion cause health?': Differing interpretations and diverse meanings. *Journal of Health Psychology*, *7*(4), 365–380. doi:10.1177/1359105302007004326 PMID:22112748

Ong, J., Ulmer, C. S., & Manber, R. (2012). Improving sleep with mindfulness andacceptance: A metacognitive model of insomnia. *Behaviour Research and Therapy*, *50*(11), 651–660. doi:10.1016/j.brat.2012.08.001 PMID:22975073

Oni, T., Youngblood, E., Boulle, A., McGrath, N., Wilkinson, R. J., & Levit, N. S. (2015). Patterns of HIV, TB, and noncommunicable disease multi-morbidity in peri-urban South Africa – a cross sectional study. *BMC Infectious Diseases*, *15*(1), 20. doi:10.1186/s12879-015-0750-1 PMID:25595711

Ontario Human Rights Commission [OHRC]. (2017). Specific issues facing older persons. Retrieved May 19, 2017 from http://www.ohrc.on.ca/en/consultation-paper-changing-face-ontario-discrimination-and-our-aging-population/specific-issues-facing-older-persons

Orr, W. C., & Sohal, R. S. (1994). Extension of life-span by overexpression of superoxidedismutase and catalase in *Drosophila melanogaster. Science*, *263*(5150), 1128–1130. doi:10.1126/science.8108730 PMID:8108730

Ortman, J. M., Velkoff, V. A., & Hogan, H. (2014). An aging nation: The older population in the United States. Retrieved from https://www.census.gov/prod/2014pubs/p25-1140.pdf

Orzan, F., Brusca, A., Conte, M. R., Presbitero, P., & Figliomeni, M. C. (1993). Severe coronary artery disease after radiation therapy of the chest and mediastinum: Clinical presentation and treatment. *British Heart Journal*, *69*(6), 496–500. doi:10.1136/hrt.69.6.496 PMID:8343315

Oster, G.V., & Maskides, K.S (2005). Obesity & health conditions in elderly Mexican Americans. the Hisposic EPSESE, Established populator epidemiological studies of elderly. Ethn D's, 10(1), 318.

Osterberg, L., & Blaschke, T. (2005). Adherence to medication. *The New England Journal of Medicine*, *353*(5), 487–497. doi:10.1056/NEJMra050100 PMID:16079372

Ostro, B., Hu, J., Goldberg, D., Reynolds, P., Hertz, A., Bernstein, L., & Kleeman, M. J. (2015). Associations of mortality with long-term exposures to fine and ultrafine particles, species and sources: Results from the California Teachers Study Cohort. *Environmental Health Perspectives*, *123*(6), 549–556.

Ott, A., Stolk, R. P., Hofman, A., van Harskamp, F., Grobbee, D. E., & Breteler, M. M. (1996). Association of diabetes mellitus and dementia: The Rotterdam Study. *Diabetologia*, *39*(11), 1392–1397. doi:10.1007/s001250050588 PMID:8933010

Over, R., Mannan, S., Nsouli-Marktabi, H., Burman, K. D., & Jonklaas, J. (2010). Age and the thyrotropin response to hypothyroxinemia. *The Journal of Clinical Endocrinology and Metabolism*, *95*(8), 3675–3683. doi:10.1210/jc.2010-0281 PMID:20484476

Owen, D. C. (1989). Nurses' perspectives on the meaning of hope in patients with cancer: A qualitative study. *Oncology Nursing Forum*, *16*(1), 75–79. PMID:2911530

Ownby, R. L., Crocco, E., Acevedo, A., John, V., & Loewenstein, D. (2006). Depression and risk for Alzheimer disease: Systematic review, meta-analysis, and metaregression analysis. *Archives of General Psychiatry*, *63*(5), 530–538. doi:10.1001/archpsyc.63.5.530 PMID:16651510

Padoani, W. S. P. (2001). Attempted and completed suicide in older subjects: Results from the WHO/EURO Multicentre Study of Suicidal Behaviour. *International Journal of Geriatric Psychiatry*, *16*(3), 300–310. doi:10.1002/gps.337 PMID:11288165

Padula, W. V. (1982). Low vision related to function and service delivery for the elderly. In *Ageing and Human Visual Function* (pp. 315–322). Alan R Lis Color Inc.

Padwal, R.S., & Majumdar, S.R. (2007). Drug treatments for obesity: orlistat, sibutramine, and rimonabant. *Lancet, 369,* 71–77. 104.

Palazzolo, J. (2015). Cognitive Behavioral Therapy for Depression and Anxiety in the Elderly. *Ann Depress and Anxiety, 2*(6), 1063.

Palmer, B. W., Heaton, S. C., & Jeste, D. V. (1999). Older patients with schizophrenia: Challenges in the coming decades. *Psychiatric Services (Washington, D.C.), 50*(9), 1178–1183. doi:10.1176/ps.50.9.1178 PMID:10478904

Palmer, K., Berger, A. K., Monastero, R., Winblad, B., Bäckman, L., & Fratiglioni, L. (2007). Predictors of progression from mild cognitive impairment to Alzheimer disease. *Neurology, 68*(19), 1596–1602. doi:10.1212/01.wnl.0000260968.92345.3f PMID:17485646

Pal, R. (2010). *Analysing catastrophic OOP health expenditure in India: Concepts, determinants and policy implications.* Mumbai, India: Indira Gandhi Institute of Development Research.

Pandharipande, P. P., Girard, T. D., Jackson, J. C., Morandi, A., Thompson, J. L., Pun, B. T., ... Ely, E. W. (2013). Brain ICU study investigators: Long term cognitive impairment after critical illness. *The New England Journal of Medicine, 369*(14), 1306–1316. doi:10.1056/NEJMoa1301372 PMID:24088092

Pandya, S. Y., Lacritz, L. H., Weiner, M. F., Deschner, M., & Woon, F. L. (2017). Predictors of Reversion from Mild Cognitive Impairment to Normal Cognition. *Dementia and Geriatric Cognitive Disorders, 43*(3-4), 204–214. doi:10.1159/000456070 PMID:28301848

Panza, F., Frisardi, V., Capurso, C., D'Introno, A., Colacicco, A. M., Imbimbo, B. P., ... Solfrizzi, V. (2010). Late-life depression, mild cognitive impairment and dementia: Possible continuum? *The American Journal of Geriatric Psychiatry, 18*(2), 98–116. doi:10.1097/JGP.0b013e3181b0fa13 PMID:20104067

Paolo, A. M., Troster, A. I., & Ryan, J. J. (1997). California Verbal Learning Test: Normative data for the elderly. *Journal of Clinical and Experimental Neuropsychology, 19*(2), 220–234. doi:10.1080/01688639708403853 PMID:9240482

Papadopoulos, F. C., Petridou, E., Argyropoulou, S., Kontaxakis, V., Dessypris, N., Anastasiou, A., ... Lyketsos, C. (2005). Prevalence and correlates of depression in late life: A population based study from a rural Greek town. *International Journal of Geriatric Psychiatry, 20*(4), 350–357. doi:10.1002/gps.1288 PMID:15799076

Paraskevopoulos, E., Kuchenbuch, A., Herholz, S. C., & Pantev, C. (2012). Musical expertise induces audiovisual integration of abstract congruency rules. *The Journal of Neuroscience, 32*(50), 18196–18203. doi:10.1523/JNEUROSCI.1947-12.2012 PMID:23238733

Paraskevopoulos, E., Kuchenbuch, A., Herholz, S. C., & Pantev, C. (2014). Multisensory integration during short-term music reading training enhances both Uni- and multisensory cortical processing. *Journal of Cognitive Neuroscience, 26*(10), 2224–2238. doi:10.1162/jocn_a_00620 PMID:24669793

Pardini, D., Plante, T. G., & Sherman, A. (2001). Strength of religious faith and its association with mental health outcomes among recovering alcoholics and addicts. *Journal of Substance Abuse Treatment, 19*, 347–354. doi:10.1016/S0740-5472(00)00125-2 PMID:11166499

Pargament, K. (1997). *The Psychology of Religion and Coping*. New York: Guilford Press.

Pargament, K. I. (1999). The psychology of religion and spirituality? Yes and no. *The International Journal for the Psychology of Religion, 9*(1), 3–16. doi:10.1207/s15327582ijpr0901_2

Pargament, K. I. (2001). *The psychology of religion and coping: Theory, research, practice*. Guilford Press.

Pargament, K. I. (2002). Is Religion Nothing But...? Explaining Religion Versus Explaining Religion Away. *Psychological Inquiry, 13*(3), 239–244. doi:10.1207/S15327965PLI1303_06

Pargament, K. I., Sullivan, M. S., Balzer, W. K., Haitsma, K. S., & Raymark, P. H. (1995). The Many Meanings of Religiousness: A Policy-Capturing Approach. *Journal of Personality*, *63*(4), 953–983. doi:10.1111/j.1467-6494.1995.tb00322.x

Paris, F., Fuks, Z., Kang, A., Capodieci, P., & Juan, G. (2001). Endothelial apoptosis as the primary lesion initiating intestinal radiation damage in mice. *Science*, *293*(5528), 293–297. doi:10.1126/science.1060191 PMID:11452123

Parker, P. N. (2007, July 6). The maintenance and welfare of parents and senior citizens bill.

Park, H., Hong, Y., Lee, H., Ha, E., & Sung, Y. (2004). Individuals with type 2 diabetes and depressive symptoms exhibited lower adherence with self-care. *Journal of Clinical Epidemiology*, *57*(9), 978–984. doi:10.1016/j.jclinepi.2004.01.015 PMID:15504641

Parkin, A. (1997). *Memory and amnesia*. Oxford, UK: Blackwall.

Parks, A., & Biswas-Diener, R. (2013). Positive interventions: past, present, and future. In J. Ciarrochi (Ed.), *Mindfulness, Acceptance, and Positive Psychology: The Seven Foundations of Well-being*. Oakland, CA: New Harbinger.

Parks, F. M. (2007). Working with narratives: Coping strategies in African American folk beliefs and traditional healing practices. *Journal of Human Behavior in the Social Environment*, *15*(1), 135–147. doi:10.1300/J137v15n01_07

Park, Y. J., Lee, E. J., Choi, S. H., Park, J. H., Lee, S. B., Lim, S., ... Kim, K. W. (2010). Subclinical hypothyroidism (SCH) is not associated with metabolic derangement, cognitive impairment, depression or poor quality of life (QoL) in elderly subjects. *Achieves of Gerontololgical Geriatric*, *50*(3), e68–e73. doi:10.1016/j.archger.2009.05.015 PMID:19545916

Patane, S. (2014). Cardiotoxicity: Cisplatin and long-term cancer survivors. *International Journal of Cardiology*, *175*(1), 201–202. doi:10.1016/j.ijcard.2014.04.238 PMID:24820740

Patterson, C. (1994). Screening for visual impairment in the elderly. In Canadian Guide to Clinical Preventive Health Care (pp. 932-942). Ottawa: Health Canada.

Patterson, R. L., & Jeste, D. V. (1999). The potential impact of the babyboom generation on substance abuse among elderly persons. *Psychiatric Services (Washington, D.C.)*, *50*(9), 1184–1188. doi:10.1176/ps.50.9.1184 PMID:10478905

Patwardhan, B., & Bodeker, G. (2008). Ayurvedic genomics: Establishing genetic basis for mind-body typologies. *Journal of Alternative and Complementary Medicine*, *14*(5), 571–576. doi:10.1089/acm.2007.0515 PMID:18564959

Pauling, L. (2008). The Pauling Blog. Clarifying Three Widespread Quotes. Retrieved from https://paulingblog.wordpress.com/2008/10/28/clarifying-three-widespread-quotes/

Paveza, G. J., Cohen, D., Eisdorfer, C., Freels, S., Semla, T., Ashford, J. W., ... Levy, P. (1992). Severe family violence and Alzheimer's disease: Prevalence and risk factors. *The Gerontologist*, *32*(4), 493–497. doi:10.1093/geront/32.4.493 PMID:1427252

Payne, G., Laporte, A., Deberm, R., & Coyte, P. (2007). Counting backward to health care's future: Using time-todeath modeling to identify changes in end-of-life morbidity and the impact of aging on health care expenditures. *The Milbank Quarterly*, *85*(2), 213–257. doi:10.1111/j.1468-0009.2007.00485.x PMID:17517114

Peal, N. (2012). *The Power of Positive Thinking*. New York, NY: Random House.

Pearlin, L. I., Schieman, S., Fazio, E. M., & Meersman, S. C. (2005). Stress, health, and the life course: Some conceptual perspectives. *Journal of Health and Social Behavior*, *46*(2), 205–219. doi:10.1177/002214650504600206 PMID:16028458

Pearlin, L., & Schooler, C. (1978). The structure of coping. *Journal of Health and Social Behavior*, *19*(1), 2–21. doi:10.2307/2136319 PMID:649936

Pedersen, B. K. (2009). The diseasome of physical inactivity and the role of myokines in muscle-- fat cross talk. *The Journal of Physiology*, *587*(23), 5559–5568. doi:10.1113/jphysiol.2009.179515 PMID:19752112

Peek, R. M. Jr, & Crabtree, J. E. (2006). Helicobacter infection and gastric neoplasia. *The Journal of Pathology*, *208*(2), 233–248. doi:10.1002/path.1868 PMID:16362989

Peeters, R. P., Debaveye, Y., Fliers, E., & Visser, T. J. (2006). Changes within the thyroid axis during critical illness. *Critical Care Clinics*, *22*(1), 41–55. doi:10.1016/j.ccc.2005.08.006 PMID:16399019

Penedo, F. J., & Dahn, J. R. (2005). Psychoneuroimmunology and aging. In K. Vedhara & M. Irwin (Eds.), Human psychoneuroimmunology (pp. 81-106). New York: Oxford University Press.

Penedo, F. J., & Dahn, J. R. (2005). Exercise and well-being: A review of mental and physical health benefits associated with physical activity. *Current Opinion in Psychiatry*, *18*(2), 189–193. doi:10.1097/00001504-200503000-00013 PMID:16639173

Penke, L., Valde ́s Hernande ́z, M. C., & Maniega, S. M. (2010). Brain iron deposits are associated with general cognitive ability and cognitive aging. *Neurobiology of Aging*. PMID:20542597

Pentz, M. (2005). Resilience among older adults with cancer and the importance of social support and spirituality-faith. *Journal of Gerontological Social Work*, *44*(3-4), 3–22. doi:10.1300/J083v44n03_02

Perk, J., De Backer, G., Gohlke, H., Graham, I., & Reiner, Z. (2012). European guidelines on cardiovascular disease prevention in clinical practice (version 2012). *International Journal of Behavioral Medicine*, *19*, 403–488. doi:10.1007/s12529-012-9242-5 PMID:23093473

Perlis, M. L., & Smith, M. T. (2005). Etiology and Pathophysiology of insomnia. In Principles and practice of sleep medicine. Elsevier. doi:10.1016/B0-72-160797-7/50067-7

Peters, A., & Laffel, L. (2011). Diabetes care for emerging adults: Recommendations for transition from pediatric to adult diabetes care systems. *Diabetes Care*, *34*(11), 2477–2485. doi:10.2337/dc11-1723 PMID:22025785

Petersen, R. C. (2004). Mild cognitive impairment as a diagnostic entity. *Journal of Internal Medicine*, *256*(3), 183–194. doi:10.1111/j.1365-2796.2004.01388.x PMID:15324362

Petersen, R. C. (2011). Clinical practice. Mild cognitive impairment. *The New England Journal of Medicine*, *364*(23), 2227–2234. doi:10.1056/NEJMcp0910237 PMID:21651394

Petersen, R. C., Caracciolo, B., Brayne, C., Gauthier, S., Jelic, V., & Fratiglioni, L. (2014). Mild cognitive impairment: A concept in evolution. *Journal of Internal Medicine*, *275*(3), 214–228. doi:10.1111/joim.12190 PMID:24605806

Petersen, R. C., Doody, R., Kurz, A., Mohs, R. C., Morris, J. C., Rabins, P. V., ... Winblad, B. (2001). Current concepts in mild cognitive impairment. *Archives of Neurology*, *58*(12), 1985–1992. doi:10.1001/archneur.58.12.1985 PMID:11735772

Petersen, R. C., & Morris, J. C. (2005). Mild cognitive impairment as a clinical entity and treatment target. *Archives of Neurology*, *62*(7), 1160–1163, discussion 1167. doi:10.1001/archneur.62.7.1160 PMID:16009779

Petersen, R. C., & Negash, S. (2008). Mild cognitive impairment: An overview. *CNS Spectrums*, *13*(1), 45–53. doi:10.1017/S1092852900016151 PMID:18204414

Petersen, R. C., Roberts, R. O., Knopman, D. S., Geda, Y. E., Cha, R. H., Pankratz, V. S., ... Rocca, W. A. (2010). Prevalence of mild cognitive impairment is higher in men. The Mayo Clinic Study of Aging. *Neurology*, *75*(10), 889–897. doi:10.1212/WNL.0b013e3181f11d85 PMID:20820000

Petersen, R. C., Smith, G. E., Ivnik, R. J., Tangalos, E. G., Schaid, D. J., Thibodeau, S. N., ... Kurland, L. T. (1995). Apolipoprotein E status as a predictor of the development of Alzheimer's disease in memory-impaired individuals. *Journal of the American Medical Association*, *273*(16), 1274–1278. doi:10.1001/jama.1995.03520400044042 PMID:7646655

Petersen, R. C., Smith, G. E., Waring, S. C., Ivnik, R. J., Tangalos, E. G., & Kokmen, E. (1999). Mild cognitive impairment: Clinical characterization and outcome. *Archives of Neurology*, *56*(3), 303–308. doi:10.1001/archneur.56.3.303 PMID:10190820

Petersen, R. C., Thomas, R. G., Grundman, M., Bennett, D., Doody, R., Ferris, S., ... Thal, L. J. (2005). Vitamin E and donepezil for the treatment of mild cognitive impairment. *The New England Journal of Medicine*, *352*(23), 2379–2388. doi:10.1056/NEJMoa050151 PMID:15829527

Peters, R. (2006). Ageing and the brain. *Postgraduate Medical Journal*, *82*(964), 84–88. doi:10.1136/pgmj.2005.036665 PMID:16461469

Pettersson, A. F., Olsson, E., & Wahlund, L. O. (2005). Motor function in subjects with mild cognitive impairment and early Alzheimer's disease. *Dementia and Geriatric Cognitive Disorders*, *19*(56), 299–304. doi:10.1159/000084555 PMID:15785030

Pfeffer, R. I., Kurosaki, T. T., Harrah, C. H., Chance, J. M., & Filos, S. (1982). Measurement of Functional Activities in Older Adults in the Community. *Journal of Gerontology*, *37*(3), 323–329. doi:10.1093/geronj/37.3.323 PMID:7069156

Phillips, B. A., Young, T., Finn, L., Asher, K., Hening, W. A., & Purvis, C. (2000). Epidemiology of restless legs symptoms in adults. *Archives of Internal Medicine*, *160*(14), 2137–2141. doi:10.1001/archinte.160.14.2137 PMID:10904456

Phillips, L. R. (1983). Theoretical explanations of elder abuse. In *Elder abuse: Conflict in the family* (pp. 197–217). Dover, UK: Auburn House.

Phillips, M. R., Yang, G., Zhang, Y., Wang, L., Ji, H., & Zhou, M. (2002). Risk factors for suicide in China: A national case-control psychological autopsy study. *Lancet*, *360*(9347), 1728–1736. doi:10.1016/S0140-6736(02)11681-3 PMID:12480425

Phillips, R. E. III, Lakin, R., & Pargament, K. I. (2002). Brief report: Development and implementation of a spiritual issues psychoeducational group for those with serious mental illness. *Community Mental Health Journal*, *38*(6), 487–495. doi:10.1023/A:1020832218607 PMID:12474936

Pies, R. W., & Popli, A. P. (1995). Self-injurious behavior: Pathophysiology and implications to treatment. *Journal of Clinical Psychology*, *56*, 580–588. PMID:8530335

Piette, J. D., & Kerr, E. A. (2006). The impact of comorbid chronic conditions on diabetes care. *Diabetes Care*, *29*(3), 725–731. doi:10.2337/diacare.29.03.06.dc05-2078 PMID:16505540

Piguet, O., Grayson, D., Broe, A., Tate, R. L., Bennett, H. P., Lye, T. C., ... Ridley, L. (2002). Normal ageing and executive functions in the 'old-old' community dwellers poor performance is not an inevitable outcome. *International Psychogeriatrics*, *14*(2), 139–159. doi:10.1017/S1041610202008359 PMID:12243206

Pike, K. E., Kinsella, G. J., Ong, B., Mullaly, E., Rand, E., Storey, E., ... Parsons, S. (2013). Is the WMS-IV verbal paired associates as effective as other memory tasks in discriminating amnestic mild cognitive impairment from normal aging? *The Clinical Neuropsychologist*, *27*(6), 908–923. Retrieved https://www.ncbi.nlm.nih.gov/pubmed/23767765 doi:10.1080/13854046.2013.809149 PMID:23767765

Pillermer, K., & Finkelhor, D. (1988). Prevalence of elder abuse: A random sample survey. *The Gerontologist*, *28*(1), 51–57. doi:10.1093/geront/28.1.51 PMID:3342992

Pinto, E. (2007). Blood pressure and ageing. *Postgraduate Medical Journal*, *83*(976), 109–114. doi:10.1136/pgmj.2006.048371 PMID:17308214

Pinto, J. M., Fontaine, A. M., & Neri, A. L. (2016). The influence of physical and mental health on life satisfaction is mediated by self-rated health: A study with Brazilian elderly. *Archives of Gerontology and Geriatrics*, *65*, 104–110. doi:10.1016/j.archger.2016.03.009 PMID:27017415

Pitkälä, K., Isometsä, E. T., Henriksson, M. M., & Lönnqvist, J. K. (2000). Elderly suicide in Finland. *International Psychogeriatrics, 12*(2), 209–20. <ALIGNMENT.qj></ALIGNMENT>10.1017/S1041610200006335Plassman, B. L., Langa, K. M., Fisher, G. G., Heeringa, S. G., Weir, D. R., Ofstedal, M. B., ... Steffens, D. C. (2008). Prevalence of cognitive impairment without dementia in the United States. *Annals of Internal Medicine*, *148*(6), 427–434. doi:10.7326/0003-4819-148-6-200803180-00005 PMID:18347351

Podgorski, C. A., Langford, L., Pearson, J. L., & Conwell, Y. (2010). Suicide Prevention for Older Adults in Residential Communities: Implications for Policy and Practice Suicide in Residential Communities. *PLoS Medicine*, *7*(5), 3–7. doi:10.1371/journal.pmed.1000254 PMID:20502523

Podnieks, E. (1992). National survey on abuse of the elderly in Canada. *Journal of Elder Abuse & Neglect*, *4*(1-2), 5–58. doi:10.1300/J084v04n01_02

Pollner, M. (1989). Divine relations, social relations, and well-being. *Journal of Health and Social Behavior*, *30*(1), 92–104. doi:10.2307/2136915 PMID:2470806

Poloma, M. M., & Gallup, G. H., Jr. (1990). Religiosity, forgiveness and life satisfaction: An exploratory study. In *Proceedings of the annual meeting of the Society for the Scientific Study of Religion,* Virginia Beach, VA.

Poloma, M. M., & Pendleton, B. F. (1989). Exploring types of prayer and quality of life: A research note. *Review of Religious Research*, *31*(1), 46–53. doi:10.2307/3511023

Poloma, M. M., & Pendleton, B. F. (1991). The effects of prayer and prayer experiences on measures of general well-being. *Journal of Psychology and Theology*, *1*, 71–83.

Posner, R. (1995). *Aging and Old Age*. University of Chicago Press.

Potter, G. G., & Steffens, D. C. (2007). Contribution of depression to cognitive impairment and dementia in older adults. *The Neurologist*, *13*(3), 105–117. doi:10.1097/01.nrl.0000252947.15389.a9 PMID:17495754

Potts, A., Grace, V. M., Vares, T., & Gavey, N. (2006). Sex for life"?Men's counter-stories on "erectile dysfunction", male sexuality and ageing. *Sociology of Health & Illness*, *28*(3), 306–329. doi:10.1111/j.1467-9566.2006.00494.x PMID:16573718

Pouwer, F., Nefs, G., & Nouwen, A. (2013). Adverse effects of depression on glycemic control and health outcomes in people with diabetes: A review. *Endocrinology and Metabolism Clinics of North America*, *42*(3), 529–544. doi:10.1016/j.ecl.2013.05.002 PMID:24011885

Powdthavee, N. (2009). What happens to people before and after disability? Focusing effects, lead effects, and adaptation in different areas of life. *Social Science & Medicine*, *69*(12), 1834–1844. doi:10.1016/j.socscimed.2009.09.023 PMID:19833424

Powell, R. R. (1974). Psychological effects of exercise therapy in institutionalized geriatric mental patients. *Journal of Gerontology*, *29*(2), 157–164. doi:10.1093/geronj/29.2.157 PMID:4811950

Prakash, R., Rastogi, P., Dubey, I., Abhishek, P., Chaudhury, S., & Small, B. J. (2012). Long-term concentrative meditation and cognitive performance among older adults. *Neuropsychology Developmental Cognitive Behaviour Aging Neuropsychological Cognition*, *19*(4), 479–494. doi:10.1080/13825585.2011.630932 PMID:22149237

Prati, G., & Pietrantoni, L. (2009). Optimism, social support, and coping strategies as factors contributing to posttraumatic growth: A meta-analysis. *Journal of Loss and Trauma*, *14*, 364–388.

Prentice, A. M., & Jebb, S. A. (1995). Obesity in Britain: Gluttony or sloth? *BMJ: British Medical Journal*, *311*(7002), 437–439. doi:10.1136/bmj.311.7002.437 PMID:7640595

Pressman, S. D., & Cohen, S. (2005). Does positive affect influence health? *Psychological Bulletin*, *131*(6), 925–971. doi:10.1037/0033-2909.131.6.925 PMID:16351329

Priestley, J. G. (1985). Towards finding the hidden curriculum: A consideration of the spiritual dimension of experience in curriculum planning. *British Journal of Religious Education*, *7*(3), 112–119. doi:10.1080/0141620840070303

Prince, M., Bryce, R., Albanese, E., Wimo, A., Ribeiro, W., & Ferri, C. P. (2013). The global prevalence of dementia: A systematic review and meta-analysis. *Alzheimer's & Dementia*, *9*(1), 63–75. doi:10.1016/j.jalz.2012.11.007 PMID:23305823

Pruchno, R. A., Blow, F. C., & Smyer, M. A. (1984). Life events and interdependent lives: Implications for research and intervention. *Human Development*, *27*(1), 31–41. doi:10.1159/000272901 PMID:6698531

Pruyser, P. W. (1986). Maintaining hope in adversity. *Pastoral Psychology*, *35*(2), 120–131. doi:10.1007/BF01768711

Puts, M. T., Deeg, D. J., Hoeymans, N., Nusselder, W. J., & Schellevis, F. G. (2008). Changes in the prevalence of chronic disease and the association with disability in the older Dutch population between 1987 and 2001. *Age and Ageing*, *37*(2), 187–193. doi:10.1093/ageing/afm185 PMID:18250095

Pyne, J. M., Patterson, T. L., & Kaplan, R. M. (1997). Assessment of quality of life of patients with major depression. *Psychiatric Services (Washington, D.C.)*, *48*(2), 224–230. doi:10.1176/ps.48.2.224 PMID:9021855

Qualls, S. H., & Noecker, T. L. (2009). Caregiver family therapy for conflicted families. In S. H. Qualls & S. H. Zarit (Eds.), *Aging families and caregiving: A clinician's guide to research, practice, and technology* (pp. 155–188). Hoboken, NJ: John Wiley & Sons, Inc.

Qualls, S. H., & Smyer, M. A. (1995a). Mental health. In G. L. Maddox (Ed.), *The encyclopaedia of aging* (2nd ed.; pp. 629–631). New York: Springer.

Quan, H., Arboleda-Flórez, J., Fick, G. H., Stuart, H. L., & Love, E. J. (2002). Association between physical illness and suicide among the elderly. *Social Psychiatry and Psychiatric Epidemiology*, *37*(4), 190–197. doi:10.1007/s001270200014 PMID:12027246

Quan, S. F., Katz, R., Olson, J., Bonekat, W., Enright, P. L., Young, T., & Newman, A. (2005). Factors associated with incidence and persistence of symptoms of disturbed sleep in an elderly cohort: The Cardiovascular Health Study. *The American Journal of the Medical Sciences*, *329*(4), 163–172. doi:10.1097/00000441-200504000-00001 PMID:15832098

Radhakrishnan, R., & Andrade, C. (2012). Suicide: An Indian perspective. *Indian Journal of Psychiatry*, *54*(4), 304–319. doi:10.4103/0019-5545.104793 PMID:23372232

Radulovacki, M., Virus, R. M., Djuricic-Nedelson, M., & Green, R. D. (1984). Adenosine analogs and sleep in rats. *The Journal of Pharmacology and Experimental Therapeutics*, *228*, 268–274. PMID:6694111

Rahimi, J., & Kovac, G. G. (2014). Prevalence of mixed pathologies in the aging brain. *Alzheimer's Research & Therapy*, *6*(9), 82. doi:10.1186/s13195-014-0082-1 PMID:25419243

Rahimi, R., Ali, N., Md Noor, S., Mahmood, M. S., & Zainun, K. A. (2015). Suicide in the elderly in Malaysia. *The Malaysian Journal of Pathology*, *37*(3), 259–263. doi:10.1097/00001504-200107000-00027 PMID:26712672

Raina, P., Wong, M., Dukeshire, S., Chambers, L. W., & Lindsay, J. (2000). Prevalence, risk factors and self-reported medical causes of seeing and hearing-related disabilities among older adults. *Canadian Journal on Aging*, *19*(02), 260–278. doi:10.1017/S0714980800014045

Rajkamal, R., Singh, Z., Stalin, P., & Muthurajesh, E. (2015). Prevalence and determinants of overweight and obesity among elderly population in an urban area of Puducherry. *International Journal of Medical Science and Public Health*, *4*(3), 369–372. doi:10.5455/ijmsph.2015.3110201477

Raju, S. (2006). *Ageing in India in the 21st Century: A Research Agenda*. Mumbai: The Harmony Initiative.

Ramamurthi, P. V. (1970). Life Satisfaction in the older Years. *Indian Journal of Gerontology*, *2*, 68–70.

Ramamurthi, P. V. (1978). *The sixth decade and after. Tirupati.* S.V. University.

Ramamurti, P. V. (2008). Perspectives of Research on Aging in India. *Journal of Aging & Social Policy*, *15*(2-3). PMID:14696688

Ramlall, S., Chipps, J., Bhigjee, A. I., & Pillay, B. J. (2014). Sensitivity and specificity of neuropsychological tests for dementia and mild cognitive impairment in a sample of residential elderly in South Africa. *South African Journal of Psychiatry*, *20*(4), 153–159. doi:10.4102/sajpsychiatry.v20i4.558

Ramscar, M., Hendrix, P., Shaoul, C., Milin, P., & Baayen, H. (2014). The myth of cognitive decline: Non-linear dynamics of lifelong learning. *Cognitive Science*, *6*(1), 5–42. PMID:24421073

Ramsey, J. L., & Blieszner, R. (2013). *Spiritual resiliency and aging: hope, relationality, and the creative self.* Amityville, NY: Baywood.

Raschetti, R., Albanese, E., Vanacore, N., & Maggini, M. (2007). Cholinesterase inhibitors in mild cognitive impairment: A systematic review of randomised trials. *PLoS Medicine*, *4*(11), e338. doi:10.1371/journal.pmed.0040338 PMID:18044984

Raskin, A., Friedman, A. S., & DiMascio, A. (1982). Cognitive and performance deficits in depression. *Psychopharmacology Bulletin*, *18*(4), 196–202. PMID:7156290

Rasmussen, U. F. (2011). Subclinical Hypothyroidism and Cardiovascular Risk –An Overview of Current Understanding: Thyroid disorder. *European Endocrinology*, *27*(1), 53–57.

Raviglione, M. C., Narain, J. P., & Kochi, A. (1992). HIV-associated tuberculosis in developing countries: Clinical features, diagnosis, and treatment. *Bulletin of the World Health Organization*, *70*(4), 515. PMID:1394786

Raymond, A. (2011). *Never Fear Cancer Again: How to Prevent & Reverse Cancer* (p. 14). Health Communications Inc.

Reeves, R. R., & Brister, J. C. (2008). Psychosis in late life: Emerging issues. *Journal of Psychosocial Nursing and Mental Health Services*, *46*(11), 45–52. doi:10.3928/02793695-20081101-09 PMID:19051578

Reid, M. J. A., Tsima, B. M., & Kirk, B. (2012). HIV and diabetes in Africa. *African Journal of Diabetes Medicine*, *20*(2), 28–32.

Reifler, B. V. (2000). A case of mistaken identity: Pseudodementia is really predementia. *Journal of the American Geriatrics Society*, *48*(5), 593–594. doi:10.1111/j.1532-5415.2000.tb05010.x PMID:10811557

Reisberg, B., Ferris, S., de Leon, M. J., Franssen, E. S. E., Kluger, A., Mir, P., ... Cohen, J. (1988). Stage-specific behavioral, cognitive, and in vivo changes in community residing subjects with age-associated memory impairment and primary degenerative dementia of the Alzheimer type. *Drug Development Research*, *15*(2-3), 101–114. doi:10.1002/ddr.430150203

Reischies, F. M., & Neu, P. (2000). Comorbidity of mild cognitive disorder and depression–a neuropsychological analysis. *European Archives of Psychiatry and Clinical Neuroscience*, *250*(4), 186–193. doi:10.1007/s004060070023 PMID:11009071

Reuben, D. B., Mui, S., Damesyn, M., Moore, A. A., & Greendale, G. A. (1999). The prognostic value of sensory impairment in older persons. *Journal of the American Geriatrics Society*, *47*(8), 930–935. doi:10.1111/j.1532-5415.1999.tb01286.x PMID:10443852

Reynolds, K., Lewis, B., Nolen, J.D., Kinney, G.L., & Sathya, B., & He, J. (2003). Alcohol consumption and risk of stroke: a meta-analysis. *Journal of the American Medical Association, 5*;289(5):579-88.

Richards, P. S., & Bergin, A. E. (1997). A spiritual strategy for counseling and psychotherapy.

Richmond, C. A., Ross, N. A., & Egeland, G. M. (2007). Social support and thriving health: A new approach to understanding the health of indigenous Canadians. *American Journal of Public Health*, *97*(10), 1827–1833. doi:10.2105/AJPH.2006.096917 PMID:17761564

Riekkinen, P. Jr, Soininen, H., Helkala, E.-L., Partanen, K., Laakso, M. P., VanHanen, M., & Riekkinen, P. J. Sr. (1995). Hippocampal atrophy, acute THA treatment and memory in Alzheimer's disease. *Neuroreport*, *6*(9), 1297–1300. doi:10.1097/00001756-199506090-00017 PMID:7669991

Ries, L. A., Kosary, C. L., Hankey, B. F., Harras, A., Miller, B. A., & Edwards, B. K. (1996). *SEER cancer statistics review, 1973–1993: tables and graphs.* Bethesda, MD: National Institutes of Health.

Ritchie, K., Artero, S., & Touchon, J. (2001). Classification criteria for mild cognitive impairment A population-based validation study. *Neurology*, *56*(1), 37–42. doi:10.1212/WNL.56.1.37 PMID:11148233

Rivallan, A. (2006). Suicide and attempted suicide in France. *Soins. Psychiatrie, 19*(246), 18–9.

Rivas-Vazquez, R. A., Mendez, C., Rey, G. J., & Carrazana, E. J. (2004). Mild cognitive impairment: New neuropsychological and pharmacological target. *Archives of Clinical Neuropsychology*, *19*(1), 11–27. doi:10.1093/arclin/19.1.11 PMID:14670376

Riza, A. L., Pearson, F., Ugarte-Gil, C., Alisjahbana, B., van de Vijver, S., Panduru, N. M., ... van Crevel, R. (2014). Clinical management of concurrent diabetes and tuberculosis and the implications for patient services. *The Lancet. Diabetes & Endocrinology*, *2*(9), 740–753. doi:10.1016/S2213-8587(14)70110-X PMID:25194887

Rizzuto, A. M. (1991). Religious development: A psychoanalytic point of view. *New Directions for Child and Adolescent Development*, *1991*(52), 47–60. doi:10.1002/cd.23219915205 PMID:1956547

Roberts, L. M., Pattison, H., Roalfe, A., Franklyn, J., Wilson, S., Hobbs, F. D. R., & Parle, J. V. (2006). Is subclinical thyroid dysfunction in the elderly associated with depression or cognitive dysfunction? *Annals of Internal Medicine*, *145*(8), 573–581. doi:10.7326/0003-4819-145-8-200610170-00006 PMID:17043339

Robinson, L., Benedictis, T. D., & Segal, J. (2012). Elder abuse and neglect: Warning signs, risk factors, prevention, and help.

Robinson, A. (2004). A personal exploration of the power of poetry in palliative care, loss and bereavement. *International Journal of Palliative Nursing*, *10*(1), 32–39. doi:10.12968/ijpn.2004.10.1.12017 PMID:14966443

Robnett, R. H., & Chop, W. C. (2010). Medications. In *Gerontology for the Health Care Professional* (p. 119). Boston: Jones and Bartlett publishers.

Rodondi, N., Bauer, D.C., & Cappola, A.R. (2008). Subclinical thyroid dysfunction, cardiac function, and the risk of heart failure. The Cardiovascular Health study. *Journal of American College of Cardiology, 30*, 1152–9.

Rodondi, N., den Elzen, W. P., Bauer, D. C., Cappola, A. R., Razvi, S., Walsh, J. P., ... Gussekloo, J. (2010). Thyroid Studies Collaboration: Subclinical hypothyroidism and the risk of coronary heart disease and mortality. *Journal of the American Medical Association, 304*(12), 1365–1374. doi:10.1001/jama.2010.1361 PMID:20858880

Roepke, S. K., & Ancoli-Israel, S. (2010). Sleep disorders in the elderly. *The Indian Journal of Medical Research, 131*, 302–310.

Roger, V.L., Go, A.S., Lloyd-Jones, D.M., Adams, R.J., Berry, J.D., Brown, T.M., ... Wylie-Rosett, J. (2011). Heart Disease and Stroke Statistics--2011 Update: A Report From the American Heart Association. *Circulation*. CIR.0b013e3182009701.

Rogers, K., Sacher, G. A., Shock, N. W., Simic, P., & Guarente, L. P. (2016). *Ageing*. Encyclopaedia Britannica.

Rogers, T. (1976). Manifestations of religiosity and the aging process. *Religious Education (Chicago, Ill.), 71*(4), 405–415. doi:10.1080/0034408760710406

Roger, V. L., Go, A. S., Lloyd-Jones, D. M., Adams, R. J., Berry, J. D., Brown, T. M., ... Turner, M. B. (2011). Statistical Update Heart Disease and Stroke Statistics—2011 Update: A Report from the American Heart Association. *Circulation, 123*(4), e18–e209. doi:10.1161/CIR.0b013e3182009701 PMID:21160056

Roh, S., Burnette, C. E., Lee, K. H., Lee, Y. S., Easton, S. D., & Lawler, M. J. (2014). Risk and protective factors for depressive symptoms among American Indian older adults: Adverse childhood experiences and social support. *Aging & Mental Health*. doi:10.1080/13607863.2014.938603 PMID:25070293

Rolls, B. A., & Drewnowski, A. (1996) Diet and nutrition. In Encyclopedia of Gerontology (vol. 1, pp. 429-440). Academic Press.

Ron, B., Elizabeth, J., Kathryn, Z., & Michael, A. H. (2007). Forecasting the global burden of Alzheimer's disease ELSEVIER. *Alzheimer's & Dementia*, 3186–3191.

Roof, W. C. (1993). *A generation of seekers: The spiritual journeys of the baby boom generation*. Harper Collins.

Rosen, R., Leiblum, S., & Spector, I. (1994). Psychologically based treatment for male erectile disorder: A cognitive-interpersonal model. *Journal of Sex & Marital Therapy, 20*(2), 67–85. doi:10.1080/00926239408403419 PMID:8035472

E. Rosowsky, J. Casciani, & M. Arnold (Eds.). (2008). *Geropsychology and long-term care: A practitioner's guide*. New York: Springer.

Ross, C. E., & Mirowsky, J. (1989). Explaining the social patterns of depression: Control and problem solving or support and talking? *Journal of Health and Social Behavior, 30*(2), 206–219. doi:10.2307/2137014 PMID:2738367

Rossi, D. J., Jamieson, C. H., & Weissman, I. L. (2008). Stems cells and the pathways to aging and cancer. *Cell, 132*(4), 681–696. doi:10.1016/j.cell.2008.01.036 PMID:18295583

Rowe, J. W., & Kahn, R. L. (1987). Human aging: Usual and successful. *Science, 237*, 143–149. doi:10.1093/geront/37.4.433 PMID:9279031

Rowe, J. W., & Kahn, R. L. (1998). *Successful aging*. New York: Pantheon/ Random House.

Rowland, D. L., & McMohan, C. (2008). Premature Ejaculation. In D. L. Rowland & L. A. Incrocci (Eds.), *Sexual and Gender Identity Disorders* (pp. 68–99). John Wiley & Sons. doi:10.1002/9781118269978

Roy, T., & Lloyd, C. E. (2012). Epidemiology of depression and diabetes: a systematic review. *Journal of Affective Disorders, 142*(Suppl.), S8-21.

RPD Act. (2016). The Rights of Person with Disabilities Act, Ministry of Law and Justice. *The Gazette of India*, p. 3.

Rubenowitz, E., Waern, M., Wilhelmson, K., & Allebeck, P. (2001). Life events and psychosocial factors in elderly suicides--a case-control study. *Psychological Medicine*, *31*(7), 1193–1202. doi:10.1017/S0033291701004457 PMID:11681545

Rubin, D. C. (2000). Autobiographical memory and aging.

Rubin, R. R., & Peyrot, M. (1999). Quality of life and diabetes. *Diabetes/Metabolism Research and Reviews*, *15*(3), 205–218. doi:10.1002/(SICI)1520-7560(199905/06)15:3<205::AID-DMRR29>3.0.CO;2-O PMID:10441043

Rudolph, J. L., Inouye, S. K., Jones, R. N., Yang, F. M., Fong, T. G., Levkoff, S. E., & Marcantonio, E. R. (2010). Delirium: An independent predictor of functional decline after cardiac surgery. *Journal of the American Geriatrics Society*, *58*(4), 643–649. doi:10.1111/j.1532-5415.2010.02762.x PMID:20345866

Rugulies, R. (2002). Depression as a predictor for coronary heart disease. *American Journal of Preventive Medicine*, *23*(1), 51–61. doi:10.1016/S0749-3797(02)00439-7 PMID:12093424

Rukhman, N., & Silverberg, A. (2011). Thyroid cancer in older men. *The Aging Male*, *14*(2), 91–98. doi:10.3109/13685538.2010.529195 PMID:21087173

Ryan, R. (1997). Cancer Research-A super fraud? Retrieved from http://www.pnc.com.au/~cafmr/online/research/cancer.html

Ryan, S. M., & Nolan, Y. M. (2016). Neuroinflammation negatively affects adult hippocampal neurogenesis and cognition: Can exercise compensate? *Neuroscience and Biobehavioral Reviews*, *61*, 121–131. doi:10.1016/j.neubiorev.2015.12.004 PMID:26695382

Rybash, J. W., Roodin, P. A., & Santrock, J. W. (1991). Adult development and aging (2nd ed.). Dubuque, IA: Wm C. Brown Publishers.

Ryff, C. D. (1995). Psychological well-being in adult life. *Current Directions in Psychological Science*, *4*(4), 99–104. doi:10.1111/1467-8721.ep10772395

Ryff, C. D. (2003). Corners of Myopia in the Positive Psychology Parade. *Psychological Inquiry*, *14*(2), 153–159.

Ryff, C. D., & Keyes, C. L. (1995). The structure of psychological well-being revisited. *Journal of Personality and Social Psychology*, *69*(4), 719–727. doi:10.1037/0022-3514.69.4.719 PMID:7473027

Ryff, C. D., Singer, B. H., & Love, G. D. (2004). Positive health: Connecting well-being with biology. *Philosophical Transactions of the Royal Society of London. Series B, Biological Sciences*, *359*(1449), 1383–1394. doi:10.1098/rstb.2004.1521 PMID:15347530

Rystedt, I. B., & Bartels, S. J. (2008). Medical comorbidity. In K. T. Mueser & D. V. Jeste (Eds.), *Clinical handbook of schizophrenia* (pp. 424–436). New York: Guilford.

Ryu, S. H., Katona, C., & Rive, B. (2005). Persistence of and changes in neuropsychiatric symptoms in Alzheimer disease over 6 months: The LASER-AD study. *The American Journal of Geriatric Psychiatry*, *13*, 976–983. PMID:16286441

Sachdev, P. S., Lipnicki, D. M., Crawford, J., Reppermund, S., Kochan, N. A., Trollor, J. N., ... Team, A. S. (2013). Factors Predicting Reversion from Mild Cognitive Impairment to Normal Cognitive Functioning: A Population-Based Study. *PLoS One*, *8*(3), e59649. doi:10.1371/journal.pone.0059649 PMID:23544083

Saczynski, J., Marcantonio, E. R., Quach, L., Fong, T. G., Gross, A., Inouye, S. K., & Jones, R. N. (2012). Cognitive trajectories after postoperative delirium. *The New England Journal of Medicine, 367*(1), 30–39. doi:10.1056/NEJMoa1112923 PMID:22762316

Sajatovic, M., Blow, F. C., & Ignacio, R. V. (2006). Psychiatric comorbidity in older adults with bipolar disorder. *International Journal of Geriatric Psychiatry, 21*(6), 582–587. doi:10.1002/gps.1527 PMID:16783798

Sakamoto, A., & Tsutou, A. (2013). Comparing the effects of different individualized music interventions for elderly individuals with severe dementia. *International Psychogeriatric, 25,* 775–784.

Salami, & Samuel, O. (2010). Retirement context and psychological factors as predictors of wellbeing among retired teachers. *Europe's Journal of Psychology, 6*(2), 47-64.

Salat, D. H., Kaye, J. A., & Janowsky, J. S. (2002). Greater orbital prefrontal volume selectively predicts worse working memory performance in older adults. *Cerebral Cortex, 12*(5), 494–505. doi:10.1093/cercor/12.5.494 PMID:11950767

Salihu, H. M., Bonnema, S. M., & Alio, A. P. (2009). Obesity: What is an elderly population growing into? *Maturitas, 63*(1), 7–12. doi:10.1016/j.maturitas.2009.02.010 PMID:19328637

Salthouse, T. A. (1984). Effects of age and skill in typing. *Journal of Experimental Psychology. General, 113*(3), 345.

Salthouse, T. A. (2010). Selective review of cognitive aging. *Journal of the International Neuropsychological Society: JINS, 16*(5), 754–760. doi:10.1017/S1355617710000706 PMID:20673381

Salthouse, T. A., Fristoe, N. M., Lineweaver, T. T., & Coon, V. E. (1995). Aging of attention: Does the ability to divide decline? *Memory & Cognition, 23*(1), 59–71. doi:10.3758/BF03210557 PMID:7885266

Sands, L. P., Wang, Y., McCabe, G. P., Jennings, K., Eng, C., & Covinsky, K. E. (2006). Rates of acute care admissions for frail older people living with met versus unmet activity of daily living needs. *Journal of the American Geriatrics Society, 54*(2), 339–344. doi:10.1111/j.1532-5415.2005.00590.x PMID:16460389

Santini, Z. I., Koyanagi, A., Tyrovolas, S., & Haro, J. M. (2015). The association of relationship quality and social networks with depression, anxiety, and suicidal ideation among older married adults: Findings from a cross-sectional analysis of the Irish Longitudinal Study on Ageing (TILDA). *Journal of Affective Disorders, 179,* 134–141. doi:10.1016/j.jad.2015.03.015 PMID:25863909

Saposnik, G., Cote, R., Phillips, S., Gubitz, G., Bayer, N., Minuk, J., & Black, S. (2008). Stroke outcome in those over 80: A multicenter cohort study across Canada. *Stroke, 39*(8), 2310–2317. doi:10.1161/STROKEAHA.107.511402 PMID:18556583

Sarason, I. G., Sarason, B. R., & Pierce, G. (1994). Social support: Global and relationship-based levels of analysis. *Journal of Social and Personal Relationships, 11*(2), 295–312. doi:10.1177/0265407594112008

Saraswati, S. N. (1999, January). Yogic Management of Ageing.Magazine of Bihar School of Yoga. Retrieved from http://www.yogamag.net/archives/1999/ajan99/ageing.shtml

Sateia, M. J. (2014). International Classification of Sleep Disorders-third edition: Highlights and modifications. *Chest, 146*(5), 1387–1394. doi:10.1378/chest.14-0970 PMID:25367475

Sathyanarayana Rao, T. S. (2015). Sexual disorder among elderly: An epidemiological study in South Indian rural population. *Indian Journal of Psychiatry, 57*(3), 236–241. doi:10.4103/0019-5545.166618 PMID:26600575

Sathyanarayana, Rao, T.S., Ismail, S., Darshan, M.S., & Tandon, A. (2015). Sexual disorders among elderly: Anepidemiological study in south Indian rural population. *Indian Journal of Psychiatry*, *57*, 236–241. doi:10.4103/0019-5545.158143 PMID:26600575

Sato, T., Kishi, R., Suzukawa, A., Horikawa, N., Saijo, Y., & Yoshioka, E. (2008). Effects of social relationships on mortality of the elderly: How do the influences change with the passage of time? *Archives of Gerontology and Geriatrics*, *47*(3), 327–339. doi:10.1016/j.archger.2007.08.015 PMID:17936379

Satre, D., Knight, B. G., & David, S. (2006). Cognitive behavioural interventions with older adults: Integrating clinical and gerontological research. *Professional Psychology, Research and Practice*, *37*(5), 489–498. doi:10.1037/0735-7028.37.5.489

Saunders, G. H., & Echt, K. V. (2007). An overview of dual sensory impairment in older adults: Perspectives for rehabilitation. *Trends in Amplification*, *11*(4), 243–258. doi:10.1177/1084713807308365 PMID:18003868

Saunders, N. L., & Summers, M. J. (2010). Attention and working memory deficits in mild cognitive impairment. *Journal of Clinical and Experimental Neuropsychology*, *32*(4), 350–357. doi:10.1080/13803390903042379 PMID:19787522

Sawin, C. T., Castelli, W. P., Hershman, J. M., McNamara, P., & Bacharach, P. (1985). The aging thyroid. Thyroid deficiency in the Framingham study. *Archieves International Medicinie*, *145*(8), 1386–1388. doi:10.1001/archinte.1985.00360080056006 PMID:4026469

Sawin, C. T., Chopra, D., & Azizi, F. (1979). The aging thyroid. Increased prevalence of elevated serum thyrotropin levels in the elderly. *Journal of the American Medical Association*, *242*(3), 247–250. doi:10.1001/jama.1979.03300030019013 PMID:448912

Sawin, C. T., Geller, A., Wolf, P., Belanger, A., Baker, E., Bacharach, P., ... D'agostino, R. B. (1994). Low serum thyrotropin concentrations as a risk factor for atrial fibrillation inolder persons. *The New England Journal of Medicine*, *331*(19), 1249–1252. doi:10.1056/NEJM199411103311901 PMID:7935681

Saxena, S., & Lawley, D. (2009). Delirium in the elderly: A clinical review. *Postgraduate Medical Journal*, *85*(1006), 405–413. doi:10.1136/pgmj.2008.072025 PMID:19633006

Scarmeas, N., Albert, S. M., Manly, J. J., & Stern, Y. (2006). Education and rates of cognitive decline in incident Alzheimer's disease. *Journal of Neurology, Neurosurgery, and Psychiatry*, *77*(3), 308–316. doi:10.1136/jnnp.2005.072306 PMID:16484637

Scarmeas, N., Levy, G., Tang, M.-X., Manly, J., & Stern, Y. (2001). Influence of leisure activity on the incidence of Alzheimer's disease. *Neurology*, *57*(12), 2236–2242. doi:10.1212/WNL.57.12.2236 PMID:11756603

Scarmeas, N., & Stern, Y. (2004). Cognitive reserve: Implications for diagnosis and prevention of Alzheimer's disease. *Current Neurology and Neuroscience Reports*, *4*(5), 374–380. doi:10.1007/s11910-004-0084-7 PMID:15324603

Scarmeas, N., Stern, Y., Mayeux, R., Manly, J. J., Schupf, N., & Luchsinger, J. A. (2009). Mediterranean diet and mild cognitive impairment. *Archives of Neurology*, *66*(2), 216–225. doi:10.1001/archneurol.2008.536 PMID:19204158

Schaie, K. W. (2008). Historical processes and patterns of cognitive ageing. In S. M. Hofer & D. F. Alwin (Eds.), *Handbook of Cognitive Aging: Interdisciplinary Perspectives* (pp. 368–383). Thousand Oaks, CA: Sage Pub. Inc. doi:10.4135/9781412976589.n23

Schaie, K. W., & Hofer, S. M. (2001). Longitudinal studies in research of ageing. In J. E. Birren & K. W. Schaie (Eds.), *Handbook of the Psychology of ageing* (5th ed., pp. 55–77). San Diego, CA: Academic Press.

Schaie, K. W., & Willis, S. L. (1991). Adult personality and psychomotor performance: Cross-sectional and longitudinal analyses. *Journal of Gerontology*, *46*(6), 275–P284. doi:10.1093/geronj/46.6.P275 PMID:1940082

Scheen, A. J. (2003). Pathophysiology of type 2 diabetes. *Acta Clinica Belgica*, *58*(6), 335–341. doi:10.1179/acb.2003.58.6.001 PMID:15068125

Schellevis, F. G., van der Velden, J., van de Lisdonk, E., van Eijk, J. T., & van Weel, C. (1993). Comorbidity of chronic diseases in general practice. *Journal of Clinical Epidemiology*, *46*(5), 469–473. doi:10.1016/0895-4356(93)90024-U PMID:8501473

Scherder, E. J. A., Bouma, A., & Steen, A. M. (1998). Isolated transcutaneous electrical nerve stimulation in Alzheimer's disease. *Biological Psychiatry*, *43*, 417–424. doi:10.1016/S0006-3223(97)00208-4 PMID:9532346

Scherder, E. J. A., Van Someren, E. J. W., & Swaab, D. F. (1999). Transcutaneous electrical nerve stimulation (TENS) improves the rest–activity rhythm in midstage Alzheimer's disease. *Behavioural Brain Research*, *101*(1), 105–107. doi:10.1016/S0166-4328(98)00150-8 PMID:10342404

Schiavi, R.C., & Rehman. (1995). Sexuality and aging. *The Urologic Clinics of North America*, *22*, 711–726. PMID:7483124

Schiff, B., & Cohler, B. J. (2001). Telling survival backwards: Holocaust survivors narrate the past. In G. M. Kenyon, P. G. Clark, & B. de Vries (Eds.), *Narrative gerontology: Theory research, and practice* (pp. 113–136). New York: Springer.

Schiller, J. S., Lucas, J. W., & Peregoy, J. A. (2012). Summary health statistics for U.S. adults: National health interview survey. *Vital and Health Statistics*, *10*(252), 1–207. PMID:22834228

Schlauch, C. R. (2006). Deeper affinities: Fundamental resonances between psychoanalysis and religion. *Pastoral Psychology*, *55*(1), 61–80. doi:10.1007/s11089-006-0032-3

Schlebusch, L. (2005). *Suicidal behaviour in South Africa*. Pietermaritzburg: University of KwaZulu-Natal Press.

Schneidman, E. (1985). *Definition of Suicide*. New York: John Wiley & Sons Inc.

Schoenberg, M. R., & Scott, J. G. (2011). *The little black book of neuropsychology: A syndrome-based approach*.

Schönknecht, P. (2011). Neurobiological and psychological aspects of mild cognitive impairment Bridging the gap.

Schow, R. L., & Nerbonne, M. A. (1980). Hearing levels among elderly nursing home residents. *The Journal of Speech and Hearing Disorders*, *45*(1), 124–132. doi:10.1044/jshd.4501.124 PMID:7354624

Schram, M. T., Baan, C. A., & Pouwer, F. (2009). Depression and quality of life in patients with diabetes: A systematic review from the European depression in diabetes (EDID) research consortium. *Current Diabetes Reviews*, *5*(2), 112–119. doi:10.2174/157339909788166828 PMID:19442096

Schroder, K., Schwarzer, R., & Endler, N. S. (1997). Predicting cardiac patients' quality of life from the characteristics of their spouses. *Journal of Health Psychology*, *2*(2), 231–244. doi:10.1177/135910539700200219 PMID:22013006

Schroots, J. J. F. (1996). Theoretical Developments in the Psychology of Aging. *The Gerontologist, 36*(6), 742-748. Retrieved from http://gerontologist.oxfordjournals.org/content/36/6/742.full.pdf

Schueller, S. M., & Seligman, M. E. (2010). Pursuit of pleasure, engagement, and meaning: Relationships to subjective and objective measures of well-being. *The Journal of Positive Psychology*, *5*(4), 253–263. doi:10.1080/17439761003794130

Schuessler, W. H. (2013). The *Biochemic Handbook*. CMG Archives. Retrieved from http://www.campbellmgold.com

Schulze, M. B., Rimm, E. B., Li, T., Rifai, N., Stampfer, M. J., & Hu, F. B. (2004). C-reactive protein and incident cardiovascular events among men with diabetes. *Diabetes Care*, *27*(4), 889–894. doi:10.2337/diacare.27.4.889 PMID:15047644

Schure, M. B., Conte, K. P., & Goins, R. T. (2015). Unmet Assistance Need Among Older American Indians: The Native Elder Care Study. *The Gerontologist*, *55*(6), 920–928. doi:10.1093/geront/gnt211 PMID:24451895

Schuster, J. P., Hoertel, N., Le Start, Y., Manetti, A., & Limoson, F. (2013). Personality disorders in older adults: Findings from the National Epidemiological Survey on Alcohol and Related Conditions. *The American Journal of Geriatric Psychiatry*, *21*(8), 757–768. doi:10.1016/j.jagp.2013.01.055 PMID:23567365

Schwartz, A. V., Hillier, T. A., Sellmeyer, D. E., Resnick, H. E., Gregg, E., Ensrud, K. E., ... Cummings, S. R. (2002). Older women with diabetes have a higher risk of falls: A prospective study. *Diabetes Care*, *25*(10), 1749–1754. doi:10.2337/diacare.25.10.1749 PMID:12351472

Schwartz, A. V., Sellmeyer, D. E., Ensrud, K. E., Cauley, J. A., Tabor, H. K., Schreiner, P. J., ... Cummings, S. R. (2001). Older women with diabetes have an increased risk of fracture: A prospective study. *The Journal of Clinical Endocrinology and Metabolism*, *86*(1), 32–38. doi:10.1210/jcem.86.1.7139 PMID:11231974

Schwarzer, R., & Leppin, A. (1992). Possible impact of social ties and support on morbidity and mortality. In H.O.F. Veiel & U. Baumann (Eds.), The meaning and measurement of social support (pp. 65-83). Washington, DC: Hemisphere.

ScienceDaily. (2016). The Endocrine Society: Older overweight and obese adults with diabetes benefit from better diet and exercise. Retrieved July 11, 2017 from www.sciencedaily.com/releases/2016/04/160401130616.htm

Scocco, P., & De Leo, D. (2002). One-year prevalence of death thoughts, suicide ideation and behaviours in an elderly population. *International Journal of Geriatric Psychiatry*, *17*(9), 842–846. doi:10.1002/gps.691 PMID:12221658

Scott, D., & Donnelly, M. (2005). The early identification of cognitive impairment. A stakeholder evaluation of a 'Dementia Awareness Service' in Belfast. *Dementia (London)*, *4*(2), 207–232. doi:10.1177/1471301205051093

Seaberg, E. C., Wiley, D., Martinez-Maza, O., Chmiel, J. S., Kingsley, L., Tang, Y., ... Jacobson, L. P. (2010). Cancer incidence in the multicentre AIDS cohort study before and during HAART era: 1984 to 2007. *Cancer*, *116*(23), 5507–5516. doi:10.1002/cncr.25530 PMID:20672354

Seal, E. C., Metz, J., Flicker, L., & Melny, J. (2002). A randomized, double-blind, placebo-controlled study of oral vitamin B12 supplementation in older patients with subnormal or borderline serum vitamin B12 concentrations. *Journal of the American Geriatrics Society*, *50*(1), 146–151. doi:10.1046/j.1532-5415.2002.50020.x PMID:12028259

Seelye, A. M., Schmitter-Edgecombe, M., & Flores, J. (2010). Episodic memory predictions in persons with amnestic and nonamnestic mild cognitive impairment. *Journal of Clinical and Experimental Neuropsychology*, *32*(4), 433–441. doi:10.1080/13803390903201751 PMID:20397298

Seeman, T. E., & Robbins, R. J. (1994). Aging and hypothalamic-pituitary-adrenal response to challenge in humans. *Endocrine Reviews*, *15*, 233–260. PMID:8026389

Seidel, D., Jagger, C., Brayne, C., Matthews, F. E., & Cfas, M. (2009). Recovery in instrumental activities of daily living (IADLs): Findings from the Medical Research Council Cognitive Function and Ageing Study (MRC CFAS). *Age and Ageing*, *38*(6), 663–668. doi:10.1093/ageing/afp128 PMID:19633320

Seifert, L. S. (2002). Toward a psychology of religion, spirituality, meaning-search, and aging: Past research and a practical application. *Journal of Adult Development*, *9*(1), 61–70. doi:10.1023/A:1013829318213

Seinfeld, S., Figueroa, H., Ortiz-Gil, J., & Sanchez-Vives, M. V. (2013). Effects of music learning and piano practice on cognitive function, mood and quality of life in older adults. *Frontiers in Psychology*, *4*, 810. doi:10.3389/fpsyg.2013.00810 PMID:24198804

Seligman, M. E. (2004). *Authentic Happiness: Using the New Positive Psychology to Realize Your Potential for Lasting Fulfillment*. New York: The Free Press.

Seligman, M. E. P. (2002). *Authentic happiness: using the new positive psychology to realize your potential for lasting fulfillment*. New York: Free Press.

Seligman, M. E. P., Steen, T. A., Park, N., & Peterson, C. (2005). Positive psychology progress -Empirical validation of interventions. *The American Psychologist*, *60*(5), 410–421. doi:10.1037/0003-066X.60.5.410 PMID:16045394

Seligman, M. E., Rashid, T., & Parks, A. C. (2006). Positive psychotherapy. *The American Psychologist*, *61*(8), 774–788. doi:10.1037/0003-066X.61.8.774 PMID:17115810

Sethi, B. B., & Trivedi, J. K. (1979). Drug abuse in rural population. *Indian Journal of Psychiatry*, *21*, 211–216.

Seuring, T., Archangelidi, O., & Suhrcke, M. (2015). The economic costs of type 2 diabetes: A global systematic review. *PharmacoEconomics*, *33*(8), 811–831. doi:10.1007/s40273-015-0268-9 PMID:25787932

Shah, A. S., Lee, K. K., McAllister, D. A., Hunter, A., Nair, H., Whiteley, W., & Mills, N. L. (2015). Short term exposure to air pollution and stroke: systematic review and meta-analysis. *BMJ*, 24 350. PMID:25633926

Shah, K., Stufflebam, A., Hilton, T. N., Sinacore, D. R., Klein, S., & Villareal, D. T. (2009). Diet and exercise interventions reduce intrahepatic fat content and improve insulin sensitivity in obese older adults. *Obesity (Silver Spring, Md.)*, *17*(12), 2162–2168. doi:10.1038/oby.2009.126 PMID:19390517

Shahrawat, R., & Rao, K. D. (2011). Insured yet vulnerable: Out-of-pocket payments and India's poor. *Health Policy and Planning*, czr029. PMID:21486910

Shankar, R., & Tondon, J. (2006). Health status of elderly population in rural area of Varanasi district. *Indian Journal of Public Health*, *51*(1), 56–58. PMID:18232146

Shaw, A. C., Goldstein, D. R., & Montgomery, R. R. (2013). Age-dependent dysregulation of innate immunity. *Nature Reviews. Immunology*, *13*(12), 875–887. doi:10.1038/nri3547 PMID:24157572

Sheldrake, P. (1992). *Spirituality and History: Christian living and the Doctrine of God*. New York: Marykmoll.

Shelly, J. A., & Fish, S. (1988). *Spiritual care: The nurse's role*. Inter Varsity Press.

Shelton, P. S. (2002). Disease management programs. *Disease Management & Health Outcomes*, *10*(8), 461–467. doi:10.2165/00115677-200210080-00001

Shenkin, S. D., Bastin, M. E., Macgillivray, T. J., Deary, I. J., Starr, J. M., & Wardlaw, J. M. (2009). Birth parameters are associated with late-life white matter integrity in community-dwelling older people. *Stroke*, *40*(4), 1225–1228. doi:10.1161/STROKEAHA.108.527259 PMID:19213950

Sherr, C. J., & Roberts, J. M. (1995). Inhibitors of mammalian G1 cyclin-dependent kinases. *Genes & Development*, *9*(10), 1149–1163. doi:10.1101/gad.9.10.1149 PMID:7758941

Sheshadri, S., Beiser, A., Kelly-Hayes, M., Kase, C. S., Au, R., Kannel, W. B., & Wolf, P. A. (2008). The lifetime risk of stroke: Estimates from the Framingham Study. *Stroke*, *37*(2), 345–350. doi:10.1161/01.STR.0000199613.38911.b2 PMID:16397184

Shettar, S. C. (2013). Problems of Aged in Changing Indian Scenario. Retrieved May 21, 2017 from http://yojana.gov.in/problems-of-aged.asp

Shibamoto, K., Mochizuki, M., & Kusuhara, M. (2010). Aroma Therapy in Anti-Aging Medicine. *Anti-Aging Medicine*, *7*(6), 55–59. doi:10.3793/jaam.7.55

Shields, G. C., King, D. A., & Wynne, L. C. (1995). Interventions with later life families. In R. H. Mikesell, D. Lusterman, & S. H. McDaniel (Eds.), *Integrating family therapy: Handbook of family psychology and systems theory* (pp. 141–158). Washington, DC: American Psychological Association. doi:10.1037/10172-008

Shilling, D. (2008). Improving the court system's response to elder abuse. *Victimization of the Elderly and Disabled, 11*, 49, 51-52, 59, 62-63.

Shimoni, Y., & Severson, D. L. (1995). Thyroid status and potassium currents in rat ventricular myocytes. *The American Journal of Physiology, 268*, H576–H583. PMID:7864182

Shukla, P. (2015). Spirituality and positive view of ageing in modern society. *Indian Journal of Positive Psychology, 6*(1), 122–126.

Simoni-Wastila, L., & Yang, H. K. (2006). Psychoactive drug abuse in older adults. *The American Journal of Geriatric Pharmacotherapy, 4*(4), 380–394. doi:10.1016/j.amjopharm.2006.10.002 PMID:17296542

Simon, N. M., Otto, M. W., & Wisniewsk, S. R. (2004). Anxiety disorder comorbidity in bipolar patients: Data from the first 500 participants in the Systematic Treatment Enhancement Program for Bipolar Disorder (STEP-BO). *The American Journal of Psychiatry, 161*(12), 2222–2229. doi:10.1176/appi.ajp.161.12.2222 PMID:15569893

Simpson, M. E., & Conklin, G. H. (1989). Socioeconomic Development, Suicide and Religion: A Test of Durkheim's Theory of Religion and Suicide. *Social Forces, 67*(4), 945–964. doi:10.1093/sf/67.4.945

Simpson, R. J., Lowder, T. W., Spielmann, G., Bigley, A. B., LaVoy, E., & Kunz, H. (2012). Exercise and the aging immune system. *Aging Research Review, 11*(3), 404–420. doi:10.1016/j.arr.2012.03.003 PMID:22465452

Singer, S., Das-Munshi, J., & Brahler, E. (2010). Prevalence of mental health conditions in cancer patients in acute care—a meta-analysis. *Annals of Oncology: Official Journal of the European Society for Medical Oncology, 21*(5), 925–930. doi:10.1093/annonc/mdp515 PMID:19887467

Singh, A. P., Kumar, K. L., & Reddy, C. P. (2012). Psychiatric morbidity in geriatric population in old age homes and community: A comparative study. *Indian Journal of Psychological Medicine, 34*(1), 39–43. doi:10.4103/0253-7176.96157 PMID:22661806

Singh, B., Parsaik, A. K., Mielke, M. M., Erwin, P. J., Knopman, D. S., Petersen, R. C., & Roberts, R. O. (2014). Association of Mediterranean diet with Mild Cognitive Impairment and Alzheimer's disease: A Systematic Review and Meta-Analysis. *Journal of Alzheimer's Disease, 39*(2), 271–282. PMID:24164735

Singh, J. G., Singh, S., & Dawara, V. (1983). Adjustment problem of old people. *Indian Journal of Clinical Psychology, 10*, 127–131.

Singh-Manoux, A., Kivimaki, M., Glymour, M. M., Elbaz, A., Berr, C., Ebmeier, K. P., ... Dugravot, A. (2012). Timing of onset of cognitive decline: Results from Whitehall II prospective cohort study. *BMJ (Clinical Research Ed.), 344*, d7622. doi:10.1136/bmj.d7622 PMID:22223828

Sin, N. L., & Lyubomirsky, S. (2009). Enhancing well-being and alleviating depressive symptoms with positive psychology interventions: A practice-friendly meta-analysis. *Journal of Clinical Psychology, 65*(5), 467–487. doi:10.1002/jclp.20593 PMID:19301241

Sivertsen, H., Bjorklof, G. H., Engedal, K., Selbaek, G., & Helvik, A. S. (2015). Depression and quality of life in older persons: A review. *Dementia Gereatria Cognition Disorder, 40*, 5–6. PMID:26360014

Sjöström, L., Peltonen, M., Jacobson, P., Sjöström, C. D., Karason, K., Wedel, H., & Bouchard, C. (2012). Bariatric surgery and long-term cardiovascular events. *Journal of the American Medical Association, 307*(1), 56–65. doi:10.1001/jama.2011.1914 PMID:22215166

Skaff, M. M. (2007). Sense of control and health: A dynamic duo in the aging process. In C. M. Aldwin, C. L. Park, & A. Spiro (Eds.), *Handbook of health psychology and aging* (pp. 186–209). New York: Guilford.

Skinner, T. R., Scott, I. A., & Martin, J. H. (2016). Diagnostic errors in older patients: A systematic review of incidence and potential causes in seven prevalent diseases. *International Journal of General Medicine, 9*, 137–146. doi:10.2147/IJGM.S96741 PMID:27284262

Skoog, I., Aevarsson, Ó., Beskow, J., Larsson, L., Palsson, S., Waern, M., ... Östling, S. (1996). Suicidal feelings in a population sample of nondemented 85-year-olds. *The American Journal of Psychiatry, 153*(8), 1015–1020. doi:10.1176/ajp.153.8.1015 PMID:8678169

Slater, C. L. (2003). Generativity versus stagnation: An elaboration of Erikson's adult stage of human development. *Journal of Adult Development, 10*(1), 53–65. doi:10.1023/A:1020790820868

Slinin, Y., Paudel, M. L., Taylor, B. C., Fink, H. A., Ishani, A., Canales, M. T., … Osteoporotic Fractures in Men (MrOS) Study Research Group. (2010). 25-Hydroxyvitamin D levels and cognitive performance and decline in elderly men. *Neurology, 74*(1), 33–41.

Sloane, P. D., Zimmermanm, S. Z., Suchindran, C., Reed, P., Wang, L., & Boustani, M. (2002). The public health impact of Alzheimer's disease, implication of treatment advances. *Annual Review of Public Health, 23*, 213–231. doi:10.1146/annurev.publhealth.23.100901.140525 PMID:11910061

Smith, G., Del Sala, S., Logie, R. H., & Maylor, E. A. (2000). Prospective and retrospective memory in normal ageing and dementia: A questionnaire study. *Memory (Hove, England), 8*(5), 311–321. doi:10.1080/09658210050117735 PMID:11045239

Smith, M. T., Perlis, M. L., & Chengazi, V. U. (2002). Neuroimaging of NREM sleep in primary insomnia: A Tc-99-HMPAO single photon emission computed tomography study. *Sleep, 25*, 325–335. PMID:12003163

Smoking and Heart Health. (2014). Centre for disease control prevention office on smoking and health. Retrieved 05.10.2017 from https://www.cdc.gov/tobacco/data_statistics/sgr/50thanniversary/pdfs/fs_smoking_CVD_508.pdf

Sodestrom, K. E., & Martinson, I. M. (1987). Patients' spiritual coping strategies: A study of nurse and patient perspectives. *Oncology Nursing Forum, 14*(2), 41–46. PMID:3644298

Sofi, F., Valecchi, D., Bacci, D., Abbate, R., Gensini, G. F., Casini, A., & Macchi, C. (2011). Physical activity and risk of cognitive decline: A meta-analysis of prospective studies. *Journal of Internal Medicine, 269*(1), 107–117. doi:10.1111/j.1365-2796.2010.02281.x PMID:20831630

Solenkova, N. V., Newman, J. D., Berger, J. S., Thurston, G., Hochman, J. S., & Lamas, G. A. (2014). Metal pollutants and cardiovascular disease: Mechanisms and consequences of exposure. *American Heart Journal, 168*(6), 812–822. doi:10.1016/j.ahj.2014.07.007 PMID:25458643

Solfrizzi, V., Capurso, C., Introno, A., D', , Colacicco, A. M., Santamato, A., & Ranieri, M. (2008). Lifestyle-related factors in predementia and dementia syndromes. *Expert Review of Neurotherapeutics, 8*(1), 133–158. doi:10.1586/14737175.8.1.133 PMID:18088206

Sommaruga, M., Tramarin, R., Angelino, E., Bettinardi, O., & Cauteruccio, M. A. (2003). Guidelines on psychological intervention in cardiac rehabilitation- methodological process. *Monaldi Archives for Chest Disease*, *60*, 40–44. PMID:12827831

Sonnen, J. A., Larson, E. B., Brickell, K., Crane, P. K., Woltjer, R., Montine, T. J., & Craft, S. (2009). Different patterns of cerebral injury in dementia with or without diabetes. *Archives of Neurology*, *66*(3), 315–322. doi:10.1001/archneurol.2008.579 PMID:19139294

Sood, R. (2000). The problem of geriatric tuberculosis. *Journal of Indian Academy of Clinical Medicine*, *5*, 157.

Sopori, M. L., Kozak, W., Savage, S. M., Geng, Y., & Kluger, M. J. (1998). Nicotine-induced modulation of T Cell function. Implications for inflammation and infection. *Advances in Experimental Medicine and Biology*, *437*, 279–289. doi:10.1007/978-1-4615-5347-2_31 PMID:9666281

Sotozaki, K. (2008). 'Fragrance' and 'healing' into the life. [in Japanese]. *Journal of Japanese Society of Aromatherapy*, *7*, 33–00.

Spaargaren, G., & VanVliet, B. (2000). Lifestyle, Consumption and the Environment: The Ecological Modernisation of Domestic Consumption. *Environmental Politics*, *9*(1), 50–75.

Spandau, U. H. M., & Rohrschneider, K. (2002). Prevalence and geographical distribution of Usher syndrome in Germany. Graefe's archive for clinical and experimental ophthalmology. *Graefes Archive for Clinical and Experimental Ophthalmology*, *240*(6), 495–498. doi:10.1007/s00417-002-0485-8

Spiegel, D. (2002). Cancer Patients: Psychotherapy. In M. Hersen & W. Sledge (Eds.), Encyclopedia of Psychotherapy (1st ed., pp. 359-364). USA: Elsevier Science, Academic Press.

Spiegel, D., Bloom, J. R., & Yalom, I. (1981). Group Support for Patients With Metastatic Cancer A Randomized Prospective Outcome Study. *Archives of General Psychiatry*, *38*(5), 527–533. doi:10.1001/archpsyc.1980.01780300039004 PMID:7235853

Spielman, A., Caruso, L., & Glovinsky, P. (1987). A behavioral perspective on insomnia treatment. *The Psychiatric Clinics of North America*, *10*, 541–553. PMID:3332317

Spijkerman, A. M., Dekker, J. M., Nijpels, G., Jager, A., Kostense, P. J., van Hinsbergh, V. W. M., ... Stehouwer, C. D. A. (2002). Impact of diabetes duration and cardiovascular risk factors on mortality in type 2 diabetes: The Hoorn Study. *European Journal of Clinical Investigation*, *32*(12), 924–930. doi:10.1046/j.1365-2362.2002.01090.x PMID:12534452

Spilka, B. (1993). Spirituality: Problems and directions in operationalizing a fuzzy concept. In *Proceedings of the annual meeting of the American Psychological Association*, Toronto.

Spilka, B., & McIntosh, D. N. (1996). Religion and spirituality: The known and the unknown. *What is the difference between religion and spirituality.*

Sprangers, M. A., Cull, A., Bjordal, K., Groenvold, M., & Aaronson, N. K. (1993). The European Organization for Research and Treatment of Cancer. Approach to quality of life assessment: Guidelines for developing questionnaire modules. EORTC Study Group on Quality of Life. *Quality of Life Research: An International Journal of Quality of Life Aspects of Treatment, Care and Rehabilitation*, *2*(4), 287–295. doi:10.1007/BF00434800 PMID:8220363

Srinivasan, K., Vaz, M., & Thomas, T. (2010). Prevalence of health related disability among community dwelling urban elderly from middle socioeconomic strata in Bangaluru, India. *The Indian Journal of Medical Research*, *131*, 515–521. PMID:20424302

Srinivasan, T., & Hannah, P. P. (2012). Bidirectional communication between the neuroendocrine system and the immune system: Relevance to health and diseases. *Annals of Neurosciences*, *19*(1), 40–46. PMID:25205962

Srivastava, S., & Kulshreshtha, N. (2000). Expression of suicidal intent in depressives. *Indian Journal of Psychiatry*, *42*, 184–187. PMID:21407933

Staffurth, J. S., Gibberd, J. S., & Tang, F. S. (1977). Arterial embolism in thyrotoxicosis with atrial fibrillation. *British Medical Journal*, *2*(6088), 688–690. doi:10.1136/bmj.2.6088.688 PMID:902055

Stahel, A. (n.d.). Healing Cancer Naturally. German New Medicine: A Revolutionary Biological Paradigm. Retrieved from http://www.healingcancernaturally.com/hamer-new-medicine-interpretation-part2.html

Stanley, I. H., Hom, M. A., Rogers, M. L., Hagan, C. R., & Joiner, T. E. Jr. (2016). Understanding suicide among older adults: A review of psychological and sociological theories of suicide. *Aging & Mental Health*, *20*(2), 113–122. doi:10.1080/13607863.2015.1012045 PMID:25693646

Starfield, B. (2007). Pathways of influence on equity in health. *Social Science & Medicine*, *64*(7), 1355–1362. doi:10.1016/j.socscimed.2006.11.027 PMID:17208343

Stefanacci, R. G., Reich, S., & Casiano, A. (2015). Application of PACE principles for population health management of frail older adults. *Population Health Management*, *18*(5), 367–372. doi:10.1089/pop.2014.0096 PMID:25647691

Steiner, V. A. G., Mansur, L. L., Brucki, S. M., & Nitrini, R. (2008). Phonemic verbal fluency and age: A preliminary study. *Dementia & Neuropsychologia*, *2*(4), 328–332. doi:10.1590/S1980-57642009DN20400017

Steinsbekk, A., Rygg, L., Lisulo, M., Rise, M. B., & Fretheim, A. (2012). Group based diabetes self-management education compared to routine treatment for people with type 2 diabetes mellitus. A systematic review with meta-analysis. *BMC Health Services Research*, *12*(1), 213. doi:10.1186/1472-6963-12-213 PMID:22824531

Stepanski, E. J. (2000). Behavioral therapy for insomnia. In M. H. Kryger, T. G. Roth, & W. C. Dement (Eds.), *Principles and Practice of Sleep Medicine* (pp. 647–656). Philadelphia: WB Saunders.

Stephen, J. M. (2012). *Current medical diagnosis & treatment 2012* (p. 430). New York: McGraw-Hill Medical.

Steptoe, A., Demakakos, P., De Oliveira, C., & Wardle, J. (2012). Distinctive biological correlates of positive psychological well-being in older men and women. *Psychosomatic Medicine*, *74*(5), 501–508. doi:10.1097/PSY.0b013e31824f82c8 PMID:22511728

Steptoe, A., O'Donnell, K., Badrick, E., Kumari, M., & Marmot, M. G. (2008). Neuroendocrine and inflammatory factors associated with positive affect in healthy men and women: Whitehall II study. *American Journal of Epidemiology*, *167*(1), 96–102. doi:10.1093/aje/kwm252 PMID:17916595

Steptoe, A., Wardle, J., & Marmot, M. (2005). Positive affect and health-related neuroendocrine, cardiovascular, and inflammatory processes. *Proceeding of the National Academy of Science United States of America*, *102*, 6508–6512. doi:10.1073/pnas.0409174102

Stern, Y., Albert, S., Tang, M.-X., & Tsai, W.-Y. (1999). Rate of memory decline in AD is related to education and occupation: Cognitive reserve? *Neurology*, *53*(9), 1942–1947. doi:10.1212/WNL.53.9.1942 PMID:10599762

Steunenberg, B., Beekman, A. T., Deeg, D. J., & Kerkhof, A. J. (2006). Personality and the onset of depression in late life. *Journal of Affective Disorders*, *92*(2-3), 243–251. doi:10.1016/j.jad.2006.02.003 PMID:16545466

Stevens, J. (2000). Impact of age on association between weight & mortality. *Nutrition Reviews*, *58*(5), 129–137. doi:10.1111/j.1753-4887.2000.tb01847.x PMID:10860392

Stoll, R. I. (1979). Guidelines for spiritual assessment. *AJN The American Journal of Nursing*, *79*(9), 1574–1577. PMID:258568

Stramba-Badiale, M., Fox, K. M., Priori, S. G., Collins, P., & Daly, C. (2006). Cardiovasculardiseases in women: A statement from the policy conference of the European Society ofCardiology. *European Heart Journal*, *27*(8), 994–1005. doi:10.1093/eurheartj/ehi819 PMID:16522654

Strang, S., & Strang, P. (2002). Questions posed to hospital chaplains by palliative care patients. *Journal of Palliative Medicine*, *5*(6), 857–864. doi:10.1089/10966210260499041 PMID:12685532

Strauss, E., Sherman, E. M. S., & Spreen, O. A. (2006). *Compendium of Neuropsychological Tests: Administration, norms, and commentary* (3rd ed.). Oxford: Oxford University Press.

Strawbridge, W. J., Wallhagen, M. I., Shema, S. J., & Kaplan, G. A. (2000). Negative consequences of hearing impairment in old age: A longitudinal analysis. *The Gerontologist*, *40*(3), 320–326. doi:10.1093/geront/40.3.320 PMID:10853526

Strecker, R. E., Morairty, S., Thakkar, M. M., Porkka-Heiskanen, T., Basheer, R., Dauphin, L. J., ... McCarley, R. W. (2000). Adenosinergic modulation of basal forebrain and preoptic/anterior hypothalamic neuronal activity in the control of behavioral state. *Behavioural Brain Research*, *115*(2), 183–204. doi:10.1016/S0166-4328(00)00258-8 PMID:11000420

Streiner, D. L., Chairney, J., & Veldhuizen, S. (2006). The epidemiology of psychological problems in the elderly. *Canadian Journal of Psychiatry*, *51*(3), 185–191. doi:10.1177/070674370605100309 PMID:16618010

Strotmeye, E. S., Cauley, J. A., Schwartz, A. V., Nevitt, M. C., Resnick, H. E., Bauer, D. C., ... Newman, A. B. (2005). Nontraumatic fracture risk with diabetes mellitus and impaired fasting glucose in older white and black adults: The health, aging, and body composition study. *Achieves International Medicine*, *165*(14), 1612–1617. doi:10.1001/archinte.165.14.1612 PMID:16043679

Subak, L. L., Wing, R., West, D. S., Franklin, F., Vittinghoff, E., Creasman, J. M., ... Macer, J. (2009). Weight loss to treat urinary incontinence in overweight and obese women. *The New England Journal of Medicine*, *360*(5), 481–490. doi:10.1056/NEJMoa0806375 PMID:19179316

Substance Abuse and Mental Health Services Administration, Office of Applied Studies. (2011). *Treatment Episode Data Set (TEDS), 1999-2009. DASIS Series: S-56, HHS Publication No. SMA 11-4646.* Rockville, MD: Substance Abuse and Mental Health Services Administration.

Substance Abuse and Mental Health Services Administration. (2012). *Results From the 2011 National Survey on Drug Use and Health: Summary of National Findings.* NSDUH Series H-44, HHS Publication No. (SMA) 12-4713. Rockville, MD: Substance Abuse and Mental Health Services Administration, The Center for Disease Control and Prevention. Medication Safety. Retrieved from http://www.cdc.gov/medicationsafety/

Suessenbacher, A., Potocnik, M., Dorler, J., Fluckinger, G., Wanitschek, M., Pachinger, O., ... Alber, H. F. (2011). Comparison of peripheral endothelial function in shift versus nonshift workers. *The American Journal of Cardiology*, *107*(6), 945–948. doi:10.1016/j.amjcard.2010.10.077 PMID:21247546

Sugisawa, A., Hidehiro, S., Yomeni, N., & Hiroshi, S. (1997). Effect of retirement on mental health and social wellbeing among elderly Japanese. *Japanese Journal of Public Health*, *44*(2), 123–130. PMID:9130849

Sullivan, P. W., Morrato, E. H., Ghushchyan, V., Wyatt, H. R., & Hill, J. O. (2005). Obesity, inactivity, and the prevalence of diabetes and diabetes-related cardiovascular comorbidities in the U.S., 2000–2002. *Diabetes Care*, *28*(7), 1599–1603. doi:10.2337/diacare.28.7.1599 PMID:15983307

Sun, J., Kale, S. P., Childress, A. M., Pinswasdi, C., & Jazwinski, S. M. (1994). Divergent roles of RAS1 and RAS2 in yeast longevity. *The Journal of Biological Chemistry*, *269*, 18638–18645. PMID:8034612

Sun, Z. (2015). Aging, arterial stiffness, and hypertension. *Hypertension*, *65*(2), 252–256. doi:10.1161/HYPERTENSIONAHA.114.03617 PMID:25368028

Surks, M. I., & Boucai, L. (2010). Age- and race-based serum thyrotropin reference limits. *The Journal of Clinical Endocrinology and Metabolism*, *95*(2), 496–502. doi:10.1210/jc.2009-1845 PMID:19965925

Surks, M. I., & Hollowell, J. G. (2007). Age-specific distribution of serum thyrotropin and antithyroid antibodies in the US population: Implications for the prevalence of subclinical hypothyroidism. *The Journal of Clinical Endocrinology and Metabolism*, *92*(12), 4575–4582. doi:10.1210/jc.2007-1499 PMID:17911171

Surks, M. I., Ortiz, E., Daniels, G. H., Sawin, C. T., Col, N. F., Cobin, R. H., ... Weissman, N. J. (2004). Subclinical thyroid disease: Scientific review and guidelines for diagnosis and management. *Journal of the American Medical Association*, *291*(2), 228–238. doi:10.1001/jama.291.2.228 PMID:14722150

Susan, K. R., & Israel, S. A. (2010). Sleep Disorders in the Elderly. *The Indian Journal of Medical Research*, *131*, 302–310. PMID:20308755

Svansdottir, H. B., & Snaedal, J. (2006). Music therapy in moderate and severe dementia of Alzheimer's type: A case-control study. *International Psychogeriatrics*, *18*(04), 613–621. doi:10.1017/S1041610206003206 PMID:16618375

Svare, S., Nilsen, T. I. L., Bjoro, T., Forsmo, S., Schei, B., & Langhammer, A. (2009). Hyperthyroid levels of TSH correlate with low bone mineral density: The HUNT 2 study. *European Journal of Endocrinology*, *161*(5), 779–786. doi:10.1530/EJE-09-0139 PMID:19671706

Swaab, D. F. (1999). Biological rhythms in health and disease: the suprachiasmatic nucleus and the autonomous system. In P.J. Vinken and G.W. Bruyn, O. Appenzeller (Eds.), Handbook of Clinical Neurology (pp. 467–521). Amsterdam: Elsevier.

Swaab, D. F. (1991). Brain aging and Alzheimer's disease: 'wear and tear' versus 'use it or lose it'. *Neurobiology of Aging*, *12*(4), 317–324. doi:10.1016/0197-4580(91)90008-8 PMID:1755879

Swaab, D. F., Lucassen, P. J., Salehi, A., Scherder, E. J. A., Van Someren, E. J. W., & Verwer, R. W. H. (1998). Reduced neuronal activity and reactivation in Alzheimer's disease. In J. Verhaagen, F. W. Van Leeuwen, & A. Salehi et al. (Eds.), Progress in Brain Research (pp. 343–377). Amsterdam: *Elsevier*. doi:10.1016/S0924-977X(98)80078-3

Swain, L. (2015). Human reproductive biology: Changes through life. In Developmental perspectives on human sexuality (pp. 29-34) Bhubaneshwar: Indian Institute of Sexology.

Swami, H. M., Bhatia, V., Dutt, R., & Bhatia, S. P. (2002). A community based study of the morbidity profile among the elderly in Chandigarh, India. *Bahrain Medical Bulletin*, *24*, 13–16.

Swami, H. M., Bhatia, V., Gupta, A. K., & Bhatia, S. P. S. (2005). An epidemiological study of obesity among elderly in Chandigarh. *Indian Journal of Community Medicine*, *30*(3), 255–258.

Swedish National Institute of Public Health (SNIPH). (2007). Healthy Ageing, A Challenge for Europe. Retrieved from www.healthyageing.eu)

Sweeney, C., Blair, C. K., Anderson, K. E., Lazovich, D., & Folsom, A. R. (2004). Risk factors for breast cancer in elderly women. *American Journal of Epidemiology*, *160*(9), 868–875. doi:10.1093/aje/kwh276 PMID:15496539

Swenor, B. K., Ramulu, P. Y., Willis, J. R., Friedman, D., & Lin, F. R. (2013). The prevalence of concurrent hearing and vision impairment in the United States. Investigative Ophthalmology and Visual Science, 54(12), 7683-7690.

Swinton, J. (2001). *Spirituality and mental health care: Rediscovering a 'forgotten' dimension*. Jessica Kingsley Publishers.

Szewczyk-Krolikowski, K., Tomlinson, P., Nithi, K., Wade-Martins, R., Talbot, K., Ben-Shlomo, Y., & Hu, M. T. M. (2014). The influence of age and gender on motorand non-motor features of early Parkinson's disease: Initial findings from the Oxford Parkinson Disease Center (OPDC) discovery cohort. *Parkinsonism & Related Disorders*, *20*(1), 99–105. doi:10.1016/j.parkreldis.2013.09.025 PMID:24183678

Tailor, A., & Gosney, M. A. (2011). Sexuality in older age: Essential considerations for health care professionals. *Age and Ageing*, *40*(5), 538–543. doi:10.1093/ageing/afr049 PMID:21778176

Talbot, F., & Nouwen, A. (2000). A review of the relationship between depression and diabetes in adults: Is there a link? *Diabetes Care*, *23*(10), 1556–1562. doi:10.2337/diacare.23.10.1556 PMID:11023152

Taler, V., & Phillips, N. A. (2008). Language performance in Alzheimer's disease and mild cognitive impairment: A comparative review. *Journal of Clinical and Experimental Neuropsychology*, *30*(5), 501–556. doi:10.1080/13803390701550128 PMID:18569251

Talwar, P., Sinha, J., Grover, S., Rawat, C., Kushwaha, S., Agarwal, R., & Taneja, V. (2015). *Dissecting complex and multifactorial nature of Alzheimer's disease pathogenesis: A clinical, genomic, and systems biology perspective*. Academic Press.

Tam, C. W. C., & Chiu, H. F. K. (2011). Depression and suicide in the elderly. *Zeitschrift für Gerontologie*, *16*(9), 13–16.

Tang, M. X., Jacobs, D., Stern, Y., Marder, K., Schofield, P., Surland, B., ... Mayeux, R. (1996). Effect of estrogen during menopause on risk and age of onset of Alzheimer's disease. *Lance*, *348*(9025), 429–432. doi:10.1016/S0140-6736(96)03356-9 PMID:8709781

Tang-Wai, D. F., Knopman, D. S., Geda, Y. E., Edland, S. D., Smith, G. E., Ivnik, R. J., ... Petersen, R. C. (2003). Comparison of the short test of mental status and the mini-mental state examination in mild cognitive impairment. *Archives of Neurology*, *60*(12), 1777–1781. doi:10.1001/archneur.60.12.1777 PMID:14676056

Taphoorn, M. J., Sizoo, E. M., & Bottomley, A. (2015). Review on quality of life issues in patients with primary brain tumors. *The Oncologist*, *15*(6), 618–626. doi:10.1634/theoncologist.2009-0291 PMID:20507891

Tart, C. T. (1983). Information acquisition rates in forced-choice ESP experiments: Precognition does not work as well as present-time ESP. *Journal of the American Society for Psychical Research*, *77*, 293–310.

Taylor, D., Gehrman, P., Dautovich, N. D., Lichstein, K. L., & McCrae, C. S. (2014). Causes of Insomnia. In Handbook of insomnia. Springer Healthcare Communitation. DOI. doi:10.1007/978-1-907673-73-3-2

Taylor, P. R., Reid, M. M., & Stark, A. N. (1995). *De novo* acute myeloid leukaemia in patients over 55-years-old: A population-based study of incidence, treatment and outcome. *Leukemia*, *9*, 231–237. PMID:7532766

Taylor, T. N., Munoz-Plaza, C. E., Goparaju, L., Martinez, O., Holman, S., Minkoff, H. L., ... Wilson, T. E. (2016). The Pleasure Is Better as I've Gotten Older": Sexual Health, Sexuality, and Sexual Risk Behaviors Among Older Women Living With HIV. *Archives of Sexual Behavior*. PMID:27220311

Teachman, B. A., Siedlecki, K. L., & Magee, J. C. (2007). Aging and symptoms of anxiety and depression: Structural invariance of the tripartite model. *Psychology and Aging*, *22*(1), 160–170. doi:10.1037/0882-7974.22.1.160 PMID:17385992

Tekkalaki, B. (2015). Issues of sexuality in geriatric population. In Developmental perspectives on human sexuality (pp. 36-43) Bhubaneshwar: Indian Institute of Sexology.

Tellez-Plaza, M., Jones, M. R., Dominguez-Lucas, A., Guallar, E., & Navas-Acien, A. (2013). Cadmium exposure and clinical cardiovascular disease: A systematic review. *Current Atherosclerosis Reports*, *15*(10), 356. doi:10.1007/s11883-013-0356-2 PMID:23955722

Teng, E., Tassniyom, K., & Lu, P. H. (2012). Reduced quality-of-life ratings in mild cognitive impairment: Analyses of subject and informant responses. *The American Journal of Geriatric Psychiatry*, *20*(12), 1016–1025. doi:10.1097/JGP.0b013e31826ce640 PMID:23018474

Tepper, L., Rogers, S. A., Coleman, E. M., & Malony, H. N. (2001). The prevalence of religious coping among persons with persistent mental illness. *Psychiatric Services (Washington, D.C.)*, *52*(5), 660–665. doi:10.1176/appi.ps.52.5.660 PMID:11331802

Thal, L. J., Ferris, S. H., Kirby, L., Block, G. A., Lines, C. R., Yuen, E., ... Reines, S. A. (2005). A randomized, double-blind study of rofecoxib in patients with mild cognitive impairment. *Neuropsychopharmacology*, *30*(6), 1204–1215. doi:10.1038/sj.npp.1300690 PMID:15742005

Thapliyal, G., Halder, S., & Mahato, A. (2016). Memory, verbal fluency and response inhibition in normal aging. *Journal of Geriatric Mental Health*, *3*(2), 145–149. doi:10.4103/2348-9995.195636

Thatcher, A. (1991). A critique of inwardness in religious education. *British Journal of Religious Education*, *14*(1), 22–27. doi:10.1080/0141620910140105

Thaut, M. H. (2005). *Rhythm, music and the brain: scientific foundations and clinical applications*. New York: Routledge.

The American Speech-Language-Hearing Association. (ASHA) (2016). Hearing Screening. Retrieved from http://www.eventsinamerica.com/events/2016-asha-convention-american-speech-language-hearing-association/ev51362a573a0ed/

The human brain: From neurons to nervous system (n.d) Sleep Disorder (online image) Retrived 27 August, 2017 from neurons co.uk/Neurosciences/Chapter/%206/P.6%20Sleep%20 Disorders.html.

The ICD-10 Classification of Mental and Behavioural Disorders. (n.d.). *Clinical descriptions and diagnostic guidelines*. World Health Organization.

Theis, W., & Bleiler, L. (2013). Alzheimer's association: Alzheimer's disease facts and figures. *Alzheimer's & Dementia*, *9*(2), 208–245. PMID:23507120

Thoits, P. A. (2006). Personal agency in the stress process. *Journal of Health and Social Behavior*, *47*(4), 309–323. doi:10.1177/002214650604700401 PMID:17240922

Thomas, F. B., Mazzaferri, E. L., & Skillman, T. G. (1970). Apathetic thyrotoxicosis: A distinctive clinical and laboratory entity. *Annals of Internal Medicine*, *72*(5), 679–685. doi:10.7326/0003-4819-72-5-679 PMID:4194420

Thomas, K. S., Baier, R., Kosar, C., Ogarek, J., Trepman, A., & Mor, V. (2017). Individualized Music Program is Associated with Improved Outcomes for U.S. Nursing Home Residents with Dementia. *The American Journal of Geriatric Psychiatry*, *25*(9), 931–938. doi:10.1016/j.jagp.2017.04.008 PMID:28483436

Thomas, P. A. (2011). Trajectories of social engagement and limitations in late life. *Journal of Health and Social Behavior*, *52*(4), 430–443. doi:10.1177/0022146511411922 PMID:22144732

Thomas, R. J., & King, M. (2010). Writing Committee to Develop Clinical Performance Measures for Cardiac Rehabilitation. AACVPR/ACCF/AHA 2010 update. *Circulation*, *122*, 1342–1350. doi:10.1161/CIR.0b013e3181f5185b PMID:20805435

Thomas, T. Y., & Rajagopalan, S. (2001). Tuberculosis and aging: A global health problem. *Clinical Infectious Diseases*, *33*(7), 1034–1039. doi:10.1086/322671 PMID:11528577

Thoresen, C. E. (1999). Spirituality and health: Is there a relationship? *Journal of Health Psychology*, *4*(3), 291–300. doi:10.1177/135910539900400314 PMID:22021598

Timonen, M., Viilo, K., Väisänen, E., Räsänen, P., Hakko, H., & Särkioja, T. (2002). Burden of illness and suicide in elderly people. *BMJ: British Medical Journal*, *325*(7361), 441. doi:10.1136/bmj.325.7361.441/a PMID:12193366

Tison, F., Mons, N., Geffard, M., & Henry, P. (1991). The metabolism of exogenous L-dopa in the brain: An immune histochemical study of its conversion to dopamine in non-catecholaminergic cells of the rat brain. *Journal of Neural Transmission. Parkinson's Disease and Dementia Section*, *3*(1), 27–39. doi:10.1007/BF02251134 PMID:2064729

Tkatch, R., Musich, S., MacLeod, S., Alsgaard, K., Hawkins, K., & Yeh, C. S. (2016). Population Health Management for Older Adults: Review of Interventions for Promoting Successful Aging Across the Health Continuum. *Gerontology & Geriatric Medicine*, *2*, 1–13. PMID:28680938

Tombaugh, T. N. (2004). Trail Making Test A and B: Normative data stratified by age and education. *Archives of Clinical Neuropsychology*, *19*(2), 203–214. doi:10.1016/S0887-6177(03)00039-8 PMID:15010086

Toniato, A., Bernardi, C., Piotto, A., Rubello, D., & Pelizzo, M. R. (2011). Features of papillary thyroid carcinoma in patients older than 75 years. *Updates in Surgery*, *63*(2), 115–118. doi:10.1007/s13304-011-0060-0 PMID:21416286

Tornstam, L. (1989). Gero-transcendence: A meta-theoretical reformulation of the disengagement theory. *Aging*, *1*, 55–63. PMID:2488301

Tornstam, L. (1996). Gerotranscendence- a theory about maturing into old age. *Journal of Aging and Identity*, (1): 37–50.

Tornstam, L. (1999). Transcendence in later life. *Generations (San Francisco, Calif.)*, *23*(4), 10.

Touitou, Y. (2001). Human aging and melatonin. Clinicalrelevance. *Experimental Gerontology*, *36*(7), 1083–1100. doi:10.1016/S0531-5565(01)00120-6 PMID:11404053

Troll, L. E., & Bengtson, V. L. (1993). The oldest-old in families: An intergenerational perspective. In L. Burton (Ed.), *Families and ageing* (pp. 70–89). Amityville, NY: Baywood Press.

Tsugane, S., & Inoue, M. (2010). Insulin resistance and cancer: Epidemiological evidence. *Cancer Science*, *101*(5), 1073–1079. doi:10.1111/j.1349-7006.2010.01521.x PMID:20345478

Tugade, M. M., & Fredrickson, B. L. (2004). Resilient individuals use positive emotions to bounce back from negative emotional experiences. *Journal of Personality and Social Psychology*, *86*(2), 320–333. doi:10.1037/0022-3514.86.2.320 PMID:14769087

Turner, R. P., Lukoff, D., Barnhouse, R. T., & Lu, F. G. (1995). A culturally sensitive diagnostic category in the DSM-IV. *The Journal of Nervous and Mental Disease*, *183*(7), 435–444. doi:10.1097/00005053-199507000-00003 PMID:7623015

Turvey, C. L., Conwell, Y., Jones, M. P., Phillips, C., Simonsick, E., Pearson, J. L., & Wallace, R. (2002). Risk factors for late-life suicide: A prospective, community-based study. *The American Journal of Geriatric Psychiatry : Official Journal of the American Association for Geriatric Psychiatry*, *10*(4), 398–406. doi:10.1097/00019442-200207000-00006 PMID:12095899

Twelfree, H., & Qazi, A. (2006). Relationship between anxiety and agitation in dementia. *Aging & Mental Health*, *10*(4), 362–367. doi:10.1080/13607860600638511 PMID:16798628

U.S. Department of Health and Human Services. (1995). Vital and health statistics, Current estimates from the National Health Interview Survey.

United Nation Population Assessment. (1992). In: WHO Technical Report Series 853. Geneva, p. 4.

United Nations demographic yearbook, special issue: Population ageing and the situation of elderly persons. (1993). New York: United Nations.

United Nations Department of Economic and Social Affairs, Population Division. (2008). World Population Prospects (2008 Revision). Retrieved from http://esa.un.org/unpp/index.asp?panel=2

United Nations Population Division (UN). (2011). World Population Prospects: The 2010 Revision. In Population Reference Bureau. Retrieved from http://www.prb.org/pdf12/TodaysResearchAging25.pdf

United Nations, Department of Economic and Social Affairs, Population Division. (2015). *World Population Ageing 2015* (ST/ESA/SER.A/390).

United Nations. (n.d.). *World population ageing 2009*. Retrieved from www.un.org/esa/population/publications/WPA2009/WPA2009_WorkingPaper.pdf

University of California at San Francisco. (2013, November 14). *Estimating prognosis for elders*. Retrieved from http://eprognosis.ucsf.edu/calculators

Unützer, J., Patrick, D. L., Diehr, P., Simon, G., Grembowski, D., & Katon, W. (2000). Quality adjusted life years in older adults with depressive symptoms and chronic medical disorders. *International Psychogeriatrics*, *12*(1), 15–33. doi:10.1017/S1041610200006177 PMID:10798451

Vagefi, P. A., & Longo, W. E. (2005). Colorectal cancer in patients with inflammatory bowel disease. *Clinical Colorectal Cancer*, *4*(5), 313–319. doi:10.3816/CCC.2005.n.003 PMID:15663834

Vaidya, A. B., & Vaidya, R. A. (1997). Ancient insights and modern discoveries in the process of aging—an overview. *Indian Journal of Medical Sciences*, *51*, 10,349–363. PMID:9567510

Vakil, E., Greenstein, Y., & Blachstein, H. (2010). Normative data for composite scores for children and adults derived from the Rey Auditory Verbal Learning Test. *The Clinical Neuropsychologist*, *24*(4), 662–677. doi:10.1080/13854040903493522 PMID:20155574

Valderas, J.M., Starfield, B.&Roland, M. (2007). Multimorbidity's many challenges: A research priority in the UK. *British Medical Journal, 334*(7604), 1128.

Valderas, J. M., Starfield, B., Sibbald, B., Salisbury, C., & Roland, M. (2009). Defining Comorbidity: Implications for Understanding Health and Health Services. *Annals of Family Medicine*, *7*(4), 357–363. doi:10.1370/afm.983 PMID:19597174

Valerie, K. S., & Margory, A. M. (2015). Aging and obesity: General assessment and management considerations. *Geriatric Nursing*, *36*(5), 407–409. doi:10.1016/j.gerinurse.2015.08.008 PMID:26734699

Van Alphen, S. P. J., Derksen, J. J., Sadavoy, J. J., & Rosowsky, E. E. (2012). Features and challenges of personality disorders in late life. *Aging & Mental Health*, *16*(7), 805–810. doi:10.1080/13607863.2012.667781 PMID:22417221

Van Beljouw, I. M., van Exel, E., de Jong Gierveld, J., Comijs, H. C., Heerings, M., Stek, M. L., & van Marwijk, H. W. J. (2014). Being all alone makes me sad": Loneliness in older adults with depressive symptoms. *International Psychogeriatrics*, *9*, 1–11. doi:10.1017/S1041610214000581 PMID:24717770

Van Crevel, R., & Dockrell, H. M. (2014). TANDEM: Understanding diabetes and tuberculosis. *The Lancet. Diabetes & Endocrinology*, *2*(4), 270–272. doi:10.1016/S2213-8587(14)70011-7 PMID:24703039 van de Beek, D., de Gans, J., Tunkel, A. R., & Wijdicks, E. F. M. (2006). Community-acquired bacterial meningitis in adults. *The New England Journal of Medicine*, *354*(1), 44–53. doi:10.1056/NEJMra052116 PMID:16394301

Van den Akker, M., Buntinx, F., Metsemakers, J. F. M., Roos, S., & Knottnerus, J. A. (1996). Multimorbidity in general practice: Prevalence, incidence, and determinants of co-occurring chronic and recurrent diseases. *Journal of Clinical Epidemiology*, *51*(5), 367–375. doi:10.1016/S0895-4356(97)00306-5 PMID:9619963

Van Den Beld, A. W., Visser, T. J., Feelders, R. A., Grobbee, D. E., & Lamberts, S. W. J. (2000). Thyroid hormone concentrations, disease, physical function and mortality in elderly men. *The Journal of Clinical Endocrinology and Metabolism*, *90*(12), 6403–6409. Retrieved from https://www.ncbi.nlm.nih.gov/pubmed/16174720. doi:10.1210/jc.2005-0872 PMID:16174720

Van Dooren, F. E. P., Denollet, J., Verhey, F. R. J., Stehouwer, C. D. A., Sep, S. J. S., Henry, R. M., ... Schram, M. T. (2016). Psychological and personality factors in type 2 diabetes mellitus, presenting the rationale and exploratory results from The Maastricht Study, a population-based cohort study. *BMC Psychiatry*, *16*(1), 17. doi:10.1186/s12888-016-0722-z PMID:26817600

Van Dooren, F. E., Nefs, G., Schram, M. T., Verhey, F. R., Denollet, J., & Pouwer, F. (2013). Depression and risk of mortality in people with diabetes mellitus: A systematic review and meta-analysis. *PLoS One*, *8*(3), e57058. doi:10.1371/journal.pone.0057058 PMID:23472075

Van Orden, K., & Conwell, Y. (2011). Suicides in late life. *Current Psychiatry Reports*, *13*(3), 234–241. doi:10.1007/s11920-011-0193-3 PMID:21369952

Van Orden, K., Witte, A., Tracy, K., Cukrowicz, K. C., Braithwaite, S. R., Selby, E. A., & Joiner, T. E. (2010). The interpersonal theory of suicide. *Psychological Review*, *117*(2), 575–600. doi:10.1037/a0018697 PMID:20438238

Van Someren, E. J. W., Lijzenga, C., Mirmiran, M., & Swaab, D. F. (1997b). Long-term fitness training improves the circadian rest–activity rhythm in healthy elderly males. *Journal of Biological Rhythms*, *12*(2), 146–156. doi:10.1177/074873049701200206 PMID:9090568

Van Tilburg, T. (1998). Losing and gaining in old age: Changes in personal network size and social support in a four-year longitudinal study. *The Journals of Gerontology. Series B, Psychological Sciences and Social Sciences*, *53*(6), S313–S323. doi:10.1093/geronb/53B.6.S313 PMID:9826973

van Uffelen, J. G. Z., Chinapaw, M. J. M., van Mechelen, W., & Hopman-Rock, M. (2008). Walking or vitamin B for cognition in older adults with mild cognitive impairment? A randomised controlled trial. *British Journal of Sports Medicine*, *42*(5), 344–351. doi:10.1136/bjsm.2007.044735 PMID:18308888

van Weel, C., & Schellevis, F. G. (2006). Comorbidity and guidelines: Conflicting interests. *Lancet*, *367*(9510), 550–551. doi:10.1016/S0140-6736(06)68198-1 PMID:16488782

Vanlaere, L., Bouckaert, F., & Gastmans, C. (2007). Care for suicidal older people: Current clinical-ethical considerations. *Journal of Medical Ethics*, *33*(7), 376–381. doi:10.1136/jme.2006.017897 PMID:17601861

Varjassyová, A., Hořínek, D., Andel, R., Amlerova, J., Laczó, J., Sheardová, K., ... Geda, Y. E. (2013). Recognition of facial emotional expression in amnestic mild cognitive impairment. *Journal of Alzheimer's Disease*, *33*(1), 273–280. PMID:22954669

Vaughan, F. (1991). Spiritual issues in psychotherapy. *Journal of Transpersonal Psychology*, *23*(2), 105.

Vaughan, F., Wittine, B., & Walsh, R. (1998). Transpersonal psychology and the religious person. In P. Shafranske (Ed.), *Religion and the Clinical Practice of Psychology* (pp. 483–509). Washington, DC: American Psychological Association.

Vaughn, B. V., & Giallanza, P. (2008). Technical review of polysomnography. *Chest*, *134*, 1310–1319.

Veenhoven, R. (2005). Average happiness in 90 nations in the early 2000s.World Database of Happiness, Distributional Findings in Nations (Rank report 2005/1). Retrieved from http://worlddatabaseofhappiness.eur.nl/hap_nat/findingreports/

Veenhoven, R. (2000). Wellbeing in the welfare state, level not higher, distribution not more equitable. *Journal of Comparative Policy Analysis*, *2*(1), 91–125. doi:10.1080/13876980008412637

Veiel, H. O. (1997). A preliminary profile of neuropsychological deficits associated with major depression. *Journal of Clinical and Experimental Neuropsychology*, *19*(4), 587–603. doi:10.1080/01688639708403745 PMID:9342691

Veinot, J. P., & Edwards, W. D. (1996). Pathology of radiation-induced heart disease: A surgical and autopsy study of 27 cases. *Human Pathology*, *27*(8), 766–773. doi:10.1016/S0046-8177(96)90447-5 PMID:8760008

Velayudhan, L., Poppe, M., Archer, N., Proitsi, P., Brown, R. G., & Lovestone, S. (2010). Risk of developing dementia in people with diabetes and mild cognitive impairment. *The British Journal of Psychiatry*, *196*(1), 36–40. doi:10.1192/bjp.bp.109.067942 PMID:20044657

Velayutham, B. R. V., Nair, D., Chandrasekaran, V., Raman, B., Sekar, G., Watson, B., & Swaminathan, S. (2014). Profile and response to anti-tuberculosis treatment among elderly tuberculosis patients treated under the TB Control programme in South India. *PLoS One*, *9*(3), e88045. doi:10.1371/journal.pone.0088045 PMID:24618888

Velden, P. G., Kleber, R. J., Fournier, M., Grievink, L., Drogendijk, A., & Gersons, B. P. (2007). The association between dispositional optimism and mental health problems among disaster victims and a comparison group: A prospective study. *Journal of Affective Disorders*, *102*(3), 35–45. doi:10.1016/j.jad.2006.12.004 PMID:17239959

Venkoba Rao, A. (1992). Suicide. In *Postgraduae Psychiatry*. New Delhi: BI Churchil Livingstone.

Verduin, M. L., Carter, R. E., Brady, K. T., Myrick, H., & Timmerman, M. A. (2005). Health service use among persons with comorbid bipolar and substance use disorders. *Psychiatric Services (Washington, D.C.)*, *56*(4), 475–480. doi:10.1176/appi.ps.56.4.475 PMID:15812100

Vestergaard, P., & Mosekilde, L. (2003). Hyperthyroidism, bone mineral, fracture risk-a meta-analysis. *Thyroid*, *13*(6), 585–593. doi:10.1089/105072503322238854 PMID:12930603

Vijaykumar, L. (2009). Religion-A protective factor in suicide. In A. Sharma (Ed.), Spirituality and mental health (pp. 357–367). Mount Abu: Indian Psychiatric Society.

Vijayshri. (2015). Optimistic and Pessimistic Attitude Influencing Depressive Symptoms in Older Age. *International Research Journal of Social Sciences*, *4*(5), 52-58.

Villareal, D. T., Apovian, C. M., Kushner, R. F., & Klein, S. (2005). American Society for Nutrition; NAASO, The Obesity Society. Obesity in older adults: Technical review and position statement of the American Society for Nutrition and NAASO, The Obesity Society. *The American Journal of Clinical Nutrition*, *82*(5), 923–934. PMID:16280421

Villareal, D. T., Apovian, C. M., Kushner, R. F., & Klein, S. (2005). Obesity in older adults: Technical review and position statement of the American Society for Nutrition and NAASO, The Obesity Society. *Obesity (Silver Spring, Md.)*, *13*(11), 1849–1863. PMID:16339115

Villareal, D. T., Chode, S., Parimi, N., Sinacore, D. R., Hilton, T., Armamento-Villareal, R., & Shah, K. (2011). Weight loss, exercise, or both and physical function in obese older adults. *The New England Journal of Medicine*, *364*(13), 1218–1229. doi:10.1056/NEJMoa1008234 PMID:21449785

Vink, A. C., Bruinsma, M. S., & Scholten, R. J. (2011). Music therapy for people with dementia. *Cochrane Database of Systematic Reviews*, *3*, CD003477. PMID:15266489

Vinkers, D. J., Gussekloo, J., Stek, M. L., Westendorp, R. G., & van der Mast, R. C. (2004). Temporal relation between depression and cognitive impairment in old age: Prospective population based study. *British Medical Journal*, *329*(7471), e881. doi:10.1136/bmj.38216.604664.DE PMID:15345599

Visser, P. J., Verhey, F., Knol, D. L., Scheltens, P., Wahlund, L.-O., Freund-Levi, Y., ... Blennow, K. (2009). Prevalence and prognostic value of CSF markers of Alzheimer's disease pathology in patients with subjective cognitive impairment or mild cognitive impairment in the DESCRIPA study: A prospective cohort study. *Lancet Neurology*, *8*(7), 619–627. doi:10.1016/S1474-4422(09)70139-5 PMID:19523877

Viticchi, G., Falsetti, L., Buratti, L., Sajeva, G., Luzzi, S., Bartolini, M., ... Silvestrini, M. (2017). Framingham Risk Score and the Risk of Progression from Mild Cognitive Impairment to Dementia. *Journal of Alzheimer's Disease*, *59*(1), 67–75. doi:10.3233/JAD-170160 PMID:28582863

Vitiello, M. V. (1996). Sleep disorders and aging. *Current Opinion in Psychiatry*, *9*(4), 284–289. doi:10.1097/00001504-199607000-00011

Vitiello, M. V. (2009). *Sleep and Circadian rhythms disorders in human ageing and dementia. University of Washington.* Seattle, WA, USA: Elsevier Ltd.

Vitry, A., & Zhang, Y. (2008). Quality of Australian clinical guidelines and relevance to the care of older people with multiple comorbid conditions. *The Medical Journal of Australia*, *189*(7), 360–365. PMID:18837677

Vogeli, C., Shields, A. E., Lee, T. A., Gibson, T. B., Marder, W. D., Weiss, K. B., & Blumenthal, D. (2007). Multiple chronic conditions: Prevalence, health consequences, and implications for quality care management, and costs. *Journal of General Internal Medicine*, *22*(S3), 391–395. doi:10.1007/s11606-007-0322-1 PMID:18026807

Volker, H. (2016). *Lies in the Medical Profession* (Vol. 2).

Volpato, S., Bianchi, L., Lauretani, F., Lauretani, F., Bandinelli, S., Guralnik, J. M., ... Ferrucci, L. (2012). Role of muscle mass and muscle quality in the association between diabetes and gait speed. *Diabetes Care*, *35*(8), 1672–1679. doi:10.2337/dc11-2202 PMID:22596176

Volpato, S., Ferrucci, L., Blaum, C., Ostir, G., Cappola, A., Fried, L. P., ... Guralnik, J. M. (2003). Progression of lower-extremity disability in older women with diabetes: The Women's Health and Aging Study. *Diabetes Care*, *26*(1), 70–75. doi:10.2337/diacare.26.1.70 PMID:12502660

Volzke, H., Alte, D., Kohlmann, T., Lüdemann, J., Nauck, M., John, U., & Meng, W. (2005). Reference intervals of serum thyroid function tests in a previously iodine-deficient area. *Thyroid*, *15*(3), 279–285. doi:10.1089/thy.2005.15.279 PMID:15785248

Voyer, P., Preville, M., Roussel, M. E., Berbiche, D., & Beland, S. G. (2009). Factors associated with benzodiazepine dependence among community-dwelling seniors. *Journal of Community Health Nursing*, *26*(3), 101–113. doi:10.1080/07370010903034375 PMID:19662558

Wærn, M. (2003). Physical illness and depression in the elderly. *Geriatrics & Aging*, *6*, 56–59.

Waern, M., Rubenowitz, E., & Wilhelmson, K. (2003). Predictors of suicide in the old elderly. *Gerontology*, *49*(5), 328–334. doi:10.1159/000071715 PMID:12920354

Walsh, R., & Shapiro, S. L. (2006). The meeting of meditative disciplines and Western psychology: A mutually enriching dialogue. *The American Psychologist*, *61*(3), 227–239. doi:10.1037/0003-066X.61.3.227 PMID:16594839

Wand, A.P.F., Peisah, C., Draper, B., Jones, C., & Brodaty, H. (2016). *Case Report Rational Suicide, Euthanasia, and the Very Old: Two Case Reports*. Academic Press.

Wang, V., Depp, C. A., Ceglowski, J., Thompson, W. K., Rock, D., & Jeste, D. V. (2015). Sexual health and function in later life: A population-based study of 606 olderadults with a partner. *The American Journal of Geriatric Psychiatry*, *23*(3), 227–233. doi:10.1016/j.jagp.2014.03.006 PMID:24840610

Warburton, D. E., Nicol, C. W., & Bredin, S. S. (2006). Health benefits of physical activity: The evidence. *Canadian Medical Association Journal*, *174*(6), 801–809. doi:10.1503/cmaj.051351 PMID:16534088

Ward, A., Arrighi, H. M., Michels, S., & Cedarbaum, J. M. (2012). Mild cognitive impairment: Disparity of incidence and prevalence estimates. *Alzheimer's & Dementia*, *8*(1), 14–21. doi:10.1016/j.jalz.2011.01.002 PMID:22265588

Ward, B. W., & Schiller, J. S. (2013). Prevalence of multiple chronic conditions among US adults: Estimates from the National Health Survey 2010. *Preventing Chronic Disease*, *10*, 120203. doi:10.5888/pcd10.120203 PMID:23618545

Ware, J. E., & Sherbourne, E. C. (1992). The MOS 36-Item Short Form Health Survey 1: Conceptual framework and item selection. *Medical Care*, *30*, 473–483. doi:10.1097/00005650-199206000-00002 PMID:1593914

Warren, M. (1988). Catechesis and spirituality. *Religious Education (Chicago, Ill.)*, *83*(1), 116–132. doi:10.1080/0034408880830109

Warren, M. F., Serby, M. J., & Roane, D. M. (2008). The effects of testosterone on cognition in elderly men: A review. *CNS Spectrums*, *13*(10), 887–897. doi:10.1017/S1092852900016990 PMID:18955944

Wasserman, D., & Ringskog, S. (2001). Suicide among elderly in Sweden. Stockholm: Academic Press.

Watanabe, S., & Imanishi, J. (2009). Aromatherapy. [in Japanese]. *Anti-Aging Igaku*, *5*, 375–379.

Watson, G. R. (2001). Low vision in the geriatric population: Rehabilitation and management. *Journal of the American Geriatrics Society*, *49*(3), 317–330. doi:10.1046/j.1532-5415.2001.4930317.x PMID:11300245

Watters, C., Owen, M., & Munroe, S. (2005). *A Study of Deaf-Blind Demographics and Services in Canada*. North York, ON: Canadian National Society of the Deaf Blindness.

WeeksMD. (2011). Sober Reflection up on Chemotherapy……? The Economist! Retrieved from http://weeksmd.com/2011/12/sober-reflection-upon-chemotherapy-source-the-economist/

Weiss, B. D. (2007). *Health Literacy and Patient Safety: Help Patients Understand. Manual for Clinicians* (2nd ed.). AMA Foundation.

Weissberg-Benchell, J., & Antisdel-Lomaglio, J. (2011). Diabetes-specific emotional distress among adolescents: Feasibility, reliability, and validity of the problem areas in diabetes-teen version. *Pediatric Diabetes*, *12*(4 Pt 1), 341–344. doi:10.1111/j.1399-5448.2010.00720.x PMID:21443583

Wells, K. B., & Sherbourne, C. D. (1999). Functioning and utility for current health of patients with depression or chronic medical conditions in managed primary care practices. *Archives of General Psychiatry*, *56*(10), 897–904. doi:10.1001/archpsyc.56.10.897 PMID:10530631

Wells, K. B., Stewart, A., & Hays, R. D. (1989). The functioning and well-being of depressed patients: Results from the Medical Outcomes Study. *Journal of the American Medical Association*, *262*(7), 914–919. doi:10.1001/jama.1989.03430070062031 PMID:2754791

Wells, M. (2010). Resilience in older adults living in rural, suburban, and urban areas. *Online Journal of Rural Nursing and Health Care: the Official Journal of the Rural Nurse Organization*, *10*(2), 4554.

Wendler, D. S. (2013). Problems with the consensus definition of the therapeutic misconception. *The Journal of Clinical Ethics*, *24*(4), 387–394. doi:10.1038/jid.2014.371 PMID:24597427

Westendorp, R. (2006). What is healthy aging in the 21st century? *The American Journal of Clinical Nutrition*, *83*(2), 404–409. PMID:16470003

West, R., Herndon, R. W., & Covell, E. (2003). Neural correlates of age-related declines in the formation and realization of delayed intentions. *Psychology and Aging*, *18*(3), 461–473. doi:10.1037/0882-7974.18.3.461 PMID:14518808

Wethington, E., & Kessler, R. C. (1986). Perceived support, received support, and adjustment to stressful life events. *Journal of Health and Social Behavior*, *27*(1), 78–89. doi:10.2307/2136504 PMID:3711634

Whalley, L. J. (2001). *The aging brain*. New York: Columbia University Press.

Whalley, L. J., Deary, I. J., Appleton, C. L., & Starr, J. M. (2004). Cognitive reserve and the neurobiology of cognitive aging. *Ageing Research Reviews*, *3*(4), 369–382. doi:10.1016/j.arr.2004.05.001 PMID:15541707

Whitbeck, L. B., McMorris, B. J., Hoyt, D. R., Stubben, J. D., & LaFromboise, T. (2002). Perceived discrimination, traditional practices, and depressive symptoms among American Indians in the upper midwest. *Journal of Health and Social Behavior*, *43*(4), 400–418. doi:10.2307/3090234 PMID:12664673

White, C. (2011). Brain circuitry model for mental illness will transform management, NIH mental health director says. *British Medical Journal*, *343*(2), d5581. doi:10.1136/bmj.d5581 PMID:21885534

White, C. A., & Macleod, U. (2002). Cancer. *BMJ (Clinical Research Ed.)*, *325*(7360), 377–380. doi:10.1136/bmj.325.7360.377 PMID:12183312

Whitmer, R. A., Karter, A. J., Yaffe, K., Quesenberry, C. P., & Selby, J. V. (2009). Hypoglycemic episodes and risk of dementia in older patients with type 2 diabetes mellitus. *Journal of the American Medical Association*, *301*(15), 1565–1572. doi:10.1001/jama.2009.460 PMID:19366776

WHO MONICA Project Investigators. (1988). The World Health Organization MONICA Project (Monitoring trends and determinants in cardiovascular disease. *Journal of Clinical Epidemiology*, *41*(2), 105–114. doi:10.1016/0895-4356(88)90084-4 PMID:3335877

WHO. (1992). *International Classification of Diseases, Clinical descriptions and diagnostic guidelines 1992*. Geneve: World Health Organization.

WHO. (2000). Obesity: Preventing and managing the global epidemic. Report of a WHO Consultation. WHO Technical Report.

WHO. (2007). Age-Friendly Cities: A Guide.

WHO. (2016). Cancer. Retrieved from http://www.who.int/cancer/en/

WHO. (n.d.). WHO/NMH/NPH/02.2.

WHO/INPEA (2002b).*Missing voices: views of older persons on elder abuse.*

WHO/INPEA. (2001a). *Daichman, L., Guido, O., Aguas, S., &Bertone, M. National report on elder abuse in Argentina*. Geneva: WHO.

WHO/INPEA. (2001b). *L. Machado, National report on elder abuse in Brazil*. Geneva: WHO.

WHOQOL Group. (1998). The World Health Organization Quality of Life Assessment (WHOQOL): Development and general psychometric properties. *Social Science & Medicine*, *46*(12), 1569–1585. doi:10.1016/S0277-9536(98)00009-4 PMID:9672396

Widerlöv, E., Bråne, G., Ekman, R., Kihlgren, M., Norberg, A., & Karlsson, I. (1989). Elevated CSF somatostatin concentrations in demented patients parallel improved psychomotor functions induced by integrity-promoting care. *Acta Psychiatrica Scandinavica*, *79*(1), 41–47. doi:10.1111/j.1600-0447.1989.tb09232.x PMID:2564721

Wild, S. H., Morling, J. R., McAllister, D. A., Kerssens, J., Fischbacher, C., Parkes, J., ... Byrne, C. D. (2016). Type 2 diabetes and risk of hospital admission or death for chronic liver diseases. *Journal of Hepatology*, *64*(6), 1358–1364. doi:10.1016/j.jhep.2016.01.014 PMID:26812073

Wilhemson, K., Andersson, C., Waern, M., & Allebeck, P. (2005). Elderly people's perspectives on quality of life. *Ageing and Society*, *25*(04), 585–600. doi:10.1017/S0144686X05003454

Williams, B. W., Mack, W., & Henderson, V. W. (1989). Boston naming test in Alzheimer's disease. *Neuropsychologia*, *27*(8), 1073–1079. doi:10.1016/0028-3932(89)90186-3 PMID:2797414

Williams, J., Lyons, B., & Rowland, D. (1997). Unmet long-term care needs of elderly people in the community: A review of the literature. *Home Health Care Services Quarterly*, *16*(1-2), 93–119. doi:10.1300/J027v16n01_07 PMID:10168492

Williams, R. B., & Schneiderman, N. (2002). Resolved: Psychosocial interventions can improve clinical outcomes in organic disease (pro). *Psychosomatic Medicine*, *64*, 552–557. PMID:12140342

Wilson, R. S., Krueger, K. R., Gu, L., Bienias, J. L., Mendes de Leon, C. F., & Evans, D. A. (2005). Neuroticism, extraversion, and mortality in a defined population of older persons. *Psychosomatic Medicine*, *67*(6), 841–845. doi:10.1097/01.psy.0000190615.20656.83 PMID:16314587

Wimo, A., Jonsson, L., & Winblad, B. (2006). An estimate of the worldwide prevalence and direct costs of dementia in 2003. *Dementia and Geriatric Cognitive Disorders*, *21*(3), 175–181. doi:10.1159/000090733 PMID:16401889

Windle, G., Hughes, D., Linck, P., Russell, I., & Woods, B. (2010). Is exercise effective in promoting mental well-being in older age? A systematic review. *Aging & Mental Health*, *14*(6), 652–669. doi:10.1080/13607861003713232 PMID:20686977

Windle, G., Woods, R. T., & Markland, D. A. (2010). Living with Ill-Health in Older Age: The Role of a Resilient Personality. *Journal of Happiness Studies*, *11*(6), 763–777. doi:10.1007/s10902-009-9172-3

Wing, R. R., & Hill, J. O. (2001). Successful weight loss maintenance. *Annual Review of Nutrition*, *21*(1), 323–341. doi:10.1146/annurev.nutr.21.1.323 PMID:11375440

Winnicott, D. W. (1971). *Playing and reality*. Psychology Press.

Wolff, J. L., Starfiled, B., & Anderson, G. F. (2002). Prevalence, expenditures, and complications of multiple chronic conditions in the elderly. *Archives of Internal Medicine*, *162*(20), 2269–2276. doi:10.1001/archinte.162.20.2269 PMID:12418941

Wolf, R. (2000). Introduction: The nature and scope of elder abuse. *Generations (San Francisco, Calif.)*, *24*, 6–11.

Wolk, A., Gridley, G., Svensson, M., Nyrén, O., McLaughlin, J. K., Fraumeni, J. F., & Adami, H. O. (2001). A prospective study of obesity and cancer risk (Sweden). *Cancer Causes & Control*, *12*(1), 13–21. doi:10.1023/A:1008995217664 PMID:11227921

Wolk, D. A., Mancuso, L., Kliot, D., Arnold, S. E., & Dickerson, B. C. (2013). Familiarity-based memory as an early cognitive marker of preclinical and prodromal AD. *Neuropsychologia*, *51*(6), 1094–1102. doi:10.1016/j.neuropsychologia.2013.02.014 PMID:23474075

Wolters, F. J., Van der Lee, S. J., Koudstaal, P. J., Van Duijn, C. M., Hofman, A., & Ikram, M. K. …Ikram, M. A. (2017). Parental family history of dementia in relation to subclinical brain disease and dementia risk [Abstract]. *Neurology*. Retrieved from http://www.neurology.org/content/early/2017/03/29/WNL.0000000000003871.abstract

Wong, N. (2003). Reducing Suicide: A National Imperative. American Journal of Psychiatry, 160. doi:10.1176/appi.ajp.160.8.1534

Wong, P. T. (1989). Personal meaning and successful aging. *Canadian Psychology*, *30*(3), 516–525. doi:10.1037/h0079829

Wong, P. T. P. (1998). Spirituality, meaning, and successful aging. In P. T. P. Wong & P. Fry (Eds.), *The human quest for meaning: A handbook of psychological research and clinical applications* (pp. 359–394). Mahwah, NJ: Erlbaum.

Woodward, M., Lam, T. H., Barzi, F., Patel, A., Gu, D., Rodgers, A., & Suh, I. (2005). Asia Pacific Cohort Studies Collaboration. Smoking, quitting, and the risk of cardiovascular disease among women and men in the Asia-Pacific region. *International Journal of Epidemiology*, *34*(5), 1036–1045. doi:10.1093/ije/dyi104 PMID:15914503

Woolf, A.D., & Pfleger, B., (2003). Burden of major musculoskeletal conditions. *Bulletin of the World Health Organization, 81*, 646–656.

World Health Organisation. (1968). *Prevention of suicide*. Geneva: WHO.

World Health Organization (2004). *Global Burden of Disease*. WHO.

World Health Organization (WHO). (2010). *Global recommendations on physical activity for health*. Geneva.

World Health Organization (WHO). (2014). Visual Impairment and Blindness. Retrieved from http://www.who.int/mediacentre/factsheets/fs282/en/

World Health Organization (WHO). (2016). *Global report on diabetes*. Geneva.

World Health Organization [WHO]. (2005). *Global strategy on diet, physical activity, and health.* Retrieved July 24, 2008, from www.who.int/dietphysicalactivity/publications/facts/obesity/en/

World Health Organization WHO. (2015). Aging and Health. Retrieved from http://www.who.int/mediacentre/factsheets/fs404/en/

World Health Organization WHO. (2016). Mental health and older adults. Extracted from http://www.who.int/mediacentre/factsheets/fs381/en/*)*

World Health Organization. (1948). *Constitution of the World Health Organization.* Available at: http//www.who.int/governance/eb/who_constitution_en.pdf

World Health Organization. (1992). *The ICD-10 Classification of mental and behavioral disorders: clinical descriptions and diagnostic guidelines*. Geneva: World Health Organization.

World Health Organization. (1999). *Facts and figures about suicide.* Geneva: World Health Organisation Press Office. Retrieved from http://scholar.google.com/scholar?hl=en&btnG=Search&q=intitle:Facts+and+Figures+About+Suicide#2

World Health Organization. (2002). *Active ageing: A policy framework.* Report No: WHO/NMH/NPH/02.8. Geneva: World Health Organisation. Retrieved from http://whqlibdoc.who.int/hq/2002/WHO_NMH_NPH_02.8.pdf

World Health Organization. (2005). *Affordable technology. Blood pressure measuring devices for low resource settings.* Geneva: WHO.

World Health Organization. (2008). Molecular line probe assays for rapid screening of patients at risk of multidrug-resistant tuberculosis (MDR-TB). *Policy Statement, 27.*

World Health Organization. (2011). Same-day diagnosis of tuberculosis by microscopy. *Policy statement. World Health Organization Document WHO/HTM/TB/2011.7, 1*(11).

World Health Organization. (2012). *Good health adds life to years: global brief for World Health day 2012.* Geneve: World Health Organization. Retrieved on January 6, 2012 from http:// www.who.int/world_ health_day/2012

World Health Organization. (2013). *United Nations. World Population Aging*. WHO.

World Health Organization. (2014). Global Atlas on Cardiovascular Disease Prevention and Control 2011. Retrieved from www.who.int

World Health Organization. (2014a). *Preventing suicide: a global imperative*. Geneva: WHO.

World Health Organization. (2014b). Preventing suicide. A global imperative. *Journal de l'Association Medicale Canadienne, 143*(7), 609–610.

World Health Organization. (2015). *World Report on Ageing and Health.* Geneva: WHO.

World Health Organization. (2017). *Ageing and Health.* WHO.

World Health Organization. (Ed.). (2013). *Global tuberculosis report 2013.* World Health Organization.

World Report on Disability. (2011). World Health Organization.

Worrall, L., & Hickson, L. M. (2003). Theoretical foundations of communication disability in aging. In L.E. Worrall & L.M. Hickson (Eds.), Communication disability in aging: from prevention to intervention.

Wortman, J., Lucas, R. E., & Donnellan, M. B. (2012). Stability and change in the Big Five personality domains: Evidence from a longitudinal study of Australians. *Psychology and Aging, 27*(4), 867–874. doi:10.1037/a0029322 PMID:22775362

Wright, L. K. (1998). Affection and sexuality in the presence of Alzheimer's disease: A longitudinal study. *Sexuality and Disability, 16*(3), 167–179. doi:10.1023/A:1023042924997

Wu, L. T., & Blazer, D. G. (2011). Illicit and nonmedical drug use among older adults: A review. *Journal of Aging and Health, 23*(3), 481–504. doi:10.1177/0898264310386224 PMID:21084724

Wu, L. T., Woody, G. E., Yang, C., Mannelli, P., & Blazer, D. G. (2011). Differences in onset and abuse/dependence episodes between prescription opioids and heroin: Results from the National Epidemiologic Survey on Alcohol and Related Conditions. *Substance Abuse and Rehabilitation, 2*, 77–88. doi:10.2147/SAR.S18969 PMID:21686045

Wurm, S., Tesch-Römer, C., & Tomasik, M. J. (2007). Longitudinal findings on aging-related cognitions, control beliefs, and health in later life. *The Journals of Gerontology. Series B, Psychological Sciences and Social Sciences, 62B*(3), 156–164. doi:10.1093/geronb/62.3.P156 PMID:17507583

Wurm, S., Tomasik, M. J., & Tesch-Römer, C. (2010). On the importance of a positive view on ageing for physical exercise among middle-aged and older adults: Cross-sectional and longitudinal findings. *Psychology & Health, 25*(1), 25–42. doi:10.1080/08870440802311314 PMID:20391205

Yaffe, K., Kanaya, A., Lindquist, K., Simonsick, E. M., Harris, T., Shorr, R. I., ... Newman, A. B. (2004). The metabolic syndrome, inflammation, and risk of cognitive decline. *Journal of the American Medical Association, 292*(18), 2237–2242.

Yaffe, K., Blackwell, T., Kanaya, A. M., Davidowitz, N., Barrett-Connor, E., & Krueger, K. (2004). Diabetes, impaired fasting glucose, and development of cognitive impairment in older women. *Neurology*, *63*(4), 658–663. doi:10.1212/01.WNL.0000134666.64593.BA PMID:15326238

Yaffé, K., Krueger, K., Sarkar, S., Grady, D., Barrett-Connor, E., Cox, D. A., & Nickelsen, T. (2001). Cognitive function in postmenopausal women treated with raloxifene. *The New England Journal of Medicine*, *344*(16), 1207–1213. doi:10.1056/NEJM200104193441604 PMID:11309635

Yancy, C. W., Jessup, M., & Bozkurt, B. (2013). ACCF/AHA guideline for the management of heart failure. *Journal of the American College of Cardiology*, *62*, e147–e239. doi:10.1016/j.jacc.2013.05.019 PMID:23747642

Yanhong, O., Chandra, M., & Venkatesh, D. (2013). Mild cognitive impairment in adult: A neuropsychological review. *Annals of Indian Academy of Neurology*, *16*(3), 310. doi:10.4103/0972-2327.116907 PMID:24101808

Yeap, B. B. (2012). (in press). Hormones and health outcomes in aging men. *Experimental Gerontology*. doi:10.1016/j.exger.2012.07.012 PMID:22884846

Yee, L., & Yee, L. (2010). Aging and sexuality. *American Family Physician, 39*(10), 8–11.

Yeh, E. T., Tong, A. T., Lenihan, D. J., Yusuf, S. W., & Swafford, J. (2004). Cardiovascular complications of cancer therapy. *Circulation*, *109*(25), 3122–3131. doi:10.1161/01.CIR.0000133187.74800.B9 PMID:15226229

Yesavage, J. A., Brink, T. L., Rose, T. L., Lum, O., Huang, V., Adey, M. B., & Leirer, V. O. (1983). Development and validation of a geriatric depression screening scale: A preliminary report. *Journal of Psychiatric Research*, *17*(1), 37–49. doi:10.1016/0022-3956(82)90033-4 PMID:7183759

Yoshikawa, T. T. (1992). Tuberculosis in aging adults. *Journal of the American Geriatrics Society*, *40*(2), 178–187. doi:10.1111/j.1532-5415.1992.tb01941.x PMID:1740604

Young, J. (2008). Supporting health and physical well-being. In M. Downs & B. Bowers (Eds.), *Excellence in Dementia Care: Research into Practice* (pp. 256–257). Berkshire, UK: Open University Press.

Young, T., Shahar, E., Nieto, F. J., Redline, S., Newman, A. B., & Gottlieb, D. J. (2002). Predictors of sleep-disordered breathing in community-dwelling adults: The Sleep Heart Health Study. *Archives of Internal Medicine*, *162*, 893–900. doi:10.1001/archinte.162.8.893 PMID:11966340

Yu, C. E., Oshima, J., Fu, Y. H., Wijsman, E. M., Hisama, F., Alisch, R., ... Schellenberg, G. D. (1996). Positional cloning of the Werner's syndrome gene. *Science*, *272*(5259), 258–262. doi:10.1126/science.272.5259.258 PMID:8602509

Yu, C. E., Oshima, J., Wijsman, E. M., Nakura, J., Miki, T., & Piussan, C. (1997). Mutations in the consensus helicase domains of the Werner syndrome gene. Werner's Syndrome Collaboration Group. *American Journal of Human Genetics*, *60*, 330–341. PMID:9012406

Yu-Shiun, C. H., Chyn-Yng, C., Yang Jui-Chen, T., Min-Huey, C., Yuan-Mei, L., Mei-ju, C., & Liu Kuei-Ru, C. (2015). The efficacy of music therapy for people with dementia: A meta-analysis of randomised controlled trials. *Journal of Clinical Nursing*. PMID:26299594

Yusuf, S., Pfeffer, M. A., Swedberg, K., Granger, C. B., Held, P., McMurray, J. J., ... Östergren, J. (2003). Effects of candesartan in patients with chronic heart failure and preserved leftventricular ejection fraction: The CHARM-Preserved Trial. *Lancet*, *362*(9386), 777–781. doi:10.1016/S0140-6736(03)14285-7 PMID:13678871

Zakzanis, K., Leach, L., & Kaplan, E. (1998). On the nature and pattern of neurocognitive function in major depressive disorder. *Cognitive and Behavioral Neurology*, *11*(3), 111–119. PMID:9742509

Zanetti, O., Frisoni, G. B., De Leo, D., Della Buono, M., Bianchetti, A., & Trabucchi, M. (1995). Alzheimer Disorder. *Related Disorders*, *9*, 132–138.

Zarit, S. H., & Zarit, J. M. (2007). *Mental disorders in older adults (2nd ed.)*. Guilford.

Zautra, A. J., Reich, J. W., & Newsom, J. T. (1995). Autonomy and sense of control among older adults: An examination of their effects on mental health. In L. A. Bond, S. J. Cutler, & A. Grams (Eds.), *Promoting successful and productive aging* (pp. 153–170). Thousand Oaks, CA: Sage.

Zekry, D., Herrmann, F. R., Grandjean, R., Meynet, M.-P., Michel, J.-P., Gold, G., & Krause, K.-H. (2008). Demented versus non-demented very old inpatients: The same comorbidities but poorer functional and nutritional status. *Age and Ageing*, *37*(1), 83–89. doi:10.1093/ageing/afm132 PMID:17971391

Zhang, Z., & Hayward, M. (2001). Childlessness and the psychological well-being of older persons. *The Journals of Gerontology. Series B, Psychological Sciences and Social Sciences*, *56B*(5), S311–S320. doi:10.1093/geronb/56.5.S311 PMID:11522813

Zheng, D., Dong, X., Sun, H., Xu, Y., Ma, Y., & Wang, X. (2012). The overall impairment of core executive function components in patients with amnestic mild cognitive impairment: A cross-sectional study. *BMC Neurology*, *12*(1), 138. doi:10.1186/1471-2377-12-138 PMID:23164134

Zheng, T., Holford, T. R., Chen, Y., Ma, J. Z., Flannery, J., Liu, W., ... Boyle, P. (1996). Time trend and age-period-cohort effect on incidence of thyroid cancer in Connecticut, 1935–1992. *International Journal of Cancer*, *67*(4), 504–509. doi:10.1002/(SICI)1097-0215(19960807)67:4<504::AID-IJC7>3.0.CO;2-W PMID:8759608

Zillmer, E. A., Spiers, M. V., & Culbertson, W. (2007). *Principles of neuropsychology*. Nelson Education.

Zinnbauer, B. J., Pargament, K. I., Cole, B., Rye, M. S., Butter, E. M., Belavich, T. G., ... Kadar, J. L. (1997). Religion and spirituality: Unfuzzying the fuzzy. *Journal for the Scientific Study of Religion*, *36*(4), 549–564. doi:10.2307/1387689

Zinnbauer, B. J., Pargament, K. I., & Scott, A. B. (1999). The emerging meanings of religiousness and spirituality: Problems and prospects. *Journal of Personality*, *67*(6), 889–919. doi:10.1111/1467-6494.00077

Zucconi, M., & Ferri, R. (2014) Assessment of sleep disorders and diagnostic procedure, sleep medicine Textbook. *European Sleep Research Society*. Reterived from www.esrs.eu/fileadmin/user.../ESRS_Sleep_Medicine_Textbook_cChapter_b1.pdf Acesseed on 20,August,2017,95-109

About the Contributors

Barre Vijay Prasad completed Master's Degree in Psychology from Andhra University, he later went to acquire his first M Phil in Rehabilitation Psychology from National Institute for the Mentally Handicapped (NIMH). Thereafter, he went on to acquire his second M Phil in Clinical Psychology from one of the most reputed institutes in India Institute of Human Behaviour and Allied Sciences (IHBAS), Delhi. He is the first psychologist to have accreditation as a dually trained professional psychologist with qualifications as a Clinical Psychologist and a Rehabilitation Psychologist from Rehabilitation Council of India (RCI) - Delhi. He is a Professional Life Member of Indian Association of Clinical Psychology (IACP). He has awarded Doctoral Degree in Psychology from Centre for Health Psychology, University of Hyderabad. He has been awarded: Centenary Merit award during beginning of his professional psychology career. Currently he is working as Associate Professor and Head Department of Clinical Psychology at Dharwad Institute of Mental Health and Neurosciences (DIMHANS-India). He is now working to produce ways of working manuals for reducing psychological distress amongst mentally ill and patients with cancer in the field of Psycho-oncology. He is trained at conducting various assessments such as Psycho-diagnostics, neuropsychological profiling, personality assessments amongst other skills. He is trained in providing support for various initiatives disability rehabilitation, promotion of mental health and wellbeing. He specializes in cognitive behavioural therapies and behavioural interventions for various clinical disorders. He has published many articles in national and international journals, book chapters and books as well, and presented several conference papers on mental health, disability rehabilitation and psycho-oncology. He is also working on writing few other titles i.e "21st Century Eminent Psychologists- Biography", and Biological Foundations of Human Behaviour: Clinical Neuropsychology, Theories and Practices - Oxford University Press.

Shamsi Akbar completed her post-graduation in clinical psychology from Rohilkhand University Bareilly. She worked as a Clinical Psychologist Chandra Psychiatric center Bareilly. Thereafter in 2011 she moved to Lucknow and joined the Dept. of Geriatric Mental Health, King Georges Medical University Lucknow perusing research. In 2013 she got best Poster presentation award in 9th Annual National Conference of Indian Association for Geriatric Mental Health (IAGMH).In 2014 she developed a 1st scale in India for older adults "Scale for Satisfaction and Expectation of Older Adults in Old Age Homes." In 2015 she received the "Best Research Paper" among medical science section K G's Medical University Lucknow. In 2015 "Best Researcher Award " in the Department of Geriatric Mental Health K.G s Medical University Lucknow. In 2015 she got IAGMH / INTAS award in National Conference of Indian Association for Geriatric Mental Health (IAGMH)She has number of publications in National and International Journals, Chapters in Books and has enlisted many presentation / participations at national and international conferences.

* * *

N. T. Alee is a Research Scholar in the Department of Psychology, Aligarh Muslim University, Aligarh, UP, India.

Manjunath R Bajantri is currently working as Assistant professor in Department of Psychiatry Dharwad Institute of Mental Health and Neurosciences DIMHANS Dharwad. He has Articles Published in National and International Journals to his credit.His areas of research interests are psycho-social interventions: In Patients with Affective disorders, schizophrenia and their care givers. Alcohol/ Drug abuses, De-Addiction and Psychosocial Rehabilitation. Yoga intervention in Relapse Prevention. Child and Adolescents Mental Health issues: Yoga & Music therapy in ADHD. Complimentary & Alternative medicine (CAM): Promising Future of Yoga, & Music (Indian Classical Music- Instrumental & Vocal) as an intervention in Psychiatry. In this direction actively Functioning Yoga Therapy and Music Therapy Unit has been initiated at DIMHANS conducting yoga workshops and Demonstration classes at the premise of DIMHANS regularly with related research activities on music therapy.

Gagan Chooramani is currently working as a Clinical Research Coordinator at M.V. Hospital Lucknow.She has been working as Technical Officer under FIND project in TB lab (IRL Lucknow), Deptt of microbiology KGMU, Lucknow - India. She has completed her M.Phil with the project entitled "Evaluation of Nucleic Acid Amplification Method in Diagnosing of Enteric Fever in Children "as a part of dissertation project in M.Phil at KGMU, Lucknow - India. She also served as an author and co-authored in number of national and international publications.

Rishna Priya Devi has been obtaining her bachelor degree in (Genetics) from IGE (Institute of Genetic Engineering). She is also associated with Indian School of Complementary Therapy and Allied Sciences. She is interested to complete her Master degree in Forensic science.

Amit Garg completed a post graduation degree in Psychiatry from Maulana Azad Medical College, latter he joined as Senior Resident in Institute of Human Behavior and Allied Sciences (IHBAS), Delhi. After finishing his tenure, he has been selected as Assistant Professor, in department of psychiatry at IHBAS. He holds special interest in the field if De-addiction and Dual Diagnosis disorders including Psycho-pharmacology and also he is a Consultant Psychiatrist, Felicity Mindcare Clinic, Delhi.

Shobit Garg is working as Assistant Professor, Department of Psychiatry, SMI Medical College and Hospital, Dehradun. He received his DPM and MD from CIP, Ranchi. He is an assistant professor in the Department of Psychiatry, SMI Medical College and Hospital, Dehradun, since 2013. He was ex-senior residence in CIP, Ranchi. He has done various national and international publications and chapters and has presented papers on national conferences.

Srijan Goswami is the Founder Director of Indian School of Complimentary Therapy & Allied Sciences, Ichapur, India. A non-profit and non-government organization providing awareness, education and treatment on Complimentary therapies on a charitable basis. He is also associated with Shree Krishna Biochemic College, Ichapur, India as Honorary Professor of Biochemistry. He is associated as Assistant Professor, at the Department of Molecular Biology, institute of Genetic Engineering, Badu, India. He is trained in Biochemic System of Medicine from Indian Council of Biochemic Medicine & Yoga Therapy, Naihati, India. He is trained in microbiology and biochemistry from R.G. Kar Medical

College and Calcutta National Medical College, India, respectively. He is the editorial review board member of International Journal of Public Health Management & Ethics formerly known as IJDCCS. He has teaching and research experience of around five years. He has numerous international journal and conference publications.

Swagata Goswami is a student of M.Sc in Genetics from Institute of Genetic Engineering, Badu, Kolkata, India. She holds B.Sc degree in Biotechnology from University of Science and Technology, Meghalaya, India.

Garima Gupta is an Assistant Professor in Psychology at Arya Mahila P.G. College (Admitted to the privileges of Banaras Hindu University), Varanasi. She is in teaching and research from three years and has published many research articles in reputed indexed and refereed journals. She has received several best paper awards in various national and international conferences. She has received an International grant from Jacobs Center for Productive Youth Development, Switzerland to attend and participate in a summer school on Society for Longitudinal and Life Course Studies at Zurich University, Switzerland. Her research areas are hemispheric asymmetry, affect and affective disorders, and health well-being.

Susmita Halder is Clinical Psychologist with over 8 years of clinical and teaching experiences. Currently she is Associate Professor in Clinical Psychology at Institute of Psychiatry, Kolkata. Her major area of interest is cognitive assessment and training in different conditions. She is having more than 20 publications in national and international journals and member of various psychological and psychiatric associations.

Akbar Husain is Professor and Coordinator, UGC?SAP (DRS-I) at the Department of Psychology, Faculty of Social Sciences, Aligarh Muslim University, Aligarh. He received his Ph.D. Degree in Psychology from the Aligarh Muslim University, Aligarh (INDIA) in 1981. Professor Husain was awarded the D.Litt. degree in Psychology in 2015 for his work on Explorations and Applications of Spirituality in Psychology. He has over thirty-five years of teaching and research experience. He has successfully supervised 07 Research Reports to the M. Ed students at University of Malaya, Malaysia, 10 M.Phil. dissertations and 22 Ph.D. theses at the Aligarh Muslim University, Aligarh. He has authored, co-authored and edited 30 books and contributed 210 research papers, theoretical articles and book chapters in National and International Journals and Books. Prof. Husain has attended and presented papers, gave Invited Talk/Lecture and Keynote Addresses in the several National and International Conferences and Seminars. He was Editor of the Journal of the Indian Academy of Applied Psychology (2002-2005) and Journal of Educational Research, University of Malaya (2009). Prof. Husain is also reviewer of various National and International Journals of Psychology. He has standardized numerous psychological tests and completed four research projects. He is a Life Member and Annual Member of various National and International Associations. Prof. Husain was offered Founding Member of the International Board of the International Transpersonal Association, USA in 2009 and Membership of the Nyenrode Spirituality in Business Community, Netherlands in 2008. He has visited several countries for attending conferences and teaching assignments. In recent years he has been involved in conducting the researches on various topics such as spiritual values/virtues, spiritual fitness, spiritual personality, spiritual support, spiritual distress, etc. related to the area of Spiritual Psychology. In addition to this his current areas of research are: Clinical Psychology, Health Psychology, Counseling Psychology, and Positive Psychology.

Trecy Jigdung has been obtaining her bachelor degree in Genetics from IGE (Institute of Genetic Engineering). She is associated with Indian School of Complementary Therapy and Allied Sciences, India and further interested in the human genetics.

Pradeep Kallollimath is currently working as Assistant Professor of Neurology at DIMHANS/KIMS, He did his MBBS from KIMS, Hubli (1998-2004); MD in General Medicine from VIMS, Bellary (2005-2008) and DM Neurology from NIMHANS, Bangalore (2010-2013). His areas of interest are stroke, epilepsy and Wilson's disease. He is a life member of Indian medical association, life member of Indian academy of neurology and member of American academy of neurology. He presented papers in national and international conferences. He has many publication and book chapters' national and international journals and books.

Pratima Kaushik is currently working as Assistant Professor at Amity University, Noida, U.P., India for more than 6 years. Prior to this she worked as freelancing clinical psychologist at several renowned psychiatric hospitals in New Delhi. She is Gold Medalist in her Post graduation (Clinical Psychology) from Dev Sanskriti Vishwavidhyalay, Uttranchal. Later she was awarded Ph.D. degree from Delhi University in year 2012. Apart from teaching she is also specialized in psychometric assessment, psychotherapy, soft skills training and conducting workshops for students, teachers and other professionals. She is actively involved in conducting experiments and researches. She has authored one book on chronic mental illness and has seven book chapters in various edited books on related aspects of psychology. She has more than a dozen national and international research publications in her credit.

Rajpal Kaushik is currently working as consultant Clinical Psychologist at West Delhi Psychiatry Centre and various other Psychiatric centers, Nursing homes and Hospitals. He had Post graduated from Maharishi Dayanand University, Rohtak with specialization in Clinical Psychology and completed his M.Phil. from Annamalai University in Social Psychology. Later he qualified RCI recognized P.G. Diploma in Rehabilitation Psychology. He has more than a decade of experience in the field of Clinical Psychology. He has been involved in psychometric testing, Individual, Family and Group Psychotherapy for stress, work life balance, relationship issues, marital issues, childhood disorders and various psychiatric and non-psychiatric problems. Apart from these he also gives his services in conducting workshops and awareness camps in schools and hospitals for students, teachers and other professionals. He also provides training modules for students attending internship programs. He is an active member of Indian Association of Holistic Psychology.

Hitesh Khurana Graduated from Institute of Medical Sciences, BHU, Varanasi (MBBS, 1992) followed by post-graduation (MD, 1995). Completed specialist training as senior resident at Postgraduate Institute of Medical Education & Research (PGIMER), Chandigarh, India in October 1998. Registered with Medical Council if India as specialist. Taught currently working at the Institute of Mental Health, Pt BD Sharma Postgraduate Institute of Medical Sciences, Rohtak, Haryana (India). His areas of interests were including schizophrenia; Dementia; Music and art therapies; and Research Methodology and Biostatistics. Around 20 national and international publications and 8 book chapters.

Ashok S. Kori is a Psychiatric Social Worker at Dharwad Institute of Mental Health and Neurosciences (DIMHANS). He has clinical experience since 2005 in psychiatric social work field. He has completed

Master of Social Worker from Gulbarga University, Gulbarga. He has completed Postgraduate Degree in Sociology from Karnataka University, Dharwad. He has completed M.Phil in Psychiatric Social Work at National Institute of Mental Health and Neurosciences (NIMHANS), Bangalore in 2014. He has clinical skills in providing counselling, conducting Group Therapy for psychiatric patients in clinical setting. He has coordination skills to conduct awareness programs of mental illness in the community in association with different Government organizations at Dharwad District. He has presented papers in National level conference and received best presented paper award in ISPSW conference.

Kongkoan Mahanta is a student of M.Sc Genetics from Institute of Genetic Engineering, Kolkata, India. He owns a B.Sc degree in Biotechnology from University of Science and Technology, Meghalaya, India. He has one year of experience in medical research.

Akash Mahato is a registered Clinical Psychologist with Rehabilitation Council of India (RCI) and he is currently working as Associate Professor in Clinical Psychology at Department of Clinical Psychology, Amity University Kolkata. His area of interest is researching neurocognitive correlates of functioning in different clinical populations and CBT.

Pooja Mahour has done her M.phil and PhD in Clinical Psychology, currently working as Assistant Professor and Child psychologist in the department of psychiatry, King George's Medical University; in her working experience of around 9 years in different fraternities, she has earn a range of achievements. She is one of the pioneer faculty of running M.phil Clinical Psychology course in her department, she has a special interest in child and adolescent psychology, Psychotherapy and skilled at IQ assessment, Personality assessment, psychometrics, rating scales etc. In research area she has worked under ICMR funded project and is a co –guide in a project funded by DST. Her work is being published in national indexed journals, national newspapers & Souvenirs. She has attended several conferences at national / International level, she is a member of national level professional bodies like IACP & IACAP, and she herself is Hon. General Secretary of IACP – UP chapter. She has guided (9) MD, (8) M.phil and (1) Ph.D thesis. Apart from academics she has special interest in music and athletics where she has won many meddles and certificates of appreciation. She is faculty in -charge of athletic association of the university.

Lipika Malik has completed her Masters in Psychology (MA) from Jamia Millia Islamia, Delhi. Her thesis in MA was titled "Exploring Honour Killings: A Social Identity Perspective with Reference to the Village of Buana Lakhu". She has presented various research papers in areas of health psychology, well-being, social psychology and abnormal psychology at various national and international conferences. She is currently pursuing Masters of Philosophy (MPhil) in Clinical Psychology from Institute of Mental Health, Rohtak. Her areas of interest lie in the field of Child and Adolescent psychiatry, De addiction, Spirituality, Social psychology and Positive psychology.

Surendra Mattoo graduated from Government Medical College, Jammu (MBBS, 1979) followed by post-graduation (MD, 1983) and specialist training (1983-1987) in Psychiatry from Postgraduate Institute of Medical Education & Research (PGIMER), Chandigarh, India. Registered with General Medical Council, UK for Adult Psychiatry since 2002. Taught almost all through at Central Institute of Psychiatry (1987-1989) and PGIMER (1987 onward, Professor since 2007). Worked as a Consultant Psychiatrist with the North Essex Mental Health Foundation NHS Trust, UK (2003-2005) and the Institute of Mental Health, Singapore (2012-2014). Areas of interest include schizophrenia, psychosomatic disorders and addictions. Close to 200 publications.

Preeti Mishra received her Ph.D (clinical psychology) from Central Institute of Psychiatry (CIP), Ranchi in 2013. She has worked as a Research officer at CIP in a project "HIFAZAT". She has done various publications and has presented papers on national conference. She has delivered various lectures on the community level. She is now working as a clinical psychologist in the department of psychiatry at SMI Medical College and Hospital, Dehradun.

Ashima Nehra started her education in Panjab University Chandigarh, India where she did masters in Psychology (Clinical, Child, Criminal) and Post Diploma in Guidance & Counselling. She perused PhD. Clinical Psychology from Post Graduate Institute of Medical Education & Research (PGIMER), Chandigarh (U.T.) India, where she started her carrier in 1987. She worked in Stroke Rehabilitation program at George Washington University Medical Center, USA. She was recognized by Rehabilitation Council of India (RCI). Presently she is an Additional Professor (Clinical Neuropsychology) & Head, Div. Clinical Psychology at All India Institute of Medial Sciences (AIIMS), New Delhi, India. She has been actively involved in teaching & clinical work since 20 years, in research work since 30 years. She has had an honor of winning various awards and honors from international and national bodies. She has co-authored about 30 awards with her students. She has developed various Neuropsychological Copyrighted tests and rehabilitation packages along with her team. She has published and presented many papers in international & national forums (Publications about 100 & Presentations about 200). She has been working actively and continuously in the area of Neuropsychology since the last 17 years (2001) started Neuropsychology Services at PGI, Chandigarh which was a debut in her carrier. She has conducted many lectures, workshops and talk sessions for Post Graduate students of Psychology, Social Work and Nursing. She also offers a comprehensive internship programme to Master's students every year and is a guide and mentor to five PhD students under her.

Jyoti Mishra Pandey received her M.Phil in medical and social psychology (M.M&SP) from Central Institute of Psychiatry (CIP), Ranchi in 2011. She has been awarded as a first rank holder in her M.Phil (M&SP). She has completed her Ph.D from Ranchi Institute of Neuro-Psychiatry and Allied Sciences (RINPAS), Ranchi. She has also worked as assistant professor in the department of clinical psychology at central institute of psychiatry (CIP). She has also worked as a clinical psychologist in the department of psychiatry and pediatric at Bharati Vidyapeeth Medical College and Hospital, Pune. Professional member of IACP & registered in RCI. She has various publications and has presented papers on national conference. She has two chapters in an international index books and also two chapters are in process of publication. She has delivered lectures and conducted workshops on the academic level. Currently, she is working as a clinical psychologist at GMCH, Dept of Psychiatry, Chandigarh.

Smita Pandey is working as Assistant Professor in Clinical Psychology (M.Phil Program - RCI recognized). She has several researches on geriatric population to her credit. She has ample experience in the field and is dealing with the geriatric patients on day to day basis. She has been interested in neuropsychological assessments and cognitive rehabilitation of the patients.

Ashwini R. Patil she completed her masters in Psychology from University of Mysore and she went acquire her M. Phil in Psychology from Shri Venkateswara University from Tirupati. Currently she is working as a Clinical Psychologist at Dharwad Institute of Mental Health and Neurosciences (DIMHANS), Dharwad – India. She specializes in cognitive behavioural therapies and behavioural interventions for various clinical disorders; OCD, anxiety and depression, adaptation of integrated psychological therapy (IPT) for wives of schizophrenia. Her research interests are in the broad area of women's mental health, and family psychotherapy. She also published chapters and articles in various national and international books and journals.

Vikas Punia has completed his Masters in Psychology from Maharashi Dayanand University, Rohtak. He then went on to acquire Doctorate of Philosophy (Ph.D) in Clinical Psychology from Central Institute of Psychiatry, Ranchi. His Ph.D thesis was entitled "Electrophysiological Correlates of Craving Related Emotional and Neutral Cues Before and After Motivational Enhancement Therapy in Patients with Alcohol Dependence". He has published research in areas of substance dependence, well-being and deliberate self-harm along with other mental health issues. He is currently pursuing Masters of Philosophy in Clinical Psychology from Institute of Mental Health, Rohtak. His areas of interest lie in Cognitive Behaviour Therapy, Neuropsychological assessment, De addiction, Spirituality and well-being.

Aishwarya Raj is a Clinical Psychologist with a Master of Philosophy (M.Phil.) Clinical Psychology from Institute of Mental Health PGIMS Rohtak. Standing first in her M.Phil. Clinical psychology with thesis titled "Expressed emotions and coping strategies in caregivers of Schizophrenia and Obsessive compulsive Disorder patients she is passionate about her work. She specializes in dealing with psychological, emotional, behavioral problems. She has expertise in Psychological assessment and management for children, adults and elderly population. She is recognized by Rehabilitation Council of India(RCI) and is a lifetime member of Indian Association of Clinical Psychologists(IACP). She is currently working at Navkiran- 1 as a Clinical Psychologist which is the first half way /long stay home in Delhi under the Department of Social Welfare GNCT of Delhi. Her area of interest lies in psychotherapy primarily involved with elderly care.

Shivani Sharma has done her M.A is Psychology after which she worked as a Clinical Psychologist on a project under Cognitive Science Research Initiative, funded by the Government of India at Jai Prakash Narayan Apex Trauma Centre, All India Institute of Medical Sciences, New Delhi, India. Recently, she has cleared the National Eligibility Test, an exam for assistant professorship in India. Due to her exceptional academic performance, she has been awarded the coveted Junior Research Fellowship with a pass rate of 1-1.5% by the University Grants Commission, Government of India, to pursue her Ph.D. in Psychology. After securing the highest marks in the entrance examination across disciplines, she has now joined Ph.D. in Clinical Neuropsychology, Neurosciences Centre at the prestigious All India Institute of Medical Sciences, New Delhi, India. She is passionate about her work and committed to contributing to the scientific community. She has authored three articles in Indian and International peer-reviewed scientific journals and newsletters. An accomplished orator, she has won awards at national conferences for having the best poster, and best oral presentation.

Pooja Singh, currently working as Research Associate at Department of Biochemical Engineering & Biotechnology, IIT Delhi under a project entitled, "Development of an affordable, automated and field deployable, point of care and contained system for rapid diagnosis of TB caused by *Mycobacteriumtuberculosis*".She has completed her PhD with the thesis entitled "Mechanisms of fluoroquinolone resistance in *Mycobacterium tuberculosis*; a study on clinical isolates" at the Tuberculosis Laboratory, Department of Microbiology, King George's Medical University, Lucknow, India. She has working experience with microbial drug resistance, degree of antibiotic susceptibility and their association which furnishes implications for designing new antimicrobial drugs and also helped to implement measures to prevent the development of such resistance. As a result of her PhD research work, she served as a primary author and co-author in number of publications. She also presented research papers in various National and International conferences which were appreciated by some prestigious awards such as Prof. Archana Aayyagari Young Scientist Best Paper Award. During her PhD, she worked as Principal investigator (PI) of Women Scientist (WOS-A) funded by Department of Science and Technology (DST) Government of India, at Department of Microbiology, King George's Medical University, Lucknow, India.

Pallavi Sinha is currently working as Assistant Professor, Department of Psychiatry, NDMC Medical College and Hindu Rao Hospital, Delhi. After completing her post graduation from IHBAS, she also cleared DNB examination in Psychiatry. She worked as senior Resident in the Department of Psychiatry at Institute of Human Behavior and Allied Sciences (IHBAS). Her interests in the field of Psychiatry include De-addiction and Dual Diagnosis disorders.

Garima Srivastava is a Clinical Psychologist, registered in Rehabilitation Council of India (RCI) and currently she is a Research Scholar at Department of Psychology, Allahabad University. She completed her M.Phil in Medical and Social Psychology from Central Institute of Psychiatry (CIP), Ranchi. She has worked in the Department of Geriatric Mental Health, King's George Medical University (KGMU), Lucknow as Senior Research Fellow in ICMR funded Projects and held the post of Research Scientist in a project. She has received the award for extraordinary research contribution in the department in 2009 and the IAGMH/INTAS Award 2008 and 2009 by Indian Association of Geriatric Mental Health. She is Life Time member of Indian Association for Geriatric Mental Health (IAGMH). She has seven research papers published in national and international journals related to areas such as Cognitive disorders in old age, Impairment of sexual functioning and mental health among elderly, diabetes as risk factor of cognitive function etc. She has also worked as a counselor in the department of psychology at Allahabad University, Allahabad.

Bheemsain Tekkalaki has obtained his MBBS from KIMS Hubli and MD Psychiatry from KGMC Lucknow. He is currently working as Assistant Professor in the department of Psychiatry, K.L.E University's J.N Medical College Belagavi, Karnataka. He has published 14 research papers in both national and international journals, and has authored chapter on similar topic. His areas of interest are liaison psychiatry, psychosomatic medicine, social psychiatry and sexual medicine.

Deepa L. Tiwari has done post graduate diploma in counseling and psychotherapy from Banaras Hindu University, Varanasi. She has worked as a school counselor in the reputed school of Varanasi and presently working as a freelancer counselor. Her expertise of counseling is stress management, family and adjustment problems.

Rakesh Kumar Tripathi graduated (Psychology Honours) and post graduated in Psychology from Banaras Hindu University (BHU) Varanasi, UP, India. He completed MPhil in Medical and Social Psychology from Ranchi Institute of Neuropsychiatry and Allied Sciences (RINPAS), Ranchi and awarded PhD degree from King George's Medical University (KGMU), Lucknow, UP, India. He has worked in District Disability Rehabilitation Center and Drug Deaddiction Center, run by Indian Red Cross Society Kangra district Branch at Dharmshala (Himachal Pradesh), India. He awarded Senior Research Fellowship in different research projects funded by Indian Council of Medical Research (ICMR), New Delhi, India in the Department of Geriatric Mental Health, KGMU, Lucknow. Currently he is working as a faculty in the Department of Geriatric Mental Health, KGMU, Lucknow, India since year 2009. He has recieved 14 awards, published more than 40 papers in Indexed and Peer reviewed Journals. He is a master trainer for Adolescent's Mental Health Problems, guest speaker for communication skill, disaster management (mental health probblems), Counselling, Psychometric and Neuropsychological Assessment for Older Adults, & Psychosocial Dimensions of Aging. He is actively involved in Psychodiagnosis, Psychotherapy and Research activities. Joint Secretary IACP UP chapter, Member of Rehabilitation Council of India, Indian Association of Clinical Psychologists, Association of Industrial Psychiatry of India and Editorial Board member of Journal of Gerontology & Geriatric Research.

Neelam Verma is a Clinical Psychologist with Master of Philosophy (M.Phil) Degree in Clinical Psychology. She is recognized by Rehabilitation Council of India (RCI) and holds lifetime professional membership of Indian Association of Clinical Psychologists (IACP). She achieved her major educational milestones at Mahila PG College, Lucknow University, Banaras Hindu University, and Institute of Human Behaviour and Allied Sciences (IHBAS), Delhi University. During her professional career she has been actively dealing with individuals having psychological issues and psychiatric disorders. She has been involved in conducting brief clinical training programs for students of psychology and actively contributing to the literature of clinical psychology by writing in edited books and journal articles. She has been serving in the field of mental health since the year 2011 and her passion for this field has motivated her to expand the services and take a step forward. She has now expanded the access of counselling and psychotherapy services through electronic means and running her own mental health and wellness website www.talktocure.com.

Shailendra Prasad Verma has done MD in Medicine and specialization in Clinical Hematology. He is currently working as Assistant Professor in department of Clinical Hematology, King George's Medical University, Lucknow, India. He has done extensive work in field of haemophilia, Myeloma, and ITP. He has extensive experience in management of lymphoma and leukemias in elderly. He has more than 30 publications in various national and international journals and 4 book chapters to his credit. He has attended several conferences at national and International level including ASH update 2017 as a trainee sponsored by American Society of Hematology at Hong Kong. He is a member of national level professional bodies like ISHBT and API.He has guided 5 MD thesis as co-guide.

Index

A

B

C

D

E

G

H

I

L

M

O

P

Q

R

S

T

V

W

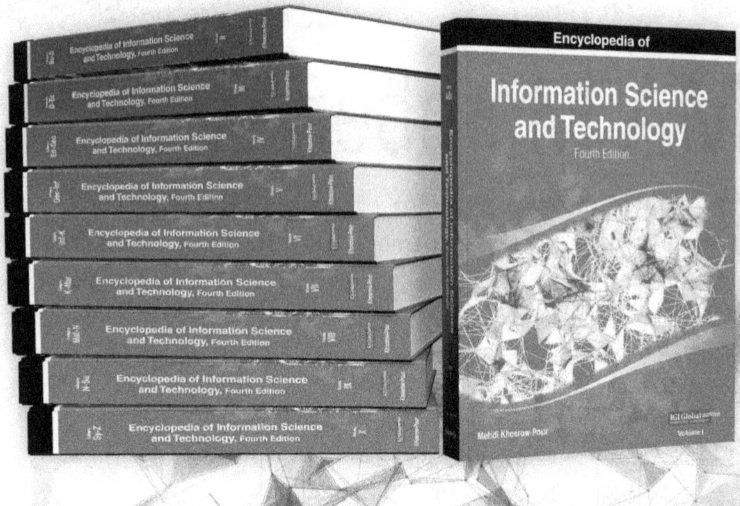
Encyclopedia of
Information Science and Technology
Fourth Edition
Mehdi Khosrow-Pour

CPSIA information can be obtained
at www.ICGtesting.com
Printed in the USA
BVHW020512030123
655399BV00004B/52

9 781522 534808